2010
YEAR BOOK OF
PEDIATRICS®

The 2010 Year Book Series

Year Book of Anesthesiology and Pain Management™: Drs Chestnut, Abram, Black, Gravlee, Lee, Mathru, and Roizen

Year Book of Cardiology®: Drs Gersh, Cheitlin, Elliott, Graham, Sundt, and Waldo

Year Book of Critical Care Medicine®: Drs Dellinger, Parrillo, Balk, Bekes, Dorman, and Dries

Year Book of Dermatology and Dermatologic Surgery™: Dr Del Rosso

Year Book of Diagnostic Radiology®: Drs Osborn, Abbara, Birdwell, Elster, Levy, Manaster, Oestreich, Offiah, Rosado de Christenson, and Walker

Year Book of Emergency Medicine®: Drs Hamilton, Bruno, Handly, Quintana, and Werner

Year Book of Endocrinology®: Drs Mazzaferri, Bessesen, Clarke, Howard, Kennedy, Leahy, Meikle, Molitch, Rogol, and Schteingart

Year Book of Gastroenterology™: Drs Lichtenstein, Dempsey, Drebin, Jaffe, Katzka, Kochman, Makar, Morris, Osterman, Rombeau, and Shah

Year Book of Hand and Upper Limb Surgery®: Drs Yao and Steinmann

Year Book of Medicine®: Drs Barkin, Berney, Frishman, Garrick, Khardori, and Loehrer

Year Book of Neonatal and Perinatal Medicine®: Drs Fanaroff, Neu, Benitz, Papile, and Donn

Year Book of Neurology and Neurosurgery®: Drs Klimo and Rabinstein

Year Book of Obstetrics, Gynecology, and Women's Health®: Drs Dungan and Shulman

Year Book of Oncology®: Drs Loehrer, Arceci, Glatstein, Gordon, Hanna, Morrow, and Thigpen

Year Book of Ophthalmology®: Drs Rapuano, Cohen, Eagle, Flanders, Hammersmith, Myers, Nelson, Penne, Sergott, Shields, Tipperman, and Vander

Year Book of Orthopedics®: Drs Morrey, Beauchamp, Huddleston, Swiontkowski, and Trigg

Year Book of Otolaryngology-Head and Neck Surgery®: Drs Sindwani, Balough, Franco, Gapany, and Mitchell

Year Book of Pathology and Laboratory Medicine®: Drs Raab, Parwani, Bejarano, and Bissell

Year Book of Pediatrics®: Dr Stockman

Year Book of Plastic and Aesthetic Surgery™: Drs Miller, Bartlett, Garner, McKinney, Ruberg, Salisbury, and Smith

2010

The Year Book of PEDIATRICS®

Editor

James A. Stockman III, MD

President, The American Board of Pediatrics; Clinical Professor of Pediatrics, University of North Carolina Medical School at Chapel Hill, and Duke University Medical Center, Durham, North Carolina

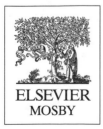

ELSEVIER
MOSBY

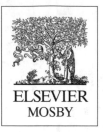

ELSEVIER
MOSBY

Vice President, Continuity: John A. Schrefer
Editor: Carla Holloway
Production Supervisor, Electronic Year Books: Donna M. Skelton
Electronic Article Manager: Jennifer C. Pitts
Illustrations and Permissions Coordinator: Linda Jones

2010 EDITION

Printed in the United States of America
Composition by TnQ Books and Journals Pvt Ltd, India
Printing/binding by Sheridan Books, Inc.

Editorial Office:
Elsevier
Suite 1800
1600 John F. Kennedy Blvd.
Philadelphia, PA 19103-2899

International Standard Serial Number: 0084-3954
International Standard Book Number: 978-0-323-06842-0

Table of Contents

JOURNALS REPRESENTED ix

INTRODUCTION xi

1. Adolescent Medicine 1
2. Allergy and Dermatology 19
3. Blood 49
4. Child Development 73
5. Dentistry and Otolaryngology (ENT) 87
6. Endocrinology 105
7. Gastroenterology 119
8. Genitourinary Tract 155
9. Heart and Blood Vessels 167
10. Infectious Diseases and Immunology 205
11. Miscellaneous 287
12. Musculoskeletal 335
13. Neurology and Psychiatry 361
14. Newborn 399
15. Nutrition and Metabolism 443
16. Oncology 475
17. Ophthalmology 505
18. Respiratory Tract 515
19. Therapeutics and Toxicology 535

ARTICLE INDEX 571

AUTHOR INDEX 583

Journals Represented

Journals represented in this YEAR BOOK are listed below.

Acta Paediatrica
American Journal of Clinical Nutrition
American Journal of Obstetrics and Gynecology
American Journal of Preventive Medicine
American Journal of Psychiatry
American Journal of Public Health
Annals of Internal Medicine
Archives of Disease in Childhood
Archives of Disease in Childhood Fetal & Neonatal Edition
Archives of General Psychiatry
Archives of Ophthalmology
Archives of Pediatrics & Adolescent Medicine
Blood
Brain
British Journal of Cancer
British Medical Journal
Canadian Journal of Psychiatry
Clinical Pediatrics
European Journal of Paediatric Neurology
Epilepsia
Gastrointestinal Endoscopy
Gut
Human Reproduction
Journal of Adolescent Health
Journal of Allergy and Clinical Immunology
Journal of Clinical Endocrinology & Metabolism
Journal of Clinical Oncology
Journal of Clinical Psychiatry
Journal of Developmental and Behavioral Pediatrics
Journal of General Internal Medicine
Journal of Pediatric Gastroenterology and Nutrition
Journal of Pediatric Hematology/Oncology
Journal of Pediatric Ophthalmology & Strabismus
Journal of Pediatric Orthopaedics
Journal of Pediatrics
Journal of Pediatric Surgery
Journal of the American Academy of Child & Adolescent Psychiatry
Journal of the American Academy of Dermatology
Journal of the American Medical Association
Journal of Thoracic and Cardiovascular Surgery
Journal of Urology
Lancet
Nature Medicine
New England Journal of Medicine
Ophthalmology
Pediatric Cardiology
Pediatric Dermatology

Pediatric Emergency Care
Pediatric Hematology and Oncology
Pediatric Infectious Disease Journal
Pediatric Neurology
Pediatric Research
Pediatrics

STANDARD ABBREVIATIONS

The following terms are abbreviated in this edition: acquired immunodeficiency syndrome (AIDS), cardiopulmonary resuscitation (CPR), central nervous system (CNS), cerebrospinal fluid (CSF), computed tomography (CT), deoxyribonucleic acid (DNA), electrocardiography (ECG), health maintenance organization (HMO), human immunodeficiency virus (HIV), intensive care unit (ICU), intramuscular (IM), intravenous (IV), magnetic resonance (MR) imaging (MRI), ribonucleic acid (RNA), ultrasound (US), and ultraviolet (UV).

NOTE

The YEAR BOOK OF PEDIATRICS® is a literature survey service providing abstracts of articles published in the professional literature. Every effort is made to assure the accuracy of the information presented in these pages. Neither the editors nor the publisher of the YEAR BOOK OF PEDIATRICS® can be responsible for errors in the original materials. The editors' comments are their own opinions. Mention of specific products within this publication does not constitute endorsement.

To facilitate the use of the YEAR BOOK OF PEDIATRICS® as a reference tool, all illustrations and tables included in this publication are now identified as they appear in the original article. This change is meant to help the reader recognize that any illustration or table appearing in the YEAR BOOK OF PEDIATRICS® may be only one of many in the original article. For this reason, figure and table numbers will often appear to be out of sequence within the YEAR BOOK OF PEDIATRICS.®

Introduction

"There are some patients that we cannot help; there are none whom we cannot harm."

Arthur L. Bloomfield (1888-1962)

Dr Arthur L. Bloomfield was a dominant figure in the history of American medicine. For most of the 28 years he was Professor of Medicine and Executive of the Department of Medicine at the Stanford Medical School, he was a leading intellectual figure in internal medicine, particularly in the western part of this country. A superb and beloved teacher, an extraordinarily wise physician and consultant, he had an amazing sense of feel for the needs of students, residents, physicians, and patients under his care. He contributed greatly to the advancement of medicine, particularly knowledge of infectious diseases, and was a pioneer in the clinical use of penicillin and other antibiotics. When Dr Bloomfield died in 1962, there was little in the way of literature about quality improvement and patient safety as we now know it. The Institute of Medicine's reports *Crossing the Quality Chasm* and *To Err is Human* were more than three decades in the offing. Nonetheless, as we see in the quote of Dr Bloomfield, the concepts of quality improvement and patient safety are not new and certainly not novel. This volume of the YEAR BOOK OF PEDIATRICS is the thirty-second that this editor has been privileged to work on. No time in the history of the YEAR BOOK OF PEDIATRICS, however, have the issues of quality improvement and patient safety been more apparent in the literature, some of which is abstracted in this edition.

In addition to the above, sprinkled elsewhere throughout the book are many other "hot topics." The following is a "baker's dozen" of subjects receiving lots of attention in the current literature these days. They are but a few among many included in this YEAR BOOK for your reading:

1. Avian influenza (HSN1)—its spread into the United States.
2. Metabolic syndrome—lots of information, some of it new, including the severity of its consequences to the growing child and adolescent.
3. Cold medication use in children—a not so benign therapy.
4. Community and hospital-acquired methicillin resistant staphylococcus aureus—a view from a pediatric research network.
5. The 80-hour work week—can residents in training acquire the requisite skills for independent practice?
6. Nut allergy—the explosion of information about the prevalence and current prognosis.
7. HIV infection—lots of new information, including updates on its incidence, relationship to breast feeding, and the effects of circumcision in its prevention.
8. Mental health issues in teens—including what appears to be almost an epidemic of depression, a not-so-new morbidity.

9. Papillomavirus infection—its consequences, prevention, and how You Tube can help educate our youth about safe sex.
10. The hospitalist movement—how it has changed the palate of pediatric practice.
11. Autism—its prevalence and origins.
12. Tainted formulas—'tain't just a problem in China.
13. Social networking—how MySpace, Facebook, You Tube, and Twitter impact our adolescents, sometimes in a not-so-healthy way.

As you will see, this YEAR BOOK has tried to evolve with the times. Ever so slowly our medical lexicon has changed and continues to do so. Not very long ago, our language did not contain words and phrases such as Twitter, Facebook, or MySpace. We try to keep up with this phenomenon and thus close this introduction with a few medical terms that have recently entered our vocabulary that you might want to be aware of.[1]

- *A 404 Moment:* The point in a hospital teaching round when despite searches of notes or electronic records, a resident cannot find the required information. (from the World Wide Web error message: 404—document not found).
- *Adminisphere:* The pleasantly decorated, often palatial, offices of the senior hospital administration.
- *Administrivia:* The flurry of pointless e-mails and paperwork that emanate from the adminisphere.
- *Agnostication:* The attempt (usually vain) to answer the question: how long have I got, doc?
- *Blamestorming:* Those tedious hospital meetings in which experts attempt to define why a "never" event occurred.
- *A Fonzie:* A physician who is seemingly unflappable in any medical emergency (based on the character Arthur "Fonzie" Fonzarelli from the sitcom *Happy Days*).
- *A Hasselhoff:* A patient presenting to an emergency room with an injury requiring a bizarre explanation (after the former *Bay Watch* actor, David Hasselhoff, who in real life suffered a freak injury when he hit his head on a chandelier while shaving; broken glass severed four tendons as well as an artery in his right arm requiring immediate surgery).
- *A Jack Bauer:* A resident still up and working after 24 hours on the job—now something of a rarity, but a condition well recognized by older physicians (from the lead in the television series *24*).
- *Testiculation:* The holding forth with expressive hand gestures (hand held supine with fingers pointing up) by a consultant on a subject on which he or she has relatively little knowledge (the term being a concatenation of testicle and gesticulate).

One wonders what Dr Bloomfield would have thought about agnosticating Fonzies. In any event, pull a Jack Bauer and read this year's YEAR BOOK OF PEDIATRICS straight through.

James A. Stockman III, MD

P.S. From time to time when reading this YEAR BOOK's commentaries you will run across a "Clinical Fact/Curio," a new feature of the YEAR BOOK OF PEDIATRICS intended to provide insights into the world of interesting, possibly offbeat aspects of medicine.

Reference

1. Keley P. Pimp my slang. *BMJ*. 2007;335:1295.

1 Adolescent Medicine

Age at Menarche in the Canadian Population: Secular Trends and Relationship to Adulthood BMI

Harris MA, Prior JC, Koehoorn M, et al (Univ of British Columbia, Vancouver, Canada; et al)
J Adolesc Health 43:548-554, 2008

Purpose.—Studies from around the world indicate a trend toward younger ages of menarche. The extent of this trend in the Canadian population is unknown, and the relationship to later-life health indicators has not yet been fully elucidated. The objective of this study is to estimate the trend in age at menarche (AAM) in the Canadian population and evaluate the relationship between AAM and adult body mass index (BMI).

Methods.—Our data source was a nationally representative survey (the Canadian Community Health Survey, 2.2), and analyses included 8080 women, aged 15 and older, who self-reported AAM. Height and weight were measured by the interviewers for the calculation of current BMI. We modeled the secular trend in AAM over time, and the relationship between current BMI and AAM.

Results.—We found a statistically significant decline in AAM in successive age cohorts, indicating a 0.73-year (8.8-month) decrease in AAM between the oldest and youngest age cohorts in the sample. A 1-year increase in AAM was associated with a decrease in mean BMI of approximately 0.5 kg/m^2, after adjustment for covariates. A current age–AAM interaction term was nonsignificant, indicating that the relationship was stable throughout increasing temporal separation from puberty.

Conclusion.—The observed trend toward earlier menarche could be an indicator of a change in insulin-related metabolism, possibly mediated by behavioral and environmental variables. This study suggests that AAM may be an important clinical and public health indicator of susceptibility to overweight and obesity and attendant morbidity.

▶ At first glance, you would think that this report does not provide particularly new information given that the bottom line is that the age of menarche has been decreasing. We all know that. What is important about this study is its design and the fact that it also correlates age at menarche with body mass index (BMI). The study emanates from Canada where 8000 Canadian females age 15 and older were the basis of this report that involved a cross-sectional analysis of women whose date of birth ranged from before 1933 to those born as late as 1990. In the 5 or more decades covered by this report, the age at menarche had decreased by 8.8 years. Importantly, the study goes beyond just reporting that age at menarche is occurring earlier. The study also focused on timing of menarche and its association with BMI and showed that earlier age of menarche is associated with a higher adult BMI. This introduces the speculation that obesity may play a significant role in this earlier age of menarche seen over the last half or more century.

Many books could be filled with the literature on puberty and timing of puberty. Nonetheless, there is no doubt that there is much more to learn about the timing of puberty. Although various explanations exist, one example of defining mechanisms associated with the timing of puberty is evidenced by a current multi-site study underway that addresses potential environmental mechanisms.[1] In the latter, a creative model that combines research in both human and lower animal models and community outreach was used. The overall topic of puberty and its timing have recently been reviewed by Dorn.[2]

J. A. Stockman III, MD

References

1. Wolff MS, Titelbaum SL, Windham G, et al. Study of urinary biomarkers of phytoestrogens, phythalates, and phenols in girls. *Environ Health Perspect.* 2007;115: 116-121.
2. Dorn LD. Another milepost on the road to understanding puberty. *J Adolesc Health.* 2008;43:525-526.

Age at Menarche and First Pregnancy Among Psychosocially At-Risk Adolescents
Dunbar J, Sheeder J, Lezotte D, et al (Univ of Colorado, Denver)
Am J Public Health 98:1822-1824, 2008

We sought to determine which factors influence the association between menarche and conception among adolescent study participants (n = 1030), who demonstrated an earlier age of menarche than did national samples. Age at first sexual intercourse (coitarche) mediated the relationship between age at menarche and first pregnancy among White girls, whereas gynecologic age at coitarche (age at coitarche minus age at menarche) and age at menarche explained the timing of the first pregnancy among Black and Hispanic girls. Pregnancy prevention interventions to delay coitarche should also include reproductive education and contraception.

▶ The findings from this report come as no surprise. American adolescents who become pregnant experience menarche at an earlier age than do their nonpregnant peers. This is particularly true for white girls. However, among black and Hispanic adolescent girls, gynecologic age is the strongest predictor of age at first pregnancy. The findings from this report also suggest that black and Hispanic girls may have a higher likelihood of conception than do white girls who engage in the same level of sexual risk taking behaviors, because they show a longer period between menarche and their first sexual experience. As such, black and Hispanic girls are more fertile when they first engage in sexual activity.

J. A. Stockman III, MD

Reducing At-Risk Adolescents' Display of Risk Behavior on a Social Networking Web Site: A Randomized Controlled Pilot Intervention Trial
Moreno MA, VanderStoep A, Parks MR, et al (Univ of Washington, Seattle)
Arch Pediatr Adolesc Med 163:35-41, 2009

Objective.—To determine whether an online intervention reduces references to sex and substance abuse on social networking Web sites among at-risk adolescents.

Design.—Randomized controlled intervention trial.

Setting.—www.MySpace.com.

Participants.—Self-described 18- to 20-year-olds with public MySpace profiles who met our criteria for being at risk (N = 190).

Intervention.—Single physician e-mail.

Main Outcome Measures.—Web profiles were evaluated for references to sex and substance use and for security settings before and 3 months after the intervention.

Results.—Of 190 subjects, 58.4% were male. At baseline, 54.2% of subjects referenced sex and 85.3% referenced substance use on their social networking site profiles. The proportion of profiles in which references decreased to 0 was 13.7% in the intervention group vs 5.3% in the control group for sex ($P = .05$) and 26.0% vs 22% for substance use ($P = .61$). The proportion of profiles set to "private" at follow-up was 10.5% in the intervention group and 7.4% in the control group ($P = .45$). The proportion of profiles in which any of these 3 protective changes were made was 42.1% in the intervention group and 29.5% in the control group ($P = .07$).

Conclusions.—A brief e-mail intervention using social networking sites shows promise in reducing sexual references in the online profiles of at-risk adolescents. Further study should assess how adolescents view different risk behavior disclosures to promote safe use of the Internet (Fig 2).

▶ A report from this same group of investigators at the University of Washington in Seattle describes how adolescents display health risk behaviors on MySpace, a social networking Internet site.[1] This report, however, takes the topic one step further by attempting to show how one might be able to mitigate some of the risk-taking behaviors on the part of adolescents who post personal information that could get them into trouble on MySpace. The investigators researched the web profiles of 18- to 20-year-olds to see if these profiles might put them at risk by revealing certain types of personal information. Those with profiles that fit these criteria were then e-mailed messages that were sent within the MySpace system from a Dr Meg. The content of the e-mailed note may be seen in Fig 2.

Hi (login name),
I'm Dr. Meg, an adolescent medicine doctor and researcher from the University of
Washington. (Really—you can check me out at http://depts.washington.edu/adolmed
/meganmoreno.htm). I'm exploring MySpace to understand how teens talk about
health, especially sexual issues. I noticed something on your MySpace profile that
concerned me. You seemed to be quite open about sexual issues or other behaviors
such as drinking or smoking. Are you sure that's a good idea? After all, if I could see
it, nearly anybody could. That probably includes some people you do not want seeing
your profile or who would take things the wrong way. You might consider revising
your page to better protect your privacy.

I'm also concerned that you are at risk for a sexually transmitted disease, or STD
(like chlamydia or gonorrhea). Anyone who has had sex could have an STD. Many
teenagers don't know that they could have one and not have any symptoms. Since
you are probably pretty comfortable with the Internet, you may be interested in
getting more information and even free testing using the Internet. Here is the website:
www.iwantthekit.org. There are lots of other ways to get tested too: at your doctor,
the local health department, or a Planned Parenthood. If you are concerned about
getting this e-mail, please talk with your parents, health care provider, a trusted adult,
or you can e-mail back with any questions.
Regards, Dr. Meg

FIGURE 2.—E-mail message sent once to intervention group subjects' MySpace inbox. (Reprinted
from Moreno MA, VanderStoep A, Parks MR, et al. Reducing at-risk adolescents' display of risk behavior
on a social networking web site: a randomized controlled pilot intervention trial. *Arch Pediatr Adolesc
Med*. 2009;163:35-41, with permission from the American Medical Association.)

The study was designed to show whether or not such an e-mail intervention
might reduce the social networking display of risk behaviors. Indeed, this single
e-mail message proved to be both feasible and potentially effective in this
regard, at least in part. The intervention seemed to have an effect on adolescents' decision to remove sexual references from their profiles. The intervention
was not successful in reducing online references to substance abuse, a finding
without explanation.

Obviously, some teens will view Dr Meg as a peeping Tom. Others will
recognize that there is someone out there who is trying to be of help in protecting them from harm. Obviously, it is not possible to monitor the personal
profiles of the millions of adolescents and young adults who choose to post
personal information, so the real world impact of this randomized controlled
pilot intervention trial from Seattle remains speculative at best.

J. A. Stockman III, MD

Reference

1. Moreno MA, Parks MR, Zimmerman FJ, et al. Display of health risk behaviors on
MySpace by adolescents. *Arch Pediatr Adolesc Med*. 2009;163:27-34.

Display of Health Risk Behaviors on MySpace by Adolescents: Prevalence and Associations

Moreno MA, Parks MR, Zimmerman FJ, et al (Univ of Washington, Seattle, WA; et al)
Arch Pediatr Adolesc Med 163:27-34, 2009

Objective.—To determine the prevalence of and associations among displayed risk behavior information that suggests sexual behavior, substance use, and violence in a random sample of the self-reported 18-year-old adolescents' publicly accessible MySpace Web profiles.

Design.—Cross-sectional study using content analysis of Web profiles between July 15 and September 30, 2007.

Setting.—www.MySpace.com.

Participants.—A total of 500 publicly available Web profiles of self-reported 18 year olds in the United States.

Main Outcome Measures.—Prevalence and associations among displayed health risk behaviors, including sexual behavior, substance use, or violence, on Web profiles.

Results.—A total of 270 (54.0%) profiles contained risk behavior information: 120 (24.0%) referenced sexual behaviors, 205 (41.0%) referenced substance use, and 72 (14.4)% referenced violence. Female adolescents were less likely to display violence references (odds ratio [OR],0.3; 95% confidence interval [CI], 0.15-0.6). Reporting a sexual orientation other than "straight" was associated with increased display of references to sexual behavior (OR,4.48; 95% CI, 1.27-15.98). Displaying church or religious involvement was associated with decreased display of all outcomes (sex: OR, 0.32; 95% CI, 0.12-0.86; substance use: OR,0.38; 95% CI, 0.19-0.79; violence: OR,0.12; 95% CI, 0.02-0.87; any risk factor: OR,0.36; 95% CI, 0.19-0.7). Displaying sport or hobby involvement was associated with decreased references to violence (OR,0.27; 95% CI, 0.09-0.79) and any risk factor (OR,0.46; 95% CI, 0.27-0.79).

Conclusions.—Adolescents frequently display risk behavior information on public Web sites. Further study is warranted to explore the validity of such information and the potential for using social networking Web sites for health promotion.

▶ The parent of any teen or preteen worries about the exposure their youngster has when they sign on to Internet sites such as MySpace or Facebook. The report of Moreno et al reminds us that, as with any new media technology, there are potential benefits and drawbacks to such social networking opportunities. In terms of drawbacks, it is fairly clear that social networking sites are environments in which adolescents may express themselves in ways that put them at risk for victimization or personal consequence. Moreno et al found that 54% of MySpace profiles of 18-year-old individuals contained references to risky behaviors, including sexual behaviors, substance abuse, and violence. References to substance abuse in personal profiles may have long-lasting effects that adolescents may not take into consideration, such as a negative impact on future employment opportunities. Some sites, particularly MySpace, also include access to medical information provided by those who are doing the social networking—information that can be misleading or inaccurate. A report of Versteeg et al that reviewed MySpace cataloged the degree of misinformation appearing on the topic of asthma.[1] For example, one bit of advice posted on MySpace was: "Cocaine helps my asthma. I'll snort a line and my breathing gets better."

It is our role as pediatricians to be aware of what those under our care are reading on social networking sites. We must advise adolescents to be critical of what they may be viewing. It is impossible, and likely inappropriate to restrict access to such sites, and thus we must encourage parents to be familiar with the content of them. We must be sure that children are taught that harassing statements are inappropriate no matter where they originate.

To read more about teenagers wanting medical advice and the consequences of social networking on the Internet, see the excellent editorial by Mitchell and Ybarra.[2]

J. A. Stockman III, MD

References

1. Versteeg KM, Knopf JM, Posluszny S, Vockell AL, Britto MT. Teenagers wanting medical advice: is MySpace the answer? *Arch Pediatr Adolesc Med.* 2009;163: 91-92.
2. Mitchell KJ, Ybarra M. Social networking sites. Finding a balance between their risks and benefits. *Arch Pediatr Adolesc Med.* 2009;163:87-89.

The Availability and Portrayal of Stimulants Over the Internet

Schepis TS, Marlowe DB, Forman RF, et al (Yale Univ School of Med, New Haven, Connecticut; Treatment Res Inst, Philadelphia, PA; et al)
J Adolesc Health 42:458-465, 2008

Purpose.—To quantify the online availability and portrayal of amphetamine-class prescription stimulants with a focus on those medications commonly prescribed to and abused by adolescents.

Method.—The Google™ search engine was used in searches to assess the frequency of web sites offering to sell controlled stimulants (retail sites) or web sites that directly linked to retail sites (portal sites). In addition separate searches were used to evaluate the portrayal of controlled prescription stimulants by the initial 20 web sites returned by Google. Retail and portal web site frequency was collected for each search. For searches measuring the portrayal of stimulants, web pages were categorized as pro-use, anti-misuse, neutral or other, based on set criteria.

Results.—Sites offering to sell stimulants without a prescription were found for nearly all search terms. Across all searches, the Schedule III stimulants indicated for the treatment of obesity returned more sites offering to sell stimulants without a prescription than Schedule II stimulants indicated for the treatment of attention-deficit hyperactivity disorder (ADHD). Internet site portrayal of each stimulant varied; however sites that contained "methamphetamine" often included anti-misuse information.

Conclusions.—The apparent availability of stimulants over the Internet without a prescription indicates the potential for a significant public health problem. The extent to which teens are obtaining these drugs via the Internet remains unclear, but clinicians must be aware of the potential for abuse, concomitant prescription use issues, illicit sources, and diversion of these medications, which can be highly addictive. Education of consumers and physicians as well as further governmental interventions are needed to limit the potential scope of this problem.

▶ The report of Schepis et al is quite disturbing. These researchers used the Google search engine to assess the availability of web site offerings to sell controlled stimulants over the Internet, presumably without much in the way of prescription screening. They found that a range of prescription-only stimulants was indeed available to buy without any involvement from a healthcare provider. If nothing else the study illustrates that there is a potential for teens to acquire powerful stimulants in much the same way that they may order a new DVD or that "must-have" iPod accessory. Unfortunately, the study does not tell us just how often teens exercise this option for access of online stimulant purchase.

There seems to be no way to make a serious dent in the possibility of teens purchasing online drugs. Monitoring of teen Internet activity while seemingly worthwhile is likely to be doomed to fail, given the ubiquitous accessibility teens have to more than 1 computer these days. Obviously, we need further studies to determine whether effective dialog between parents and their offspring might help to address these issues. In any event, this report of Schepis et al does provide a stimulant for care providers to think more about online access to medications. The Internet can and is helpful in addressing adolescents' unmet health information needs. There is no question that teens cruise the Internet in this regard. We must work with adolescents so they can understand the positive power and danger of the Internet. There is nothing worse than anyone receiving medications online that are not good for them much less adulterated medications that can do harm. To read more about health information on the Internet, see the excellent editorial by Gray.[1]

J. A. Stockman III, MD

Reference

1. Gray NJ. Health information on the Internet – a double-edged sword? *J Adolesc Health.* 2008;42:432-433.

Noncoital Sexual Activities Among Adolescents
Lindberg LD, Jones R, Santelli JS (Guttmacher Inst, NY; et al)
J Adolesc Health 43:231-238, 2008

Purpose.—Although prior research has demonstrated that many adolescents engage in noncoital sexual behavior, extant peer-reviewed studies have not used nationally representative data or multivariate methods to examine these behaviors. We used data from Cycle 6 of National Survey of Family Growth (NSFG) to explore factors related to oral and anal sex among adolescents.

Methods.—Data come from 2,271 females and males aged 15–19 in 2002. Computer-assisted self-administered interviews were used to collect sensitive information, including whether respondents had ever engaged in vaginal, oral or anal sex. We used *t* tests and multivariate logistic regression to test for differences and identify independent characteristics associated with experience with oral or anal sex.

Results.—In all, 54% of adolescent females and 55% of adolescent males have ever had oral sex, and one in 10 has ever had anal sex. Both oral sex and anal sex were much more common among adolescents who had initiated vaginal sex as compared with virgins. The initiations of vaginal and oral sex appear to occur closely together; by 6 months after first vaginal intercourse, 82% of adolescents also engaged in oral sex. The strongest predictor of anal sex involvement was time since initiation of vaginal sex and the likelihood of anal sex increased with greater time since first vaginal intercourse. Teens of white ethnicity and higher socioeconomic status were more likely than their peers to have ever had oral or anal sex.

Conclusions.—Health professionals and sexual health educators should address noncoital sexual behaviors and risk for sexually transmitted infections risk, understanding that noncoital behaviors commonly co-occur with coital behaviors.

▶ We know a lot about oral sexual behavior in adolescents. For example, at least 1 in 5 adolescents has had oral sex by the time they have completed freshman year of high school. By graduation, this percentage has increased to 50%. Oral sexual activity is substantially more common than vaginal sex. Both males and females report receiving oral sex at about the same rate and both report receiving oral sex more than giving oral sex.

Teens do not view oral sex as a risky activity. Although oral sex certainly negates the risk of pregnancy and results in far lower likelihood of consequences compared with vaginal sex, oral sex is not risk free. There is good evidence that oral sex is associated with negative health outcomes such as sexually transmitted infections, including herpes, hepatitis, gonorrhea, chlamydia, syphilis, and HIV. Adolescents perceive that oral sex holds significantly less risk when it comes to social and emotional outcomes including feeling guilty, getting into trouble, feeling bad about themselves, and having a bad reputation. Adolescents also tend to believe that oral sex is not actually sex and that by engaging in oral sex one can still remain a virgin.

One can debate the riskiness of oral sex. The real issue, in some minds, is whether oral sex either forestalls or in fact accelerates movement toward the time of vaginal sex. Lindberg et al address this question. It was observed that adolescents who initiated vaginal sex were more likely to have had oral sex than adolescents who had delayed their vaginal sex experiences. Further, adolescents without vaginal sex experience were less likely to have had oral sex than nonvirgins. Oral sex was much more likely among youth who had already experienced vaginal sex and more likely among those who had initiated vaginal sex earlier. If one looks at these findings in greater detail, one can conclude that the onset of oral sex and vaginal sex occurs fairly close together.

The bottom line here is that oral sex is the slippery slope for many, if not most teens to more risky sexual behavior such as vaginal and anal sex. For this reason, our educational programs should focus on all forms of sexual activity since nothing is without some risks.

As this commentary closes, here's a *Clinical Fact/Curio*, this having to do remotely with adolescent medicine. A recent survey in Great Britain indicates that those in their late teens and young adults (to age 25) do not believe the term "binge drinking" is appropriate any longer. A new report based on a United Kingdom survey says that the term binge drinking is too emotive. It is suggested that the term "calculated hedonism" better describes the behavior of the young people who participated in the British survey, say the researchers.[1] Just what we need, another medical term that pretends to better inform. Is there such a disorder as "miscalculated hedonism?"

J. A. Stockman III, MD

Reference

1. Good bye binge drinking, hello calculated hedonism [editorial comment]. *BMJ*. 2008;337:a1915.

Why Do Young Women Continue to Have Sexual Intercourse Despite Pain?
Elmerstig E, Wijma B, Berterö C (Linköping Univ, Sweden; et al)
J Adolesc Health 43:357-363, 2008

Purpose.—Many young women suffer from pain and discomfort during sexual intercourse, and an increasing number of them seek help for their problems. It seems that some young women continue to have sexual intercourse despite pain. However, their motives are unclear.

Methods.—A total of 16 women, aged 14 to 20 years, with variable degrees of coital pain were selected at a youth center in a city in southeastern Sweden, to explore why they continued to have sexual intercourse despite pain. The women participated in audiotaped qualitative individual interviews, which were analyzed using the constant comparative method from grounded theory.

Results.—During the analysis we identified the core category *striving to be affirmed in their image of an ideal woman* and the categories *resignation, sacrifice,* and *feeling guilt.* The perceived ideal women had several distinct characteristics, such as willingness to have sexual intercourse, being perceptive of their partner's sexual needs, and being able to satisfy their partners. Having sexual intercourse per se was considered to be an affirmation of being a normal woman, irrespective of pain or discomfort.

Conclusions.—These young women's focus on a constructed ideal explains why they continue to have sexual intercourse despite pain. Greater awareness of these beliefs among gynecologists, sexologists, and other healthcare professionals involved in the management of young women with coital pain would be beneficial.

▶ This report appearing in the *Journal of Adolescent Health* emanates from Sweden. The findings from this report most likely do apply to young women in the United States, however. Many of the latter are concerned about their sexual health and a frequent complaint is pain during sexual intercourse. Almost nothing is known about coital pain in young women under the age of 18. In Sweden, however, a pilot study found that 34% of young women visiting an adolescent health center in Stockholm reported regular pain related to intercourse.[1] Coital pain is probably multifactorial including physical as well as psychosocial components. The DSM-IV definition of dyspareunia is far from clear, and the terminology of pain during sexual intercourse/coital pain/dyspareunia is inconsistently used in the literature. What is clear, though, is that young women, including teens, continue to have sexual intercourse despite pain and their motives have not been fully understood, the purpose of the investigation carried out by Elmerstig et al.

This report probed in some depth why young women continued to have intercourse despite having significant pain or discomfort. The data from this report provide interesting and new information on the psyche of our teen population. In this study, the young women's reason for continuing to have sexual intercourse despite pain and discomfort was not a sexual desire for sexual intercourse. Rather, the experience of coital pain in fact did decrease their sexual desire and arousal. The reason for their behavior rather was that they were striving to be affirmed in their image of an ideal woman. This striving, together with resignation to the fact they were going to have pain provides an explanation for why young women continue to have sexual intercourse. In part they want to do this to appear as a complete woman capable of satisfying their partner. The results clearly show that the partner's sexual pleasure was very important for the teen, whereas the experience of pain during sexual intercourse or their own sexual pleasure took second place. One wonders if a guy experiencing such displeasure would be as accommodating.

The women in this city were between 14 and 20 years of age. These young women clearly stated that they were preoccupied during sexual activity with trying to please, which only further contributed to their own lack of satisfaction. What is not known is what the prospect for these teens' sexual desire will be in the long run. If nothing else, this report provides us with greater insights into the mental processes women experiencing coital pain are having. This should allow us, gynecologists, and other health professionals to better assist these young women with coital pain.

This commentary closes with a question related to a *Clinical Fact/Curio* relevant to some teens and young adults. You are caring for a 17-year-old with type 2 diabetes, polycystic ovarian syndrome, and hypertension. You are using a treatment regimen that includes metformin and hydrochlorothiazide. This teen has a greater probability of what?

This young lady should be advised that her treatments can significantly increase her likelihood of pregnancy should she be sexually active. By increasing insulin sensitivity and decreasing serum insulin concentrations, these agents may decrease ovarian androgen production, potentially stimulating ovulation in women who might be otherwise thought to be infertile.[2]

J. A. Stockman III, MD

References

1. Berglund AL, Nigaard L, Rylander E. Vulvar pain, sexual behavior and genital infections in a young population: a pilot study. *Acta Obstet Gynecol Scand.* 2002;81:738-742.
2. Guirguis AB, Malone RM, Chelminski PR, et al. Conception as a potential conse quence of diabetes treatment. *Clin Diabetes.* 2008;26:83-84.

Waterpipe Tobacco Smoking on a U.S. College Campus: Prevalence and Correlates

Eissenberg T, Ward KD, Smith-Simone S, et al (Virginia Commonwealth Univ, Richmond; Syrian Ctr for Tobacco Studies, Aleppo, Syria; Princeton Univ and Robert Wood Johnson Foundation, New Jersey; et al)
J Adolesc Health 42:526-529, 2008

Purpose.—Waterpipe tobacco smoking is reported to be growing in popularity, particularly among college students. This study examined the prevalence of waterpipe tobacco smoking prevalence and perceptions in a university-based population.

Method.—This was a cross-sectional Internet-based survey of first-year university students, which examined waterpipe tobacco smoking and other tobacco use, risk perceptions, influences, and perceived social acceptability.

Results.—Waterpipe tobacco smoking within the past 30 days was reported by 20% (151/744). Relative to never users, users were more likely to perceive waterpipe tobacco smoking as less harmful than cigarette use.

Conclusions.—Because waterpipe tobacco smoking is increasing in prevalence and because it can involve toxicant inhalation at even greater levels than with cigarette smoking, it represents a growing public health issue.

▶ A waterpipe is also known as a hookah, shisha, nargile, and hubble-bubble. These are single or multi-stemmed waterpipes used for tobacco smoking. A waterpipe has a mouthpiece, hose, water bowl, body, and "head" that is filled with sweetened and flavored tobacco and then heated with charcoal. During inhalation from the mouthpiece, charcoal and tobacco smoke pass through the body, bowl, and hose into the user's lungs. Waterpipe smoking is a tradi-tional method of tobacco use, particularly in the eastern Mediterranean region. Its use is spreading worldwide, and its prevalence in the United States has been unclear. One anecdotal report suggests that it may be particularly common among college students and a recent survey of 411 first-year university students indicates that about 15% of students report waterpipe use within the last month.[1] This use may be driven by a perception of lower health risk relative to cigarette smoking.

Eissenberg et al report a nearly 50% lifetime prevalence rate and a 20% past 30-day use rate among first-year college students at the Virginia Commonwealth University. These data are particularly worrisome. Hookah smoking while delivering nicotine to young people does so in settings with pro-social and positive messages. The experience is spread through social, word of mouth use on college campuses and in "hookah bars" or cafes frequented by youth. Substantial misinformation about the smoke being "cleaner" or "natural" is being passed along without any mention of the fact that nicotine is absorbed exactly the same way as with cigarette smoking and is just as addictive.

Although the findings reported come from a single university in just one state, the chances are that the data reported are likely to be typical of most college campuses. Given the recent knowledge that even casual smoking can lead to addiction, the findings from this report should be considered quite worrisome.

This commentary closes with a *Clinical Fact/Curio* having to do with adolescent medicine. It is posed in the form of a question. Unfortunately, more and more teens are drinking hard liquor these days. The question is: Is one more likely to become drunk faster by the imbibition of a straight drink or a mixed drink with the same amount of alcohol? The answer is alcohol consumption differs person to person and the type of "mixer" consumed with alcohol is in fact one of the influencing factors for the rate of alcohol absorption. A recent study looked at volunteers who participated in a study of vodka mixed with still water, sparkling water, or no mixer at all. The drinks were consumed over 5 minutes. Alcohol concentrations in breath showed that 20 of the 21 participants absorbed vodka in a mixed drink (either type) faster than native vodka, and the absorption was significantly quicker with a mixer of carbonated water.[2]

J. A. Stockman III, MD

References

1. Smith SY, Corbow B, Stillman F. Harm perception of nicotine products in college freshman. *Nicotine Tob Res.* 2007;9:977-982.
2. Roberts C, Robinson SP. Alcohol concentration and carbonation of drinks: the effect on blood alcohol levels. *J Forensic Legal Medicine.* 2007;14:398-405.

Longitudinal Risk Factors for Persistent Fatigue in Adolescents

Viner RM, Clark C, Taylor SJC, et al (Univ College London, England; Centre for Psychiatry, Barts and the London, Queen Mary's School of Med and Dentistry; Centre for Health Sciences, Queen Mary's School of Med and Dentistry)
Arch Pediatr Adolesc Med 162:469-475, 2008

Objective.—To examine whether sedentary behavior, obesity, smoking, and depression are risk factors for persistent fatigue in adolescents.

Design.—Longitudinal population-based survey.

Setting.—Twenty-eight randomly selected schools in east London, England, in 2001 and 2003.

Participants.—A total of 1880 adolescents (49% male; 81% nonwhite British) aged 11 to 12 years and 13 to 14 years in 2000.

Intervention.—Confidential questionnaires completed in class.

Main Outcome Measures.—Persistent fatigue (extreme tiredness twice weekly or more often in the previous month at both surveys), sedentary behavior, physical activity, depressive symptoms, body mass index, and smoking.

Results.—Severe fatigue was reported in 11% of participants aged 11 to 14 years and 17% of participants aged 13 to 16 years. Eighty-four participants (4%) reported persistent fatigue. Across both surveys, only 3 pupils reported chronic fatigue syndrome. In multivariate logistic regression, risk of persistent fatigue was independently associated with being sedentary for more than 4 hours per day (odds ratio = 1.6; 95% confidence interval, 1.1-2.3; $P = .01$), being physically active (odds ratio = 1.5; 95% confidence interval, 1.1-2.3; $P = .004$), and depressive symptoms (odds ratio = 2.0; 95% confidence interval, 1.5-2.7; $P < .001$) in the first survey, after adjustment for age, sex, and socioeconomic status. Obesity and smoking were not associated with fatigue.

Conclusions.—Persistent fatigue is common. Being highly sedentary or highly active independently increased the risk of persistent fatigue, suggesting that divergence in either direction from healthy levels of activity increases the risk for persistent fatigue. Mental health is important in the etiology of persistent fatigue. To help define effective preventive strategies, further work is needed on the mechanisms by which these factors contribute to fatigue.

▶ This report by Viner shows just how common persistent fatigue is among adolescents. Previous studies done elsewhere have suggested that 1 in 5 teenage girls and slightly more than 1 in 20 teenage boys report having fatigue at a clinical level in the previous 2 weeks.[1] A study from the United Kingdom of youngsters 11 to 15 years of age suggests that 0.6% report severe fatigue lasting longer than 6 months and 0.19% fit the Centers for Disease Control and Prevention criteria for having the chronic fatigue syndrome.[2] The report of Viner et al takes this all one step further by defining in a longitudinal manner the risk factors for persistent fatigue in adolescence. Specifically, watching too much television (4 or more hours a day), and large amounts of video or computer use essentially doubles the risk of persistent fatigue. At the same time, excessive physical activity and depressive symptoms are also independent risk factors for persistent fatigue. These risk factors appear to be independent of confounding factors, including socioeconomic status, body mass index, and having an underlying chronic illness. The data from this report also suggest that 1 in 4 young teens will report having fatigue weekly or more often.

If there is any message in this report it is that during late childhood, kids have to get off the sofa and be active. Contrary to data from elsewhere, the report does suggest that being overly active may also be a risk factor for severe fatigue, a finding that does not seem to make a great deal of sense. Nonetheless, those teens who exceed the normal recommendations for physical activity (at least 20 minutes of vigorous physical activity 3 days a week and 30 minutes of moderate activity 5 days a week) do seem to have more fatigue than their peers. Maybe they are just plain tired after all that physical activity.

The finding that depressive symptoms increase the risk of persistent fatigue is consistent with a large body of literature showing that fatigue is associated with depression both in the general adult population and in those with persistent fatigue states, including the chronic fatigue syndrome. Although all these findings should be further studied in prospective investigations, the findings do suggest that the promotion of healthy levels of activity and emotional well-being in childhood may prevent the onset of fatigue-related symptoms, and possibly chronic fatigue syndrome, during the teen years and possibly later. Also, it may be worth screening kids with fatigue with laboratory studies examining serum inflammatory factors such as C-reactive protein. A recent study performed in Spain has shown that low-grade inflammation is negatively associated with muscle strength in adolescence, even in situations where there is no defined underlying disorder.[3]

J. A. Stockman III, MD

References

1. Ter Wolbeek M, van Doornen LJ, Kavelaars A, Heijnen CJ. Severe fatigue in adolescence: a common phenomenon? *Pediatrics.* 2006;117:e1078-e1086.
2. Fukuda K, Straus SE, Hickie I, Sharpe MC, Dobbins JG, Komaroff A. The chronic fatigue syndrome: a comprehensive approach to its definition and study. *Ann Intern Med.* 1994;121:953-959.
3. Ruiz JR, Ortega FE, Wärnberg J, et al. Inflammatory proteins and muscle strength in adolescents: the AVENA study. *Arch Pediatr Adolesc Med.* 2008;162:462-468.

Moderate-to-Vigorous Physical Activity From Ages 9 to 15 Years

Nader PR, Bradley RH, Houts RM, et al (Univ of California San Diego; Univ of Arkansas, Little Rock; RTI International Res Triangle Park, NC; et al)
JAMA 300:295-305, 2008

Context.—Decreased physical activity plays a critical role in the increase in childhood obesity. Although at least 60 minutes per day of moderate-to-vigorous physical activity (MVPA) is recommended, few longitudinal studies have determined the recent patterns of physical activity of youth.

Objective.—To determine the patterns and determinants of MVPA of youth followed from ages 9 to 15 years.

Design, Setting, and Participants.—Longitudinal descriptive analyses of the 1032 participants in the 1991-2007 National Institute of Child Health and Human Development Study of Early Child Care and Youth Development birth cohort from 10 study sites who had accelerometer- determined minutes of MVPA at ages 9 (year 2000), 11 (2002), 12 (2003), and 15

(2006) years. Participants included boys (517 [50.1%]) and girls (515 [49.9%]); 76.6% white (n = 791); and 24.5% (n = 231) lived in low-income families.

Main Outcome Measure.—Mean MVPA minutes per day, determined by 4 to 7 days of monitored activity.

Results.—At age 9 years, children engaged in MVPA approximately 3 hours per day on both weekends and weekdays. Weekday MVPA decreased by 38 minutes per year, while weekend MVPA decreased by 41 minutes per year. By age 15 years, adolescents were only engaging in MVPA for 49 minutes per weekday and 35 minutes per weekend day. Boys were more active than girls, spending 18 and 13 more minutes per day in MVPA on the weekdays and weekends, respectively. The rate of decrease in MVPA was the same for boys and girls. The estimated age at which girls crossed below the recommended 60 minutes of MVPA per day was approximately 13.1 years for weekday activity compared with boys at 14.7 years, and for weekend activity, girls crossed below the recommended 60 minutes of MVPA at 12.6 years compared with boys at 13.4 years.

Conclusion.—In this study cohort, measured physical activity decreased significantly between ages 9 and 15 years.

▶ If you are not familiar with the National Institute of Child Health and Human Development (NICHD) study of early child care and youth development, it is a multisite study originally designed to determine the effects of nonmaternal care on the development of children. Children began to be enrolled in this study back in 1991 and were followed from birth to 15 years with a common study protocol, including interview, home school, and neighborhood observation. This included healthy newborns of English-speaking mothers, discharged within 1 week of birth. Many things have been followed as part of this NICHD study, including the amount of physical activity each child engaged in during a typical week, as measured by using an accelerometer. Measurements of the latter were done at ages 9, 11, 12, and 15 years.

The data from this report show that age at 9, the average child did engage in moderate-to-vigorous physical activity approximately 3 hours a day on both weekends and weekdays. After age 9, there was a steady decline on a yearly basis in the level of physical activity such that by 15 years of age, adolescents were engaging in moderate-to-vigorous activity for just over 3 quarters of an hour on weekdays and just over half hour on weekend days (Fig 3).

We all know that for adults 30 minutes per day of significant physical activity is the current recommendation to maintain health. Among adults, adherence to the recommendation to obtain 30 minutes per day of physical activity is less than 5%. While there is no single accepted protocol across existing studies for setting accelerometer-based cutoff points for moderate-to-vigorous physical activity, when you are involved with no activity at all, it is fair to say that the adult, if one considers the adult an apple, does not fall far from the tree of the adolescent. At the average age of 15, a minority of adolescents are

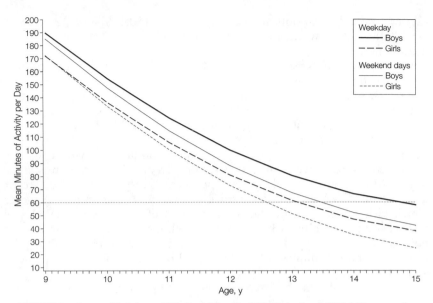

FIGURE 3.—Average Weekday and Weekend Minutes of MVPA by Sex. MVPA indicates moderate-to-vigorous physical activity. Dotted horizontal line indicates the recommended 60 minutes per day of MVPA for children.[10] Graphs were generated from estimates obtained from growth curve model 2, which included intercepts, age, sex, age × sex, and age × age to describe change in MVPA on weekdays and weekends between ages 9 and 15 years. Girls cross below the recommended 60 minutes of MVPA per day at approximately 13.1 years (95% CI, 12.9-13.3) for weekday activity and 12.6 years (95% CI, 12.3-12.8) for weekend activity; boys cross below the recommended 60 minutes of MVPA per day at approximately 14.7 years (95% CI, 14.3-15.3) for weekday activity and 13.4 years (95% CI, 13.2-13.7) for weekend activity. Editor's Note: Please refer to original journal article for full references. (Reprinted from Nader PR, Bradley RH, Houts RM, et al. Moderate-to-vigorous physical activity from ages 9 to 15 years. *JAMA*. 2008;300:295-305. Copyright 2008 American Medical Association. All rights reserved.)

meeting the recommended minutes per day of moderate-to-vigorous physical activity, even by the most liberal standards.

Despite the fact that this editor has personally espoused the belief that you are born with a finite number of heart beats and they should not be wasted on exercise, this belief is stated tongue-in-cheek. Exercise is in fact good for you. It is especially good for you if you are a child, adolescent, or adult with dyslipidemia. Physical activity primarily effects HDL and triglyceride concentrations. Improvements in LDL concentrations have also been documented. Although there have been few randomized clinical trials to document the effects of physical activity as a specific intervention for children and adolescents, supportive data are available from epidemiologic studies.[1]

J. A. Stockman III, MD

Reference

1. Strong WB, Malina RM, Blimkie CJ, et al. Evidence-based physical activity for school-aged youth. *J Pediatr.* 2005;146:732-737.

Bone Metabolism in Adolescent Boys with Anorexia Nervosa

Misra M, Katzman DK, Cord J, et al (Massachusetts Gen Hosp for Children and Harvard Med School, Boston; Division of Adolescent Medicine, Children, Toronto, Ontario, Canada)
J Clin Endocrinol Metab 93:3029-3036, 2008

Background.—Anorexia nervosa (AN) is a condition of severe undernutrition associated with low bone mineral density (BMD) in adolescent females with this disorder. Although primarily a disease in females, AN is increasingly being recognized in males. However, there are few or no data regarding BMD, bone turnover markers or their predictors in adolescent AN boys.

Hypotheses.—We hypothesized that BMD would be low in adolescent boys with AN compared with controls associated with a decrease in bone turnover markers, and that the gonadal steroids, testosterone and estradiol, and levels of IGF-I and the appetite regulatory hormones leptin, ghrelin, and peptide YY would predict BMD and bone turnover markers.

Methods.—We assessed BMD using dual-energy x-ray absorptiometry and measured fasting testosterone, estradiol, IGF-I, leptin, ghrelin, and peptide YY and a bone formation (aminoterminal propeptide of type 1 procollagen) and bone resorption (N-telopeptide of type 1 collagen) marker in 17 AN boys and 17 controls 12–19 yr old.

Results.—Boys with AN had lower BMD and corresponding Z-scores at the spine, hip, femoral neck, trochanter, intertrochanteric region, and whole body, compared with controls. Height-adjusted measures (lumbar bone mineral apparent density and whole body bone mineral content/height) were also lower. Bone formation and resorption markers were reduced in AN, indicating decreased bone turnover. Testosterone and lean mass predicted BMD. IGF-I was an important predictor of bone turnover markers.

Conclusion.—AN boys have low BMD at multiple sites associated with decreased bone turnover markers at a time when bone mass accrual is critical for attainment of peak bone mass.

▶ All of us know about the problem of bone mineral metabolism in young women with anorexia nervosa. Unfortunately, there is much less information about this problem in boys with this condition, a disorder that is being increasingly recognized in boys. There are marked differences, normally, in bone mineralization between boys and girls given the unique hormonal discrepancies between sexes. This report from Boston and Toronto provides us with a great deal of useful information about bone mineral density, body composition, gonadal steroids, and other regulatory hormones in adolescents with anorexia nervosa. In fact, this is the first time that lower bone mineral density and height adjusted measures of bone mineral density have been reported in any detail in adolescent boys with anorexia nervosa. Specifically, lower bone mineral density was clearly observed in boys with anorexia nervosa, a phenomenon associated with reduced bone turnover and low levels of testosterone. As expected, anorexia nervosa affected boys did show lower fat mass, lean mass, testosterone, estradiol, and higher peptide YY levels. Of all these variables, testosterone turns out to be the most important and independent predictor of bone mineral density. Even after adjusting for height, lower bone mineral densities were observed.

Just as with girls, boys with anorexia nervosa will grow up to be adults with poor bone mineral density and thus are at long-term risk of fractures, and other bone-related problems. It is critically important to keep on top of this complication of anorexia nervosa in both sexes.

J. A. Stockman III, MD

2 Allergy and Dermatology

Good prognosis, clinical features, and circumstances of peanut and tree nut reactions in children treated by a specialist allergy center
Clark AT, Ewan PW (Cambridge Univ Hosp Natl Health Service Found Trust, UK)
J Allergy Clin Immunol 122:286-289, 2008

Background.—The diagnosis of nut allergy causes anxiety. Few studies exist that estimate risk of reactions and inform management.

Objective.—To describe frequency and circumstances of reactions after the institution of a management plan.

Methods.—Prospective study of children with peanut/nut allergy with an allergist's management plan. Severity and circumstances of worst reaction before diagnosis (index) and follow-up reactions were evaluated.

Results.—A total of 785 children were followed for 3640 patient-years from diagnosis. Index reactions were mild in 66% (516), moderate in 29% (224), and severe in 5% (45). Fourteen percent (114/785) had follow-up reactions (3% annual incidence rate). Ninety percent had the same/reduced severity grade, and 1 of 785 (0.1%) had a severe reaction. Preschool children (n = 263) had a low incidence of reactions, and none were severe. There was a 3-fold reduction in injected epinephrine use from that used in the index reaction, required in 1 severe reaction, never twice; 14% (16/114) required no medication, 78% only oral antihistamines. Forty-eight percent reacted to the index nut type, 19% to a different nut (55% sensitized at diagnosis, 14% not sensitized, 31% not tested). Accidental versus index reactions were 4-fold more likely to be a result of contact exposure rather than ingestion. Contact reactions were always mild. Most (53%) reactions occurred at home, 5% in school, 21% at other sites (21% not recorded). The nut was given by a parent/self in 69 (61%) reactions or teacher in 5 (4%).

Conclusion.—With a comprehensive management plan, accidental reactions were uncommon and usually mild, most requiring little treatment; 99.8% self-treated appropriately and 100% effectively.

▶ This is an important report because it represents one of the largest natural history studies of children with peanut and tree nut allergy. Almost 800 youngsters with peanut and/or nut allergy were followed for an average of over

5 years. The diagnosis of peanut and/or nut allergy was made after a recent history of a typical type 1 hypersensitivity reaction (urticaria/angioedema with or without wheezing, with or without vomiting and with or without abdominal pain, and change in behavior). Evidence of sensitization to nuts was confirmed by skin-prick test. Each patient was enrolled in a comprehensive food allergy management program that provided detailed written and verbal advice on nut avoidance, provision of emergency medication, training of family members in the use of these emergency medications, and notification of each child's school or nursery of the diagnosis along with training of school personnel with respect to avoidance advice and emergency medication training.

With the aggressive approach described, the follow-up of these youngsters showed an annual incidence rate for accidental ingestion of peanut and/or tree nuts of just 3%. This is much lower than has been previously described. This study was also the first to describe whether children react to the same or a different nut type during initial and subsequent accidental reactions. Despite the advice to avoid all nut types, at least 20% reacted to a different one, not previously ingested, and at least half of those were known to have a positive skin prick test to that type at presentation.

A number of factors should go into the decision of whether to advise children to avoid all nuts, or only the kind of nut shown to cause a reaction. Children with nut allergy in fact do have a poor ability to distinguish different nut types on the basis of appearance. That can be true of all of us. Further, peanut is commonly used by manufacturers to bulk out other nut-type foods in which the nut type cannot be clearly identified, such as sauces. In 2-year-olds with peanut allergy, about 20% are sensitized to at least 2 nut types, but this rises by age 10 to over 70%. The only workable policy for most youngsters is to avoid all nut types.

This report from overseas also shows that a significant proportion of accidental reactions in school-aged children occur outside the school and home. A wide range of situations and locales were associated with accidental reactions, including parties, scout groups, aircraft, restaurants, and churches. One final comment about nut allergy. Cashew nut allergy seems to be increasing rapidly in prevalence. In this series, it was the third most common cause of initial reactions, an almost unheard of problem just 20 years ago. A greater proportion of reactions to cashew are severe. Fortunately, the frequency of accidental follow-up reactions to cashew nuts is low, presumably because cashews are relatively easy to avoid, being less often used as an ingredient or hidden in foods.

If there is any good news in this, it is that the prognosis for children with nut allergy is good if they are carefully managed. Interventions such as oral desensitization are being developed to prevent accidental reactions; however, until they are available, we should learn from these reports how to improve allergen avoidance advice. Families and schools can be reassured that simple noningestion contact reactions tend to be mild.

J. A. Stockman III, MD

Tolerance to extensively heated milk in children with cow's milk allergy

Nowak-Wegrzyn A, Bloom KA, Sicherer SH, et al (Mount Sinai School of Medicine, NY)

J Allergy Clin Immunol 122:342-347, 2008

Background.—Cow's milk allergy is the most common childhood food allergy. Previously we noted that children who outgrew their milk allergy had milk-specific IgE antibodies primarily directed against conformational epitopes; those with persistent milk allergy also had IgE antibodies directed against specific sequential epitopes.

Objective.—Because high temperature largely destroys conformational epitopes, we hypothesized that some children with milk allergy would tolerate extensively heated (baked) milk products.

Methods.—Children with milk allergy were challenged with heated milk products; heated milk–tolerant subjects were subsequently challenged with unheated milk. Heated milk–tolerant, unheated milk–reactive subjects ingested heated milk products for 3 months and were then re-evaluated. Immune responses were assessed in all subjects; growth and intestinal permeability were followed in heated milk–tolerant subjects.

Results.—One hundred children (mean age, 7.5 years; range, 2.1-17.3 years) underwent heated milk challenges. Sixty-eight subjects tolerated extensively heated milk only, 23 reacted to heated milk, and 9 tolerated both heated and unheated milk. Heated milk–reactive subjects had significantly larger skin prick test wheals and higher milk-specific and casein-specific IgE levels than other groups. At 3 months, subjects ingesting heated milk products had significantly smaller skin prick test wheals and higher casein-IgG$_4$ compared with baseline; other immunologic parameters, growth, and intestinal permeability were not significantly different. Heated milk–reactive subjects had more severe symptoms during heated milk challenge than heated milk–tolerant subjects experienced during their unheated milk challenge.

Conclusion.—The majority (75%) of children with milk allergy tolerate heated milk.

▶ There have been reports that have suggested that children with egg allergy can tolerate egg if heated, but not in the nonheated form. This is what stimulated the investigators from Mount Sinai School of Medicine to evaluate whether patients with milk allergy might possibly tolerate extensively heated milk products. You should read this report in detail to see its study design, but the bottom line was that the majority (75%) of children with a recent diagnosis of milk allergy did in fact tolerate extensively heated milk during an initial oral food challenge. This suggests the notion that children with milk allergy in fact are clinically and immunologically heterogeneous and that reactivity to heated milk proteins is a marker of this heterogeneity. It has been shown before that high heat, such as with baking, can reduce the allergenicity of many food proteins, presumably by altering the conformation of heat-labile proteins that results in loss of conformational epitopes. The classic examples are birch tree pollen allergen, and Bet v 1 cross-reactive proteins in apple and carrot that in the uncooked form cause oral symptoms (pollen-food allergy syndrome), but after heating are readily tolerated. In contrast, the Bet v 1 cross-reactive protein in soybean retains allergenicity even in heat-processed foods, suggesting that thermostability is highly variable and food-specific, even for food allergens in the same protein family. High temperature is capable of enhancing allergenicity as a result of glycation. This is especially true of peanut proteins.

Published data indicate that heating decreases but does not completely eliminate milk allergenicity. Actually there are many different potential allergens in cow milk including casein, alpha lactalbumin, and other whey proteins, including beta-lactaglobin and serum albumin. Depending on which component in cow's milk one is reactive to, since heat inactivates some of these allergens at different rates, one might expect a varying response to heat treatment of cow milk as one measure to diminish cow milk allergy.

The researchers at Mount Sinai School of Medicine suggest that there are at least two different phenotypes of IgE-milk mediated allergy in children. They define a type I individual who is eventually able to tolerate milk and experiences a "transient" food allergy. This individual is more likely not to have difficulty with heat-treated cow milk. Type II individuals are not able to down regulate their allergic response and have persistent food allergy. If the data from this report are confirmed, it could well change our approach to the diagnosis and management of milk allergy since allowing ingestion of heated milk products could dramatically improve the quality of life for the majority of subjects with milk allergy by vastly increasing the variety of food products they are able to consume.

It would be important for all of us to follow the emerging story about heat treatment as a method to reduce reactions to food products in sensitive individuals. This could be a very simple way to help our patients lead a better life.

J. A. Stockman III, MD

Birth by cesarean section, allergic rhinitis, and allergic sensitization among children with a parental history of atopy

Pistiner M, Gold DR, Abdulkerim H, et al (Children's Hosp Boston; Brigham and Women's Hosp; et al)
J Allergy Clin Immunol 122:274-279, 2008

Background.—Cesarean delivery can alter neonatal immune responses and increase the risk of atopy. Studies of the relation between cesarean delivery and allergic diseases in children not selected on the basis of a family history of atopy have yielded inconsistent findings.

Objective.—We sought to examine the relation between birth by cesarean delivery and atopy and allergic diseases in children at risk for atopy.

Methods.—We examined the relation between mode of delivery and the development of atopy and allergic diseases among 432 children with a parental history of atopy followed from birth to age 9 years. Asthma was defined as physician-diagnosed asthma and wheeze in the previous year, and allergic rhinitis was defined as physician-diagnosed allergic rhinitis and naso-ocular symptoms apart from colds in the previous year. Atopy was considered present at school age if there was 1 or more positive skin test response or specific IgE to common allergens. Stepwise logistic regression was used to study the relation between cesarean delivery and the outcomes of interest.

Results.—After adjustment for other covariates, children born by cesarean section had 2-fold higher odds of atopy than those born by vaginal delivery (odds ratio, 2.1; 95% CI, 1.1-3.9). In multivariate analyses birth by cesarean section was significantly associated with increased odds of allergic rhinitis (odds ratio, 1.8; 95% CI, 1.0-3.1) but not with asthma.

Conclusions.—Our findings suggest that cesarean delivery is associated with allergic rhinitis and atopy among children with a parental history of asthma or allergies. This could be explained by lack of contact with the maternal vaginal/fecal flora or reduced/absent labor during cesarean delivery.

▶ This is not the first report to suggest that birth by cesarean section is associated with a higher probability of developing allergic problems, including asthma. In fact, at least 2 biologically plausible hypotheses have been proposed to suggest the connection between cesarean section and asthma. The first of these relates to the "hygiene hypothesis." When a baby is born by cesarean section, that baby is colonized by bacteria, not from the birth canal, perineum, or skin of the mother, but largely from bacteria of the environment of the hospital. Gut flora have a significant impact on stimulation and maturation of an infant's immune system, and its composition varies according to the mode of delivery. This first theory says that babies therefore who are born by c-section may be colonized with the "wrong" bugs and possibly have long-term adverse effects on the immune system as a consequence, the latter triggering reactive airway disease and atopic diseases. The second hypothesis states that because cesarean section is associated with an increased risk of respiratory distress syndrome and transient tachypnea in newborns, and these conditions have been reported to be risk factors for reactive airway disease, cesarean section therefore sets an infant up for a greater risk of the development of asthma.

What we see in this report from Boston are the results of the first prospective birth cohort study of the relation between birth by cesarean section and atopy and allergic diseases at school age among children at high risk for atopy. In this study, birth by cesarean section appears to be associated with increased risks of allergic rhinitis and atopy, but not with asthma. Other studies have examined birth by cesarean section and allergic rhinitis and have shown inconclusive results. The same is true of studies that have looked at birth by cesarean section and subsequent atopy. The authors of this study previously reported preliminary findings of an association between cesarean section and increased levels of IL-13 and IFN-gamma in cord blood, which in turn have been associated with an increased risk for the development of atopy and asthma in childhood.[1]

This Boston report should not be considered definitive in its results. At the same time this report appeared, data from the Medical Birth Registry of Norway also appeared. A population-based cohort study of 1 756 700 infants reported to this registry between 1967 and 1998, followed up to age 18 years or the year 2002, showed a significant correlation between birth by cesarean section and an increased risk of asthma. Children delivered by cesarean section had a 52% increased risk of asthma compared with spontaneously vaginally delivered children. Planned and emergency cesarean section was associated with a 42% and a 59%, respectively, increased risk of asthma.[2]

So whose data are stronger, investigators from Boston looking at 432 children or investigators from Norway tracking almost 2 million live births? If you believe the latter, you see a confirmation of a moderate association between cesarean section and severe asthma, consistent with many previous studies. Because asthma constitutes an important and increasing burden in children today, and the rate of cesarean section continues to rise, you can be darn sure that you will be seeing more studies appearing in the literature explaining the putative link between the two.

J. A. Stockman III, MD

References

1. Ly NP, Ruiz-Perez B, Onderdonk AB, et al. Mode of delivery and cord blood cytokines: a birth cohort study. *Clin Mole Allergy.* 2006;4:13.
2. Tollanes MC, Moster D, Daltveit AK, Irgens LM. Cesarean section and the risk of severe childhood asthma: a population-based cohort study. *J Pediatr.* 2008;153: 112-116.

Mediterranean Diet as a Protective Factor for Wheezing in Preschool Children

Castro-Rodriguez JA, Garcia-Marcos L, Alfonseda Rojas JD, et al (Pontificia Universidad Catolica de Chile, Santiago, Chile; Univ of Murcia, Spain; Cartagena Health Ctr, Spain)
J Pediatr 152:823-828, 2008

Objective.—To test the hypothesis that the Mediterranean diet can be a protective factor for current wheezing in preschoolers.

Study Design.—Questionnaires were completed by parents of 1784 preschoolers (mean age, 4.08 ± 0.8 years). Children were stratified according to whether they experienced wheezing (20.0%) or not in the previous year. A Mediterranean diet score was built according to the intake frequency of several foods.

Results.—Age, birth by cesarean section, low birth weight, exposure to livestock during pregnancy, antibiotic use in the first year of life, acetaminophen consumption in the previous 12 months, rhinoconjunctivitis, eczema, parental asthma and tobacco consumption, maternal educational level, maternal age, physical activity, cat at home, and Mediterranean diet were associated with current wheezing but not with obesity. In the multivariate analysis, eczema, rhinoconjunctivitis, paternal asthma, and acetaminophen consumption remained risk factors for current wheezing (adjusted odds ratio [aOR] = 2.35 [95% confidence interval (CI) = 1.2 to 4.8], 2.78 [95% CI = 1.3 to 6.1], 3.89 [95% CI = 1.4 to 10.7], and 2.38 [95% CI = 1.2 to 4.6], respectively). Conversely, Mediterranean diet and older age remained protective factors (aOR = 0.54 [95% CI = 0.3 to 0.9] and 0.67 [95% CI = 0.5 to 0.9], respectively).

Conclusions.—The Mediterranean diet is an independent protective factor for current wheezing in preschoolers, irrespective of obesity and physical activity.

▶ There are various reports and references to the potential association between cesarean birth and asthma. Now we see that there is an inverse correlation between dieting on Mediterranean cuisine and wheezing. Indeed, according to the International Study of Asthma and Allergy in Childhood, asthma prevalence is lower in the Mediterranean countries.[1] One common factor in these Mediterranean countries, besides the climate, is the "Mediterranean diet." There are a number of variations of the Mediterranean diet, but common to these variants is a diet that includes a high monounsaturated/saturated fat ratio, high consumption of vegetables, fruit, legumes, and grains, and moderate consumption of milk and dairy products. In this report from Spain, the investigators tested the hypothesis that the Mediterranean diet would indeed be a protective factor for current wheezing in Spanish preschool-aged children. Some 3000 children were invited to participate in the study and almost 2000 actually completed the requisite portions of the study. The study results did suggest that the Mediterranean diet is likely to be a protective factor for current wheezing in preschool-aged children independent of other factors such as obesity and physical activity.

So what is it about the Mediterranean diet that could theoretically be protective against the development of reactive airway disease? Certainly this diet is rich in both antioxidants and monounsaturated fatty acids. Studies have previously suggested that the prevalence of allergic sensitization is lower with higher intakes of fruits and vitamins A and C as well as vegetables. The Mediterranean diet may offer protection from wheezing due to a positive balance effects of eating "protective" foods while avoiding "risky" foods. On the other hand, data have also shown that fast-food ingestion is associated with a higher probability of developing reactive airway disease.[2]

When all else fails, a little pasta, with fresh tomato sauce and a glass of wine followed by a fruit plate will do your lungs good.

This commentary closes with a *Clinical Fact/Curio* having to do with pediatric allergy and is posed in the form of a question. For years you have been recommending using mattress protectors as an intervention in the management of asthma for those patients with the latter condition who are sensitive to house dust mites. Just how good has your advice been? The answer is that there is no evidence that interventions, such as using mattress protectors and removing soft toys from beds, are beneficial in the management of asthma in youngsters who are sensitive to house dust mites. This is the conclusion based on the latest evidence from the Cochrane Collaboration on Physical and Chemical Measures to Control Dust-Mite Levels. The review was of pooled data from 54 trials of 3002 patients with asthma. Interventions included spray chemicals and powders, mattress encasings, vacuuming, frequent washing of linen at high temperatures, and removal of soft toys from beds. Outcomes were measured as improvements in asthma symptom scores, medication usage, FEV_1 levels, and peak-flow measurements. The results confirm those from the Cochrane Collaboration's earlier 2004 review of 49 trials, so these conclusions do not come as a surprise. The issue is why no one is listening. The United States National Heart Lung and Blood Institute's 2007 guidelines for the treatment and management of asthma continue to recommend encasement of mattresses and pillows in allergen-impermeable covers. Overseas, such guidelines are considered with some degree of skepticism. For example, the British Thoracic Society acknowledges that the clinical benefit of these interventions has yet to be proven. Virtually all patient information groups, Web sites, etc use the National Heart Lung and Blood Institute's guidelines for providing management strategies for those with asthma.

Life would be so simple if we could merely cover over the little mite creatures that so commonly either cause or exacerbate episodes of asthma.[3,4]

J. A. Stockman III, MD

References

1. Worldwide variations in the prevalence of asthma symptoms. International Study of Asthma and Allergy in Childhood (ISAAC). *Euro Respir J.* 1998;12:315-335.
2. Wickens K, Barry D, Friezema A, et al. Fast-foods: are they are risk factor for asthma? *Allergy.* 2005;60:1537-1541.
3. Dust-mite control measures are of no use [editorial comment]. *Lancet.* 2008;371: 1390.
4. Gøtzsche PC, Johansen HK. House dust mite control measures for asthma. *Cochrane Database Syst Rev.* 2008;2: CD001187.

Wheezing and bronchial hyper-responsiveness in early childhood as predictors of newly diagnosed asthma in early adulthood: a longitudinal birth-cohort study

Stern DA, Morgan WJ, Halonen M, et al (Univ of Arizona, Tucson)
Lancet 372:1058-1064, 2008

Background.—Incidence of asthma increases during early adulthood. We aimed to estimate the contributions of sex and early life factors to asthma diagnosed in young adults.

Methods.—1246 healthy newborn babies were enrolled in the Tucson Children's Respiratory Study. Parental characteristics, early-life wheezing phenotypes, airway function, and bronchial hyper-responsiveness to cold dry air and sensitisation to *Alternaria alternata* were determined before age 6 years. Physician-diagnosed asthma, both chronic and newly diagnosed, and airway function were recorded at age 22 years.

Findings.—Of 1246 babies enrolled, 849 had follow-up data at 22 years. Average incidence of asthma at age 16–22 years was $12 \cdot 6$ per thousand person-years. 49 (27%) of all 181 cases of active asthma at 22 years were newly diagnosed, of which 35 (71%) were women. Asthma remittance by 22 years was higher in men than in women (multinomial odds ratio [M-OR] $2 \cdot 0$, 95% CI $1 \cdot 2$–$3 \cdot 2$, p=$0 \cdot 008$). Age at diagnosis was linearly associated with the ratio of forced expiratory volume at 1 s to forced vital capacity at age 22 years. Factors independently associated with chronic asthma at 22 years included onset at 6 years ($7 \cdot 4$, $3 \cdot 9$–$14 \cdot 0$) and persistent wheezing ($14 \cdot 0$, $6 \cdot 8$–$28 \cdot 0$) in early life, sensitisation to A *alternata* ($3 \cdot 6$, $2 \cdot 1$–$6 \cdot 4$), low airway function at age 6 years ($2 \cdot 1$, $1 \cdot 1$–$3 \cdot 9$), and bronchial hyper responsiveness at 6 years ($4 \cdot 5$, $1 \cdot 9$–$10 \cdot 0$). Bronchial hyper-responsiveness ($6 \cdot 9$, $2 \cdot 3$–$21 \cdot 0$), low airway function at 6 years ($2 \cdot 8$, $1 \cdot 1$–$6 \cdot 9$), and late-onset ($4 \cdot 6$, $1 \cdot 7$–$12 \cdot 0$) and persistent wheezing ($4 \cdot 0$, $1 \cdot 2$–$14 \cdot 0$) predicted newly diagnosed asthma at age 22 years.

Interpretation.—Asthma with onset in early adulthood has its origins in early childhood.

▶ This is an interesting report and a powerful one in that over 12 000 healthy newborns were evaluated over time having been enrolled in the Tucson Children's Respiratory Study. The investigators designed a study to determine whether potential risk factors for asthma measured during preschool years would predict the prevalence and incidence of asthma and asthma-like symptoms in early adulthood. The information provided from this study is quite potent, illustrating that over 70% of young adults with current asthma and 63% of those with newly-diagnosed asthma at age 22 years had episodes of wheezing in the first 3 years of life or were reported by parents at 6 years of age to have had wheezing. The findings unequivocally support the belief that most forms of asthma have their origins early in life on our watch as care providers. The data also show that women are more likely to have had early onset wheezing and that asthma in children is more likely to not result in asthma during adulthood if the affected individual is male. One of the greatest risk factors for wheezing in young adulthood and a strong predictor is active smoking.

Although no real cure for reactive airway disease exists, early identification of patients at risk of disease progression could lead to better treatment opportunities and, hopefully, improved outcomes in adulthood. Nevertheless, early intervention has not yet been shown to be beneficial in terms of disease modification, which might be because of the failure to identify appropriate subgroups of responders. Studies during early childhood have not shown a clear benefit of early anti-inflammatory treatment in terms of symptom-free days after the treatment period in preschool children. However, inhaled steroids do seem to reduce the accelerated decline. Enforced expiratory volume could be of benefit on the long haul in terms of minimizing the adult expression of asthma.

One other diagnosis also predicts the adult onset or exacerbation of asthma and that is the presence of allergic rhinitis in childhood. A recent report shows that many young adults with asthma had the asthma preceded by episodes of allergic rhinitis in childhood.[1] This report suggests that rather than simply using agents that reduce nasal symptoms (topical steroids, leukotriene antagonist, etc), which basically simply produce symptomatic relief from allergic rhinitis, we might think about actually trying to interfere with the basic cause of allergic rhinitis by immunotherapy approaches. Symptomatic treatment has no role in the secondary prevention of asthma, whereas immunotherapy might very well.

While the cure of allergic rhinitis might only prevent some cases of new onset asthma in young adults, the goal of achieving even that is laudable. To say this differently, allergic rhinitis is more than simply a runny nose. It can be a setup for asthma later in life.

J. A. Stockman III, MD

Reference

1. Shaaban R, Zureik M, Soussan D, et al. Rhinitis and the onset of asthma: a longitudinal population-based study. *Lancet.* 2008;372:1049-1057.

Childhood eczema and asthma incidence and persistence: A cohort study from childhood to middle age
Burgess JA, Dharmage SC, Byrnes GB, et al (Univ of Melbourne, Carlton; et al)
J Allergy Clin Immunol 122:280-285, 2008

Background.—The association between eczema and asthma is well documented, but the temporal sequence of this association has not been closely examined.

Objectives.—To examine the association between childhood eczema and asthma incidence from preadolescence to middle age, and between childhood eczema and asthma persisting to middle age. A further aim was to examine any effect modification by nonallergic childhood exposures on the association between childhood eczema and both childhood asthma and later life incident asthma.

Methods.—Data were gathered from the 1968, 1974, and 2004 surveys of the Tasmanian Longitudinal Health Study. Multivariable logistic regression examined the association between childhood eczema and childhood asthma. Cox regression examined the association between childhood eczema and asthma incidence in preadolescence, adolescence, and adult life. Binomial regression examined the association between childhood eczema and childhood asthma persisting to age 44 years.

Results.—Childhood eczema was significantly associated with childhood asthma and with incident asthma in preadolescence (hazard ratio [HR], 1.70; 95% CI, 1.05-2.75), adolescence (HR, 2.14; 95% CI, 1.33-3.46), and adult life (HR, 1.63; 95% CI, 1.28-2.09). Although childhood eczema was significantly associated with asthma persisting from childhood to middle age (relative risk, 1.54; 95% CI, 1.17-2.04), this association was no longer evident when adjusted for allergic rhinitis.

Conclusion.—Childhood eczema increased the likelihood of childhood asthma, of new-onset asthma in later life and of asthma persisting into middle age.

► All those involved with the care of children are aware of the relationship between childhood eczema and the likelihood of developing asthma during childhood. This report reminds us that a recent systematic review documented that about one-third of children with atopic eczema manifesting before age 4 will develop reactive airway disease by age 6 years or older.[1] In terms of the relationship between eczema and asthma, this is where our knowledge base seems to end since there is little known about childhood eczema and asthma much later in life. That is the subject of this report from Melbourne, Australia, where the association between childhood eczema and asthma from preadolescence to middle age was examined.

This report summarizes data from the Tasmanian Longitudinal Health Study (TLHS). TLHS began way back in 1968 when over 8000 7-year-old children in Tasmania were initially surveyed and then followed throughout later childhood into adulthood. Careful histories were taken of allergic problems including asthma, hayfever, eczema, food and medicine allergy, and urticaria. Several surveys were done of these children over the years and as recently as 2004, more than 80% were still able to be located. The well-recognized relationship between eczema and asthma in childhood was clearly documented, but as importantly, over time from age 8 to age 44 years, asthma incidence was nearly twice as high in those with childhood eczema, compared with those with no history of eczema. These results clearly suggest that the effect of childhood eczema on asthma risk continues well past childhood, this report being the first study to document this. The study also documented the predicted 33% likelihood that a child early in life who develops eczema will have asthma by 7 years of age.

Although we have long recognized the relationship between various forms of allergy in terms of clinical expression, the mechanism that explains the association has remained an enigma. There is good evidence supporting both genetic and environmental factors as links between eczema and asthma. Specific chromosomal markers showing this linkage have been proposed. Also proposed is the possibility that exposure of damaged skin early in life to potential allergens can be a setup by which later migration of T-memory cells from the skin to the bronchus-associated lymphoid tissue would occur such that subsequent inhalation of sensitizing allergen would cause a cellular and humoral response in the airways resulting in asthma. If this latter theory were to hold true, it might suggest that a more aggressive management of childhood eczema could modify the subsequent risk of asthma.

There is nothing quite as powerful as data derived from many thousands of study subjects. That is the case with TLHS and we should be grateful to our friends from "Down Under" for warning us about the truly long-term consequences of a common problem, eczema, in early childhood.

J. A. Stockman III, MD

Reference

1. van der Hulst AE, Klip H, Brand PL. Risk of developing asthma in young children with atopic eczema: a systematic review. *J Allergy Clin Immunol.* 2007;120: 565-569.

MAS063DP is Effective Monotherapy for Mild to Moderate Atopic Dermatitis in Infants and Children: A Multicenter, Randomized, Vehicle-Controlled Study

Boguniewicz M, Zeichner JA, Eichenfield LF, et al (Natl Jewish Med and Res Ctr and Univ of Colorado School of Medicine, Denver; Mt Sinai School of Medicine, NY; Rady Children's Hosp and Univ of California, San Diego; et al)
J Pediatr 152:854-859, 2008

Objective.—To examine the efficacy and safety of MAS063DP (Atopiclair) cream in the management of mild to moderate atopic dermatitis in infants and children.

Study Design.—One hundred forty-two patients aged 6 months to 12 years were administered MAS063DP (n = 72) or vehicle (n = 70) cream 3 times per day to affected areas and sites prone to develop atopic dermatitis. The primary endpoint for efficacy was the Investigator's Global Assessment at day 22. Secondary endpoints included Investigator's Global Assessment at other time-points, patient's/caregiver's assessment of pruritus, onset, duration of itch relief, Eczema Area and Severity Index, subject's/caregiver's assessment of global response, and need for rescue medication in the event of an atopic dermatitis flare.

Results.—MAS063DP cream was statistically more effective ($P < .0001$) than vehicle cream for the primary endpoint and all secondary endpoints. Treatment discontinuation as a result of an adverse event occurred in 9.9% of patients using MAS063DP cream and 16% of patients using vehicle cream.

Conclusion.—MAS063DP cream is effective and safe as monotherapy for the treatment of symptoms of mild to moderate atopic dermatitis in infants and children (Figs 1 and 2).

▶ It seems like you need a contemporary course in molecular biology to be able to manage allergic disorders in this day and age. That is particularly true when it comes to the management of reactive airway disease, atopic dermatitis, and allergy in general. When it comes to atopic dermatitis, a number of studies have now shown that mutations in a filaggrin gene are a major predisposing factor for the disorder. If you are not familiar with filaggrin, it is a prominent epidermal protein. This protein is a key factor for the formation of a normal

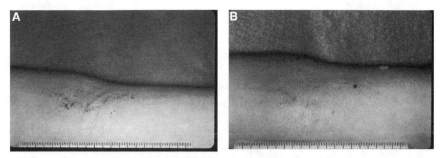

FIGURE 1.—Representative atopic dermatitis skin lesions at day 1 (A) and day 8 (B) of treatment with MAS063DP. (Reprinted from Boguniewicz M, Zeichner JA, Eichenfield LF, et al. MAS063DP is effective monotherapy for mild to moderate atopic dermatitis in infants and children: a multicenter, randomized, vehicle-controlled study. *J Pediatr.* 2008;152:854-859, with permission from Elsevier.)

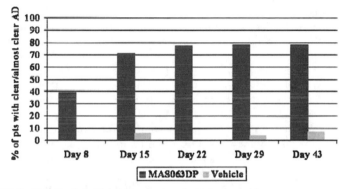

FIGURE 2.—Investigator's Global Assessment of atopic dermatitis treatment successes ("Clear" or "almost clear" ratings). MAS063DP vs Vehicle: $P < .0001$ at all time points. (Reprinted from Boguniewicz M, Zeichner JA, Eichenfield LF, et al. MAS063DP is effective monotherapy for mild to moderate atopic dermatitis in infants and children: a multicenter, randomized, vehicle-controlled study. *J Pediatr.* 2008;152:854-859, with permission from Elsevier.)

skin barrier. Patients with atopic dermatitis also show abnormalities in an important enzyme, a serine protease, located in the extracellular space of the stratum corneum. This protein is specific for cells forming keratin undergoing desquamation. Increases in the production of the enzyme protease and premature breakdown of the skin barrier are both features of atopic dermatitis.

So what does all this have to do with MAS063DP? This is also known as Atopiclair, a nonsteroidal cream that has been found to be efficacious in several studies in adults with atopic dermatitis and contact dermatitis. MAS063DP contains glycyrrhetinic acid, a grapevine extract, and telmestine. Glycyrrhetinic acid comes from licorice root and has been known for some time to have anti-inflammatory and anti-itch activity. It also blocks the breakdown of endogenous cortisol by inhibiting a dehydrogenase enzyme. The grapevine extract has antioxidant and antiprotease activity, both properties of which protect against the breakdown of the epidermis. It also has antiprotease activity and inhibits a number of different enzymes that tend to be overexpressed at high levels in the skin of patients with atopic dermatitis. The report abstracted gives us the results of the potential benefits of MAS063DP cream as part of the management of mild to moderate atopic dermatitis in children and adolescents. Youngsters 6 months to 12 years of age were given the cream 3 times a day to affected areas and sites prone to the development of atopic dermatitis. After 22 days, the patients were compared with a matched set of patients who were receiving a placebo. The study was particularly powerful because a total of 142 subjects were enrolled.

So is MAS063DP effective? You bet. A highly significant difference was found between MAS063DP and placebo treatment groups with 77% of subjects receiving the new agent responding extremely well. Skin improvement was seen with MAS063DP as early as the eighth day of treatment. Also, in comparison with subjects receiving the placebo who had only a minimal improvement in their itching, those receiving MAS063DP had remarkable improvement in this regard.

Given the complexity of skin abnormalities in youngsters with atopic dermatitis, the combination of antipruritic, anti-inflammatory, hydrating, and barrier-restoring activities covers pretty much the waterfront of what needs to be provided to those affected with atopic dermatitis. Clearly, additional studies will need to be done with MAS063DP. For example, the study reported failed to do any monitoring for systemic toxicity. It is well known that the ingestion of large amounts of licorice-containing glycyrrhetinic acid can be associated with pseudohyperaldosteronism. In adults, 50 g of licorice daily for 14 days can cause a significant rise in blood pressure. It is reasonable to expect some systemic absorption of MAS063DP through inflamed skin. Despite these potential concerns, thus far side effects have not been reported as a consequence of use.

J. A. Stockman III, MD

Differences in Acne Treatment Prescribing Patterns of Pediatricians and Dermatologists: An Analysis of Nationally Representative Data
Yentzer BA, Irby CE, Fleischer AB Jr, et al (Wake Forest Univ School of Medicine, Winston-Salem, NC)
Pediatr Dermatol 25:635-639, 2008

Background.—Acne vulgaris is a very common disease process that is seen frequently by both pediatricians and dermatologists. However, treatment may be different depending on specialty.

Objectives.—To compare pediatricians' and dermatologists' patterns of treatment for acne vulgaris.

Methods.—National Ambulatory Medical Care Survey data on office visits to pediatricians and dermatologists for acne vulgaris were analyzed from 1996 to 2005.

Results.—During this 10-year time period, dermatologists managed an estimated 18.1 million acne visits and pediatricians managed an estimated 4.6 million acne visits. Dermatologists prescribed topical retinoids considerably more frequently than did pediatricians (46.1% of acne visits for dermatologists vs 12.1% for pediatricians.)

Conclusions.—There is an opportunity for pediatricians to play a greater role in the management of patients with acne. A shift toward greater use of topical retinoids by pediatricians would be more in line with the practice of dermatologists and with current acne treatment consensus guidelines.

▶ This interesting report compares how pediatricians manage patients with acne as opposed to dermatologists. The report derives information from the databases of the National Ambulatory Medical Care Survey (NAMCS). If you are not familiar with NAMCS, for over 30 years, NAMCS has obtained outpatient visit data from nonfederally employed physicians throughout the United States. Data from NAMCS provide an unbiased national estimate sample based on randomly accessed physician records recording the numbers of visits, diagnoses, services provided, medications prescribed, referral practices, and the demographic distribution for a set of randomized patients. This allowed an analysis of the numbers of acne visits to dermatologists versus pediatricians and the use of the most commonly available acne remedies by each group.

What we learn from this report is that millions of youngsters see pediatricians and dermatologists every year. By age 12, substantially more patients were being seen by dermatologists for acne than by pediatricians. When adjusted for acuity of the dermatologic problem, the top 2 medications prescribed by pediatricians are benzoyl peroxide and clindamycin. Dermatologists, on the other hand, prescribe adapalene and tretinoin most frequently. Overall, dermatologists prescribe retinoids significantly more often than do pediatricians (46.1% of acne visits to dermatologists versus 12.1% of acne visits to pediatricians) throughout the period of 1996 through 2005 (Tables 1 and 2).

It seems clear that more acne is now being managed by dermatologists than by the generalist pediatrician. Many of these visits, in fact most, are visits that

TABLE 1.—The Most Frequently Prescribed Acne Medications by Pediatricians, 1996–2005

	Medication	NAMCS Estimates	Percentage (%)
1	Benzoyl peroxide	785,415	17.1
2	Clindamycin	388,124	8.4
3	Tretinoin	340,262	7.4
4	Erythromycin	329,995	7.2
5	Benzaclin (clindamycin 1-benzoyl peroxide 5 topical gel)	224,056	4.9
6	Benzamycin (erythromycin 3-benzoyl peroxide 5 topical gel)	220,762	4.8
7	Aapalene	214,794	4.7
8	Doxycycline	204,528	4.4
9	Tetracycline	177,149	3.9
10	Minocycline	172,771	3.8

Note that percentage of acne visits was calculated by taking estimated acne visits to the pediatrician in which the medication was prescribed and dividing by the total estimated number of acne visits to pediatricians. Ex: Percentage of acne visits in which Benzoyl Peroxide was prescribed = (785,415/4,600,000).

(Reprinted from Yentzer BA, Irby CE, Fleischer AB Jr, et al. Differences in acne treatment prescribing patterns of pediatricians and dermatologists: an analysis of nationally representative data. *Pediatr Dermatol.* 2008;25:635-639.)

TABLE 2.—The Most Frequently Prescribed Acne Medications by Dermatologists, 1996–2005

	Medication	NAMCS Estimates	Percentage of Rx (%)
1	Adapalene	4,432,261	24.5
2	Tretinoin	3,911,904	21.6
3	Clindamycin	3,322,311	18.4
4	Minocycline	3,008,858	16.6
5	Benzoyl peroxide	2,043,072	11.3
6	Doxycycline	1,632,462	9.0
7	Benzamycin (erythromycin 3-benzoyl peroxide 5 topical gel)	1,327,459	7.3
8	Tetracycline	989,811	5.5
9	Benzaclin (clindamycin 1-benzoyl peroxide 5 topical gel)	937,694	5.2
10	Erythromycin	510,262	2.8

Medications listed include all name brand and formulations mentioned in the NAMCS data. Note that NAMCS estimates add up to greater than the total number of acne visits to the dermatologist (18.1 million). This is likely due to the prescribing of more than one medication at some visits. Percents are calculated by taking the number of visits in which that drug was mentioned and dividing by the total number of acne visits to dermatologists.

(Reprinted from Yentzer BA, Irby CE, Fleischer AB Jr, et al. Differences in acne treatment prescribing patterns of pediatricians and dermatologists: an analysis of nationally representative data. *Pediatr Dermatol*. 2008;25:635-639.)

are direct appointments by parents to the dermatologist without referral by the generalist. Interestingly, it appears that pediatricians are quite reluctant to prescribe topical retinoids. Some may be reluctant to prescribe topical retinoids because of the irritating side effect of the first-generation retinoids. Irritation may lead to patient dissatisfaction and poor adherence to treatment. It should be noted, however, that newer agents such as adapalene offer fewer side effects. This suggests that some may not be aware of these newer retinoids.

It has only been in the last few years that we saw a consensus set of guidelines for the treatment of acne vulgaris published.[1] These guidelines developed by an international committee recommend a common approach that targets all 3 major factors of acne pathogenesis: comedone formation and sebaceous hyperplasia, bacterial colonization, and inflammation. These largely evidence-based recommendations advocate that a topical retinoid should be used as the primary treatment for all mild to moderate acne. Oral antibiotics are the drugs of choice for moderate to severe acne, but should be used in combination with topical retinoids. Due to their comedolytic properties, topical retinoids are also essential for maintenance therapy. Topical retinoids can clear acne and can be used for long-term management without the need for an antibiotic. The tendency for the development of antibiotic-resistant bacteria has led to a shift toward greater use of non-antibiotic based treatment of acne.

With such a pervasive problem as acne, one would expect that the generalist pediatrician should be the major provider of treatment for teens and early preteens. Dermatologists are busy enough without being inundated with adolescents with acne. Time to roll up our sleeves and do more in this regard.

This commentary closes with a *Clinical Fact/Curio* about dermatology. The humble tomato, it appears, can protect the human skin from sun and oxidative damage. Researchers have found that lycopene, the powerful antioxidant found in the red pigment of tomatoes, can "quench" (neutralize) reactive oxygen species brought about by the harmful effects of ultraviolet light. Lycopene is found in highest concentration in cooked tomatoes. Compared with controls, tomato paste eaters enjoy some 33% more protection against sunburn than non-tomato paste eaters, at least in 1 study. The sun protective factor (SPF) of oral tomato paste is estimated therefore to be 1.3 (http://www.bad.org.uk).[2] Unfortunately, the tomato study did not tell us what the SPF of a tomato paste is, especially if the latter is smeared on.

J. A. Stockman III, MD

References

1. Zaenglein AL, Thiboutot DM. Expert committee recommendations for acne management. *Pediatrics.* 2006;118:1188-1199.
2. Lycopene protection [editorial comment]. *BMJ.* 2008;336:1078.

Infantile Acne: A Retrospective Study of 16 Cases

Hello M, Prey S, Léauté-Labrèze C, et al (Nantes Univ Hosp, France; Pellegrin Children's Hosp, Bordeaux, France)

Pediatr Dermatol 25:434-438, 2008

Infantile acne is a rare and poorly understood disorder. The objective of this study was to improve our knowledge about the epidemiology and clinical course of infantile acne, and evaluate approaches to treatment. This two-center retrospective study covered the period between 1985 and 2007. Inclusion criteria were: (i) age less than 24 months when lesions appeared; (ii) presence of both inflammatory and noninflammatory lesions; (iii) persistence of lesions for at least 2 months. The data were drawn from clinical and photographic records, followed by administration of a telephone questionnaire to parents. It was proposed that each case be reviewed on the basis of the child's appearance and score on an acne scar clinical grading scale. Sixteen children were included. Nine had a family history of severe adolescent acne. The average duration of disease was 22 months. Two patients had been effectively treated with oral isotretinoin. More than half of the patients exhibited scars. We re-examined five children (average acne scar clinical grading scale score = 12/540). On the basis of the frequency of scarring, and the severity and average duration of lesions, the use of oral retinoids in severe infantile acne warrants evaluation.

▶ Somewhere in my general pediatric training, I missed the lecture on infantile acne. There is an old saying that the clinician cannot diagnose a disease he or she does not know anything about. For this reason, if you do not know anything about infantile acne, chances are you have never seen it. It indeed is a relatively rare condition that in fact shares a great deal in common with the more typical adolescent acne. It is characterized by comedones, superficial inflammatory papules and pustules, and in some cases, nodulocystic lesions on the face, particularly the cheeks. It must be distinguished from more common facial rashes that can look quite similar, such as neonatal cephalic pustulosis and neonatal sebaceous gland hyperplasia, sometimes also called "neonatal acne" although incorrectly so. This report reminds us that infantile acne has to be distinguished from other dermatologic disorders including infection, benign tumors of the face (such as dermoid cysts), and other uncommon entities such as infantile rosacea.

What we learn from this report is the follow-up of fewer than a dozen cases diagnosed with infantile acne. The follow-up was quite lengthy, on average 11 years. About 70% of the children on follow-up had evidence of acne scars. These scars were typically atrophic. The treatment that these youngsters had received in infancy was quite varied and included benzoyl peroxide, topical antibiotics, topical retinoids, as well as systemic approaches including the use of oral antibiotics and isotretinoins.

The findings from this report reaffirm much of what has already been known about infantile acne. It largely affects boys and begins somewhere in the second half of the first year of life. The cheeks are mostly affected and the lesions resolve naturally, but can take several years to do so. Underlying disorders triggering the acne were found in none of the cases reported. A review of the existing cases gives no hint as to what the pathophysiological mechanisms are of infantile acne.

Just one patient at follow-up had an exacerbation of acne at the onset of puberty. Unfortunately, too few patients were seen in follow-up to be sure that there might not be more cases developing. It is also not possible to tell from this case series what the best therapy is for infantile acne. Most dermatologists use a graded approach using typical acne drugs. In the 2 cases in which oral isotretinoin was used, it was quite successful, although virtually anyone would consider this a front-line treatment. Given the fact that there are no controlled studies in the management of infantile acne, the approaches used will have to be hand-tailored and probably best done with the assistance of a pediatric dermatologist.

This commentary closes with a question related to a *Clinical Fact/Curio* having to do with the skin. You are seeing a 14-year-old youngster who has complaints of deformed nails and white horizontal lines across the nails of the lateral (ulnar side) fingers of her right hand. On examination, you find transient growth disturbances of the nails of the middle, ring, and little fingers of her right hand. What question should you ask about in the history that might explain these findings?

Injury to the nerves serving the fingers can lead to transient growth disturbances of the nails in the dermatome distribution supplied by those nerves. Recently described was a young woman who fractured her ulna resulting in injury to the ulnar nerve causing neuropraxia. This occurred while playing camogie, a team field sport played in Ireland. The fracture healed after internal fixation, but the young woman developed transient growth arrest of several of her fingernails. The nails recovered fully as her nerve injury resolved. Nails in the dermatomes supplied by a particular nerve can undergo trophic changes when the nerve is injured and recover along with the nerve.[1]

J. A. Stockman III, MD

Reference

1. Deogaonkar KJ, Elliott J. Nail changes in the dermatome supplied by the ulnar nerve. *BMJ.* 2008;336:1026.

Growth characteristics of infantile hemangiomas: implications for management
Chang LC, Haggstrom AN, Drolet BA, et al (Univ of California, San Francisco)
Pediatrics 122:360-367, 2008

Objectives.—Infantile hemangiomas often are inapparent at birth and have a period of rapid growth during early infancy followed by gradual involution. More precise information on growth could help predict short-term outcomes and make decisions about when referral or intervention, if needed, should be initiated. The objective of this study was to describe growth characteristics of infantile hemangioma and compare growth with infantile hemangioma referral patterns.

Methods.—A prospective cohort study involving 7 tertiary care pediatric dermatology practices was conducted. Growth data were available for a subset of 526 infantile hemangiomas in 433 patients from a cohort study of 1096 children. Inclusion criteria were age younger than 18 months at time of enrollment and presence of at least 1 infantile hemangioma. Growth stage and rate were compared with clinical characteristics and timing of referrals.

Results.—Eighty percent of hemangioma size was reached during the early proliferative stage at a mean age of 3 months. Differences in growth between hemangioma subtypes included that deep hemangiomas tend to grow later and longer than superficial hemangiomas and that segmental hemangiomas tended to exhibit more continued growth after 3 months of age. The mean age of first visit was 5 months. Factors that predicted need for follow-up included ongoing proliferation, larger size, deep component, and segmental and indeterminate morphologic subtypes.

Conclusions.—Most infantile hemangioma growth occurs before 5 months, yet 5 months was also the mean age at first visit to a specialist. Recognition of growth characteristics and factors that predict the need for follow-up could help aid in clinical decision-making. The first few weeks to months of life are a critical time in hemangioma growth. Infants with hemangiomas need close observation during this period, and those who need specialty care should be referred and seen as early as possible within this critical growth period.

▶ Most of us do not tend to think of infantile hemangiomas as being tumors, but indeed they are, and in fact they are the most common tumor of infancy. These hemangiomas in most instances are not readily detectable at birth, but then undergo rapid expansion in early infancy followed by involution in the first few years of life. This rapid expansion often causes alarm on the part of parents who want quick answers as to what is going on and what the natural history of these hemangiomas will be. The authors of this report assist us in addressing these concerns by describing the specific growth characteristics during infancy and the implications of these growth characteristics for management of infantile hemangiomas. More than 1000 patients were enrolled in a cooperative study at 7 pediatric dermatology centers in the United States and in Spain. Classification into 1 of 6 classic growth stages was undertaken: nascent, referring to a premonitory mark; early proliferative denoting the rapid proliferative phase; late proliferative, reflecting ongoing albeit less rapid growth; plateau phase; involution; and abortive (hemangiomas that did not undergo proliferation even over time).

The data from this report really do us all a great service. The study documents that most hemangioma growth is completed by 5 months of age, regardless of the subtype or depth. Specifically, hemangiomas reached an average of 80% of their final size during the early proliferative stage, a stage that ends at a mean age of 3.2 months, so most growth is completed by 5 months of age. Even in hemangiomas that do exhibit growth beyond 6 months of age, the most dramatic growth still occurs in the first few months of life, and the growth after 6 months of age is markedly lower than that noted in the first few months. It is also clear that hemangiomas mark out their own territory early in life. This specifically means that proliferation tends to occur within very defined anatomical areas.

Other findings from this report are that deep hemangiomas tend to appear later and grow for a longer period of time. Furthermore, the "plateau" phase of hemangiomas as we observe them may not be a true biological stage. The age of hemangiomas in this phase lies predominantly within the growth curves of late proliferative and, to a lesser extent, involuting hemangiomas. Also, recent advances in the understanding of the molecular basis of hemangioma pathogenesis raises doubts about a true static plateau phase. However, hemangiomas probably proliferate to the point at which something happens to turn the proliferation off and involution begins. We just do not see that transition and ascribe it to some sort of plateauing of a hemangioma.

One interesting finding from this report is that virtually all the hemangiomas described in this study were noted before a month of age, yet the average patient did not present to a pediatric dermatologist until 5 months of age, a time when growth of the hemangioma actually had already been completed and when complications such as ulceration or permanent skin distortion likely had already occurred. This is an important observation because current hemangioma treatments are generally much more effective in arresting growth than in causing significant involution. Thus, if treatment is going to be given it would best be done before most of the growth has already occurred.

The authors of this report do make some very specific recommendations. They suggest that follow-up intervals should be tailored to the age of the patient and the nature of the lesion. Very young patients require closer scrutiny than older infants. For example, a 1-month-old infant with a potentially site-threatening islet hemangioma needs follow-up every few weeks rather than every few months. A 2-week-old with a large, segmental facial hemangioma, even if relatively flat, requires frequent visits and consideration of systemic steroids, whereas a 5-month-old with a stable, asymptomatic hemangioma, even if bulky, may not need follow-up as often. We, as primary care physicians, should be aware of which hemangiomas are most likely to cause complications and/or need treatment. Patients with these need to have expedited referrals. At the same time, we should not plug up the referral system with unnecessary referrals of hemangiomas that are likely to remain innocuous. Also, referrals for high-risk hemangiomas that are growing should be considered urgent rather than routine by both the referring primary care physician and the consulting dermatologist. The wait list to see a dermatologist can be quite long, but these are patients who need to be "slipped in" very quickly.

Well worth your time is reading this report in detail. We guarantee you will learn a lot that will affect your practice.

This commentary closes with a *Clinical Fact/Curio* having to do with a dermatologic topic. Fingerprints on a painting from the studio of Leonardo DaVinci show the touch of the master himself and have confirmed that the artist had Arab ancestors, Italian researchers say. This was done using infrared light to study fingerprints on the *Martyrdom of St. Catherine* and *La Madone de LaRoque*—paintings attributed to Leonardo. Researchers have now matched these prints with fingerprints on *Lady with a Ermine*, unequivocally known to have been painted by Leonardo. The artist often used his fingers in place of brushes, diluting colors with saliva. Scholars have long suggested that Leonardo's mother was an Arab slave. Current research on Leonardo's fingerprints seems to confirm the artist's Middle Eastern origins. The print from his left index finger has a Y-shaped pattern, shared by a large majority of Middle Easterners, a fact confirmed by paleontologists. Fingerprints, like blood group or skin color, can be used to help determine a person's ancestral origins.

J. A. Stockman III, MD

Pediatric morphea (localized scleroderma): Review of 136 patients
Christen-Zaech S, Hakim MD, Afsar FS, et al (Northwestern Univ Feinberg School of Medicine, Chicago, IL)
J Am Acad Dermatol 59:385-396, 2008

Background.—Morphea is an autoimmune inflammatory sclerosing disorder that may cause permanent functional disability and disfigurement.

Objectives.—We sought to determine the clinical features of morphea in a large pediatric cohort.

Methods.—We conducted a retrospective chart review of 136 pediatric patients with morphea from one center, 1989 to 2006.

Results.—Most children showed linear morphea, with a disproportionately high number of Caucasian and female patients. Two patients with rapidly progressing generalized or extensive linear morphea and arthralgias developed restrictive pulmonary disease. Initial oral corticosteroid treatment and long-term methotrexate administration stabilized and/or led to disease improvement in most patients with aggressive disease.

Limitations.—Retrospective analysis, relatively small sample size, and risk of a selected referral population to the single site are limitations.

Conclusions.—These data suggest an increased prevalence of morphea in Caucasian girls, and support methotrexate as treatment for problematic forms. Visceral manifestations rarely occur; the presence of progressive problematic cutaneous disease and arthralgias should trigger closer patient monitoring.

▶ Morphea is an interesting disorder. It is also commonly known as "localized scleroderma." Despite a shared histologic appearance between systemic sclerosis and localized disease, these are certainly 2 very different disorders. Localized scleroderma, or morphea, occurs at least 10 times more commonly in children than systemic sclerosis/scleroderma. There are several different types of morphea such as plaque morphea, generalized morphea, morphea profunda, linear morphea, and pansclerotic disabling morphea as well as mixed forms. Morphea has also been seen in association with other connective tissue diseases such as lupus, rheumatoid arthritis, Sjögren's syndrome, and eosinophilic fasciitis. Plaque morphea commonly involves the trunk, whereas linear morphea usually affects the face and extremities. The diagnosis is made on its clinical presentation and biopsy is confirmatory.

This report of 136 patients with pediatric morphea from the Departments of Dermatology and Pediatrics, Northwestern University describes in some detail the course of localized scleroderma in children. The review represents the largest of its type in the literature. We learn that girls are 2 and one-half times more likely than boys to be affected. White children develop the problem 5 times more commonly than non-white children. Linear morphea is the most common presentation, usually affecting the extremities. The characteristic appearance of indurated purplish brown plaques occurs in about 90% of children presenting with morphea (Figs 1 and 2). Generalized morphea was noted to occur in just 9%. Most of the skin involvement is unilateral. One in 4 children with generalized morphea were documented to have developed contractures. Also common was undergrowth of affected extremities.

Far more than any other reports on localized scleroderma in children, this report from Chicago describes the natural course of the disease, including some of its trigger factors. For example, a number of children who developed localized scleroderma had this following a sunburn. Trauma was also commonly described. The most frequent age at presentation was between 2 and 8 years (seen in almost 50% of patients) followed by ages 8 to 14 years in 40%. The diagnosis was often missed. The mean time to diagnosis following presentation

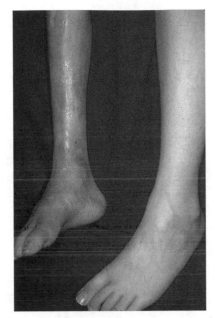

FIGURE 1.—Entire right leg was indurated with hyperpigmentation and marked reduction in both circumference and length. (Reprinted from Christen-Zaech S, Hakim MD, Afsar FS, et al. Pediatric morphea (localized scleroderma): review of 136 patients. *J Am Acad Dermatol.* 2008;59:385-396, with permission from the American Academy of Dermatology.)

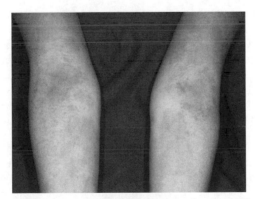

FIGURE 2.—Indurated hyperpigmented plaques covered more than 50% of body surface, including extensive involvement of arms. (Reprinted from Christen-Zaech S, Hakim MD, Afsar FS, et al. Pediatric morphea (localized scleroderma): review of 136 patients. *J Am Acad Dermatol.* 2008;59:385-396, with permission from the American Academy of Dermatology.)

was 1 year and 2 months. A number of children also developed nonskin manifestations with arthralgias being the most common noncutaneous clinical manifestation. Table 2 shows many of these noncutaneous clinical manifestations. A rare but serious complication that is restrictive pulmonary disease, of the type actually seen in those with true scleroderma.

TABLE 2.—Noncutaneous Clinical Manifestations

	Plaque	Generalized	Profunda	Linear	ECDS	PHA	Total
Total No. of patients	50*	12	5	44	23	3*	136
Musculoskeletal							
Total affected	2	5	3	18	0	0	28
Arthralgia	2	5	3	13	0	0	23
Muscular cramps	0	0	0	4	0	0	4
Scoliosis	0	0	0	2	0	0	2
Thorax asymmetry	0	1	0	0	0	0	1
Central nervous system							
Total affected	0	3	1	3	10	0	17
Headaches/migraines	0	2	1	2	6	0	11
Seizures	0	0	0	1	3	0	4
Stroke	0	0	0	0	1	0	1
Peripheral neuropathy	0	1	0	0	0	0	1
Dyspnea	0	2	1	3	0	0	6
Gastrointestinal							
No. of patients affected	0	3	1	3	0	0	7
Reflux	0	1	1	2	0	0	4
Dysphagia	0	1	0	2	0	0	3
Abdominal pain	0	1	1	1	0	0	3

ECDS, En coup de sabre; PHA, progressive hemifacial atrophy.
*One of the patients presented with both PHA and plaque type morphea.
(Reprinted from Christen-Zaech S, Hakim MD, Afsar FS, et al. Pediatric morphea (localized scleroderma): review of 136 patients. J Am Acad Dermatol. 2008;59:385-396, with permission from the American Academy of Dermatology.)

There is no "standard" treatment for morphea presenting in childhood. In this series of 136 patients, 60% could be treated with just topical medications. About one-third of children required both topical and systemic treatment. The most commonly used topical treatment was with calcipotriene ointment. Tacrolimus ointment was also used in a number of children along with topical steroids. As far as systemic therapy is concerned, the most common approach is with the use of a combination of methotrexate and corticosteroids. Most data from the literature suggest that methotrexate will suppress localized scleroderma until spontaneous improvement in disease activity occurs, typically a few years after onset. Methotrexate does not necessarily cure the condition, however.

This report reminds us that a small subset of children with morphea (just 1.5% in this series) will develop life-threatening noncutaneous manifestations of the type commonly seen in patients with progressive systemic sclerosis. The lungs, heart, esophagus or a combination of these are the organs most affected. Data from the literature suggest that the presence of serologic evidence of ANAs and rheumatoid factor should alert one to the possible development of internal organ involvement. In the series from Chicago, the patients who did develop visceral disease had both arthralgias and rapidly progressive and extensive skin disease.

We should be grateful to the pediatric dermatology group at Northwestern for providing us with a detailed update on this interesting and unusual skin disorder, a disorder that needs the expertise of our dermatology colleagues.

This commentary closes with a *Clinical Fact/Curio* regarding the skin. Bet you were not aware that tattoo inflammatory reactions are a rare but recognized manifestation of sarcoidosis. Recently a 40-year-old man presented to a rheumatology clinic with polyarthralgia, chest pain, and malaise. He also complained of tenderness of the "tree trunk only" portion of a 20-year-old tattoo. This tattoo was of a naked woman lying against a palm tree. Only the palm tree had a red pigment. A granulomatous reaction confined to the colored portion of the tattoo was observed on biopsy. A CT of his chest showed hilar lymphadenopathy with early interstitial lung involvement. Biopsies were consistent with sarcoidosis.

Chances are you will never see a tattoo reaction presenting as the initial manifestation of sarcoidosis. Nonetheless, this is very interesting.[1]

J. A. Stockman III, MD

Reference

1. Ramabhadran B, Merry P. Tattoo reactions in a case of sarcoidosis. *BMJ.* 2009; 338:b168.

Adjuvant therapy with pegylated interferon alfa-2b versus observation alone in resected stage III melanoma: final results of EORTC 18991, a randomised phase III trial

Eggermont AMM, for the EORTC Melanoma Group (Erasmus Univ Med Ctr, Rotterdam, Netherlands; et al)

Lancet 372:117-126, 2008

Background.—Any benefit of adjuvant interferon alfa-2b for melanoma could depend on dose and duration of treatment. Our aim was to determine whether pegylated interferon alfa-2b can facilitate prolonged exposure while maintaining tolerability.

Methods.—1256 patients with resected stage III melanoma were randomly assigned to observation (n=629) or pegylated interferon alfa-2b (n=627) 6 μg/kg per week for 8 weeks (induction) then 3 μg/kg per week (maintenance) for an intended duration of 5 years. Randomisation was stratified for microscopic (N1) versus macroscopic (N2) nodal involvement, number of positive nodes, ulceration and tumour thickness, sex, and centre. Randomisation was done with a minimisation technique. The primary endpoint was recurrence-free survival. Analyses were done by intention to treat. This study is registered with ClinicalTrials.gov, number NCT00006249.

Findings.—All randomised patients were included in the primary efficacy analysis. 608 patients in the interferon group and 613 patients in the observation group were included in safety analyses. The median length of treatment with pegylated interferon alfa-2b was 12 (IQR 3·8–33·4) months. At 3·8 (3·2–4·2) years median follow-up, 328 recurrence events had occurred in the interferon group compared with 368 in the observation group (hazard ratio 0·82, 95% CI 0·71–0.96; p=0·01); the 4-year rate of recurrence-free survival was 45·6% (SE 2·2) in the interferon group and 38·9% (2·2) in the observation group. There was no difference in overall survival between the groups. Grade 3 adverse events occurred in 246 (40%) patients in the interferon group and 60 (10%) in the observation group; grade 4 adverse events occurred in 32 (5%) patients in the interferon group and 14 (2%) in the observation group. In the interferon group, the most common grade 3 or 4 adverse events were fatigue (97 patients, 16%), hepatotoxicity (66, 11%), and depression (39, 6%). Treatment with pegylated interferon alfa-2b was discontinued because of toxicity in 191 (31%) patients.

Interpretation.—Adjuvant pegylated interferon alfa-2b for stage III melanoma has a significant, sustained effect on recurrence-free survival.

▶ There has not been a clear-cut agent that significantly improves survivorship in patients with nonlocalized melanoma. Interferon alfa-2b has been the most widely studied agent in this regard. Trials of both high and intermediate doses of interferon for patients at high risk of recurrence after resection have shown improvements in recurrence-free survival, but without showing consistent effects on overall survival compared with observation alone. It has been estimated that based on data from randomized trials, interferon reduces a risk of recurrence of death by just about 13% for recurrence-free survival and the risk of death by only 10% compared with observation alone. Other studies have suggested that the effect of interferon on recurrence-free survival is rapidly lost after stopping treatment. In addition, one has to consider the toxicity of interferon and a patient's acceptance of this toxicity. Pegylated interferon, widely used for the treatment of hepatitis, seems at least as equally efficacious as standard recombinant interferon without as much toxicity. For these reasons, it is reasonable that investigators would have looked at this variety of interferon to see what benefit it might afford patients with nonlocalized melanoma.

Eggermont et al have shown in a large well-conducted trial from the European Organization for Research and Treatment of Cancer that pegylated interferon alfa-2b improves recurrence-free survival in patients with resected stage III (positive lymph nodes) cutaneous melanoma. The question is: Is this the result that everyone has been waiting for? Recurrence-free survival is an appropriate endpoint—many patients with melanoma are willing to accept significant toxicity in exchange for a modest improvement in recurrence-free survival, even in the absence of an overall survival effect, but is the lesser toxicity of pegylated interferon compared with the high-dose interferon regimen currently used in the United States sufficient to persuade skeptical clinicians who demand an overall survival benefit? Will patients accept 5 years of treatment for an absolute benefit in recurrence-free survival of about 6%? If one digs deeply into the data, however, what one sees is that a strong case can be made in favor of treatment for those patients whose metastatic melanoma was discovered on sentinel-node biopsy rather than as a clinically palpable node.

While we are awaiting for the true magic bullet that will make a truly remarkable difference in the survivorship of patients with locally metastatic melanoma, pegylated interferon may be the best that we have, for now. Its toxicity is less than that of standard varieties of interferon and disease-free survival is a tad better. Patients as young as 18 were included in this European study. Absent additional information about younger patients, there seems to be little reason not to believe that similar effects would be seen in the later age group, although clinical trials would seem to be in order.

This commentary closes with a *Clinical Fact/Curio* in the form of a clinical scenario. You are seeing a college student in your office for a routine checkup. On physical examination you find slightly painful lumps in the patient's axilla. These appear to be 25 mm in size. Because it is summer vacation, and the patient is at home for a couple of months, you schedule a revisit in several weeks. At that time, the physical findings remain the same. You draw some routine laboratory tests looking for a possible etiology and finding none you refer for biopsy. This is performed as an outpatient. You drop by to watch the short surgical procedure. Both you and the surgeon are alarmed when the lymph nodes that are removed on gross examination show dark, almost black areas consistent with metastatic melanoma. You reexamine the patient carefully and find nothing on the skin except for a tattoo over the deltoid area on the same side as the excised lymph nodes. What is your diagnosis?

This is a true scenario except for the age of the patient. A 38-year-old man in fact did present with painful, sometimes tender lumps in his axillae. He had a number of tattoos placed on his arms as well as chest, abdomen, and back. The man also had lymph nodes excised and on gross examination they were dark grey, indicating the possibility of melanoma. However, histopathological analysis showed reactive follicular hyperplasia and sinus histiocytosis, implying reactive lymphadenopathy rather than cancer. Many histiocytes contained dense black pigment. The pathological diagnosis was reactive lymphadenopathy caused by tattoo pigment.[1]

Tattoo pigments are taken up by macrophages, which migrate through lymph vessels to lymph nodes, some of which can be very distant from a tattoo.[2] Such lymph nodes can reach a diameter of 3 cm, which might ordinarily make one suspicious of a cancer. Macrophages within these lymph nodes can take up 18-fluorodeoxyglucose, causing cancer to be wrongly suspected on PET scanning.

Please note that the onset of lymphadenopathy can be quite delayed so care providers should not forget to ask, if no tattoo is found on physical examination, whether a patient might have had a tattoo removed. Needless to say, lymphadenopathy caused by tattoos remains a diagnosis of exclusion because tattoo reactive lymphadenopathy has also been described in a patient with a melanoma.

J. A. Stockman III, MD

References

1. Kluger N, Cohen-Valensi R, Nezri M. Black lymph nodes–and a colourful skin. *Lancet.* 2008;371:1214.
2. Mangas C, Fernandez-Figueras MT, Carrascosa JM, et al. A tattoo reaction in a sentinel lymph node from a patient with melanoma. *Derm Surg.* 2007;33: 766-767.

Outbreak of rash in children associated with recreational mud exposure

Turabelidze G, Tucker A, Butler C, et al (Missouri Dept of Health and Senior Services, Jefferson City; St. Louis Country Health Dept, Clayton, Missouri)
Pediatr Dermatol 25:643-644, 2008

We conducted an investigation of a rash outbreak in children who attended the "Mud Mania Festival." The mean incubation period of illness was 26 hours, and mean duration was 4.3 days. Time spent in mud was associated with the extent of rash in a dose–response fashion. The cultures from lesions of two unrelated cases yielded *Enterobacter cloacae*.

▶ This case report, albeit a very brief one, describes an outbreak of a rash illness that affected hundreds of children participating in the "Mud Mania Festival." This took place in July 2006 in Missouri. More than 5000 children attended the event, which occurred over 2 days. The event consisted of youngsters being allowed to play in wet mud similar in consistency to that employed for mud wrestling. After the event, about 1 in 10 youngsters reported having developed a rash. The median incubation of this rash was 26 hours (longest 56 hours). The mean duration of the rash was 4.3 days. The most common locations of the rash were the torso, legs, and arms. About 6% had a rash over the entire body. The dermatologic findings were also associated with itching (47%), fatigue (7%), muscle aches (4%), and swollen lymph nodes (2%). For those children who received treatment, antibiotics were the option of choice. Only 2 children had skin cultures performed and both yielded *Enterobacter cloacae*. *E cloacae* are part of the normal flora of the human intestinal tract and rarely cause disease in a healthy human. The only previously reported outbreak of rash due to *E. cloacae* was among mud-wrestling adults.[1]

It is hypothesized that bacteria entered the skin while wallowing in the mud if the skin had been injured. Those who simply were wallowing in the mud without wrestling had no evidence of rash. It should be noted that *Enterobacteriaceae* are widely distributed in soil and it is likely that the causative bacteria were present in soil, rather than in stool.

Fortunately, all the patients reported in this study recovered completely within several days. Remember this report, however, the next time some smart individual comes up with the idea of a community mudfest. Also be wary of taking a therapeutic mud bath. The latter are still popular in many parts of the world.

This commentary closes with a *Clinical Fact/Curio* about skin rashes. Bet you were not aware that up to 50% of hair dressers develop dermatitis of the hand within 3 years of starting work. This is the result of either irritant contact dermatitis resulting from chemical damage or allergic contact dermatitis from a delayed (type IV) hypersensitivity reaction. Distinguishing between these is difficult but important because of a worse prognosis in the allergic form if exposure to the allergen is not eliminated. These types of skin conditions have also been seen in teens who frequently dye their hair.[2] Separating contact dermatitis from an allergic hypersensitivity can usually be done with a referral for patch skin testing. A patch test will help to determine the cause of the individual's problem and involves a battery of patch tests against hair dyes, ammonium persulphate, aminophenol, and surfactant. These tests are negative in irritant dermatitis. Also, skin prick tests or the radioallergosorbent tests do not become positive with simple irritant dermatitis. The simple wearing of gloves when mixing and applying chemicals should markedly reduce the "hair dresser's dermatitis."

J. A. Stockman III, MD

References

1. Adler AI, Altman J. An outbreak of mud-wrestling-induced pustular dermatitis in college students. Dermatitis plaestrae limosae. *JAMA.* 1993;269:502-504.
2. Worth A, Arshad SH, Sheikh A. Occupational dermatitis in a hairdresser. *BMJ.* 2007;335:399.

3 Blood

Dyshemoglobinemias and pulse oximetry: a therapeutic challenge
Hladik A, Lynshue K (Baylor College of Medicine, Houston, TX)
J Pediatr Hematol Oncol 30:850-852, 2008

Pulse oximetry normally provides a reliable indicator of arterial blood oxygen saturation. Individuals with a variant hemoglobin with low oxygen affinity would exhibit pulse oximetry values consistent with hypoxemia despite maintaining adequate oxygen delivery to tissues. We describe a patient we diagnosed with hemoglobin Rothschild and his mother. He presented with SpO_2 81% on pulse oximetry and PaO_2 on arterial blood gas of 47 mm Hg, while his mother had SpO_2 87%. These values were significantly lower than physical examination suggested. A possible dyshemoglobinemia should be suspected when discordance exists between pulse oximetry readings and physical examination findings.

▶ This is an interesting report. Kudos should be given to the nurse who triggered the correct diagnosis in this 8-year-old youngster. The patient in question was a Sicilian boy with a 2-day history of cough and fever who upon presentation to his physician had a routine pulse oximetry performed showing a reading of 81%. Despite the fact that he had little or no respiratory distress and a chest X-ray that showed a fairly modest left lower lobe pneumonia, a decision was made to admit to hospital for the management of a pneumonia associated with hypoxia. The nurse that took care of this youngster noted that he had no real distress, although he was slightly febrile (38.4°C). His arterial oxygen saturation, measured by pulse oximetry, was 81%. Suspecting that the pulse oximeter was malfunctioning, the nurse measured her own SpO_2, which was 99%. She then measured the patient's mother's SpO_2, which was 87%. Meanwhile, the youngster had no retractions, no clubbing or cyanosis of the extremities, and relatively normal chest findings. On reviewing the past medical history, it was noted that following minor surgery in another hospital, the SpO_2 was also shown to be low. A workup revealed no cause for this. An abnormal hemoglobin was suspected as a cause of all this, and further testing performed at the Mayo Clinic confirmed this to be hemoglobin Rothschild.

Hemoglobin Rothschild is a low oxygen affinity hemoglobin variant first described in 1977. It represents a beta chain mutation where there is a substitution of tryptophan for arginine at position 37. One of the consequences of having this hemoglobinopathy is that the oxygen dissociation curve is significantly shifted to the right in comparison with that of normal hemoglobin. In some respects, this represents a "super" hemoglobin in that the hemoglobin

49

releases oxygen very freely to tissues, and therefore patients with this have no real functional impairment.

This report highlights the well-established but frequently overlooked deficiencies of pulse oximetry. Pulse oximetry uses the differing light absorption characteristics exhibited by oxygenated and deoxygenated hemoglobin and the knowledge that the concentration of a light-absorbing substance in a solution can be determined from the intensity of light of a specific wavelength transmitted through the solution, if the characteristic absorbance of that substance at that wavelength is known. The accuracy of pulse oximetry relies upon the assumption of a patient's similarity to the individuals used to create the calibration curves — a similarity precluded by the presence of hemoglobin with an abnormal oxygen binding behavior. To say this differently, pulse oximetry isn't worth a darn in patients with certain forms of hemoglobinopathies. The bottom line is that we should suspect a dyshemoglobinemia in anyone who has an oxygen saturation that is out of line with what one expects to see clinically. Patients with such "super" hemoglobins that release oxygen related to tissues will show such discrepancies, but otherwise are clinically quite normal.

This commentary closes with a *Clinical Fact/Curio* about pulse oximeters. What would happen if you take a pulse oximeter probe (intended to be clipped onto a finger) and clipped it onto the drip chamber of an IV infusion set with a drip rate of 75 per minute? The answer to this query appears in an interesting short article by Kopa.[1] If the infusion set is dripping lactated Ringer's solution, the pulse oximeter machine will show a heart rate of 75 per minute with an oxygen saturation of 99. Ringer's solution with a lactate component (about 28 mmol/l) of the balanced crystalloid is the likely culprit, causing signal extinction (thus the heart rate) and the generation of a numerical value for "oxygen saturation." If there is a lesson to be learned in any of this, it is that if you ever are hospitalized and want to sneak out of bed for a period of time, clip your pulse oximeter to your IV bag's drip chamber. The nurses will never know the difference.

J. A. Stockman III, MD

Reference

1. Kopa A. Ghost in the machine? A pulse oximeter clipped to a drip chamber seemed to conjure up life. *BMJ.* 2007;335:1298.

An Economic Analysis of Anemia Prevention during Infancy

Shaker M, Jenkins P, Ullrich C, et al (Children's Hosp at Dartmouth, Lebanon, NH; the Dana Farber Cancer Inst, Boston, MA; et al)
J Pediatr 154:44-49, 2009

Objective.—To compare the cost-benefit profile of reticulocyte hemoglobin content (CHr) with hemoglobin (Hb) alone and Hb as a component of the complete blood count (CBC) for detection and treatment of iron deficiency in 9- to 12-month-old infants.

Study Design.—Cohort simulations were used to compare CHr with Hb from a societal perspective. Assumptions included a 9% prevalence of iron deficiency and testing characteristics/costs of CHr, Hb, and CBC (CHr <27.5 pg: sensitivity 83%, specificity 72%, $11; Hb <11 g/dL: sensitivity 26%, specificity 95%, $5; CBC Hb <11 g/dL, $15), as well as cost of iron therapy ($61 for established anemia). Sensitivity analyses were performed.

Results.—Under current market conditions, the incremental cost to diagnose and treat iron deficiency, compared with diagnosing and treating anemia by Hb, was only $22 per patient screened ($440 per case of anemia prevented; number needed to treat = 20). With a 10-year time horizon incorporating risks and costs of neurocognitive delays associated with untreated iron deficiency, the cost of the CHr strategy was $280 per case of anemia prevented.

Conclusions.—CHr is an affordable strategy to prevent anemia in infants with possible iron deficiency (Fig 1 and Table 1).

▶ This is a report that is quite interesting to read if you have time to do so. It is actually necessary to read the report in detail to get its full drift. The bottom line is that reticulocyte hemoglobin content (CHr) is an affordable strategy to prevent the anemia associated with iron deficiency in infants.

By way of background, there are a number of different ways to screen for iron deficiency in the 9- to 12-month-old infants (and beyond). Many simply do a hemoglobin as a screening test. The problem with using a hemoglobin

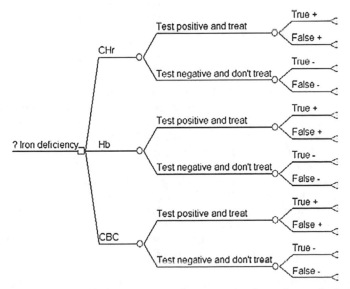

FIGURE 1.—Decision model: decision tree to evaluate competing diagnostic strategies for iron deficiency. (Reprinted from Shaker M, Jenkins P, Ullrich C, et al. An economic analysis of anemia prevention during infancy. *J Pediatr.* 2009;154:44-49, with permission from Elsevier.)

TABLE 1.—Baseline Assumptions and Probabilities

Name	Value
Costs*	
CHr screening test[15]	$11
Hb screening test[15]	$5
Complete blood count[15]	$15
Treatment cost of anemia (3 month course)*	$61
Treatment cost iron deficiency (3 month course)*	$61
Treatment cost of iron deficiency for (1 month course)*	$20
Probabilities	
CHr screening test < 27.5 pg[13]	
Sensitivity	83%
Specificity	72%
Hb screening test < 11 g/dL[13]	
Sensitivity	26%
Specificity	95%
Additional Assumptions in 10 year time horizon	
Second test probability (independent testing characteristics, Hb test performed)[17]	60%
Annual attributable risk of neurocognitive disability requiring services	
Untreated anemia[7]	10%
Treated anemia	0%
Annual (transient) charges of services† for neurocognitive delays, if required	$500

Editor's Note: Please refer to original journal article for full references.

*Local cost estimates.

†Costs of cognitive delay were derived from local charges[18] published by the Dartmouth-Hitchcock Medical Center (Lebanon, NH) of physician visits (CPT 99213 charge $118 per visit) and potential developmental assessment (CPT 99243 charge $335 per visit or 99244 charge $412 per visit).

(Reprinted from Shaker M, Jenkins P, Ullrich C, et al. An economic analysis of anemia prevention during infancy. *J Pediatr.* 2009;154:44-49, with permission from Elsevier.)

(with a lower limit of normal of 11 g/dL) is its sensitivity, which is just 26%. There are many reasons for this low sensitivity in part having to do with the overlap between abnormal and normal ranges of hemoglobin concentration in the otherwise noniron deficient child. Also, a fall in hemoglobin concentration occurs only after iron stores have been completely exhausted and the effects of the iron deficiency have been around for a while. Another screening alternative is a complete blood count (CBC) looking at the red cell indices, including the mean corpuscular volume (MCV). This is certainly better than simply measuring a hemoglobin alone, but is a bit more expensive. Some have suggested that the CHr should be the preferred test. CHr is a measure of the concentration of hemoglobin in reticulocytes, the latter being the first red blood cell to show the effects of iron deficiency, thus allowing the CHr to be an early detection technique.

The report of Shaker et al was designed to use a computer-based mathematical model that performed cohort simulations of competing diagnostic strategies used to evaluate for the presence of iron deficiency (Fig 1). The strategies employed used certain cost assumptions seen in Table 1. While the CHr would result in the treatment of 33% of children in this theoretical model assuming a 9% prevalence of iron deficiency, the use of the CHr for the prevention of the consequences of iron deficiency appears to be quite affordable. One can worry about the consequences of unnecessary treatment in so many children, and there are some, but the trade-off of this approach would be a much lower risk of the presence of cognitive problems related to missed iron deficiency.

Unfortunately, most pediatricians are not that familiar with CHr as a screening technique, largely because most laboratories have not yet routinely provided it as a separate screening test. If you read the literature carefully, you will see that you should lobby your laboratory to make this test available to you.

J. A. Stockman III, MD

Reticulocyte hemoglobin content for the diagnosis of iron deficiency
Mateos ME, De-la-Cruz J, López-Laso E, et al (Univ Hosp Reina Sofía, Córdoba, Spain)
J Pediatr Hematol Oncol 30:539-542, 2008

Summary.—Identification of iron deficiency (ID) is essential to initiate early treatment to prevent long-term systemic complications of ID anemia. This study was undertaken to evaluate the efficiency of the parameter reticulocyte hemoglobin content (CHr) compared with other laboratory parameters in the assessment of ID in a pediatric population. Blood samples were obtained for 237 children who received routine pediatric care visits in a primary care clinic (mean age: 63.7 mo; male:female ratio: 1.08:1). A multiple stepwise logistic regression analysis identified CHr as the most accurate marker independently associated to ID. A CHr cutoff value of 25 pg (sensitivity: 94%; specificity: 80%) proved an optimal performance predicting ID. Therefore, we conclude that the hematologic parameter CHr constitutes a valuable screening tool for the identification of ID with or without anemia in childhood.

▶ This is not the first study to look at the use of reticulocyte haemoglobin content (CHr) in the assessment of iron deficiency and iron deficiency anemia in children, but it is among the very largest study undertaken to date. The CHr is increasingly being recognized as a promising diagnostic tool to provide an early indicator of iron deficiency. Most tests for iron deficiency depend on hematologic studies of a mixed age population of red cells (hemoglobin, hematocrit, MCV, and RDW). Unfortunately, such studies fail to pick up iron deficiency in its early stages because it takes some time for these parameters to change after the first iron deficient red cells are produced. However, if one looks at the hemoglobin content of the reticulocyte, this begins to change quite promptly as soon as iron deficiency starts to affect red cell production. Reticulocytes allow a real time evaluation of the bone marrow erythropoietic activity, improving our ability to detect iron deficiency even before anemia is present.

The introduction of flow cytometric methods has improved the precision and accuracy of reticulocyte counting. The parameter of CHr can be incorporated into the automatic hematology analyzing equipment commonly available. Specifically, as soon as iron deficiency affects erythropoietic activity, one would expect that the youngest of red blood cells, the reticulocyte, would begin to be poorly hemoglobinized.

In the report of Mateos et al, the CHr emerged as the strongest independent indicator of iron deficiency and iron deficiency anemia. The mean CHr level was 3.09 to 3.25 pg lower in the groups with iron deficiency or iron deficiency anemia in comparison with children with noniron deficient anemia or with a normal iron status. The investigators found that a CHr cutoff value of 25 pg had the best overall sensitivity and specificity to detect iron deficiency and iron deficiency anemia in the pediatric age population.

Most now agree that deleterious effects of iron deficiency seem to begin before anemia develops. CHr is a sensitive marker for iron deficiency in children still asymptomatic whose diagnosis would not otherwise occur this early with routine testing (Fig 2 in the original article). Unfortunately, CHr's specificity is limited by other conditions such as thalassemia and the "functional" iron deficiency seen in association with infection and chronic illness. However, one can use other parameters to distinguish iron deficiency from thalassemia disorders using the Mentzer index (MCV divided by red cell blood count). In iron deficiency, red cell blood count number tends to be diminished while it remains normal in thalassemia trait disorders. This results in a high Mentzer index (> 14) in the presence of iron deficiency.

All in all, CHr is quickly emerging as a relatively simple and useful method to detect iron deficient red cell production. If the laboratory you use does not provide a CHr in addition to other red blood cell parameters, you might begin to ask when the equipment will either be replaced or modified to include this.

J. A. Stockman III, MD

Long-Term Outcome of Pediatric Patients with Severe Aplastic Anemia Treated with Antithymocyte Globulin and Cyclosporine
Scheinberg P, Wu CO, Nunez O, et al (Natl Insts of Health, Bethesda, MD)
J Pediatr 153:814-819, 2008

Objective.—To determine the long-term outcomes in children with severe aplastic anemia (SAA) treated with antithymocyte globulin (ATG) and cyclosporine (CsA) through a retrospective analysis of the pediatric patients treated at our institution in all protocols that included horse ATG (h-ATG) and CsA.

Study Design.—Between 1989 and 2006, a total of 406 patients, 20% of whom were children under age 18 years, received an initial course of immunosuppressive therapy (IST) at our institution. Here we report the outcome of 77 children who were treated with an h-ATG plus CsA–based regimen during this period.

Results.—The overall response rate at 6 months was 74% (57/77); the cumulative incidence of relapse at 10 years was 33%, and the median time to relapse was 558 days. The cumulative incidence of evolution after IST was 8.5%; all 3 such events occurred in partial responders. Overall, there were 13 deaths (17%), with 4 occurring within the 3 months after IST in patients who had a pretreatment absolute neutrophil count of $< 100/\mu L$ and the other 9 occurring more than 6 months after initiation of IST. The median time to death was 570 days. The overall 10-year survival for the entire cohort was 80%; long-term survival in the children who responded to IST was 89%.

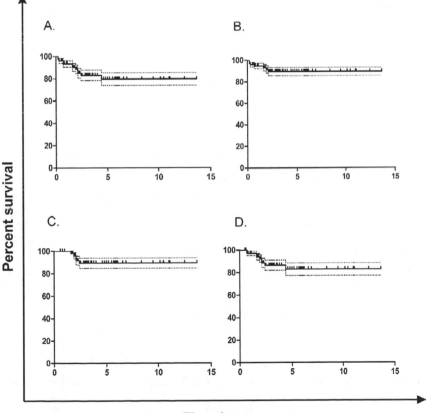

Time in years

FIGURE 4.—Overall survival (with 95% CIs) for the entire cohort, including A, those who underwent HSCT, B, of patients who underwent HSCT censored at the time of transplant, C, of patients who responded to IST and D, of patients who completed 6 months of IST regardless of response status. (Reprinted from Scheinberg P, Wu CO, Nunez O, et al. Long-term outcome of pediatric patients with severe aplastic anemia treated with antithymocyte globulin and cyclosporine. *J Pediatr.* 2008;153:814-819, with permission from Elsevier.)

Conclusions.—The long-term survival in pediatric patients who respond to IST is excellent, at about 90%. IST remains a good alternative in pediatric patients who lack an HLA-matched sibling donor and should be offered as initial therapy before possible hematopoietic stem cell transplantation from an unrelated donor.

▶ More often than not research articles dealing with aplastic anemia in children have tended to appear in scientific journals that are not commonly seen by the average pediatric practitioner. The report of Scheinberg et al is different in this regard in that it is presented in a widely read journal and provides a clear and unambiguous set of findings interpretable readily by all of us.

While aplastic anemia is not a common problem in childhood, when it does occur, it puts the fear of God into us given its natural history and lethality. Regardless of its etiology (congenital or acquired with its various causes), the outcome of untreated aplastic anemia is fairly dismal. Regardless of etiology, patients are currently treated either with immunosuppressive therapy (IST) or hematopoietic stem cell transplantation (HSCT). Children tend to fare far better than adults when it comes to outcomes after HSCT, with less frequent and less severe graft-versus-host disease and better overall survival. Unfortunately, most children with severe aplastic anemia lack an HLA-histocompatible sibling; thus, IST is often administered by default as the first therapy. Current standard IST regimens consist of antithymocyte globulin (ATG) plus cyclosporine. The investigators from the National Institutes of Health do us a service by telling us the outcomes of treatment of more than 400 patients with newly diagnosed aplastic anemia who received IST. We learn that 3 out of 4 children with severe aplastic anemia will respond to ATG plus cyclosporine and that the overall long-term survival is 80%. For those who initially respond to ATG and cyclosporine, the long-term survival is 90%. What this means is that although HLA-matched sibling bone marrow transplantation remains the therapeutic procedure of choice, we should defer to IST over unrelated donor HSCT as the backup for those who do not have a matched sibling donor, the outcomes are that good with immunosuppressive therapy.

When this editor was a resident in training, more than 3 decades ago, a diagnosis of aplastic anemia almost always meant a death sentence. This is no longer true with improved techniques involving bone marrow transplantation and immunosuppressive therapies (Fig 4).

J. A. Stockman III, MD

Systematic Review: Hydroxyurea for the Treatment of Adults with Sickle Cell Disease

Lanzkron S, Strouse JJ, Wilson R, et al (Johns Hopkins Univ, Baltimore, MD)
Ann Intern Med 148:939-955, 2008

Background.—Hydroxyurea is the only approved drug for treatment of sickle cell disease.

Objective.—To synthesize the published literature on the efficacy, effectiveness, and toxicity of hydroxyurea when used in adults with sickle cell disease.

Data Sources.—MEDLINE, EMBASE, TOXLine, and CINAHL were searched through 30 June 2007.

Study Selection.—Randomized trials, observational studies, and case reports evaluating efficacy and toxicity of hydroxyurea in adults with sickle cell disease, and toxicity studies of hydroxyurea in other conditions that were published in English.

Data Extraction.—Paired reviewers abstracted data on study design, patient characteristics, and outcomes sequentially and did quality assessments independently.

Data Synthesis.—In the single randomized trial, the hemoglobin level was higher in hydroxyurea recipients than placebo recipients after 2 years (difference, 6 g/L), as was fetal hemoglobin (absolute difference, 3.2%). The median number of painful crises was 44% lower than in the placebo group. The 12 observational studies that enrolled adults reported a relative increase in fetal hemoglobin of 4% to 20% and a relative reduction in crisis rates by 68% to 84%. Hospital admissions declined by 18% to 32%. The evidence suggests that hydroxyurea may impair spermatogenesis. Limited evidence indicates that hydroxyurea treatment in adults with sickle cell disease is not associated with leukemia. Likewise, limited evidence suggests that hydroxyurea and leg ulcers are not associated in patients with sickle cell disease, and evidence is insufficient to estimate the risk for skin neoplasms, although these outcomes can be attributed to hydroxyurea in other conditions.

Limitation.—Only English-language articles were included, and some studies were of lower quality.

Conclusion.—Hydroxyurea has demonstrated efficacy in adults with sickle cell disease. The paucity of long-term studies limits conclusions about toxicity.

▶ The exact prevalence of sickle cell disease here in the United States is not known, but somewhere between 50 000 and 1 00 000 individuals are estimated to have the disorder. About 2000 babies are born each year with sickle cell disease in the United States. This disorder was the first disease for which a specific molecular defect in a gene was identified and it remains the most common genetic disease identified as part of the Newborn Screening Program in the United States. Approximately 2 million Americans have the sickle cell trait, in which a parent passes along to the infant the gene for sickle hemoglobin. In addition to sickle cell disease, a number of other sickling disorders have been identified. Until the last 15 years or so, the management of sickle cell disease included fluid hydration and transfusion or exchange transfusion as needed along with pain control for painful crises. More recently, hydroxyurea has been added to treatment regimens.

Most do not know it, but hydroxyurea was initially synthesized in Germany back in 1869. Nearly 50 years ago, it was experimented with as an anticancer drug and has been used to treat myeloproliferative syndromes, some types of leukemia, melanoma, and ovarian cancer. It has also been used to treat psoriasis. Back in 1984, the first attempts to see what hydroxyurea might do in sickle cell disease patients was undertaken. Initial studies showed that it acts to increase the production of fetal hemoglobin-containing red blood cells and to dilute the number of sickled cells in the circulation. In the mid-1990s, investigators of a major study randomly assigned 300 adults with sickle cell disease who had more than 3 severe painful crises or episodes per year to hydroxyurea or a placebo.[1] This study clearly showed that this agent did reduce the number and severity of pain episodes in patients with sickle cell disease compared with placebo. In 1998, the United States Food and Drug Administration approved hydroxyurea for prevention of pain crises in adults with sickle cell anemia. Although the efficacy of hydroxyurea has been established in adults, the evidence of its efficacy in children is not as strong, but emerging data are supportive.

Although hydroxyurea has been useful in some patients with sickle cell disease, several issues about use of the drug are unresolved. These issues include patient and health practitioner concerns about the overall safety and effectiveness of hydroxyurea, as well as a lack of providers expert in the treatment of patients with sickle cell disease. In order to more carefully examine these issues, the National Heart Lung and Blood Institute in the Office of Medical Applications of Research of the National Institutes of Health convened a consensus conference from February 25 to 27, 2008, to assess the available scientific evidence related to the following questions:

- What is the efficacy (from clinical studies) of hydroxyurea treatment for patients with sickle cell disease in infants, preadolescents, adolescents, and adults?
- What is the effectiveness (in everyday practice) of hydroxyurea treatment for patients who have sickle cell disease?
- What are the short- and long-term harms of hydroxyurea treatment?
- What are the barriers to hydroxyurea treatment for patients who have sickle cell disease, and what are the potential solutions?
- What are the future research needs?

The report of Lanzkron addresses the first 3 of these questions and does so by producing a systematic review of the world's literature on the subject of hydroxyurea treatment. The bottom line is that hydroxyurea does increase fetal hemoglobin in adults with sickle cell disease. It reduces the frequency of pain crises, reduces the frequency and/or duration of hospitalization and minimizes the need for transfusions. Dismayingly, far less evidence is available regarding the clinically relevant outcomes of hospitalization, stroke, and pain crises, the acute chest syndrome, and death. Although the evidence is sparse, it does suggest that hydroxyurea in adults is not associated with leukemia. Evidence with respect to the fostering of other malignancies is less clear, at least to date. Also, no trial data are available with which to comment on effectiveness of this drug in a population that may take the medication for many years with less supervision and encouragement than occurs in a typical high efficiency clinical trial carried out at sickle cell centers. This latter statement has particular relevance when it comes to outcomes in children. It must also be said that the conclusions from this report cannot be generalized to all patients with variations of sickle cell disease because the data examined related only to patients with sickle cell disease. Many subgroups require further study, particularly patients with hemoglobin SC, and the second most common genotype of sickle cell disease. We also know very little about the effects of hydroxyurea in sickle cell disease patients who have comorbid diseases, specifically HIV or hepatitis C. The interactions between hydroxyurea and these underlying diseases must be clarified.

This report gives us limited insights about the use of hydroxyurea in children. The National Toxicology Program of the National Institute of Environmental Health Sciences has a center for the evaluation of risks to human reproduction. In 2007 this center reported on the effect of hydroxyurea on growth and development. The panel concluded that nursing infants of women taking hydroxyurea may be exposed to 1 mg to 6 mg of hydroxyurea daily. The expert panel found no data on the effects of hydroxyurea on female human or animal reproductive processes. Likewise, no data were available on the effect of germ cell exposure to hydroxyurea. Reproductive toxicities have been found in mice. Based on animal studies, the expert panel did express concerns about the adverse effects of hydroxyurea on spermatogenesis in men receiving hydroxyurea at therapeutic doses. Whether or not such effects are seen later in life in treated children remains an unknown.

As of this writing, hydroxyurea is the only United States Food and Drug Administration-approved medication for the treatment of sickle cell disease. Given the fact that it treats a disease that has great morbidity and is capable of seriously shortening life span, the potential toxicities of hydroxyurea have to be weighed against its documented benefits. For more on the topic of the National Institutes of Health Consensus Development Conference on hydroxyurea treatment for sickle cell disease, see the official conference statement.[2]

J. A. Stockman III, MD

References

1. Charache S, Barton FB, Moore RD, et al. Hydroxyurea and sickle cell anemia. Clinical utility of myelosuppressive "switching" agent. The Multicenter Study of Hydroxyurea in Sickle Cell Anemia. *Medicine (Baltimore)*. 1996;75:300-326.
2. Brawley OW, Cornelius LJ, Edwards LR, et al. National Institutes of Health Consensus Development Conference Statement: hydroxyurea treatment for sickle cell disease. *Ann Intern Med*. 2008;148:932-938.

Cell-Free Hemoglobin-Based Blood Substitutes and Risk of Myocardial Infarction and Death: A Meta-analysis

Natanson C, Kern SJ, Lurie P, et al (Natl Insts of Health, Bethesda, MD; Health Res Group, Public Citizen, Washington, DC)
JAMA 299:2304-2312, 2008

Context.—Hemoglobin-based blood substitutes (HBBSs) are infusible oxygen-carrying liquids that have long shelf lives, have no need for refrigeration or cross-matching, and are ideal for treating hemorrhagic shock in remote settings. Some trials of HBBSs during the last decade have reported increased risks without clinical benefit.

Objective.—To assess the safety of HBBSs in surgical, stroke, and trauma patients.

Data Sources.—PubMed, EMBASE, and Cochrane Library searches for articles using *hemoglobin* and *blood substitutes* from 1980 through March 25, 2008; reviews of Food and Drug Administration (FDA) advisory committee meeting materials; and Internet searches for company press releases.

Study Selection.—Randomized controlled trials including patients aged 19 years and older receiving HBBSs therapeutically. The database searches yielded 70 trials of which 13 met these criteria; in addition, data from 2 other trials were reported in 2 press releases, and additional data were included in 1 relevant FDA review.

Data Extraction.—Data on death and myocardial infarction (MI) as outcome variables.

Results.—Sixteen trials involving 5 different products and 3711 patients in varied patient populations were identified. A test for heterogeneity of the results of these trials was not significant for either mortality or MI (for both, $I^2 = 0\%$, $P \geq .60$), and data were combined using a fixed-effects model. Overall, there was a statistically significant increase in the risk of death (164 deaths in the HBBS-treated groups and 123 deaths in the control groups; relative risk [RR], 1.30; 95% confidence interval [CI], 1.05-1.61) and risk of MI (59 MIs in the HBBS-treated groups and 16 MIs in the control groups; RR, 2.71; 95% CI, 1.67-4.40) with these HBBSs. Subgroup analysis of these trials indicated the increased risk was not restricted to a particular HBBS or clinical indication.

Conclusion.—Based on the available data, use of HBBSs is associated with a significantly increased risk of death and MI.

▶ Chances are that you have heard a lot of negativity about the use of hemoglobin substitutes. Ever since the first complications of standard transfusion began to be noted more than a hundred years ago, pursuit of an artificial blood substitute became the equivalent of the search for the Holy Grail. The flurry of activities in the 1980s and 1990s to develop a viable and universal hemoglobin-based oxygen carrier that was free of red blood cells was largely based on concerns about the adequacy of the blood supply and real or perceived deleterious effects of standard transfusions of red blood cells. The concern at the time was that increasingly refined and limiting donor selection criteria would increase transfusion safety, but at the same time would decrease the blood donor pool. This was also about the time that HIV transmission via blood component products became apparent.

What Natanson et al have done is to report a systematic review intended to identify all published and unpublished clinical trials of hemoglobin-based oxygen carrier blood substitutes. The review documented a clinically important increase in the risk of mortality and risk of myocardial infarction in adults in trials of hemoglobin-based oxygen carrier substitutes. These findings cast serious doubt on the safety and effectiveness of such products. Specifically, the meta-analysis showed a 30% increase in the risk of death and a nearly 3-fold increased risk of myocardial infarction when all hemoglobin-based oxygen carrier blood substitute trials were pooled.

Please do not think that the findings from the report of Natanson et al are surprising. Animal evidence and early clinical trials did demonstrate that blood substitutes were associated with risks such as renal dysfunction and untoward vascular effects.

In an editorial that accompanied this report in *JAMA* one written by Fergusson and McIntyre,[1] it was stated that based on the findings of the Natanson et al report and the consistency of these results with preclinical evidence of potential toxicity, further trials of hemoglobin-based blood substitutes of these types should not be conducted. The meta-analysis seems to be bulletproof enough to support this clear-cut statement. Given the continuously improving safety of the United States blood supply, the availability of blood component products, and the technologies to minimize the need for transfusion, it does indeed not seem prudent to continue to study the use of hemoglobin-based blood substitutes developed thus far. Many of these trials have taken place in situations in which patients received the substitutes in elective surgical procedures. Unfortunately, some recipients died as a consequence. Whether or not you consider the attempt to find an adequate blood substitute a noble effort, the time has come to call a halt to the effort until some new ideas surface.

J. A. Stockman III, MD

Reference

1. Fergusson DA, McIntyre L. The future of clinical trials evaluating blood substitutes. *JAMA*. 2008;299:2324-2326.

Adverse Reactions to Allogeneic Whole Blood Donation by 16- and 17-Year-Olds

Eder AF, Hillyer CD, Dy BA, et al (American Red Cross, Washington, DC; et al)
JAMA 299:2279-2286, 2008

Context.—Donations by minors (16- and 17-year olds) now account for approximately 8% of the whole blood collected by the American Red Cross, but young age and first-time donation status are known to be independent risk factors for donation-related complications.

Objective.—To evaluate adverse reactions to allogeneic whole blood donation by 16- and 17-year-olds compared with older donors in American Red Cross blood centers.

Design, Setting, and Participants.—Prospective documentation of adverse events among 16- and 17-year-old donors using standardized collection protocols, definitions, and reporting methods in 2006. Data were from 9 American Red Cross blood centers that routinely collect from 16- and 17-year-olds, a population that provides 80% of its donations at high school blood drives.

Main Outcome Measures.—Rate of systemic (syncopal-type) and phlebotomy-related donor complications per 10 000 collections.

Results.—In 2006, 9 American Red Cross regions collected 145 678 whole blood donations from 16- and 17-year-olds, 113 307 from 18- and 19-year-olds, and 1 517 460 from donors aged 20 years or older. Complications were recorded in 15 632 (10.7%), 9359 (8.3%), and 42 987 (2.8%) donations in each corresponding age group. In a multivariate logistic regression model, young age had the strongest association with complications (odds ratio [OR], 3.05; 95% confidence interval [CI], 2.52-3.69; $P < .001$), followed by first-time donation status (OR, 2.63; 95% CI, 2.24-3.09; $P < .001$) and female sex (OR, 1.87; 95% CI, 1.62-2.16; $P < .001$). Infrequent but medically relevant complications, in particular physical injury from syncope-related falls, were significantly more likely in 16- and 17-year-old donors (86 events; 5.9/10 000 collections) compared with 18- and 19-year-old donors (27 events; 2.4/10 000 collections; OR, 2.48; 95% CI, 1.61-3.82) or adults aged 20 years or older (62 events; 0.4/10 000 collections; OR, 14.46; 95% CI, 10.43 -20.04). Sixteen-year-old donors who experienced even a minor complication were less likely to return to donate within 12 months than 16-year-olds who experienced uncomplicated donations (52% vs 73% return rate; OR, 0.40; 95% CI, 0.36-0.44).

Conclusions.—A higher incidence of donation-related complications and injury occurs among 16- and 17-year-old blood donors compared with older donors. The increasing dependence on recruiting and retaining young blood donors requires a committed approach to donor safety, especially at high school blood drives.

▶ Current estimates are that only about 38% of the US adult population is eligible to provide a blood donation. Over the last 20 years, there have been increasing restrictions on the use of certain types of donors related to age, risk of infection, and a number of other items. The latter include restrictions imposed on donor eligibility related to perceived or proven risks of transfusion-related malaria, and bovine spongiform encephalopathy, and the introduction of additional infectious disease tests, including those for Chagas disease and West Nile virus. To compensate for these restrictions, blood centers have endeavored to recruit more eligible donors by targeting underrepresented racial groups, streamlining donor history screening, eliminating unnecessary questions, obtaining variances from the United States Food and Drug Administration regulations to collect blood from individuals with hereditary hemachromatosis, relaxing the upper and lower limitations for blood donation, and advocating for state legislation to collect blood from 16- and 17-year-old high school students. Indeed, most state regulations now allow blood collection from 17-year-old donors without parent permission. At the time the report of Eder et al was published, 22 states or United States territories allowed donation by 16-year-olds with parent consent. Two states allow donation by 16-year-olds without parent consent. California allows donation by 15-year-olds with written permission of a parent or a guardian plus the written authorization of a physician or surgeon. The American Red Cross requires parent consent for all 16-year-old donors, does not collect from 15-year-olds, and follows state regulations or variances applicable to parent consent for collection from 17-year olds.

As of now, teenagers age 16 or 17 donate almost a tenth of the whole blood collected by the American Red Cross. What we see in this report of Eder et al is that these teens have a significantly high risk of complications related to donation in comparison with older teenagers and adults. In blood centers run by the Red Cross, 10.7% of 16- and 17-year-olds, 8.3% of 18- and 19-year-olds, and 2.8% of adults had some kind of complication, usually minor bruising, pallor, or lightheadedness. Far fewer lost consciousness and fewer still sustained injuries or needed outside medical help, but the risks were still highest in the youngest of donors. The data show that the rates of injury secondary to fainting were 5.9 per 10 000 donations in 16- and 17-year-olds, 2.4 per 10 000 in 18- and 19-year-olds, and just 0.4 per 10 000 in adults aged at least 20. Doing the math, the odds of injury are 14 times higher for the youngest donors relative to adults. As one might suspect, this report also shows that a 16-year-old who has even a minor complication is much less likely to donate blood again.

Although the absolute magnitudes of the differences between teens and older age groups in terms of complications of blood donation are relatively small, the differences are statistically significant. Young age is the strongest predictor of major complications and 16- and 17-year-old donors currently account for half of the syncope-related injuries, even though these teens account for only about 10% of all blood donations.

It is a bit difficult to tell what should be done with the information provided by the American Red Cross. Teens do supply a fair amount of the blood needed here in the United States. If there is a lesson to be learned from the data of the American Red Cross, it is that teens do require much more attention than older adults at the time of blood donation. Clearly there will never be a zero risk of blood donation, but we must do the most that we can to reduce these documented risks in the 16-year-olds and 17-year-olds in our blood donor population.

J. A. Stockman III, MD

A Syndrome with Congenital Neutropenia and Mutations in *G6PC3*

Boztug K, Appaswamy G, Ashikov A, et al (Hannover Med School, Germany; et al)

N Engl J Med 360:32-43, 2009

Background.—The main features of severe congenital neutropenia are the onset of severe bacterial infections early in life, a paucity of mature neutrophils, and an increased risk of leukemia. In many patients, the genetic causes of severe congenital neutropenia are unknown.

Methods.—We performed genomewide genotyping and linkage analysis on two consanguineous pedigrees with a total of five children affected with severe congenital neutropenia. Candidate genes from the linkage interval were sequenced. Functional assays and reconstitution experiments were carried out.

Results.—All index patients were susceptible to bacterial infections and had very few mature neutrophils in the bone marrow; structural heart defects, urogenital abnormalities, and venous angiectasia on the trunk and extremities were additional features. Linkage analysis of the two index families yielded a combined multipoint lod score of 5.74 on a linkage interval on chromosome 17q21. Sequencing of *G6PC3*, the candidate gene encoding glucose-6-phosphatase, catalytic subunit 3, revealed a homozygous missense mutation in exon 6 that abolished the enzymatic activity of glucose-6-phosphatase in all affected children in the two families. The patients' neutrophils and fibroblasts had increased susceptibility to apoptosis. The myeloid cells showed evidence of increased endoplasmic reticulum stress and increased activity of glycogen synthase kinase 3β (GSK-3β). We identified seven additional, unrelated patients who had severe congenital neutropenia with syndromic features and distinct biallelic mutations in *G6PC3*.

Conclusions.—Defective function of glucose-6-phosphatase, catalytic subunit 3, underlies a severe congenital neutropenia syndrome associated with cardiac and urogenital malformations.

▶ When this editor was a resident (more than 35 years ago), we frequently used the term "Kostmann syndrome" as a substitute for any form of severe congenital neutropenia. This was based on the fact that back in 1956, Rolf Kostmann, a Swedish pediatrician, described an autosomal recessive disorder that he called infantile genetic agranulocytosis. In the interim several decades, the eponym has been dropped and we simply call the disorder severe congenital neutropenia. The disorder is caused by disabling mutations in the *HAX1* gene, which encodes HAX1, a mitochondrial protein that inhibits apoptosis. We now know that there are both autosomal dominant and sporadic forms of severe congenital neutropenia, which are caused by mutations in the *ELA2* gene that encodes the serine protease, neutrophil elastase. The latter mutations account for approximately 50% to 60% of cases at the present time. There are other rare forms of congenital neutropenia as well. For example, the Wiskott-Aldrich syndrome can be associated with neutropenia.

Neutropenia of varying severity occurs in association with complex congenital disorders, such as the Shwachman-Diamond syndrome (a rare, autosomal recessive multisystem disorder primarily featuring digestive enzyme insufficiency, skeletal abnormalities, and often neutropenia), the Barth syndrome (an X-linked genetic disorder of lipid metabolism causing cellular lipid deficiency, with cardiomyopathy, neutropenia, muscular hypoplasia or weakness, and growth delay), the WHIM syndrome (an autosomal dominant disorder causing warts, hypogammaglobulinemia, recurrent bacterial infection, myelokathexis, and severe chronic leukopenia and neutropenia), and the Chediak-Higashi syndrome (an autosomal recessive multisystem disorder causing hypopigmentation of the skin, eyes, and hair, prolonged bleeding time, easy bruising, peripheral neuropathy, and recurrent infection secondary to neutropenia). It is also important to note that many patients with congenital neutropenia will have their disease transformed into a malignant disorder. This occurs in about 20% of patients, and usually results in the development of acute myeloid leukemia.

The most important diagnostic test for evaluating severe congenital neutropenia is a bone marrow examination, which typically shows an ample number of early myeloid precursors, but a paucity of mature neutrophils. Treatment with granulocyte colony-stimulating factor (G-CSF) has changed the natural history of the disease. More than 90% of patients will have a clinical response with an increase in numbers of circulating neutrophils with G-CSF treatment. The advent of G-CSF has revolutionized the management of these patients.

The report of Boztug et al tells us about mutations in the gene for glucose-6-phosphatase and its association with a newly discovered form of severe congenital neutropenia. In contrast to other forms of severe neutropenia, children with mutations in the gene for glucose-6-phosphatase also show cardiac abnormalities, thrombocytopenia, and urogenital abnormalities. The report reminds us that not all forms of severe congenital neutropenia are the same. As noted above, there are a wide variety of forms of severe congenital neutropenia, many associated with differing phenotypic physical findings. These tend to be mutation specific, meaning that we should be trying to define the genotype of all patients with congenital neutropenia to be sure of exactly which type each patient has. The hope is that with this better understanding of the molecular pathogenesis of the disorder, more effective targeted therapies will be developed.

To read more about the many causes of severe congenital neutropenia, see the excellent editorial by Dale and Link.[1]

J. A. Stockman III, MD

Reference

1. Dale DC, Link DC. The many causes of severe congenital neutropenia. *N Engl J Med.* 2009;360:3-5.

Severe hemorrhage in children with newly diagnosed immune thrombocytopenic purpura

Neunert CE, Buchanan GR, Imbach P, et al (Univ of Texas Southwestern Med Ctr at Dallas; Univ Children's Hosp, Basel, Switzerland; et al)
Blood 112:4003-4008, 2008

Controversy exists regarding management of children newly diagnosed with immune thrombocytopenic purpura (ITP). Drug treatment is usually administered to prevent severe hemorrhage, although the definition and frequency of severe bleeding are poorly characterized. Accordingly, the Intercontinental Childhood ITP Study Group (ICIS) conducted a prospective registry defining severe hemorrhage at diagnosis and during the following 28 days in children with ITP. Of 1106 ITP patients enrolled, 863 were eligible and evaluable for bleeding severity assessment at diagnosis and during the subsequent 4 weeks. Twenty-five children (2.9%) had severe bleeding at diagnosis. Among 505 patients with a platelet count less than or equal to 20 000/mm^3 and no or mild bleeding at diagnosis, 3 (0.6%), had new severe hemorrhagic events during the ensuing 28 days. Subsequent development of severe hemorrhage was unrelated to initial management ($P = .82$). These results show that severe bleeding is uncommon at diagnosis in children with ITP and rare during the next 4 weeks irrespective of treatment given. We conclude that it would be difficult to design an adequately powered therapeutic trial aimed at demonstrating prevention of severe bleeding during the first 4 weeks after diagnosis. This finding suggests that future studies of ITP management should emphasize other outcomes.

▶ All of us know of the controversies that have ensued during the last several decades regarding the management of childhood immune thrombocytopenic purpura (ITP). Drug treatment of ITP is often used to prevent serious bleeding, and the initial platelet count is assumed to be a surrogate for bleeding potential, especially for those who present with minimal bleeding. By all accounts; however, life-threatening hemorrhage, especially intracranial or central nervous system (CNS) bleeding, is quite rare (approximately 1 in 800 cases). Nonetheless, anxiety on a family's part and on a care provider's part is what frequently triggers treatment. The study by Neunert et al is the first to prospectively chronicle the severity of hemorrhage at diagnosis and in the 4 weeks postdiagnosis as well as the relationship of clinical symptoms to platelet count and treatment intervention in children with ITP.

In this study, 863 of 1106 children with ITP were fully evaluable and the large majority had no or mild bleeding at diagnosis with a platelet count of less than 20 000 mm^3. Therapy aimed at raising the platelet count was left to the provider's discretion. As you see in this report, about one-third of children received no drug therapy with the remainder receiving intravenous immunoglobulin (IVIG), steroids, or anti-D immunoglobulin (in approximately proportionate amounts). There was no difference in subsequent severe bleeding in those with mild or moderate bleeding at diagnosis, whether or not treatment was given. The prevalence of severe bleeding (including CNS) was found to be 3%, a finding similar to other large studies.

As the authors of this report suggest, serious bleeding in childhood acute ITP is quite rare, making the design and completion of a definitive drug intervention trial that might show differences in bleeding rates quite difficult. Accordingly, future studies in childhood ITP would likely best be aimed at investigating quality of life issues (focusing on both treatment side effects/adverse events and the troublesome symptoms of bleeding without treatment), the cost of treatment, and identifying clinical or laboratory markers that may predict the development of severe bleeding during the first 28 days of life.

Currently, most clinicians still use a platelet count of less than or equal to 20 000 to institute therapy, regardless of the severity of bleeding symptoms. The data in this report, however, would support allowing platelet counts to dive below this level and to treat based on clinical bleeding severity, thus avoiding costly and sometimes toxic treatment for patients who have only mild clinical bleeding at presentation.

For more on the topic of childhood ITP and its management, see the review by Abshire.[1]

J. A. Stockman III, MD

Reference

1. Abshire T. Childhood ITP: can we venture below 20,000? *Blood*. 2008;112: 3918-3919.

Effect of eltrombopag on platelet counts and bleeding during treatment of chronic idiopathic thrombocytopenic purpura: a randomised, double-blind, placebo-controlled trial

Bussel JB, Provan D, Shamsi T, et al (Cornell Univ, NY; Barts and The London School of Medicine, UK; Bismillah Taqee Inst of Health Sciences and Blood Disease Ctr, Karachi, Pakistan; et al)
Lancet 373:641-648, 2009

Background.—Eltrombopag is an oral, non-peptide, thrombopoietin-receptor agonist that stimulates thrombopoiesis, leading to increased platelet production. This study assessed the efficacy, safety, and tolerability of once daily eltrombopag 50 mg, and explored the efficacy of a dose increase to 75 mg.

Methods.—In this phase III, randomised, double-blind, placebo-controlled study, adults from 63 sites in 23 countries with chronic idiopathic thrombocytopenic purpura (ITP), platelet counts less than 30 000 per µL of blood, and one or more previous ITP treatment received standard care plus once-daily eltrombopag 50 mg (n = 76) or placebo (n = 38) for up to 6 weeks. Patients were randomly assigned in a 2:1 ratio of eltrombopag:placebo by a validated randomisation system. After 3 weeks, patients with platelet counts less than 50 000 per µL could increase study drug to 75 mg. The primary endpoint was the proportion of patients achieving platelet counts 50 000 per μL or more at day 43. All participants who received at least one dose of their allocated treatment were included in the analysis. This study is registered with ClinicalTrials.gov, number NCT00102739.

Findings.—73 patients in the eltrombopag group and 37 in the placebo group were included in the efficacy population and were evaluable for day-43 analyses. 43 (59%) eltrombopag patients and six (16%) placebo patients responded (ie, achieved platelet counts ≥50 000 per μL; odds ratio [OR] 9·61 [95% CI 3·31–27·86]; p<0·0001). Response to eltrombopag compared with placebo was not affected by predefined study stratification variables (baseline platelet counts, concomitant ITP drugs, and splenectomy status) or by the number of previous ITP treatments. Of the 34 patients in the efficacy analysis who increased their dose of eltrombopag, ten (29%) responded. Platelet counts generally returned to baseline values within 2 weeks after the end of treatment. Patients receiving eltrombopag had less bleeding at any time during the study than did those receiving placebo (OR 0·49 [95% CI 0·26–0·89]; p=0·021). The frequency of grade 3–4 adverse events during treatment (eltrombopag, two [3%]; placebo, one [3%]) and adverse events leading to study discontinuation (eltrombopag, three [4%]; placebo, two [5%]), were similar in both groups.

Interpretation.—Eltrombopag is an effective treatment for managment of thrombocytopenia in chronic ITP.

▶ No one will argue that the primary treatment goal of chronic idiopathic thrombocytopenic purpura (ITP) is the prevention of bleeding complications. This is an unusual but not rare complication of childhood acute ITP. Chronic ITP, of course, occurs much more frequently in adults. The treatment of this problem has largely focused on the inhibition of platelet destruction by use of steroids, intravenous immunoglobulin, intravenous anti-D, immunosuppressive drugs, splenectomy, and monoclonal antibodies directed at B-cells. While these treatments are useful, not all patients will respond to them. An interesting alternative, albeit theoretical treatment could be the use of agents to stimulate platelet production. It has been shown that an important component of the pathophysiology of ITP is the absence of a substantial compensatory increase in thrombopoietin levels despite severe thrombocytopenia. Stimulation of thrombopoiesis was explored some years ago with first-generation recombinant thrombopoietins that were tested in clinical trials primarily in healthy people and in patients with chemotherapy-induced thrombocytopenia. Unfortunately, the development of antibodies cross-reactive to endogenous thrombopoietin prevented their further use. This is where eltrombopag comes in.

Eltrombopag is an oral, small molecule, nonpeptide thrombopoietin receptor agonist that interacts with the transmembrane domain of the thrombopoietin receptor. The drug stimulates the proliferation and differentiation of megakaryocytes in the bone marrow, resulting in a dose-dependent increase in normally functioning platelets. The drug was given by subcutaneous injection. The report of Bussel et al tells us the effect of eltrombopag on platelet counts and bleeding as part of the treatment of chronic ITP in adults with the disorder. The youngest patient treated was age 19. When compared with controls who were receiving a placebo, almost 60% of those receiving eltrombopag responded with a platelet count of 50 000 per μL or more in comparison with controls who had a 16% response rate. Clinical bleeding was also improved.

In this and other studies, eltrombopag was well tolerated with an adverse event profile that was virtually similar to placebo. It should be noted that the drug does not work quickly and the absence of evidence of a platelet increase within the first week of treatment and the presumed kinetics of stimulating platelet production do not lend support to the use of eltrombopag when an urgent platelet increase is required.

Chances are you will be hearing more about the use of eltrombopag in children. It will take quite some time to accumulate information about the value of this drug in youngsters given the infrequent nature of acute ITP converting to chronic ITP however. Stay tuned.

J. A. Stookman III, MD

Inflammation induces hemorrhage in thrombocytopenia

Goerge T, Ho-Tin-Noe B, Carbo C, et al (Immune Disease Inst, Harvard Med School, Boston, MA)
Blood 111:4958-4964, 2008

The role of platelets in hemostasis is to produce a plug to arrest bleeding. During thrombocytopenia, spontaneous bleeding is seen in some patients but not in others; the reason for this is unknown. Here, we subjected thrombocytopenic mice to models of dermatitis, stroke, and lung inflammation. The mice showed massive hemorrhage that was limited to the area of inflammation and was not observed in uninflamed thrombocytopenic mice. Endotoxin-induced lung inflammation during thrombocytopenia triggered substantial intra-alveolar hemorrhage leading to profound anemia and respiratory distress. By imaging the cutaneous Arthus reaction through a skin window, we observed in real time the loss of vascular integrity and the kinetics of skin hemorrhage in thrombocytopenic mice. Bleeding—observed mostly from venules—occurred as early as 20 minutes after challenge, pointing to a continuous need for platelets to maintain vascular integrity in inflamed microcirculation. Inflammatory hemorrhage was not seen in genetically engineered mice lacking major platelet adhesion receptors or their activators (αIIbβ3, glycoprotein Ibalpha [GPIbα], GPVI, and calcium and diacylglycerol-regulated guanine nucleotide exchange factor I [CalDAG-GEFI]), thus indicating that firm platelet adhesion was not necessary for their supporting role. While platelets were previously shown to promote endothelial activation and recruitment of inflammatory cells, they also appear indispensable to maintain vascular integrity in inflamed tissue. Based on our observations, we propose that inflammation may cause life-threatening hemorrhage during thrombocytopenia.

▶ This report reminds us how tightly inflammation and hemostasis are intertwined. At sites of vascular injury, platelets adhere and aggregate to the exposed subendothelial matrix to form a platelet plug. This together with the coagulation system will seal the blood vessel and limit blood loss. It has been known for sometime, however, that 2 patients with equally low numbers of platelets will differ in their tendency to spontaneously bleed. The differences between these 2 patients have remained elusive probably because in most patients, thrombocytopenia is considered a sufficient explanation for the actual bleeding and further studies are then not performed. The study of Goerge et al provides experimental evidence that inflammation turns out to be a potent trigger of hemorrhage in the presence of thrombocytopenia. Add inflammation to any given level of platelet count and the likelihood of bleeding increases dramatically.

These findings translate nicely to the clinical situation. How many times have you seen a patient, say with leukemia, with a low platelet count who shows no evidence of bleeding? If that patient, however, say, becomes infected, bleeding in the presence of thrombocytopenia almost seems to be inevitable.

Thus, it is that platelets and intact vascular endothelium, free of inflammation, are the yin and yang of the initial process that establishes hemostasis. Either thrombocytopenia alone, or inflammation alone, may not cause bleeding, but put the 2 of them together and you have a problem. The report of Goerge et al does not clarify how platelets contribute to the maintenance of vascular integrity, but the authors propose an involvement of locally derived vasoactive mediators released from storage granules of platelets during transient interaction with the inflamed vessel wall. The authors also clearly show that inflammatory hemorrhage in the presence of thrombocytopenia is not restricted to the skin and its microcirculation. The data indicate that hemorrhage can occur at any inflamed site, including the gastrointestinal tract and the brain. While platelets have been shown in other experiments to promote recruitment of inflammatory cells and thus stimulate the inflammatory response to hasten healing, they additionally do prevent the deleterious consequences of inflammation of the vasculature. Identification of the protective factor or factors provided by platelets could be of major clinical importance if we can only determine what these are.

This commentary closes with a Clinical Fact/Curio about bleeding. It is presented in the form of a question. You care for a youngster who is on an anticoagulant. The flu season is about to begin. Is there a significant risk of giving this vaccine intramuscularly? Patients taking warfarin and other anticoagulants are often given flu vaccinations subcutaneously to reduce the risk of bleeding, but new evidence suggests that this practice is not necessary. One report now shows that intramuscular administration has no more side effects than the subcutaneous administration. In fact, the subcutaneous route actually resulted in more local reactions.[1]

J. A. Stockman III, MD

Reference

1. Casajuana J, Iglesias B, Fàbregas M, et al. Safety of intramuscular influenza vaccine in patients receiving oral anticoagulation therapy: a single blinded multi-centre randomized controlled clinical trial. *BMC Blood Disorders.* 2008;8:1.

4 Child Development

Predicting Stuttering Onset by the Age of 3 Years: A Prospective, Community Cohort Study
Reilly S, Onslow M, Packman A, et al (Univ of Melbourne, Australia; Univ of Sydney, Australia; et al)
Pediatrics 123:270-277, 2009

Objectives.—Our goals were to document (1) the onset of stuttering and (2) whether specific child, family, or environmental factors predict stuttering onset in children aged up to 3 years.

Methods.—Participants included a community-ascertained cohort of 1619 2-year-old Australian children recruited at 8 months of age to study the longitudinal development of early language. The main outcome measure was parental telephone report of stuttering onset, verified by face-to-face expert diagnosis. Preonset continuous measures of the child's temperament (approach/withdrawal) and language development were available. Information on a range of predictor measures hypothesized to be associated with stuttering onset was obtained (maternal mental health and education levels, gender, premature birth status, birth weight, birth order, twinning, socioeconomic status, family history of stuttering).

Results.—By 3 years of age, the cumulative incidence of stuttering onset was 8.5%. Onset often occurred suddenly over 1 to 3 days (49.6%) and involved the use of word combinations (97.1%). Children who stuttered were not more shy or withdrawn. Male gender, twin birth status, higher vocabulary scores at 2 years of age, and high maternal education were associated with stuttering onset. The multivariable model, however, had low predictive strength; just 3.7% of the total variation in stuttering onset was accounted for.

Conclusions.—The cumulative incidence of stuttering onset was much higher than reported previously. The hypothesized risk factors for stuttering onset together explained little of the variation in stuttering onset up to 3 years of age. Early onset was not associated with language delay, social and environmental factors, or preonset shyness/withdrawal. Health professionals can reassure parents that onset is not unusual up to 3 years of age and seems to be associated with rapid growth in language development.

▶ Most studies suggest that the cumulative incidence of stuttering up to 5 years of age runs about 3.5% in an overall population of children. Slightly under half of these youngsters will recover from stuttering naturally without any particular interference by about 6 years of age. This still leaves a fair number of children at long-term risk with this problem. A number of factors have been thought to increase the risk of stuttering including certain temperament charac-teristics (shyness, sensitivity, problems with adaptability, and vulnerability). Unfortunately, it is not at all clear whether these factors are truly associated with the onset of stuttering or whether they precede or develop as a result of stuttering. This is why the report of Reilly et al is so helpful because it seems to shed new information on this topic.

The authors followed a group of more than 1600 2-year-old children in an Australian community who were recruited at 8 months of age to study the longitudinal development of early language. The cumulative incidence of stut-tering onset by 3 years of age in this group was much higher than expected at 8.5%, almost twice the percentage reported in most other studies. The study in fact is the largest epidemiological investigation of early stuttering onset to date. Some of the findings from the study confirmed earlier reports about early stut-tering, including, for example, that boys are much more likely to stutter than girls. Also, there was a much higher positive family history of stuttering in those children affected with the problem. Three factors other than gender were significantly associated with stuttering onset. Mothers with a degree or postgraduate qualification were more likely to have children that stuttered by 3 years. It is possible that well-educated mothers are more likely to be aware of (and therefore to report) stuttering onset. It is also possible that the associ-ation with maternal education could be an artifact; stuttering onset typically occurs with the development of 3-word combinations, and such combinations may simply occur earlier in children of more highly educated mothers. Also, vocabulary scores at 2 years were more significantly associated with onset of stuttering, but not with maternal education. This unexpected association requires additional study. Another interesting finding is that temperament as measured did not predict stuttering onset. Children who started to stutter were neither shy nor more outgoing than their peers who did not stutter. The last association was that of twinning and that was an expected finding.

While on the topic of stuttering, an article recently appeared showing the effects of bilingualism on stuttering rates in childhood. In a report emanating from England, investigators did observe bilingualism to be a risk factor for stut-tering.[1] Children who are bilingual were usually found to stutter in both their languages (rather than just one). If a minority language alone is used in the home up to 5 years of age, the chance of starting to stutter is lower and the recovery rate is higher than for children who acquire English and a minority language during this period. The statistics from this study supported the posi-tion that bilingual children learning a second language in the home had a lower change of recovery as opposed to those children who were learning a second language at school. Overall, the findings from this British report suggest that if a child uses a language other than English in the home, deferring the time when they learn English reduces the chance of starting to stutter and aids the chances of recovery later in childhood. Another important finding was that stuttering in no way affected school performance.

J. A. Stockman III, MD

Reference

1. Howell P, Davis S, Williams R. The effects of bilingualism on stuttering during late childhood. *Arch Dis Child*. 2007;94:42-46.

Prevalence of Autism Among Adolescents With Intellectual Disabilities

Bryson SE, Bradley EA, Thompson A, et al (Dalhousie Univ–IWK Health Centre, Halifax, Nova Scotia; Univ of Toronto, Ontario; McMaster Univ, Hamilton, Ontario; et al)
Can J Psychiatry 53:449-459, 2008

Objective.—To estimate the prevalence of autism in an epidemiologically-derived population of adolescents with intellectual disabilities (ID).

Method.—The prevalence of autism was examined using the Autism Diagnostic Interview—Revised, with appropriate care taken in assessing lower functioning individuals and those with additional physical and sensory impairments. Individual assessment during psychological evaluation, and consensus classification of complex cases, involving clinicians experienced in the assessment of autism, contributed to the identification of autism.

Results.—Overall, 28% of individuals, or 2.0 of the 7.1/1000 with ID in the target population (as we have previously identified in another study), were identified with autism. Autism rates did not differ significantly across severe ID (32.0%) and mild ID (24.1%); males predominated (2.3 males to 1 female), but less so for severe ID (2 males to 1 female, compared with 2.8 males to 1 female for mild ID). Socioeconomic status did not distinguish the groups with and without autism. Less than one-half of the adolescents who met diagnostic criteria for autism were previously diagnosed as such.

Conclusions.—Our overall prevalence estimate for autism is in the higher range of estimates reported in previous studies of ID (more so for mild ID). This likely reflects the changes in diagnostic criteria for autism that have subsequently occurred. Discussion focuses on the identification of autism in the population with ID, and on the implications for service delivery and clinical training.

▶ This is an important report, showing that more than a quarter of a population of adolescents with intellectual disabilities can be identified to have a diagnosis of autism. Consistent with a large volume of literature on autism, the study also found that autism predominates in males, particularly those with mild intellectual disability (2.8-1 female, compared with 2.0-1 for severe intellectual disability). Interestingly, these findings support that while autism is less common among girls, when girls are affected, they will be more likely than boys to be severely intellectually impaired. An important other finding of this report is that less than one-half of adolescents who met the criteria for autism had been previously diagnosed. This underdiagnosis of autism is of considerable concern. If nothing else, undiagnosed autism in individuals with intellectual disability may also result in misdiagnosis of adult psychiatric disorders.

While on the topic of autism, the relationship between autism and vaccine administration never seems to have a close to its debate. The debate reemerged recently around Hanna Poling. When she was 19 months old, Hanna, the daughter of Jon and Terry Poling, received 5 vaccines—combined diphtheria, tetanus, acellular pertussis, *Haemophilus influenzae* type b, measles-mumps-rubella, varicella, and inactivated polio. At the time of the vaccine administration, Hanna was interactive, playful, and communicative. Two days later, she was lethargic, irritable, and febrile. Ten days after vaccination she developed a rash consistent with vaccine-induced varicella. Months later, with delays in neurologic and psychological development, Hanna was diagnosed with encephalopathy caused by a mitochondrial enzyme deficit. Hanna's signs included problems with language, communication, and behavior—all features of autism spectrum disorder. Although it is not unusual for children with mitochondrial enzyme deficiencies to develop neurologic signs between their first and second years of life, Hanna's parents believed that vaccines had triggered her encephalopathy. They sued the Department of Health and Human Services (DHHS) for compensation under the Vaccine Injury Compensation Program (VICP) and won. On March 6, 2008, the Polings took their case to the public. Standing before a bank of microphones with several major news organizations looking on, Jon Poling said that: "The results in this case may very well signify a landmark decision with children developing autism following vaccinations." For years, federal health agencies and professional organizations had reassured the public that vaccines did not cause autism. Now, with DHHS making this concession in a federal claims court, the government appears to be saying exactly the opposite. Caught in the middle, clinicians were at a loss to explain the reasoning behind the VICP's decision.

A recent editorial suggests that the VICP's concession to Hanna Poling was poorly reasoned.[1] It is noted that while it is clear that natural infections can exacerbate symptoms of encephalopathy in patients with mitochondrial enzyme deficiencies, there is no clear evidence that vaccines cause similar exacerbations. Indeed, because children with such deficiencies are particularly susceptible to infections, it is strongly recommended that they receive all vaccines. Although experts testifying on behalf of the Polings could reasonably argue that the development of fever and a varicella-vaccine rash after the administration of 9 vaccines was enough to stress a child with mitochondrial enzyme deficiency, Hanna Poling had other immunologic challenges that were not related to vaccines given her history of frequent episodes of fever and otitis media. Also, such a medical history is not at all unusual. Children typically have 4 to 6 febrile illnesses each year during their first few years of life, and vaccines are a miniscule contributor to this antigenic challenge. One could argue that children with mitochondrial enzyme deficiencies might have a lower risk of exacerbation of their underlying disorder if vaccines were withheld, delayed, or separated, but such an approach would come at a price. Even spacing out vaccinations would increase the period during which children were susceptible to natural infections. These diseases are not merely historical given the prevalence of pneumococcal, varicella, and pertussis infection in the United States. Recent outbreaks of measles infection also demonstrate the need for this vaccine.

It should be noted that governmental agencies are attempting to make it absolutely clear that the compensation provided to the Poling family was not on the basis of vaccines possibly causing autism. In fact, given the global encephalopathy caused by the known mitochondrial enzyme deficit, a diagnosis of autism would be next to impossible to make. Rett's syndrome, tuberous sclerosis, fragile X syndrome, and Down syndrome in children can also mimic features of autism.

Unfortunately, the VICP does not vigorously define the criteria by which it determines that a vaccine has caused harm. Prospectively, this should be done so there is no confusion in the public or in the practitioner's mind about why decisions are made to make awards following untoward events related to vaccine use.

This commentary closes with a *Clinical Fact/Curio*, a query having to do with one aspect of child development. Does breastfeeding improve academic performance? The answer is that while breastfeeding does not improve the academic performance of babies, it certainly may increase one's IQ as measured later in life. A Canadian study of about 14 000 children in 31 hospitals and clinics in Belarus conducted over more than 6 years has shown that prolonged and exclusive breastfeeding improves a child's cognitive ability.[2] It appears that the IQ of children in a breastfeeding promotion intervention was documented to be on average 3 to 4 points higher in comparison with a control group.

J. A. Stockman III, MD

References

1. Offit PA. Vaccines and autism revisited – the Hanna Poling case. *N Engl J Med.* 2008;358:2089-2091.
2. Kramer MS, Aboud F, Mironova E, et al. Breastfeeding and child cognitive development: new evidence from a large randomized trial. *Arch Gen Psychiatr.* 2008; 65:578-584.

Autism prevalence and precipitation rates in California, Oregon, and Washington counties
Waldman M, Nicholson S, Adilov N, et al (Cornell Univ, Ithaca, NY)
Arch Pediatr Adolesc Med 162:1026-1034, 2008

Objective.—To investigate empirically the possibility of an environmental trigger for autism among genetically vulnerable children that is positively associated with precipitation.

Design.—We used regression analysis to investigate autism prevalence rates and counts first in relation to mean annual county-level precipitation and then to the amount of precipitation a birth cohort was exposed to when younger than 3 years, controlling for time trend, population size, per capita income, and demographic characteristics. In some models, we included county fixed-effects rather than a full set of covariates.

Setting.—Counties in California, Oregon, and Washington.

Participants.—Children born in California, Oregon, and Washington between 1987 and 1999. Main Exposure: County-level precipitation.

Main Outcome Measures.—County-level autism prevalence rates and counts.

Results.—County-level autism prevalence rates and counts among school-aged children were positively associated with a county's mean annual precipitation. Also, the amount of precipitation a birth cohort was exposed to when younger than 3 years was positively associated with subsequent autism prevalence rates and counts in Oregon counties and California counties with a regional developmental services center.

Conclusions.—These results are consistent with the existence of an environmental trigger for autism among genetically vulnerable children that is positively associated with precipitation. Further studies focused on establishing whether such a trigger exists and identifying the specific trigger are warranted.

▶ One might have thought that the editors of the *Archives of Pediatrics and Adolescent Medicine* must have lost their marbles when they accepted for publication this report suggesting there is a correlation between the amount of rainfall in a particular region and the prevalence of autism. When you think about it, however, is it not possible that there could be a relationship based on factors such as increased television watching, reduced vitamin D levels, and perhaps even increased exposure to indoor chemicals in wet climates? A commentary on this report by Weiss does suggest the findings do warrant publication.[1] Weiss believes the primary target of this report is not the public at large or the practitioner, but rather the researcher interested in the causes of autism who will follow through on the findings of this report and attempt to find out why there is a link, if there is one, between precipitation rates and autism.

For now, we won't have to say there is not call for alarm if you live in Seattle as opposed to Miami Beach, but it does seem worthwhile to see what the follow-up will be to this interesting study. This commentary closes with another *Clinical Fact/Curio*, this having to do with nutrition and intelligence. For some time it has been thought that breast-fed babies were smarter. Now we see recent data that may explain why this observation is true, at least in some babies. Breast-fed infants with at least one copy of a common variant of the gene *FADS2* have IQ scores that are 6 to 7 points higher than those of non-nursed infants with similar genetics. Breastfeeding, however, does not appear to affect those children (10% of the study population) with only a less common version of *FADS2*. The gene variants may affect the conversion of dietary precursors to long-chain polyunsaturated fatty acids, which aggregate in the brain after birth. Alternatively, the fatty acids may act on the gene itself, causing it to affect the metabolic processing of the acids.[2]

J. A. Stockman III, MD

References

1. Weiss NS. Precipitation and autism. Do these results warrant publication? *Arch Pediatr Adolesc Med.* 2008;162:1095-1096.
2. Swaminathan N. Mother's milk and IQ. *Scientific American.* January, 2008;32.

A Functional Genetic Link between Distinct Developmental Language Disorders

Vernes SC, Newbury DF, Abrahams BS, et al (Univ of Oxford, UK; Univ of California, Los Angeles)
N Engl J Med 359:2337-2345, 2008

Background.—Rare mutations affecting the FOXP2 transcription factor cause a monogenic speech and language disorder. We hypothesized that neural pathways downstream of FOXP2 influence more common phenotypes, such as specific language impairment.

Methods.—We performed genomic screening for regions bound by FOXP2 using chromatin immunoprecipitation, which led us to focus on one particular gene that was a strong candidate for involvement in language impairments. We then tested for associations between single-nucleotide polymorphisms (SNPs) in this gene and language deficits in a well-characterized set of 184 families affected with specific language impairment.

Results.—We found that FOXP2 binds to and dramatically down-regulates *CNTNAP2*, a gene that encodes a neurexin and is expressed in the developing human cortex. On analyzing *CNTNAP2* polymorphisms in children with typical specific language impairment, we detected significant quantitative associations with nonsense-word repetition, a heritable behavioral marker of this disorder (peak association, $P = 5.0 \times 10^{-5}$ at SNP rs17236239). Intriguingly, this region coincides with one associated with language delays in children with autism.

Conclusions.—The *FOXP2–CNTNAP2* pathway provides a mechanistic link between clinically distinct syndromes involving disrupted language.

▶ One in 20 otherwise healthy-appearing children will have difficulty achieving basic competence in one or more aspects of our spoken language by the age of entry into school. It is believed that genetic factors have an important role in many cases. This statement is based on the fact that children with specific language impairment are 4 times as likely to have a family history of the disorder as are children who have no such impairment. Also, in monozygotic twins the concordance rate for language impairment is almost twice as great as that observed in dizygotic twins. Although the data from the literature are somewhat open to interpretation, more than 10 susceptibility genetic loci have been identified that affect language development.

It is generally recognized that cases of familial language impairment have a multifactorial and polygenetic basis. It was back in 1990 that Hurst et al discovered a 3-generation British family with autosomal dominant transmission of oral motor and speech dyspraxia.[1] Affected members of this family were shown to carry a mutation in the gene *FOXP2*, which encodes a transcription factor. The FOXP2 protein has many transcription targets in the brain. The report of Vernes et al documents that FOXP2 down-regulates the expression of *CNTNAP2*, a gene that encodes a neurexin protein. The investigators showed that a particular *CNTNAP2* variant is associated with specific language impairment. As noted by Vernes et al, variants of *CNTNAP2* have been associated with neurodevelopmental disorders whose primary manifestation is not linguistic. There has also been an association observed between *CNTNAP2* variants and autism.

An editorial by Stromswold reminds us that according to the common variant-multiple disease hypothesis, common alleles that contribute to a particular disease under particular genetic and environmental conditions may result in a different disease (or no disease) under other genetic and environmental conditions.[2] For a group of related disorders, some etiologic factors are unique to a particular disease and other factors are shared by several diseases. This hypothesis explains why several loci associated with spoken language disorders are also linked with other neurodevelopmental disorders, why different people with the same genetic mutation have different clinical pictures, and why linkage analyses of people with familial language disorders often do not identify susceptibility loci, including those previously identified.

The developmental language disorders thus can be placed in a larger class of neurodevelopmental disorders. This report and similar studies to those of Vernes et al help us begin to understand how genetic and environmental factors significantly affect language and language disorders.

This commentary closes with a *Clinical Fact/Curio* dealing with one aspect of child development. It is presented in the form of a question. Does sex ratio in preschool classes influence girls' and boys' mental, social, and motor development? Here is some news preschool boys may not want to hear: those who attend classes with a majority of girls receive an intellectual boost by the end of the preschool year. Conversely, preschool boys who attend majority-boy classes fall increasingly behind girls on measures of learning skills and other developmental feats. Note, however, class sex ratio has no effect on a girl's learning. These provocative findings come from the first large-scale investigation of how sex ratio in preschool classes influences girls' and boys' mental, social, and motor development. Investigators performing a study in Rochester, New York found that girls display generally good progress during the school year on teacher-related measures of thinking skills, social abilities, and motor proficiency whether in classes of mostly boys or girls. Boys, however, develop more slowly than girls on several measures, particularly on thinking skills, if they attend classes with a surplus of boys. In majority-girl classes, boys develop at the same rate as girls.[3]

J. A. Stockman III, MD

References

1. Lai CSL, Fisher SE, Hurst JA, Vargha-Khadem F, Monaco AP. A forkhead-domain gene is mutated in a severe speech and language disorder. *Nature*. 2001;413: 519-523.
2. Stromswold K. The genetics of speech and language impairments. *N Engl J Med*. 2008;359:2381-2383.
3. Bower D. Girls could give preschool boys learning boost. *Sci News*. July 19, 2008; 14.

Early head injury and attention-deficit/hyperactivity disorder: retrospective cohort study
Keenan HI, Hall GC, Marshall SW, et al (Univ of Utah, Salt Lake City; Ravenscroft Park, Barnet, Hertfordshire, ENS; Univ of North Carolina at Chapel Hill, NC)
BMJ 337:a1984, 2008

Objective.—To explore the hypothesis that medically attended head injury in young children may be causal in the later development of attention-deficit/hyperactivity disorder.

Design.—Retrospective cohort study.

Setting.—Health improvement network database (1988-2003), a longitudinal UK general practice dataset.

Participants.—All children registered in the database from birth until their 10th birthday.

Main Outcome Measures.—Risk of a child with a head injury before age 2 developing attention-deficit/hyperactivity disorder before age 10 compared with children with a burn injury before age 2 and children with neither a burn nor a head injury.

Results.—Of the 62 088 children who comprised the cohort, 2782 (4.5%) had a head injury and 1116 (1.8%) had a burn injury. The risk of diagnosis of attention-deficit/hyperactivity disorder before 10 years of age after adjustment for sex, prematurity, socioeconomic status, and practice identification number was similar in the head injury (relative risk 1.9, 95% confidence interval 1.5 to 2.5) and burn injury groups (1.7, 1.2 to 2.5) compared with all other children.

Discussion.—Medically attended head injury before 2 years of age does not seem to be causal in the development of attention-deficit/hyperactivity disorder. Medically attended injury before 2 years of age may be a marker for subsequent diagnosis of attention-deficit/ hyperactivity disorder.

▶ It is pretty well known that youngsters with attention-deficit/hyperactivity disorder (ADHD) tend to injure themselves more frequently than those who do not have this problem. Some have also suggested that moderate to severe traumatic brain injury in school age children can actually result in the development of ADHD (secondary ADHD).[1] Keenan et al designed a study to see if the latter is actually true. The study comprised 62 088 children from the database of the Health Improvement Network in Great Britain. The network information base contains data from 308 general practitioner practices and goes back to 1988. To ascertain whether head injury increases the incidence of ADHD occurring after a head injury, the investigators compared children with head injuries (2782) with noninjured controls (58190) and added another injury comparison group—children with burns (1116). Children in either injury group were identified as having a "medically attended" head injury or a burn, and the injury had to occur before 2 years of age and with ADHD diagnosed before 10 years. The control group was used to tease out head injury as a key factor from the influences of injury itself.

The results of this study showed no significant association between head injury and an increase in ADHD symptoms. The results also indicate that young children who get injured might have more behavioral traits that subsequently attract a diagnosis of ADHD.

The conclusions of this report are fairly clear. Trauma does not cause ADHD. ADHD can predispose some children to hurting themselves, however. To say this differently, one might think about ADHD in children who tend to injure themselves, knowing that most children in the latter category do not in fact have ADHD.

J. A. Stockman III, MD

Reference

1. Levin H, Hanten G, Max J, et al. Symptoms of attention-deficit/hyperactivity disorder following traumatic brain injury in children. *J Dev Behav Pediatr.* 2007;28:108-118.

Toilet training of healthy young toddlers: a randomized trial between a daytime wetting alarm and timed potty training
Vermandel A, Weyler J, De Wachter S, et al (Univ Antwerp, Edegem, Belgium)
J Dev Behav Pediatr 29:191-196, 2008

Objective.—Toilet training (TT) is important for every child, but there is no agreement on what is the best training method. We evaluated in a randomized way the comprehensive use of a daytime wetting alarm at home for 5 days in healthy children and compared it with timed potty training.

Methods.—Thirty-nine children, between 20 and 36 months of age, were randomized to wetting alarm diaper training (WAD-T; n = 20) or timed potty training (TP-T; n = 19). Toilet behavior was observed by parents and independent observers before, at the end, and after 2 weeks of training. Late evaluation at 1 month was done by telephone.

Results.—The WAD-T group did significantly better than the TP-T group at the end training (p = .041), at 14 days (p = .027), and 1 month after training (p = .027). Independent bladder control was achieved in 88.9% of the WAD-T group.

Conclusions.—The WAD-T method is a structured, child-friendly, highly effective option for TT young healthy children. It offers the parents clear guidelines, a limited time needed to complete TT, a high success rate, and minor emotional conflicts. Results must now be confirmed in a larger sample size.

▶ The science underscoring how we recommend toilet training for otherwise healthy toddlers is not replete with hard science. For the last 100 years or so, recommended toilet training methods have oscillated between rigid and permissive programs. Mainly, 2 methods have been applied in the last 50 years: the method by Foxx and Azrin and the method described by Brazelton.[1,2] The highly structured behavioral method designed by Foxx and Azrin consists of a single 1-day training program first described back in 1974. The training is intensive in an environment free from distractions and includes very specific maneuvers, including checking for a dry diaper every 5 minutes, prompting a trial on the potty every 15 minutes, sitting on the potty for 10 minutes, and giving the child fluids to drink every 5 minutes. Brazelton described a more "child-oriented" approach with the basic idea being that children must gently, but systematically, be encouraged to experiment with toileting behavior. This approach suggests beginning toilet training only after certain physiologic and behavioral criteria of readiness are met. It stresses the importance of permitting the child the freedom to master each step at his or her own pace with minimal conflict. Current guidelines of the American Academy of Pediatrics dealing with toilet training are based on this latter approach.

Into the gruel of potential toilet training options, Vermandel et al add a new one, that of employing a daytime wetting alarm as part of the toilet training process. The procedure described involves a training period that is undertaken for 5 consecutive days. For children who appear to be just about ready for toilet training (using the Brazelton criteria), a 5-day condensed training program using a diaper wetting alarm was described. The alarm device consists of a specially made mini-auditory box (4.0 × 3.9 × 1.9 cm) fixed to the diaper via a self-adhesive strip. The strip has a moisture sensitive component that starts a gentle ringing sound when the diaper becomes wet. If this happens, the child is put immediately on the potty and is encouraged to finish voiding there. The device is not used at nighttime. Use of the alarm methodology was compared with a timed potty training method consisting of scheduled toilet visits where the child is placed on the potty, twice in the morning and twice in the afternoon for 5 minutes each time and is encouraged to void. The toilet visits were not at fixed times, but roughly at 2- to 3-hour intervals when the parent could easily schedule it. Parents of all the toddlers were asked to use positive reinforcement with hugs, effusive praise, smiles, or applause when the child urinated in the potty.

So how well did the diaper alarm system work in potty training these toddlers? Significantly, more children in the diaper alarm group achieved complete dryness after the training period compared with children using the other methodology (77.8% vs 41.2%). For those in both groups who achieved potty training, the results were sustained for the next 2 weeks in almost 90% of those who were trained with the diaper alarm method.

The use of an auditory alarm system is a well-accepted treatment for children with enuresis. It has not been used, however, as an assist for toilet training. Although it is unlikely to catch on like wildfire, wetting alarm diaper training does combine elements of various methods previously described. Components of the Brazelton approach as approved by the American Academy of Pediatrics are still included as a readiness to start the program described. It is hard to say why toilet training is occurring at later ages than in decades past. Some have suggested that this is due to the introduction of disposable diapers and more efficient laundry facilities as well as the potential that parents lack time as both parents may be working. Others claim that the reason for postponing toilet training is that the modern parent has a different way of thinking with an increasing emphasis on a child-oriented approach to potty training. Modern diapers do not help in the sense that they absorb urine so well and keep the skin so dry that the cues to the child that the diaper is wet are not as readily obvious.

The authors of this report are very cautious about making widespread recommendations regarding the use of a diaper alarm. They do not claim that the alarm method is the best method that should be used by all parents and all children. They do, however, consider their findings important as they illustrate that bladder control can be successfully trained within a handful of days with a properly instructed set of parents using a daytime wetting alarm. You will have to be the judge of whether any of this makes sense. Currently, there are no commercial devices that are readily available to use for this type of training unless you are ready to jerry-rig some of the enuresis devices for toilet training purposes.

J. A. Stockman III, MD

References

1. Foxx RM, Azrin NH. Dry pants: a rapid method of toilet training children. *Behav Res Ther.* 1973;11:435-442.
2. Brazelton TB. A child-oriented approach to toilet training. *Pediatrics.* 1962;29: 121-128.

Like parent, like child: child food and beverage choices during role playing
Sutherland LA, Beavers DP, Kupper LL, et al (Dartmouth Med School, Lebanon, NH)
Arch Pediatr Adolesc Med 162:1063-1069, 2008

Objective.—To examine food and beverage choices of preschool-aged children.

Design.—Semistructured observational study. While pretending to be adults during a role-play scenario, children selected food and beverage items from a miniature grocery store stocked with 73 different products, of which 47 foods and beverages were examined in this analysis. Parents self-reported how frequently they purchased specific grocery items.

Setting.—A behavioral laboratory.

Participants.—One hundred twenty children, aged 2 to 6 years, and 1 parent for each child.

Main Outcome Measure.—Children's total purchases were classified according to the number of healthier and less healthy products they selected as least healthy, somewhat healthy, and most healthy choices. The same categories were used to classify parents' self-reported purchases.

Results.—Most of the children (70.8%) purchased foods that were categorized as least healthy choices. Only 13 children (10.8%) had shopping baskets consisting of the healthiest choices. On average, children in the group with the least healthy choices purchased the same number of healthier and less healthy products, whereas children in the group with most healthy choices purchased 5 healthier products for each less healthy product selected. The healthfulness of children's total purchases were significantly (P = .02) predicted by their parents' purchasing categorization.

Conclusions.—When presented with a wide array of food products, young children chose combinations of healthier and less healthy foods and beverages. The data suggest that children begin to assimilate and mimic their parents' food choices at a very young age, even before they are able to fully appreciate the implications of these choices.

▶ Like mother, like daughter. Like father, like son. Because most children are eating at least some of their meals with their parents, it is not surprising those children's diets are similar to those of their parents. To the extent, however, that these similarities are based on preference rather than simply on food availability, children may be forming dietary habits that will stay with them throughout their lives. Family dietary practices and food availability in the home have been shown to be important determinants of the quality of children's diets. If a parent is overweight as the result of their eating habits, it is likely that the child will have a much greater risk of being overweight as well.

The goal of the study of Sutherland et al was to examine young children's perceptions of adult behaviors for tobacco and alcohol use. As part of the study, however, an analysis was undertaken to identify the food preferences young children have implicitly learned through exposure to parental self-reported consumer practices, media, and other external influences. The investigators used a role-playing scenario that involved a play grocery store to determine which foods and beverages young children would choose while pretending to be adults shopping for an evening with friends. Parents were also surveyed about their own food purchasing behaviors and other factors that could potentially influence children's food and beverage choices. The play store was stocked with 133 miniature items representing 73 different products that are typically found in a grocery store. The simulation showed that even at a young age, the healthfulness of foods purchased by young children was significantly associated with the healthfulness of parent-reported food and beverage purchases.

This study suggests that preschool children are already forming food preferences and are attentive to food choices made by their parents. The findings also suggest that parent modeling of good dietary behavior goes beyond the home and may begin at the point of purchase. It would be interesting to see this simulation carried over into the real world with school-aged children who are cut loose to buy food in a supermarket for a week's worth of meals. Will it be Twinkies or green leafy vegetables? Will it be Krispy Kremes or apples and peaches? Time to check such a study out.

Here's another *Clinical Fact/Curio* about some aspects of child development. In the *Republic*, Plato states, "Imagine...a ship in which there is a captain who is taller and stronger than any of the crew, but he is a little deaf and has a similar infirmity in sight, and his knowledge of navigation is not much better."[1] Plato argues that the crew cannot select a competent captain because the crew is beguiled, in part by appearances. Plato actually is creating an allegory related to a nation's election of its leader and suggests that voters in fact lack the rational faculties to be able to judge competency and largely make decisions based on appearance. Indeed, social scientists remind us that individuals automatically infer characteristics of competency based on facial appearances.[2]

A recent commentary on predicting elections reminds us that voters may be using the same rudimentary decision heuristics that children use early in development. Facial stereotypes are well developed even in infancy.[3] Antonakis and Dalgas speculate that voters may still be using the same cues that children do to characterize an individual's competency.[4] The hypothesis was that voters pick their leaders based on the general appearance, including facial appearance, of a candidate with the latter being a substitute for a rating of competence. In their interesting study, Antonakis and Dalgas presented several thousand adults and children with pictures of the winners and runner-ups from the 2002 French Parliamentary elections. The adults and children who were studied lived in Switzerland and were unfamiliar with the French elections. Both the adults and the children were able to pick the successful candidate 75 times out of 100 based on their facial appearance!

A lot of money is spent these days on predicting election outcomes. Evidently, young children, who are less experienced than our adults in observing performance and competency will pick a winner much more often than not just by looking at who is running.

Predicting elections is child's play! This is another fascinating aspect of child development.

J. A. Stockman III, MD

References

1. Plato. The Republic. B. Jowett, Transl. New York, NY: Collier; 1901.
2. Hassin R, Trope Y. Facial appearance and competence. *J Pers Soc Psychol.* 2000;7: 201.
3. Ramsey JL, Langlois JH, Hoss RA, et al. Facial stereotypes developed during infancy. *Dev Sci.* 2004;7:201.
4. Antonakis J, Dalgas O. Predicting elections: child s play! *Science.* 2009;323:1183.

5 Dentistry and Otolaryngology (ENT)

Neonatal repair of cleft lip: a decision-making protocol
Galinier P, Salazard B, Deberail A, et al (Children's Hosp, France; Timone Hosp, France)
J Pediatr Surg 43:662-667, 2008

Purpose.—Treatment of cleft lip during the neonatal period remains a controversial subject. Those who are in favor of delayed closure argue a higher-risk general anesthesia when it was performed in neonatal period. The purpose of this study was to evaluate the complications and the feasibility of this surgery during the neonatal period.

Methods.—This was a retrospective study of 61 children with labial, labioalveolar, labio-alveolo-palatine, and labiopalatine clefts between May 2000 and November 2006. Each patient's medical file and particularly his or her anesthesia file was used to record the principal demographic data, the results of the malformation workup, and preoperative complications.

Results.—Sixty-one newborns, 20 girls and 41 boys, aged 7.5 ± 6.7 days were operated on. The mean weight on the day of surgery was 3190 ± 454 g. Fifty-four children had a malformation workup (abdominal ultrasonography, spinal bone workup, transfontanelle ultrasonography, and cardiac ultrasonography). Thirteen associated malformations (21%) were thereby detected. There were no surgical complications. The anesthesiologists did not have any real intubation problems. In 4 cases, however, intubation was only possible after several laryngoscopies and changing the type of intubation shaft. There were no major complications. However, one child did present a preoperative complication. It was an episode of desaturation with bradycardia that was quickly resolved without further consequences in a child with a ventricular septal defect and an auricular septal defect.

Conclusions.—We think that neonatal lip closure should continue to be performed. It is essential for the psychological status of the parents. We have not found any studies in the literature that reported an anesthesia risk that was greater in the neonatal period than at 3 months in patients without risk of complications.

▶ Clefting disorders have been with us since time immemorial. Archeological data and ancient historical records document the presence of cleft lip and palate and even attempts to surgically repair the cleft lip.[1] Current estimates suggest that as many as 6500 babies are born each year in the United States with orofacial clefts, including cleft palate and cleft lip with and without cleft palate. The prevalence of orofacial clefts (cleft lip and palate and cleft lip alone) has been estimated to run about 17 per 10 000 live births. Orofacial clefts are sometimes diagnosed in utero on ultrasound, although often they are not discovered until delivery. Small cleft of the lips or palate may be missed on fetal ultrasound. Clefting may occur of the lip only (unilateral or bilateral), the lip and alveolus, the lip and palate, or the palate only. More extensive facial clefting such as that sometimes seen in the frontonasal dysplasia sequence syndrome is unusual. When a diagnosis of cleft palate is made prenatally, obstetricians usually ask for a pediatrician or a neonatologist to be present at the time of delivery in case there are any unexpected respiratory difficulties or other congenital anomalies. Cleft lip and/or palate may occur in association with genetic disorders such as Velo-Cardio-Facial syndrome or Stickler's syndrome. About 1 in 5 infants identified with a cleft lip and palate will have associated malformations. Alcohol use and/or cigarette smoking during pregnancy may increase the risk of clefting, although the data on this are somewhat shaky. Almost one-half of patients with clefts present with cleft lip and palate followed by isolated cleft palate (32%) and isolated cleft lip (21%). Clefts of the palate alone are more common in females, while clefts of the lip with or without palate clefts are more common in boys. For whatever reason, left-sided unilateral cleft lips are more common than bilateral cleft lips and right-sided unilateral cleft lips are the least common. Of every 10 clefts, 6 are left sided, 3 are right sided, and 1 is bilateral. There are approximately 300 to 400 syndromes, excluding chromosomal disorders, that are associated with cleft lip and palate. In addition to those listed, other more common syndromes associated with cleft lip, with or without cleft palate, include Treacher Collins syndrome, Opitz syndrome, oral-facial-digital syndrome, Wolf-Hirschhorn syndrome, CHARGE syndrome, popliteal pterygium syndrome, Kabuki syndrome, and oculoauriculovertebral dysplasia syndrome.

The surgical treatment of cleft lip and palate deformities represents unique challenges. The surgical plan of care is obviously tailored to the specific defect involved. In most cases, the repair of the cleft lip is performed at approximately 3 months of age and the repair of the palate occurs at approximately 9 months of age. In many cases, this is just the beginning of operative procedures, as the repair may need further cosmetic refinement as the child grows. Surgery for the cleft lip corrects unilateral or bilateral incomplete or partial cleft lip, as well as correcting the associated nasal deformity and creates an aesthetically natural appearance to the patient's face. The technique most popular today for repair of the unilateral cleft lip relies on a combination of rotation and advancement flaps to achieve these goals.

While repair of a cleft lip is usually delayed until an infant is 10 weeks old and weighs approximately 10 pounds, as we see in this report from France, some pediatric plastic surgeons believe that a satisfactory repair should be undertaken, unless otherwise contraindicated, very shortly after birth. Those in favor of delayed repair suggest that better aesthetic results are obtained, better psychological acceptance of the malformation occurs on the part of the family, and the risk of general anesthesia is less later on than during the neonatal period. What we see in this report from France, however, is that there seems to be no difference in aesthetic outcomes when comparing immediate versus delayed repair. The risk of anesthesia properly administered by trained individuals appears to be small at any age. The authors argue that the issue of a better psychological acceptance of the malformation by families when the repair is delayed seems quite arguable and that many parents suffer through the first few months of life wondering if their child will ever be normal as opposed to an immediate repair where the beneficial outcome is quite obvious early on.

There is no question that pediatricians will rely on a referral center and its surgical expertise to decide when the best time is for a repair of a cleft lip. No one argues that a cleft palate should be delayed in its repair. If you want to read more about the total care of an infant with cleft lip and palate, see the excellent detailed summary of this, including the important role of the primary care provider, in a review of the topic by Kasten et al.[2]

As this commentary closes, here's another *Clinical Fact/Curio*, this having to do with dentistry. One of the truly great moments in medical history occurred on a tense fall morning in the surgical amphitheater of Boston's Massachusetts General Hospital. It was there, on October 16, 1846, that a dentist named William T. G. Morton administered an effective anesthetic to a surgical patient. Consenting to what became a most magnificent scientific revolution were John Warren, an apprehensive surgeon, and Glen Abbott, an even more nervous young man about to undergo removal of a vascular tumor on the left side of his neck. Both Warren and Abbott sailed through the procedure painlessly, although some have noted that Abbott moved a bit near the end of the procedure. Turning from the operating table toward the gallery packed with legitimately dumbstruck medical students, Warren gleefully exclaimed, "Gentlemen, this is no humbug!"[3]

Morton began his dental studies in Baltimore in 1840. Two years later he set up practice in Hartford, Connecticut, ultimately working with a dentist named Horace Wells. At this time, surgeons could offer patients little beyond opium and alcohol to endure the agonizing pain engendered by scalpels. From the late 18th century well into the 1840s, physicians and chemists experimented with agents such as nitrous oxide, ether, carbon dioxide, and other mind-altering chemicals without much success. It actually turned out to be that dentists were the individuals most in need of a good anesthetic, given the excruciating pain associated with dental extractions. Morton and Wells conducted the numerous experiments using nitrous oxide, including a demonstration at Harvard Medical School in 1845 that failed to completely squelch the pain of a student submitting to a tooth-pulling, thus publicly humiliating both dentists. This did not deter Morton, who attended the lectures of Harvard chemistry professor, Charles Jackson, including a lecture on the common organic solvent sulfuric ether. Morton purchased bottles of the stuff from his local chemist and began exposing himself and a menagerie of pets to ether fumes. Satisfied with both the safety and reliability of ether, he began using ether on dental patients. Soon, mobs of toothaching, dollar-waving Bostonians beat a pathway to his office door, garnering enormous financial success on Morton.

William Morton named his ether "creation" letheon, after the Lethe River of Greek mythology. Drinking its waters, the ancients contended, erased painful memories. Where Morton got into trouble in the medical community was his application for an exclusive patent on letheon. In the United States of the mid-19th century, it was considered unseemly, if not greedy, for members of the medical profession to profit from discoveries that universally benefited mankind, particularly from a patent for what turned out to be easily acquired sulfuric ether. When he crossed the line from practicing dentistry to "medicine," the medical community came down on him quickly and very hard. Vigorously combatting the whispered and shouted campaigns against him, the dentist spent his remaining days trying to restore his sullied reputation. Morton died broke and embittered in 1868.[4]

J. A. Stockman III, MD

References

1. Kirschner RE, LaRossa D. Cleft lip and palate. *Otolaryngol Clin North Am.* 2000; 33:1191-1215.
2. Kasten EF, Schmidt SP, Zickler CF, et al. Team care of the patient with cleft lip and palate. *Curr Probl Pediatr Adolesc Healthcare.* 2008;38:138-158.
3. Fulop-Miller R. Triumph over pain. In: Paul E. Paul C, eds. *Transactions.* New York, NY: Literary Guild of America; 1938.
4. Markel H: Not so great moments. The "discovery"of ether anesthesia and its "rediscovery" by Hollywood. *JAMA.* 2008;300:2188-2190.

Sudden oronasal bleeding in a young child

Hey E (Northern Neonatal Network, UK)
Acta Paediatr 97:1327-1330, 2008

Sudden severe upper-airway obstruction occurring in a hospital setting can sometimes precipitate an episode of acute haemorrhagic pulmonary oedema. A review of 197 published case reports shows that the presenting feature is almost always the sudden appearance of blood stained fluid coming up through the larynx or out through the mouth and nose of an adult or child in obvious respiratory distress. Such overt features are seen in 10-15% of cases of sudden severe, but sub-lethal, upper-airway obstruction. Signs normally appear within minutes once the obstruction is relieved but are occasionally only recognized after 1-4 h. All signs and symptoms usually resolve within 12-24 h. Other causes of acute pulmonary haemorrhage are rare in young children.

Conclusion.—If what looks like blood is seen in, or coming from, the mouth or nose of a previously healthy young child who has suddenly become distressed and started to struggle for breath, that child has most probably suffered an episode of acute pulmonary oedema, and the commonest precipitating cause is sudden upper-airway obstruction.

▶ Whereas nosebleeds in older children are relatively common, simple nosebleeds are rare in the first year of life. Nosebleeds that cannot be explained as due to accidental trauma and are not the first manifestation of some overt hemostatic disorder are even rarer. If what looks like blood is seen in, or coming from, the nose or mouth of a young child who has become pale, restless, and distressed, and suddenly starts to struggle for breath, that child almost certainly has experienced an episode of acute hemorrhagic pulmonary edema, based on data from the literature. In the older child, epistaxis usually occurs from the anterior portion of the nasal septum (Little's area), which has a rich blood supply. Such nosebleeds are common, frequently resulting from nose picking and a dry atmosphere. When a young baby, however, bleeds from the nose, or is reported to have had a nosebleed, the event raises the strong possibility in the minds of some experts that the child may have experienced abuse in the form of attempted suffocation. Hey suggests that if there is no suggestion that the child has been living in a damp, fungus-infected house, and all the signs and symptoms, including hypoxemia, resolve within hours rather than days, then the presumption should be that the child has experienced an acute episode of sudden upper airway obstruction, be that accidental or intentional. There is strong indirect evidence that unwitnessed smothering, both accidental and intentional, can elicit a similar response in infancy to what is well known in adults, that being that upper airway obstruction can cause hemorrhagic pulmonary edema, presenting either as blood in the mouth or blood emanating from the nose.

The next time you see an infant with a nosebleed, think of the potential possibility of accidental or nonaccidental upper airway obstruction. A careful social history should be in order.

This commentary closes with a *Clinical Fact/Curio* having to do in general with the nose. You may not have noticed, but not infrequently, you will see coffee beans placed on perfume counters. Retailers seem to have recognized that a whiff of a coffee bean somehow clears the nostrils of odors and allows one to distinguish between different fragrances. Aware too of the tendency to lose their appetites after cooking, scientists are now proposing that coffee might be useful in refreshing the olfactory receptors after a stint in the kitchen. It has now been reported that sniffing coffee beans after cooking does in fact improve the appetites of the cook. One theory is that of the 28 different odorants in coffee, one or more may be sufficiently intense to detach food odorants from their receptors, thus restimulating one's appetite.[1]

One wonders if some of the more corpulent TV chefs were onto this theory long before scientists were. While on the topic of coffee, the caffeine hit is experienced by most coffee drinkers, but it seems that caffeine may offer more than just a transient psychostimulant effect. Evidence from a sample of adults in the community aged at least 65 shows that caffeine intake seems to reduce cognitive decline in women who do not have dementia, especially so in older women.[2] No effect on the incidence of dementia was seen, but drinking more than three cups of coffee a day may yet prove useful for prolonging the period of mild cognitive impairment in women before a formal diagnosis of dementia.

One final fast fact: do you know the technical term for nose-picking? It is "rhinotillexis."

J. A. Stockman III, MD

References

1. Coffee as a means to restimulate appetite [editorial comment]. *BMJ.* 2007;335: 456.
2. Ritchie K, Carrière I, de Mendonca A, et al. The neuroprotective effects of caffeine: a prospective population study (the Three City Study). *Neurology.* 2007;69:536-545.

Tooth Extraction Socket Healing in Pediatric Patients Treated with Intravenous Pamidronate

Chahine C, Cheung MS, Head TW, et al (Shriners Hosp for Children; McGill Univ, Montréal, Québec, Canada)
J Pediatr 153:719-720, 2008

Osteonecrosis of the jaw (ONJ) has been described as a complication of bisphosphonate therapy in adults. In the present study, we did not find a case of ONJ among 278 pediatric patients who had received intravenous pamidronate during childhood or adolescence.

▶ This tidy little article provides important information for pediatric practitioners of medicine as well as for general dentists and pediatric dentists. All of us know about the problem of osteonecrosis of the jaw as a complication of the use of pamidronate, which is used to strengthen bone. In adults it helps manage those with poor bone mineralization. In children, its intravenous use is employed to strengthen the bones of children and adolescents with skeletal fragility, particularly those with osteogenesis imperfecta. Pamidronate, of course, is best known as "bisphosphonate therapy" and there are a number of reports of osteonecrosis of the jaw associated with bisphosphonate use. This is clinically visible as exposed bone in the maxillofacial area. Currently the diagnosis of osteonecrosis of the jaw is made when there is no evidence of healing after 2 months of appropriate dental care and in the absence of any other cause such as metastatic disease or radiation of the jaw.

The report of Chahine et al is important because many dentists will not be desirous of extracting teeth in someone who has been treated with a bisphosphonate largely based on the concern that osteonecrosis of the jaw and poor healing of an extraction site might occur. Dental extraction during bisphosphonate therapy does increase the risk of osteonecrosis of the jaw in adults by some

8-fold to 10-fold. What we learn from the report of Chahine et al, however, is that among 338 patients of pediatric age treated at one institution in Montreal, not a single case of osteonecrosis of the jaw was observed. Healing of the tooth socket was not different in those treated with bisphosphonates in comparison with otherwise healthy children. The singular message is that osteonecrosis of the jaw in the pediatric age group must be an exceedingly rare problem and that dental extraction should not be withheld because of previous treatment with agents such as pamidronate.

J. A. Stockman III, MD

Dexamethasone and Risk of Nausea and Vomiting and Postoperative Bleeding After Tonsillectomy in Children: A Randomized Trial

Czarnetzki C, Elia N, Lysakowski C et al, (Univ Hosps of Geneva, Switzerland)
JAMA 300:2621-2630, 2008

Context.—Dexamethasone is widely used to prevent postoperative nausea and vomiting (PONV) in pediatric tonsillectomy.

Objective.—To assess whether dexamethasone dose-dependently reduces the risk of PONV at 24 hours after tonsillectomy.

Design, Setting, and Patients.—Randomized placebo-controlled trial conducted among 215 children undergoing elective tonsillectomy at a major public teaching hospital in Switzerland from February 2005 to December 2007.

Interventions.—Children were randomly assigned to receive dexamethasone (0.05, 0.15, or 0.5 mg/kg) or placebo intravenously after induction of anesthesia. Acetaminophen-codeine and ibuprofen were given as postoperative analgesia. Follow-up continued until the 10th postoperative day.

Main Outcome Measures.—The primary end point was prevention of PONV at 24 hours; secondary end points were decrease in the need for ibuprofen at 24 hours and evaluation of adverse effects.

Results.—At 24 hours, 24 of 54 participants who received placebo (44%; 95% confidence interval [CI], 31%-59%) had experienced PONV compared with 20 of 53 (38%; 95% CI, 25%-52%), 13 of 54 (24%; 95% CI, 13%-38%), and 6 of 52 (12%; 95% CI, 4%-23%) who received dexamethasone at 0.05, 0.15, and 0.5 mg/kg, respectively ($P<.001$ for linear trend). Children who received dexamethasone received significantly less ibuprofen. There were 26 postoperative bleeding episodes in 22 children. Two of 53 (4%; 95% CI, 0.5%-13%) children who received placebo had bleeding compared with 6 of 53 (11%; 95% CI, 4%-23%), 2 of 51 (4%; 95% CI, 0.5%-13%), and 12 of 50 (24%; 95% CI, 13%-38%) who received dexamethasone at 0.05, 0.15, and 0.5 mg/kg, respectively ($P=.003$). Dexamethasone, 0.5 mg/kg, was associated with the highest bleeding risk (adjusted relative risk, 6.80; 95% CI, 1.77-16.5). Eight children had to undergo emergency reoperation because of bleeding, all of whom had received dexamethasone. The trial was stopped early for safety reasons.

Conclusion.—In this study of children undergoing tonsillectomy, dexamethasone decreased the risk of PONV dose dependently but was associated with an increased risk of postoperative bleeding.

Trial Registration.—clinicaltrials.gov Identifier: NCT00403806.

▶ Nausea, vomiting, and bleeding tend to be among the most common complications of tonsillectomy in children. Tonsillectomy remains one of the most frequently performed surgical procedures in youngsters. It has been estimated that almost 200 000 tonsillectomies are performed each year in the United States. Prophylactic dexamethasone has become a standard of care in many countries for children undergoing tonsillectomy. The rationale is to decrease the amount of emesis. It is also believed that dexamethasone has some analgesic effects. The trial reported from Geneva showed that dexamethasone significantly and dose-dependently decreases the incidence of postoperative nausea and vomiting in children undergoing tonsillectomy. Dexamethasone also decreases the need for rescue analgesia with ibuprofen. However, dexamethasone is associated with a significant increase in the risk of postoperative bleeding.

The association described between dexamethasone and an increased risk of bleeding in those who have undergone tonsillectomy is an unexpected finding in this study. Chance alone is unlikely to explain the finding given the solid nature of the statistics associated with the study. The magnitude of the association is extremely strong. Also, the effects seem to be dose dependent with the highest dose of dexamethasone having the greatest risk of bleeding (approximately 4 times higher than the risk associated without dexamethasone use).

Exactly why the risk of bleeding would be increased with dexamethasone given postoperatively remains unexplained although the most convincing biological explanation might be related to inhibition of surgical wound repair processes by glucocorticosteroids and to delayed ulcer healing. The repair of a tonsillectomy lesion is a complex repair process that could be inhibited by dexamethasone. This would explain why the bleeding observed in this report sometimes occurred several days following the surgical procedure. Tonsillectomy is not comparable with most other surgical interventions because the wound created by the excision of the tonsils is neither sutured nor covered by sealant or hemostatic material. It remains a large wound surface, which is covered by crusting and is exposed to food, air, and saliva.

Post-tonsillectomy hemorrhage is a potentially lethal complication because the upper airways are unprotected and manual compression is nearly impossible. If hemorrhage does not stop spontaneously, reintervention is unavoidable. Unfortunately, blood loss becomes evident in many only when the child is hemodynamically unstable or vomits swallowed blood.

Yes, dexamethasone does have a significant and dose-dependent antiemetic effect and a solid analgesic effect. However, it can, as we see in this report, increase the risk of postoperative bleeding. How important this added risk is will need to be determined in future studies.

J. A. Stockman III, MD

Respiratory Viruses in Laryngeal Croup of Young Children

Rihkanen H, Rönkkö E, Nieminen T, et al (Hosp for Children and Adolescents, Helsinki, Finland; Natl Public Health Inst, Helsinki, Finland; et al)

J Pediatr 152:661-665, 2008

Objectives.—To determine the viral cause of laryngeal croup by use of highly sensitive methods, and including recently recognized viruses in the analysis.

Study Design.—One hundred forty-four consecutive children with hoarse voice and inspiratory stridor attending the emergency department were enrolled. Age- and season-matched children presenting with a wheezing illness served as control subjects (n = 76). Nasopharyngeal swabs were analyzed by polymerase chain reaction for rhinovirus and enterovirus, coronavirus, respiratory syncytial virus (RSV), parainfluenza virus (PIV), influenza A and B virus, human bocavirus, human metapneumovirus, adenovirus, and *Mycoplasma pneumoniae*.

Results.—Virus infection was documented in 80% of patients with croup and 71% of control subjects. Children with croup had significantly more positive test results for PIV 1 and 2 (31% vs 4% and 6% vs 0%, respectively) and significantly fewer positive test results for RSV (15% vs 28%) than wheezing children. Rhinoviruses and enteroviruses were present equally in both groups (21% vs 25%). There was no significant difference in the frequency of influenza A virus or human bocavirus. Few subjects with adenovirus or *M. pneumoniae* were detected.

Conclusion.—Acute laryngeal croup is most often associated with PIV, RSV, rhinovirus, and enterovirus. Rhinovirus and enterovirus appeared equally often in croup and in wheezing illness. During late fall, they were found in 39% and 40%, respectively, of the tested samples (Table 3).

▶ I am not sure that there is truly any new information provided by this report, but it is always good to hear updates on the causes of common pediatric problems, in this case that being croup. It is also nice to see a systematic study using modern microbiologic tools. In this report, 80% of children presenting with croup had a common respiratory virus genome in their nasopharynx as determined by polymerase chain reaction (PCR) assay. The figure of 80% is higher than previous studies, likely because of the sensitivity of the PCR assay. Dr Floyd Denny, a pioneer in pediatric infectious diseases, reported more than 25 years ago that only about one-third of children presenting with croup could be found to be virus-positive when using typical viral culture techniques available at that time.[1] In this contemporary study, parainfluenza virus types 1 to 3 were detected in just over 40% of children with croup. This is consistent with earlier reports. Rhinoviruses and enteroviruses were the second most viruses identified in children with croup and bronchitis. This latter finding is similar to that found in bronchiolitis, which is most often caused by respiratory syncytial virus (RSV) infections.

See the table for the common viruses causing croup and viral associated reactive airway disease with wheezing. With current molecular techniques

TABLE 3.—Virus Findings Among Children With Laryngeal Croup and Acute Wheezing Illness During the 1-Year Study

	Croup n = 144		Wheezing n = 76	
Parainfluenza virus 1*	44	30.6%	3	3.9%
Parainfluenza virus 2†	7	4.9%	0	0.0%
Parainfluenza virus 3	9	6.3%	1	1.3%
Respiratory syncytial virus‡	21	14.6%	21	27.6%
Human bocavirus	18	12.5%	8	10.5%
Rhinovirus	17	11.8%	9	11.8%
Enterovirus	13	9.0%	10	13.2%
Influenza A	13	9.0%	10	13.2%
Coronavirus	3	2.1%	1	1,3%
Adenovirus	2	1.4%	0	0.0%
M.pneumoniae	1	0.7%	1	1.3%
Human metapneumovirus	0	0.0%	2	2.6%
Influenza B	0	0.0%	0	0.0%
No. of detected viruses§	148		66	
Virus positive	115	79.9%	54	71.1%
Virus negative	29	20.1%	22	28.9%

*$P < .001$ between croup and wheezy bronchitis (χ^2 test).
†$P < .05$ between croup and wheezy bronchitis (χ^2 test).
‡$P < .01$ between croup and wheezy bronchitis (χ^2 test).
§Some samples harbored more than 1 virus type.
(Reprinted from Rihkanen H, Rönkkö E, Nieminen T, et al. Respiratory viruses in laryngeal croup of young children. J Pediatr. 2008;152:661-665, with permission from Elsevier.)

available these days, we should be able to find the cause of these respiratory illnesses, if we need to, in the significant majority of cases.

J. A. Stockman III, MD

Reference

1. Denny FW, Murphy TF, Clyde WA Jr, Collier AM, Henderson FW. Croup: an 11-year study in pediatric practice. *Pediatrics*. 1983;71:871-876.

Pathogens Causing Recurrent and Difficult-to-Treat Acute Otitis Media, 2003-2006

Pichichero ME, Casey JR, Hoberman A, et al (Univ of Rochester Med Ctr and Legacy Pediatrics, NY; Children's Hosp of Pittsburgh, PA; et al)
Clin Pediatr 47:901-906, 2008

This study sought to determine the microbiology of recurrent acute otitis media (AOM) and AOM treatment failure (AOMTF) in the context of widespread use of heptavalent pneumococcal conjugate vaccine (PCV7). In this retrospective cohort study, 244 AOM isolates obtained by tympanocentesis during 3 respiratory seasons—2003-2004 (n = 126), 2004-2005 (n = 52), 2005-2006 (n = 66)—from three geographically diverse pediatric populations were compared. Most isolates were from children less than 2 years old, who had received PCV7. For the 3 seasons the proportion of *Streptococcus pneumoniae* isolates was 35%, 35%, and 46% and for *Haemophilus influenzae* was 55%, 58%, and 39%,

TABLE 2.—Distribution of AOM Pathogens Isolated from Middle Ear Fluid of Children With AOM According to Time Period and Site

Isolate	2003-2004				2004-2005				2005-2006				2003-2006			
	NY	PA	VA	Total	NY	PA	VA	Total	NY	PA	VA	Total	NY	PA	VA	Total
S. pneumoniae[a]	26	13	5	44 (35%)	12	1	5	18 (35%)	18	6	6	30 (46%)	56	20	16	92 (38%)
PSSP	14	9	5	28 (64%)	6	0	5	11 (54%)	5	4	6	15 (50%)	25	13	11	49 (56%)
PISP	4	2	0	6 (14%)	2	0	0	2 (11%)	5	2	0	7 (23%)	11	4	0	15 (17%)
PRSP	8	2	0	10 (23%)	4	1	0	5 (28%)	8	0	0	8 (27%)	20	3	0	23 (26%)
H. influenzae[b]	44	18	7	69 (55%)	28	1	1	30 (58%)	22	3	1	26 (39%)	94	22	9	125 (51%)
β-Lactamase +	26	7	0	33 (48%)	19	1	0	20 (67%)	12	0	1	13 (50%)	57	8	1	66 (53%)
β-Lactamase –	18	11	7	36 (52%)	9	0	1	10 (33%)	10	3	0	13 (50%)	37	14	8	59 (47%)
M. catarrhalis	3	0	5	8 (6%)	1	1	2	4 (3%)	3	0	5	8 (12%)	7	1	12	20 (8%)
2 pathogens	3	2		5 (4%)					1	1		2 (3%)	4	3		7 (3%)
Total[c]	76	33	17	126	41	3	8	52	44	10	12	66	161	46	37	244

Note: AOM = acute otitis media; NY = Rochester, New York; PA = Pittsburgh, Pennsylvania; VA = Vienna, Virginia; PSSP = penicillin susceptible S. pneumoniae; PISP = penicillin intermediately resistant S. pneumoniae; PRSP = penicillin resistant S. pneumoniae.

[a] Significant difference between sites in 2005-2006 in isolation of PSSP organisms; NY versus VA, P = .006.

[b] Significant difference among sites in 2003-2004 in isolation of β-lactamase + H. influenzae, NY versus VA, P = .01.

[c] The proportion of isolates that were S. pneumoniae versus the proportion that were H. influenzae for the 2003-2005 respiratory seasons pooled versus the proportions in 2005-2006 when compared P = .07; for the change in trend for the proportions across all 3 respiratory seasons, P = .09.

(Reprinted from Pichichero ME, Casey JR, Hoberman A, et al. Pathogens causing recurrent and difficult-to-treat acute otitis media, 2003-2006. Clin Pediatr. 2008;47:901-906.)

respectively (change in trend, $P = .09$). A total of 37%, 39%, and 50% of *S. pneumoniae* were penicillin nonsusceptible (PNSP) and 48%, 67%, and 50% of *H. influenzae* produced β-lactamase, respectively. Although *H. influenzae* remains the most frequently isolated pathogen in children with AOMTF or recurrent AOM, *S. pneumoniae* that are PNSP are reemerging as important organisms.

▶ This report reminds us that the more things change, the more they change when it comes to the etiology of difficult-to-treat acute otitis media (AOM). With the introduction of the conjugated heptavalent pneumococcal conjugate vaccine (PCV7), there has been a shift in the frequency of the pathogens causing AOM. Unlike when the pneumococcus was the predominant cause of AOM, the predominant pathogen now is beta-lactamase-producing *Haemophilus influenzae*, which accounts for almost 60% of cases of AOM in which the organism is identified on tympanocentesis. What we have also seen is that since the introduction of the PCV7, there has been an increase in invasive pneumococcal disease caused by *Streptococcus pneumoniae* with capsular types not covered in PCV7.

In this study, Pichichero et al report the distribution of otopathogens obtained from children undergoing tympanocentesis for recurrent AOM or AOM treatment failures. The table shows the distribution of AOM pathogens (Table 2). The data from this report provide useful information in guiding antibiotic selection in children with recurrent AOM or those who are failing current management of AOM. It would appear that such infections will be caused by *S pneumoniae* in about 50% of cases, and 50% of these strains will be penicillin nonsusceptible. About 50% of such infections will be caused by *H influenzae*, and 50% of these strains will be beta-lactamase producing. High-dose amoxicillin/clavulanate, or alternatively, cefuroxime, cefpodoxime, cefdinir, and ceftriaxone are the drugs of choice as recommended by the American Academy of Pediatrics for children with recent AOM or AOM refractory to initial therapy. For what it is worth, these are the same antibiotics endorsed for the management of pediatric otitis media.

Although the information from this report does not provide profoundly new insights into the treatment of AOM, given the fact that this field is emerging rapidly as the result of changes in the natural history of infection and influences of current vaccines, we all need to be updated on a regular basis.

J. A. Stockman III, MD

Overuse of tympanostomy tubes in New York metropolitan area: evidence from five hospital cohort
Keyhani S, Kleinman LC, Rothschild M, et al (Mount Sinai School of Med, NY; et al)
BMJ 337:a1607, 2008

Objectives.—To compare tympanostomy tube insertion for children with otitis media in 2002 with the recommendations of two sets of expert guidelines.
Design.—Retrospective cohort study.

Setting.—New York metropolitan area practices associated with five diverse hospitals.

Participants.—682 of 1046 children who received tympanostomy tubes in the five hospitals for whom charts from the hospital, primary care physician, and otolaryngologist could be accessed.

Results.—The mean age was 3.8 years. On average, children with acute otitis media had fewer than four infections in the year before surgery. Children with otitis media with effusion had less than 30 consecutive days of effusion at the time of surgery. Concordance with recommendations was very low: 30.3% (n = 207) of all tympanostomies were concordant with the explicit criteria developed for this study and 7.5% (n = 13) with the 1994 guideline from the American Academy of Pediatrics, American Academy of Family Medicine, and American Academy of Otolaryngology–Head and Neck Surgery. Children who had previously had tympanostomy tube surgery, who were having a concomitant procedure, or who had "at risk conditions" were more likely to be discordant.

Conclusions.—A significant majority of tympanostomy tube insertions in the largest and most populous metropolitan area in the United States were inappropriate according to the explicit criteria and not recommended according to both guidelines. Regardless of whether current practice represents a substantial overuse of surgery or the guidelines are overly restrictive, the persistent discrepancy between guidelines and practice cannot be good for children or for people interested in improving their health care.

▶ If you consider circumcision a surgical procedure, then the second most common operation performed in the world after circumcision is the placement of tympanostomy tubes for the management of otitis media with effusion. The report of Keyhani et al examines the clinical characteristics of children with otitis media in New York who had ventilation tubes placed and compared the clinical indications for these with the recommendations of 2 sets of expert guidelines and a set of RAND appropriateness criteria.[1] The findings of the report showed that only 30% of tympanostomies were performed in accordance with current recommendations for tube placement.

It is easy to see why there is a continuing overuse of tympanostomy tubes as part of the management of otitis media with effusion. It was pointed out more than 20 years ago that placement of ventilation tubes for otitis media with effusion possesses most of the drivers of over intervention—a complex presentation; low-risk; not overly costly; and definite and immediate, albeit very short-lived, subjective improvement leading to parent satisfaction.[2] In the intervening quarter of a century since these characteristics were articulated, it has been documented that the natural history of otitis media with effusion hardly requires intervention with a surgical procedure, nor does the surgical procedure significantly improve language and other development in the young growing child.

Hopefully in the not widely distant future, we will see another report that re-examines the frequency with which tympanostomy tubes are placed, a study that documents an improvement from the current situation. The tide against this surgical procedure has long since turned in other countries that have national systems of health care. Great Britain is one such example. We should learn from these experiences.

J. A. Stockman III, MD

References

1. Boston M, McCook J, Burke B, Derkay C. Incidence of and risk factors for additional tympanostomy tube insertion in children. *Arch Otolaryngol Head Neck Surg.* 2003;129:293-296.
2. Black N. Surgery for glu ear - a modern epidemic. *Lancet.* 1984;1:835-837.

Lateral Sinus Thrombosis as a Complication of Otitis Media: 10-Year Experience at the Children's Hospital of Philadelphia

Bales CB, Sobol S, Wetmore R, et al (Children's Hosp of Philadelphia, PA; Emory Univ Hosp, Atlanta, GA)
Pediatrics 123:709-713, 2009

Objectives.—Lateral sinus thrombosis is a rare intracranial complication of otitis media that is traditionally described in countries with poor access to medical care. Our goal was to describe the clinical presentation, management, and outcome of patients diagnosed with lateral sinus thrombosis in a US tertiary care center and to highlight the clinically relevant differences in presentation between these patients and those described in previous reports.

Patients and Methods.—The medical charts of 13 patients diagnosed with otogenic lateral sinus thrombosis were reviewed. These patients were identified from a manual search of 156 subjects with *International Classification of Diseases, Ninth Revision* codes corresponding with a diagnosis of mastoiditis or thromboembolism over a 10-year period (1997–2007) at the Children's Hospital of Philadelphia.

Results.—In contrast to previous reports in the literature, the majority of patients in this series exhibited cranial neuropathies and signs of raised intracranial pressure. Nearly all of the patients had a history of acute otitis media treated with antibiotics in the weeks preceding admission. However, many patients denied high fevers or active otomastoid symptoms, which are classically associated with lateral sinus thrombosis. The diagnosis was made in all of the children by using computed tomography and MRI/venography. Treatment strategies included myringotomy tube placement, simple mastoidectomy, intravenous antibiotics, and anticoagulation. Posthospitalization follow-up data revealed no significant long-term complications.

Conclusions.—Despite appropriate antibiotic therapy, lateral sinus thrombosis and other intracranial complications of otitis media are still a threat to children in the modern era. Neurologic, rather than otologic, symptoms may dominate the presentation of otogenic lateral sinus thrombosis. Thus, a high index of suspicion may be critical for ensuring timely diagnosis of this rare condition.

▶ Many of us do not recall the intimate anatomical components related to the middle ear and mastoid area, including the fact that this area can be the site of a lateral sinus thrombosis, a rare but particularly problematic complication, at times, of otitis media and mastoiditis. These thrombi originate in the sigmoid sinus just inside the mastoid region. A thrombus can form when the sinus wall becomes inflamed as a result of middle ear infection spreading to the mastoid bone. The major concern with a lateral sinus thrombosis is that it can spread to other venous sinuses and also to the internal jugular vein, resulting in obstruction of cerebrospinal fluid drainage leading to elevations in intracranial pressure and a resultant hydrocephalus. Emboli can break off from these thrombi; many of which are infected.

The report abstracted from the Children's Hospital of Philadelphia is an extremely important one because it gives us information about lateral sinus thrombosis occurring in children in the United States. With most cases of this problem occurring outside the United States, it is unusual to see a report on this topic originating within our borders. Between 1997 and 2007, 10 boys and 3 girls with lateral sinus thrombosis presented to the Children's Hospital of Philadelphia, allowing us to see what the risk factors are for this disorder and the course of the illness. What is a bit unusual about these patients is that they all came from families that have health insurance and were being adequately managed otherwise by their primary care providers, all pediatricians.

The 13 children (ages 2-16 years) in this series did have a typical presentation with headache (11 of 13). Current ear complaints, however, were infrequent. The patients in the sample, however, did relay a history of acute otitis media in the weeks preceding admission, but by the time they presented with lateral sinus thrombosis, their ear complaints had pretty much resolved. The majority of patients had sixth or seventh cranial nerve neuropathies, accompanied by signs and symptoms of raised intracranial pressure, including headache, nausea, and vomiting, photophobia, nuchal rigidity, and/or ataxia.

If there is one message to be taken away from what we learn from this series of patients, it is that when a child presents with a certain set of neurologic complaints, including diplopia and a sixth- or seventh-nerve palsy, we should be suspicious of a lateral sinus thrombosis related to previous ear infection even if there are no symptoms of the latter present. A careful ear exam, however, should still show evidence of abnormal tympanic membrane findings.

You may want to read this report in greater detail. It talks about the evaluation for lateral sinus thrombosis using a CT scan or MRI scan. It also talks about the value of collecting fluid for culture from the middle ear cavity. In most instances the fluid will be found to be sterile, given the fact that the majority of children presenting with lateral sinus thrombosis have been previously treated with antibiotics for their episode of acute otitis media. Treatment in this series consisted of culture to direct antibiotic therapy, myringotomy with tube placement, and mastoidectomy. There are few data available to tell us about the value of anticoagulation, but the authors of this report suggest the literature does support anticoagulation in select patients who have higher theoretical risk for infarction, embolization, or persistent septic thrombus. In particular, the authors suggest consideration of anticoagulation in patients in whom the thrombus extends beyond the sigmoid sinus, and when there are neurologic changes or with embolic events.

Chances are you will not see many cases of lateral sinus thrombosis in your practice. Remember, however, the bottom line and that is that if there is a history of acute otitis media followed by neurologic signs a week or 2 later, think lateral sinus thrombosis.

J. A. Stockman III, MD

Etiologic and Audiologic Evaluations After Universal Neonatal Hearing Screening: Analysis of 170 Referred Neonates

Declau F, Boudewyns A, Van den Ende J, et al (Univ Hosp Antwerp, Belgium)
Pediatrics 121:1119-1126, 2008

Objective.—The goal was to clarify the audiologic aspects and causes of congenital hearing loss in children who failed universal neonatal hearing screening.

Methods.—A prospective analysis of 170 consecutive records of neonates referred to a tertiary center after universal neonatal hearing screening failure, between 1998 and 2006, was performed. The data presented here represent the equivalent of ~87 000 screened newborns. The screening results were validated with a clinical ear, nose, and throat examination and electrophysiological testing, including diagnostic auditory brainstem response, automated steady state response, and/or behavioral testing. A diagnostic evaluation protocol for identification of the cause of the hearing loss was also implemented, in collaboration with the departments of genetics and pediatrics.

Results.—Permanent hearing loss was confirmed in 116 children (68.2%). Bilateral hearing loss was diagnosed in 68 infants (58.6%) and unilateral hearing loss in 48 infants (41.4%). Median thresholds for the neonates with confirmed hearing loss were severe in both unilateral and bilateral cases, at 70 dB nHL and 80 dB nHL, respectively. In 55.8% of those cases, no risk factors for hearing loss were found. In 60.4%, the initial automated auditory brainstem response diagnosis was totally in agreement with the audiologic evaluation results. In 8.3% of the cases, however, a unilateral refer result was finally classified as bilateral hearing loss. An etiologic factor could be identified in 55.2% of the cases. Of the causes identified, a genetic mechanism was present in 60.4% of the cases, peripartal problems in 20.8%, and congenital cytomegalovirus infection in 18.8%.

Conclusions.—An etiologic factor could be identified for nearly one half of the children with confirmed congenital hearing loss referred through a universal hearing screening program.

▶ This report clearly documents the value of universal neonatal hearing screen. Although the report comes from Belgium, the data should be equally applicable to the situation here in the United States. The report is the first in the literature that provides data on audiological confirmation and etiologic assessment in a large sample of newborns referred after universal screening for hearing loss

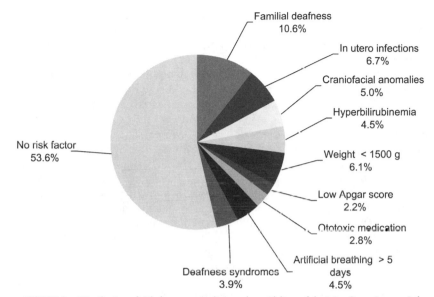

FIGURE 2.—Distribution of risk factors according to the guidelines of the Joint Committee on Infant Hearing 2000 position statement. (Reprinted from Declau F, Boudewyns A, Van den Ende J, et al. Etiologic and audiologic evaluations after universal neonatal hearing screening: analysis of 170 referred neonates. *Pediatrics.* 2008;121:1119-1126. Copyright © 2008 by the American Academy of Pediatrics.)

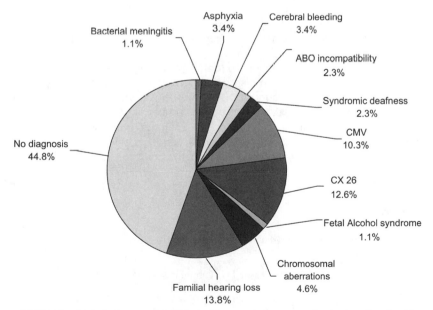

FIGURE 3.—Etiologic diagnoses for children with congenital permanent hearing loss. (Reprinted from Declau F, Boudewyns A, Van den Ende J, et al. Etiologic and audiologic evaluations after universal neonatal hearing screening: analysis of 170 referred neonates. *Pediatrics.* 2008;121:1119-1126. Copyright © 2008 by the American Academy of Pediatrics.)

in the newborn period. The study is equally important because it provides good data on the distribution of risk factors that can be a cause of hearing loss. Etiologic diagnoses were able to be obtained in more than half of children with deafness picked up by newborn hearing screening (Figs 2 and 3).

About the time that this article appeared, another emanated from Belgium that examined sensorineural hearing loss in children with congenital cytomegalovirus (CMV) infection.[1] This particular study was designed to determine whether there was any difference in the likelihood of the development of sensorineural hearing loss in children who were symptomatic at birth with CMV infection versus those who were asymptomatic at birth. Sensorineural hearing loss was found in 21% of the asymptomatic and 33% of symptomatic congenitally infected infants. Late-onset hearing loss was detected in 5%, progression in 11%, fluctuation in 16%, and improved hearing threshold in 18% of the infants with congenital CMV infection. Sensorineural hearing loss was observed in 15% of infants born after a maternal primary infection, in 7% born after a maternal recurrent infection, and in 40% after a maternal infection of indeterminate timing. These data suggest that CMV infection is the leading nongenetic cause of sensorineural hearing loss.

This comment closes with a *Clinical Fact/Curio* in the form of a question about ears. A teen in your practice presents with a blistering eruption on his ear. On physical examination the blistering is the only finding, but you note in the chart that you have observed the same condition in this youngster every year about the same time. The eruption spontaneously resolves without therapy. On careful questioning, you find that for the past several years this youngster has joined his mother, a research scientist, on visits to New Zealand during lambing season, at which time the mother engages in studies of newborn lambs. The youngster helps her mother during these activities. Your diagnosis?

If you live in New Zealand or Australia, your diagnosis would readily be lambing ears. This is a common disorder that affects individuals usually within 2 weeks of the lambing season and occurs in those who are assisting in the lambing process. If a biopsy is done of affected sites, histology will show a heavy dermal perivascular lymphocytic infiltrate with normal overlying epidermis. This unusual occupational disease occurs through close contact with the products of conception and for obvious reasons in terms of lambing ears.[2]

J. A. Stockman III, MD

References

1. Foulon I, Naessen SA, Foulon W, et al. A 10-year prospective study of sensorineural hearing loss in children with congenital cytomegalovirus infection. *J Pediatr.* 2008;153:84-88.
2. Heathcote K, Upile T, Theaker JM. Lambing ears. *BMJ.* 2008;356:780.

6 Endocrinology

Etiology of Failure to Thrive in Infants and Toddlers Referred to a Pediatric Endocrinology Outpatient Clinic

Daniel M, Kleis L, Cemeroglu AP (Helen DeVos Children's Hosp at Spectrum Health, Grand Rapids, MI)
Clin Pediatr 47:762-765, 2008

The aim of this study is to determine the underlying etiology of failure to thrive (FTT) in infants and toddlers referred to an outpatient pediatric endocrinology clinic. A chart review was done on FTT referrals to a pediatric endocrinology outpatient clinic between 2002 and 2005. Majority of patients (51.5%) had a purely nutritional deficiency. The endocrine etiologies included short stature due to being small for gestational age, constitutional or familial short stature (28.9%). The third most common etiology was gastrointestinal disease. Endocrine causes of FTT seem to be rare even in the selected population of patients referred to pediatric endocrine outpatient clinics. In the primary care setting, nutritional assessment and consultation seem to be adequate in the majority of cases. Only a small percentage of the patients with FTT will require a multidisciplinary approach and more extensive work-up (Table 3).

▶ Failure to thrive remains a common problem in infancy and childhood. A fair percentage of these youngsters will wind up in the hospital undergoing long and expensive diagnostic procedures. The numerous previous studies have documented that laboratory testing yields positive results leading to a diagnosis in only a small minority of children. In this regard, if one looks at all previous studies, nonorganic failure to thrive accounts for up to 80% of cases. This category of failure to thrive described a group of infants who failed to thrive because they have not consumed normal caloric intake in the absence of organic disease or any demonstrable abnormalities of swallowing mechanisms. A few organic conditions are occult and are detected only by laboratory investigation, but the vast majority is suspected either on the basis of history or physical examination especially when symptoms are correlated with growth chart abnormalities. A recent study looked at the predictive value of predefined symptoms and signs for allocating children with failure to thrive into 1 of 2 groups, organic and nonorganic failure to thrive.[1] Detection of at least one nonorganic symptom or sign and the absence of any truly organic symptom invariably predicts a diagnosis of nonorganic failure to thrive. The report of Panetta et al also reminds us that one better be careful about weight gain during hospitalization as a diagnostic tool. I recall during residency training that many youngsters with nonorganic failure

TABLE 3.—Etiology of Failure to Thrive

Diagnosis	n	%
Pure nutritional deficit	50	51.5
Endocrine etiology	28	28.9
Short stature due to small for gestational age[a]	11	
Constitutional short stature	3	
Familial short stature	5	
Familial and nutritional short stature	4	
Constitutional and nutritional short stature	5	
Gastrointestinal disease	15	15.5
Gastroesophageal reflux	7	
Multiple food allergies	4	
IgA deficiency[a]	2	
Celiac disease	1	
Pyloric stenosis	1	
Neurodevelopmental /syndromic	5	5.1
Developmental delay	3	
Syndromic	2	

[a]One patient had IgA deficiency and was small for gestational age and is therefore listed under both diagnoses.

to thrive actually lose weight during a hospitalization as a result of procedures requiring fasting, the simple trauma of being in a hospital, and hospital-acquired illness. Also, some youngsters with low total serum albumins will have some degree of water retention. Refeeding results in an increase in serum albumin and diuresis body water, actually causing a reduction in total weight.

The study of Daniel et al, also looking at the etiology of failure to thrive in infants, examines a select group of such infants who were referred to pediatric endocrinologists for evaluation. The table lists the causes of failure to thrive in this select population. Nonorganic failure to thrive still remains the most common etiology. The next most common set of diagnoses in this unique group include failure to thrive secondary to being born small for gestational age, having familial short stature, or constitutional short stature. The latter 2 conditions, obviously, are not a "true" cause of failure to thrive. The third most common cause reported in these referred patients was gastrointestinal disease. The list of etiologies of nonorganic and organic failure to thrive is quite extensive. It often requires the diagnostic wisdom of Osler to sort things out.

This commentary closes with a *Clinical Fact/Curio* in the form of a question, an endocrinology-related query. How has the height of Greek men changed in recent years? Has it gone up or stayed flat and what are the likely underlying reasons? Investigators in the Department of Pediatrics at the University of Athens School of Medicine decided to look at the height of young Greek males in order to see what the influence of various socioeconomic factors is on growth. The easiest way to assess this was to look at the height records of thousands of Greek military conscripts, aged 18 to 26 years. The mean height ($\pm$ SD) of the conscripts was 175.7 cm in 1990, and this height gradually increased to 178.06 cm by 2006, corresponding to a height increase of 1.4 cm per decade. If one goes way back to look at the heights of Greek conscripts from 1968 to 1990, the mean height increased by almost 8 cm. These data show that young adult Greek males present a secular trend toward greater height and that this height statistically is correlated with socioeconomic status changes. Authors of this report suggest that Greece spent most of the 20th century as a developing country. In the 1970s, the country began to enjoy socioeconomic prosperity. This degree of prosperity directly correlates with the significant increase in height, suggesting that nutrition, and perhaps hygienic improvements, account for the advancing height. It should be noted that this study of Greek conscripts found no correlation between height and BMI, suggesting that childhood overweight is not the cause of the increasing height in recent decades.[2]

J. A. Stookman III, MD

References

1. Panetta F, Mazazzu D, Sferlass C, Lombardo M, Magazzu G, Lucanto MC. Diagnosis on a positive fashion of nonorganic failure to thrive. *Acta Paediatr.* 2008;97:1281-1284.
2. Papadimitriou A, Fytanidis G, Douros K, et al. Greek young men grow taller. *Acta Paediatr.* 2008;97:1105-1107.

Mutations in the Idotyrosine Deiodinase Gene and Hypothyroidism

Moreno JC, Klootwijk W, van Toor H, et al (Erasmus Univ, Rotterdam, The Netherlands; et al)
N Engl J Med 358:1811-1818, 2008

DEHAL1 has been identified as the gene encoding iodotyrosine deiodinase in the thyroid, where it controls the reuse of iodide for thyroid hormone synthesis. We screened patients with hypothyroidism who had features suggestive of an iodotyrosine deiodinase defect for mutations in *DEHAL1*. Two missense mutations and a deletion of three base pairs were identified in four patients from three unrelated families; all the patients had a dramatic reduction of in vitro activity of iodotyrosine deiodinase. Patients had severe goitrous hypothyroidism, which was evident in infancy and childhood. Two patients had cognitive deficits due to late diagnosis and treatment. Thus, mutations in *DEHAL1* led to a deficiency in iodotyrosine deiodinase in these patients. Because infants with *DEHAL1* defects may have normal thyroid function at birth, they may be missed by neonatal screening programs for congenital hypothyroidism.

▶ Thyroid hormones are essential for normal brain development, growth, and metabolism. Hypothyroidism is the most common congenital endocrine disorder, occurring in 1 in 3000 newborns and results from complete or partial failure of thyroid development or thyroid hormone production. The synthesis of thyroid hormones is dependent on a normally developed thyroid gland, an adequate nutritional intake of iodide, and a series of biochemical steps to organify iodide. In many countries, newborns are screened for congenital hypothyroidism and detected cases are immediately treated, which can prevent the development of retardation. The report of Moreno et al describes the identification of defects in iodotyrosine dehalogenase 1 (*DEHAL1*) that produce a severe form of hypothyroidism, goiter, excessive levels of iodotyrosine in serum and urine, and variable mental defects. In order to understand what these authors are describing to us, it is important to understand the big picture of how hypothyroidism develops in utero and in early infancy.

The first step in thyroid-hormone biosynthesis consists of iodide uptake in the thyroid gland. Iodide is then released into the follicular lumen of the thyroid, presumably in part by a transporter mechanism, which also oxidizes the iodide. This oxidation requires the presence of hydrogen peroxide, which is generated by an enzyme that requires a maturation factor. The subsequent iodination of the products within thyroglobulin leads to the synthesis of monoiodotyrosine and diiodotyrosine. The next step involves a fusion of these molecules in a coupling reaction to form either triiodothyronine (T3) or thyroxine (T4). Eventually, T4 and T3 are engulfed by thyrocytes through pinocytosis, then are digested into lysosomes and subsequently are secreted into the bloodstream as 80% T4 and 20% T3.

Back in 2001, Moreno et al cloned novel genes that are relevant to thyroid function. One of the 4 genes that they identified has been referred to as *DEHAL1*. Moreno et al now provide definitive evidence that this gene is essential to the metabolism of iodide in the thyroid. The authors describe 4 patients homozygous for mutations in the *DEHAL1* gene in whom radioiodine uptake and organification of iodide were found to be normal, but in whom there was a dramatic reduction of in vitro activity of iodotyrosine deiodinase. In all 4 patients, severe hypothyroidism that was associated with large goiters developed only later in infancy and childhood. Cognitive defects did develop in 2 of the patients because of delayed onset of therapy.

These observations of Moreno et al are important from a clinical perspective. Two of the 4 patients were tested as newborns and had normal screening results with the hypothyroidism developing later in life, emphasizing that neonatal screening may not detect all patients who are affected by congenital hypothyroidism. Careful observation of a child's development is essential to avoid the deleterious consequences of hypothyroidism on brain development as was seen in 2 of the patients. Moreover, the age of onset of hypothyroidism varied significantly in affected subjects and could be confused easily with common acquired hypothyroidism.

Thus we now know 1 new form of congenital hypothyroidism, one that may not present clinically until beyond the neonatal period. Worse yet, this entity still is associated with cognitive deficiencies, and even worse yet, may not be picked up with routine neonatal screening. The importance of this article is this lesson that we still have to be on guard when it comes to looking for the signs of hypothyroidism in infancy and early childhood.

This commentary closes with a *Clinical Fact/Curio* regarding endocrinology. Seven physicians and pharmacists went on trial in February 2008 over the death of at least 110 people who became infected with Creutzfeldt-Jakob disease after being given tainted human growth hormone when they were children. The United States, Britain, and other countries halted the distribution of growth hormone in 1985, after it was discovered that 3 people died after being given the product. Growth hormone at that time was extracted from pituitary glands removed from corpses. The cause of some subsequent deaths was Creutz-feldt-Jakob disease. Doctors in France, however, continued to use the hormone for several years, treating thousands of children, before turning to a synthetic substitute in 1988. After the first death in France was recorded in 1991, the patient's family took to court the company responsible for collecting the pituitary glands, France-Hypophyse, along with the Pasteur Institute, which prepared the treatment, and the Pharmacie Centrale des Hôpitaux de Paris, which distributed the treatment. Some 250 people took out lawsuits. The defendants in this case were charged with "involuntary homicide" and "aggravated deception."

Nearly 60% of worldwide deaths caused by the administration of Creutzfeldt-Jakob disease transmitted by human growth hormone occurred in France. Among the cumulative factors in this health catastrophe is thought to be the product of French hypercentralization, which obligated the children to follow a treatment provided by France-Hypophyse, while during the same period 3 industrial firms produced and sold human growth hormone throughout the world–and none of those had cases of Creutzfeldt-Jakob disease.[1]

J. A. Stockman III, MD

Reference

1. Spurgeon B. French doctors are tried for treating children with infected human growth hormone. *BMJ*. 2008;336:348-349.

Inaccurate hemoglobin A(1C) levels in patients with type 1 diabetes and hereditary persistence of hemoglobin F

Felner EI, McGrath M (Emory Univ School of Medicine, Atlanta, GA)
J Pediatr 153:137-139, 2008

We report 2 African-American boys with type 1 diabetes and hereditary persistence of hemoglobin F. The diagnosis came to light after both patients exhibited inconsistent hemoglobin A(1C) (HbA(1C)) levels with respect to serum glucose measurements. This demonstrates the importance of frequent glucose monitoring and interpreting the HbA(1C) level in light of serum glucose measurements.

▶ Virtually all clinicians monitor hemoglobin A_{1C} to follow long-term glycemic control in diabetics. The American Diabetes Association recommends a hemoglobin A_{1C} goal of less than 7% for adults and 8% for children with diabetes. For otherwise normal individuals, the normal hemoglobin A_{1C} should be below 6%. The reason hemoglobin A_{1C} is valued for these purposes is that glucose will irreversibly and nonenzymatically result in glycation of the NH_2-terminal valines of the β chain of the hemoglobin molecule. Because hemoglobin A_{1C} forms over the average lifespan of the red blood cell, the amount of hemoglobin A_{1C} reflects average glucose concentrations over the preceding 2 to 3 months.

What most pediatricians, and internists, do not recognize, however, is the fact that there are circumstances in which hemoglobin A_{1C} as normally measured does not reflect glucose control very well. Broadly speaking, this occurs in 3 circumstances: in the presence of hemoglobinopathies, when red cell survival is short, and as the result of assay issues. In those with sickle cell disease variants (HbSS, HbSC, HbCC, etc), measurement of A_{1C} is unreliable because red cell life is shortened. The same would be true of subjects with hereditary spherocytosis. In such circumstances, there will be discordance in the measured hemoglobin A_{1C} and other measures of glycemic control, such as data from self-glucose monitoring. Shortened red cell survival results in a low hemoglobin A_{1C} because the red blood cell is not around long enough to reach equilibrium with recent glycemia control. As we note in this report of Felner et al, high levels of fetal hemoglobin will also result in artificially low levels of hemoglobin A_{1C} because current assays for hemoglobin A_{1C} measure only the effect of glucose on hemoglobin A and its variants.

In an excellent editorial on hemoglobin A_{1C} discordance, Cohen et al remind us that there are other ways of determining long-term glucose control. A particularly good one is a measurement of glycated serum fructosamine. Virtually all proteins in blood become glycosylated, and fructosamine is a particularly easy one to measure. We do not substitute a fructosamine for a hemoglobin A_{1C} in the normal setting because this protein survives in the circulation only about 2 weeks before it is turned over and therefore is not a standard monitor of long-term glucose control. However, if a patient is in a steady state of glucose control (good or bad) fructosamine measurements should be quite adequate.[1]

Remember the reasons why hemoglobin A_{1C} may not reflect glucose control in any accurate way. Patients with common hemoglobinopathy such as sickle cell disease are not immune to having diabetes. Recognize in such cases that hemoglobin A_{1C} may not be the way to go to know how well that patient's diabetic management is going.

J. A. Stockman III, MD

Reference

1. Cohen RM, Joiner CH, Franco RS. Discordant hemoglobin A1C results: the hoofbeats increase. *J Pediatr.* 2008;153:7-9.

Role of blood pressure in development of early retinopathy in adolescents with type 1 diabetes: prospective cohort study
Gallego PH, Craig ME, Hing S, et al (Children's Hospital at Westmead, Australia, et al)
BMJ 337:a918, 2008

Objective.—To examine the relation between blood pressure and the development of early retinopathy in adolescents with childhood onset type 1 diabetes.

Design.—Prospective cohort study.

Setting.—Diabetes Complications Assessment Service at the Children's Hospital at Westmead, Sydney, Australia.

Participants.—1869 patients with type 1 diabetes (54% female) screened for retinopathy with baseline median age 13.4 (interquartile range 12.0-15.2) years, duration 4.9 (3.1-7.0) years, and albumin excretion rate of 4.4 (3.1-6.8) µg/min plus a subgroup of 1093 patients retinopathy-free at baseline and followed for a median 4.1 (2.4-6.6) years.

Main Outcome Measures.—Early background retinopathy; blood pressure.

Results.—Overall, retinopathy developed in 673 (36%) participants at any time point. In the retinopathy-free group, higher systolic blood pressure (odds ratio 1.01, 95% confidence interval 1.003 to 1.02) and diastolic blood pressure (1.01, 1.002 to 1.03) were predictors of retinopathy, after adjustment for albumin excretion rate (1.27, 1.13 to 1.42), haemoglobin A_{1c} (1.08, 1.02 to 1.15), duration of diabetes (1.16, 1.13 to 1.19), age (1.13, 1.08 to 1.17), and height (0.98, 0.97 to 0.99). In a subgroup of 1025 patients with albumin excretion rate below 7.5 µg/min, the cumulative risk of retinopathy at 10 years' duration of diabetes was higher for those with systolic blood pressure on or above the 90th centile compared with those below the 90th centile (58% v 35%, P=0.03). The risk was also higher for patients with diastolic blood pressure on or above the 90th centile compared with those below the 90th centile (57% v 35%, P=0.005).

Conclusions.—Both systolic and diastolic blood pressure are predictors of retinopathy and increase the probability of early retinopathy independently of incipient nephropathy in young patients with type 1 diabetes.

▶ It should come as no surprise that both systolic and diastolic blood pressures would be predictive of retinopathy in youngsters with type 1 diabetes. The eyes and the kidneys are the 2 organs that are at greatest risk over the lifespan of children and adults affected by type 1 diabetes.

On a related topic, it was recently reported that a tweak to a diabetic's DNA could tip the balance toward blindness and kidney failure.[1] A natural variation in just a single DNA base pair raises levels of erythropoietin. Erythropoietin, as we all know, stimulates red blood cell production, but it also increases blood vessel growth. The higher the erythropoietin level, the higher the risk that a diabetic will develop diabetic retinopathy and end-stage kidney disease. Theoretically, controlling erythropoietin levels or blocking its activity could help diabetics stave off complications or halt the progression of diseases already attacking the eyes and kidneys. Diabetic retinopathy generally results when excessive blood vessel formation occurs within the retina leading to tears in eye tissue or detachment of the retina. Diabetic retinopathy is the leading cause of new cases of blindness in the United States and is responsible for about 10% of blindness overall. A change in a particular spot in a stretch of DNA that controls whether erythropoietin gene is switched on or off may affect the probability that a diabetic will develop retinopathy.[1] Patients with the variety of gene encoding DNA that produces erythropoietin at higher levels have a higher risk of developing eye and kidney complications.

Please be aware that when diabetes is not in good control, elevated levels of hemoglobin A_{1C} will result in high erythropoietin levels. Hemoglobin A_{1C} does not carry oxygen well. A hemoglobin A_{1C} level of 9% effectively means that the measured hemoglobin level is 9% less effective, causing the body to produce more erythropoietin to make new red blood cells to compensate for this. One of the side effects is that the amounts of erythropoietin produced will also stimulate blood vessel formation in the eyes, and possibly the kidneys. Thus, it is mandatory to gain the best possible control of blood sugar in order to prevent this secondary complication.

A recent report showed that if you stress men with mental arithmetic tests, you can predict the later onset of hypertension by their adrenergic findings during such testing. This study looked at arterial catecholamine concentrations in 99 men at rest and after performing mental arithmetic testing. Their resting blood pressures were taken 18 years later. The researchers found that sympathetic nervous activity during mental arithmetic predicts future blood pressure, a finding completely independent of baseline blood pressure readings and family history![2] Remember the rapid pulse rate you got in college at the time the blue books were passed out? Well, the more rapid your heart rate in those days, the more likely it is that you have hypertension now.

This commentary closes with a *Clinical Fact/Curio* regarding diabetes. A dip in the hot tub, heat therapy, can improve insulin sensitivity in individuals with diabetes.[3] Researchers have found that obese, insulin-resistant humans have low levels of heat-shock protein 72 (HSP72) in skeletal muscle, and that, in mice, heat therapy can induce HSP72. When HSP72 is genetically overexpressed, mice have been shown to be protected from insulin resistance after consuming a high-fat diet. Researchers next found that HSP72 affects the activation of the serine-threonine kinase c-jun amino terminal kinase (JNK), affecting insulin signaling. Mice expressing high levels of HSP72 have been shown to have reduced JNK activation, which allows the insulin pathway to continue signaling despite a high-fat diet. The HSP72-overexpressing mice also have increased energy expenditure and reduced fat stores compared to wild-type mice fed a high-fat diet.

Inducing HSP72 expression in obese mice with a small molecule results in improved insulin sensitivity throughout the body. The drug is now in human clinical trials. As far as diabetes is concerned, perhaps at some point in the future it will be more common than not that "when you're hot, you're hot."

J. A. Stockman III, MD

References

1. Saey TH. DNA change no good for diabetics: increased protein production stimulates blood vessel growth and may lead to blindness and kidney failure. *Sci News.* May 24, 2008;9.
2. Flaa A, Eide IK, Kjeldsen SE, Rostrup M. Sympathoadrenal stress reactivity is a predictor of future blood pressure: an 18-year follow-up study. *Hypertension.* 2008;52:336-341.
3. Chung J, Nguyen A-K, Henstridge DC, et al. HSP72 protects against obesity-induced insulin resistance. *Proc Natl Acad Sci U S A.* 2008;105:1735-1744.

Shared and Distinct Genetic Variants in Type 1 Diabetes and Celiac Disease
Smyth DJ, Plagnol V, Walker NM, et al (Univ of Cambridge, UK; et al)
N Engl J Med 359:2767-2777, 2008

Background.—Two inflammatory disorders, type 1 diabetes and celiac disease, cosegregate in populations, suggesting a common genetic origin. Since both diseases are associated with the HLA class II genes on chromosome 6p21, we tested whether non-HLA loci are shared.

Methods.—We evaluated the association between type 1 diabetes and eight loci related to the risk of celiac disease by genotyping and statistical analyses of DNA samples from 8064 patients with type 1 diabetes, 9339 control subjects, and 2828 families providing 3064 parent–child trios (consisting of an affected child and both biologic parents). We also investigated 18 loci associated with type 1 diabetes in 2560 patients with celiac disease and 9339 control subjects.

Results.—Three celiac disease loci — *RGS1* on chromosome 1q31, *IL18RAP* on chromosome 2q12, and *TAGAP* on chromosome 6q25 — were associated with type 1 diabetes (P<1.00×10^{-4}). The 32-bp insertion–deletion variant on chromosome 3p21 was newly identified as a type 1 diabetes locus (P = 1.81×10^{-8}) and was also associated with celiac disease, along with *PTPN2* on chromosome 18p11 and *CTLA4* on chromosome 2q33, bringing the total number of loci with evidence of a shared association to seven, including *SH2B3* on chromosome 12q24. The effects of the *IL18RAP* and *TAGAP* alleles confer protection in type 1 diabetes and susceptibility in celiac disease. Loci with distinct effects in the two diseases included *INS* on chromosome 11p15, *IL2RA* on chromosome 10p15, and *PTPN22* on chromosome 1p13 in type 1 diabetes and *IL12A* on 3q25 and *LPP* on 3q28 in celiac disease.

Conclusions.—A genetic susceptibility to both type 1 diabetes and celiac disease shares common alleles. These data suggest that common biologic mechanisms, such as autoimmunity-related tissue damage and intolerance to dietary antigens, may be etiologic features of both diseases.

▶ A number of reports have indicated there is a possible correlation between diabetes mellitus type 1 and the incidence of other autoimmune disorders, particularly thyroid and celiac diseases. According to various data, somewhere between 1% and 10% of children diagnosed with diabetes mellitus type 1 will develop celiac disease. The variation is largely related to age and diagnostic methods used to describe the association. The etiopathogenesis of celiac disease development in diabetic children is not fully understood. One argument in favor of the relationship being real is the fact that the same alleles of the genes HLA-DQA1 and DQB2 predispose to development of both celiac disease and diabetes mellitus type 1. A recent report from Poland suggests that tumor necrosis factor-alpha appears to be an essential component of celiac disease development, a report that also suggests that early introduction of tumor necrosis factor-alpha antagonists in the treatment of diabetes mellitus type 1 patients in whom there are elevated levels of this cytokine might help prevent the onset of celiac disease and possibly even late diabetic complications.[1]

The report of Smyth et al attempts to provide an answer to the question of why some families seem to have an undue susceptibility to type 1 diabetes mellitus and celiac disease. The study identified up to 15 genetic risk variants (or alleles) that contribute to both diseases and simultaneously demonstrated that 13 alleles were specific to one disease or the other. These observations support an emerging role of shared genetic risks for many common diseases, which may, in turn, identify previously unexpected biological pathways that link diseases together. When Smyth et al initiated their study, unequivocal associations had already been drawn between 8 alleles and the risk of celiac disease and between 15 alleles and the risk of type 1 diabetes outside of the major histocompatibility complex region. However, only 1 allele had been shown to have a definitive association with both the diseases (*SH2B3* on chromosome 12Q24). What Smyth et al attempted to do is to answer the question of whether alleles that are associated with the risk of celiac disease also confer a risk of type 1 diabetes and also whether alleles that are associated with the risk of type 1 diabetes also confer a risk of celiac disease. The answer to these questions was a definitive yes.

What this report shows is that of 8 previously validated celiac disease alleles, at least 4 also contribute to a risk of type 1 diabetes and one other allele is highly suggestive of an association. Of the 15 previously validated alleles conferring an increased risk of type 1 diabetes, at least 2 contribute to a risk of celiac disease.

As interesting as these findings are, interest will wane in the findings if they have no clinical implications. It is likely that the most important implication of the findings will be the ability to define biological pathways that can influence the course of these autoimmune diseases. On the long haul, one can look forward to novel therapies that would treat, prevent, or even cure disease. On the short haul, the most likely implication of the findings of this report is that we will soon see screening for the presence of risk alleles in asymptomatic patients with one disease (eg, celiac disease) to predict whether another disease (eg, type 1 diabetes) is likely to develop. Last, the findings of Smyth et al have implications beyond shared genetic causes of type 1 diabetes and celiac disease. A number of studies have suggested shared causes for other autoimmune diseases such as systemic lupus erythematosus and rheumatoid arthritis. Also, some autoimmune diseases are associated with a decreased risk of other problems. For example, type 2 diabetes is associated with a decreased risk of prostatic cancer over one's lifespan.

To read more about shared genetic risk factors for type 1 diabetes and celiac disease, see the excellent commentary by Plenge.[2]

J. A. Stockman III, MD

References

1. Mysliwiec M, Balcerska A, Zorena K, Myśliwska J, Wiśniewski P. Immunologic and biochemical factors of coincident celiac disease and type 1 diabetes mellitus in children. *Pediatr Res.* 2008;64:677-681.

2. Plenge RM. Shared genetic risk factors for type 1 diabetes and celiac disease. *N Engl J Med.* 2008;359:2837-2838.

Birth Weight and Risk of Type 2 Diabetes: A Systematic Review
Whincup PH, Kaye SJ, Owen CG, et al (Univ of London, UK; et al)
JAMA 300:2886-2897, 2008

Context.—Low birth weight is implicated as a risk factor for type 2 diabetes. However, the strength, consistency, independence, and shape of the association have not been systematically examined.

Objective.—To conduct a quantitative systematic review examining published evidence on the association of birth weight and type 2 diabetes in adults.

Data Sources and Study Selection.—Relevant studies published by June 2008 were identified through literature searches using EMBASE (from 1980), MEDLINE (from 1950), and Web of Science (from 1980), with a combination of text words and Medical Subject Headings. Studies with either quantitative or qualitative estimates of the association between birth weight and type 2 diabetes were included.

Data Extraction.—Estimates of association (odds ratio [OR] per kilogram of increase in birth weight) were obtained from authors or from published reports in models that allowed the effects of adjustment (for body mass index and socioeconomic status) and the effects of exclusion (for macrosomia and maternal diabetes) to be examined. Estimates were pooled using random-effects models, allowing for the possibility that true associations differed between populations.

Data Synthesis.—Of 327 reports identified, 31 were found to be relevant. Data were obtained from 30 of these reports (31 populations; 6090 diabetes cases; 152 084 individuals). Inverse birth weight–type 2 diabetes associations were observed in 23 populations (9 of which were statistically significant) and positive associations were found in 8 (2 of which were statistically significant). Appreciable heterogeneity between populations ($I^2 = 66\%$; 95% confidence interval [CI], 51%-77%) was largely explained by positive associations in 2 native North American populations with high prevalences of maternal diabetes and in 1 other population of young adults. In the remaining 28 populations, the pooled OR of type 2 diabetes, adjusted for age and sex, was 0.75 (95% CI, 0.70-0.81) per kilogram. The shape of the birth weight–type 2 diabetes association was strongly graded, particularly at birth weights of 3 kg or less. Adjustment for current body mass index slightly strengthened the association (OR, 0.76 [95% CI, 0.70-0.82] before adjustment and 0.70 [95% CI, 0.65-0.76] after adjustment). Adjustment for socioeconomic status did not materially affect the association (OR, 0.77 [95% CI, 0.70-0.84] before adjustment and 0.78 [95% CI, 0.72-0.84] after adjustment). There was no strong evidence of publication or small study bias.

Conclusion.—In most populations studied, birth weight was inversely related to type 2 diabetes risk.

▶ The bottom line of this report is that in most populations studied, birth weight is inversely related to the risk of type 2 diabetes. This may sound counterintuitive, but it is a true observation. Before the report of Whincup et al appeared, earlier reviews of the association between birth weight and type 2 diabetes were limited by being qualitative rather than quantitative or by including only a limited number of published studies, focusing on extreme birth weights rather than the birth weight distribution as a whole, and not taking account of potential confounding factors. The study of Whincup et al improved upon earlier reports by carrying out a systematic quantitative review of published studies reporting on the association between birth weight and type 2 diabetes in the adult population to establish the overall strength, consistency, and independence of the association. The investigators also examined whether the association differed among populations, notably North American populations, in which the prevalence of maternal diabetes is exceptionally high. The data from this report are consistent with several earlier studies in suggesting that low birth weights (< 2.5 kg) are associated with an increase in risk of type 2 diabetes. The study of Whincup et al also shows a relationship between birth weights less than 3 kg and a greater risk of type 2 diabetes. These same findings were found in native North American populations. The correlation between low birth weight and a risk of diabetes held up even when adjusting for socioeconomic status and other influencing and confounding factors.

Interestingly, as our obesity problem has exploded, we are seeing more pregnant women with type 2 diabetes, a pregnancy known to produce large babies. It will be interesting over time to see whether these large babies are protected from the development of type 2 diabetes simply because they are large or whether they in fact will themselves experience a higher risk of type 2 diabetes. It has been shown in previous studies of native North American populations that there is a U-shaped birth weight-type 2 diabetes association, meaning that low birth weight and high birth weight are both associated with a later risk of type 2 diabetes. Thus, it is that it is not good to be too big or too small at birth when it comes to the later development of type 2 diabetes.

This commentary closes with a *Clinical Fact/Curio* regarding a common problem. It is posed in the form of a question. You are seeing a somewhat overweight 11-year-old who entered puberty 2 years earlier. On breast examination, she has evidence of significant breast enlargement beyond that normally seen in comparable aged children. The question is, is breast size a predictor of diabetes, independent of other risk factors for this disorder? The answer is that evidence suggests that large breasts do have some predictability as a risk factor for the development of diabetes. Overweight girls tend to go through puberty earlier. This is a well-known fact. They additionally have a statistically greater probability of having larger breasts than their peers as young adults. Also, alongside greater waist circumference and body mass index, bust size has been thought to be a possible useful measure of obesity and predictor of type 2 diabetes. Findings from a cohort of women participating in the Nurses' Health Study II indicate that a large bra cup size at age 20 years predicts diabetes in middle age. This is an independent risk factor although not as strong an independent risk factor as is body mass index.[1]

Obviously it is hard to tease out the integrated risk factors that are used to predict diabetes. Only time will tell, but it is not beyond the pale to think that a risk assessment history might at some point include a question about what bra cup size a young lady might have.

J. A. Stockman III, MD

Reference

1. Ray JG, Mohllajee AP, van Dam RM, et al. Breast size and risk of type 2 diabetes mellitus. *CMAJ.* 2008;178:289-295.

7 Gastroenterology

Natural evolution of infantile regurgitation versus the efficacy of thickened formula

Hegar B, Rantos R, Firmansyah A, et al (Universitas Indonesia, Depok)

J Pediatr Gastroenterol Nutr 47:26-30, 2008

Background.—Regurgitation is frequent in infants. We evaluated changes in regurgitation among patient groups fed standard formula, standard formula subsequently thickened with cereal, or formula manufactured with bean gum as a thickening agent.

Patients and Methods.—A prospective, blinded, randomised 1-month intervention trial evaluating the efficacy of parental reassurance of the regurgitating child in combination with 3 formula interventions—standard infant formula (group A); 5 g of rice cereal added to 100 mL standard formula (group B); and formula manufactured with bean gum as a thickening agent (group C)—was performed in 60 infants presenting with more than 4 episodes of regurgitation and/or vomiting per day during the week before inclusion. Formula intake, infant comfort, stool aspects, and weight gain were evaluated. All of the infants and data recorded by parents in a diary were evaluated weekly by a blinded health care professional.

Results.—At baseline, groups A, B, and C were similar for all of the parameters. After the 1-month intervention, regurgitation/vomiting decreased significantly in all 3 groups (P < 0.0005). Although the decrease was largest in group C (-4.2 ± 2.1 episodes/day), the incidence did not differ significantly with groups A or B. At no evaluation interval was there a difference in volume of formula intake, infant comfort, stool frequency, or aspect. After 1 month, weight gain was significantly greater in group C compared with group A (19.9% vs 16.4%; P < 0.001).

Conclusions.—Thickening of formula decreases regurgitation, but not significantly. Parental reassurance remains the cornerstone of the treatment of infant regurgitation.

▶ By far, this report from Belgium is the most comprehensive update on the value of using a thickened formula to manage infants with clinically significant regurgitation. The latter is not an uncommon problem. As many as 1 in 5 infants present to their pediatric care provider with problems resulting from regurgitation. The study reported out of Belgium is of value because it tells us the natural history of regurgitation over time and the benefits in comparison with this natural history of the use of thickened formula. Two formulas were studied. The first was the use of rice cereal added to standard formula. The second was a commercially available (in Europe) formula in which the viscosity was increased by the addition of bean gum. The study reported that thickened formulas did reduce the number of episodes of regurgitation with the bean gum formula having the greater effect. However, the reduction in number of episodes did not reach statistical significance.

Most gastroenterologists if asked suggest that parental reassurance be the first step in the management of infants who regurgitate. Avoiding overfeeding has also been shown to reduce regurgitation. Volume reduction may be helpful in clearly overfed infants, but is of no or limited value for infants who are fed with a normal frequency and with normal feeding volumes. Most data have shown that milk-thickening agents do reduce regurgitation to some degree. In the United States, thickening is usually achieved with the addition of rice cereal to formula. When thickening an infant formula that has 20 kcal/oz, the addition of 1 tablespoon of rice cereal per ounce of formula increases the energy density to approximately 34 kcal/oz, whereas the addition of 1 tablespoon of rice cereal per 2 ounces of formula increases the energy density to approximately 27 kcal/oz. Adding rice starch to formula may also provide additional buffering of acid, alleviating esophageal irritability to some degree, albeit modest. With few exceptions, rice cereals have an excellent digestibility in infants as young as 1 to 3 months. Of course, when formula is thickened, it is usually necessary to crosscut the nipple to allow for adequate flow.

It has only been recently that high viscosity commercially available formulas have come onto the market in the United States. They tend to be expensive and no better than the addition of simple rice cereal to a standard formula. Many commercial antiregurgitation formulas are available in European countries that contain potato, rice or cornstarch, locust bean gum, or carboxymethylcellulose (a combination of pectin and cellulose) as thickening agents. In fact, there are many differing compositions of antiregurgitation formulas as there are formula companies. These formulas have been reported to decrease regurgitation, vomiting, and acid reflux when compared with unthickened formula, and manufacturers claim they are more effective than formula thickened with rice cereal.

Please do not think that some thickening agents are without any potential side effects. It has been suggested that thickened formulas may be associated with more coughing leading to the hypothesis that thickened formulas could theoretically worsen nonregurgitant reflux based on the possibility that a thickened formula may stay longer in the esophagus if it is refluxed. Europeans should be worried about bean gum because this is associated with malabsorption of minerals and some micronutrients. Fermentation of bean gum can cause abdominal pain, colic, and diarrhea. Although they are rare, serious complications of bean gum consumption such as acute intestinal obstruction, gastric bezoar, and necrotizing enterocolitis have been reported in a few preterms and newborns.

Half a dozen years ago, a Cochrane review was published that concluded that thickened feedings did reduce regurgitation severity and the frequency of emesis, but not that of acid reflux.[1]

J. A. Stockman III, MD

Reference

1. Craig WR, Hanlon-Dearman A, Sinclair C, Taback S, Moffatt M. Metoclopramide, thickened feedings, and positioning for gastroesophageal reflux in children under two years. *Cochrane Database Syst Rev.* 2004;4:CD003502.

14 years of eosinophilic esophagitis: clinical features and prognosis

Spergel JM, Brown-Whitehorn TF, Beausoleil JL, et al (The Children's Hosp of Philadelphia)
J Pediatr Gastroenterol Nutr 48:30-36, 2009

Objective.—To determine the natural history of treated and untreated eosinophilic esophagitis (EE) and examine the presenting symptoms of EE.

Patients and Methods.—Retrospective and prospective chart review of all patients diagnosed with EE at The Children's Hospital of Philadelphia. EE was defined as greater than 20 eosinophils per high power field after treatment with reflux medications.

Results.—We identified 620 patients in our database in the last 14 years and 330 patients with greater than 1 year of follow-up for analysis. The number of new EE patients has increased on an annual basis. Of the patients presenting with EE, 68% were younger than 6 years old. Reflux symptoms and feeding issues/failure to thrive were the most common presenting symptoms for EE. Eleven patients had resolution of all of their food allergies and 33 patients had resolutions of some of their food allergies. No patients have progression of EE into other gastrointestinal disorders.

Conclusions.—EE is a chronic disease with less than 10% of the population developing tolerance to their food allergies. EE does not progress into other gastrointestinal diseases.

▶ All of us have been hearing a lot more about the problem of eosinophilic esophagitis in the last 10 years or so. This condition is characterized by infiltration of the esophagus with eosinophils without infiltration in other parts of the gastrointestinal tract. The report abstracted emanates from the Children's Hospital of Philadelphia where a 35-fold increase in cases of eosinophilic esophagitis has been observed in the 10-year period between 1994 and 2003. The symptoms of eosinophilic esophagitis have been described as symptoms suggestive of gastroesophageal reflux not responding to standard medications. Older children sometimes present with dysphagia and younger children can present with failure to thrive. Little is known about the natural history of this disorder, but it seems to progress when left untreated. Depending on age, the most common complaints are feeding difficulties (in the very young), vomiting (in older children), abdominal pain (particularly in adolescence), dysphagia (also occurring in adolescence), along with food impaction in older adolescents.

The importance of the report from Philadelphia is that it describes the natural history of more than 600 patients with eosinophilic gastroenteritis. We learn that boys are affected with this disorder more commonly than in girls (2 to 3 times more likely to develop it). The disease tends to be one predominantly seen in the white population. Two-thirds of patients present at younger than 6 years of age. The population affected is highly atopic with two-thirds of patients having other allergic diseases. It has been suggested that one potential mechanism of eosinophilic esophagitis is the swallowing of airborne pollen that then interacts with the esophageal tissue causing a local allergic reaction and eosinophilia in the esophagus. In any event, the disorder appears to be a chronic one with periods of relapse and remission. The only way of outgrowing eosinophilic esophagitis appears to be the total avoidance of food, not an easy cure therefore. It should be noted that none of the patients with eosinophilic esophagitis have progressed to eosinophilic gastroenteritis or eosinophilic colitis.

In some respects, one should think of eosinophilic esophagitis as a chronic disease similar to asthma and allergic rhinitis. As the disease progresses over time, patients can develop esophageal thickening, leading to difficulty swallowing and eventually to food impaction.

One final comment about eosinophilic esophagitis and that is that it has been recently associated with the presence of celiac disease in some patients. Last, while a small number of children will outgrow their eosinophilic esophagitis, this should not be expected. Please note this review did not mention what the best forms of treatment are. These are actually ill defined at the present time.

J. A. Stockman III, MD

Effect of eradication of *Helicobacter pylori* on incidence of metachronous gastric carcinoma after endoscopic resection of early gastric cancer: an open-label, randomised controlled trial
Fukase K, for the Japan Gast Study Group (Yamagata Prefectural Central Hosp, Japan; et al)
Lancet 372:392-397, 2008

Background.—The relation between *Helicobacter pylori* infection and gastric cancer has been proven in epidemiological studies and animal experiments. Our aim was to investigate the prophylactic effect of *H pylori* eradication on the development of metachronous gastric carcinoma after endoscopic resection for early gastric cancer.

Methods.—In this multi-centre, open-label, randomised controlled trial, 544 patients with early gastric cancer, either newly diagnosed and planning to have endoscopic treatment or in post-resection follow-up after endoscopic treatment, were randomly assigned to receive an *H pylori* eradication regimen (n=272) or control (n=272). Randomisation was done by a computer-generated randomisation list and was stratified by whether the patient was newly diagnosed or post-resection. Patients in the eradication group received lansoprazole 30 mg twice daily, amoxicillin 750 mg twice daily, and clarithromycin 200 mg twice daily for a week; those in the control group received standard care, but no treatment for *H pylori*. Patients were examined endoscopically at 6, 12, 24, and 36 months after allocation. The primary endpoint was diagnosis of new carcinoma at another site in the stomach. Analyses were by intention to treat. This trial is registered with the UMIN Clinical Trials Registry, number UMIN000001169.

Findings.—At 3-year follow-up, metachronous gastric carcinoma had developed in nine patients in the eradication group and 24 in the control group. In the full intention-to-treat population, including all patients irrespective of length of follow-up (272 patients in each group), the odds ratio for metachronous gastric carcinoma was 0·353 (95% CI 0·161–0·775; p=0.009); in the modified intention-to treat population, including patients with at least one post randomisation assessment of tumour status and adjusting for loss to follow-up (255 patients in the eradication group, 250 in the control group), the hazard ratio for metachronous gastric carcinoma was 0·339 (95% CI 0·157–0·729; p=0.003). In the eradication group, 19 (7%) patients had diarrhoea and 32 (12%) had soft stools

Interpretation.—Prophylactic eradication of *H pylori* after endoscopic resection of early gastric cancer should be used to prevent the development of metachronous gastric carcinoma.

Funding.—Hiroshima Cancer Seminar Foundation.

▶ A good bit of the origins of *Helicobacter pylori* are found in childhood. Thus, a study of adults with gastric cancer, much of which is the consequence of longstanding *H pylori* infection, has significant relevance to those who provide care to children. Despite classification of *H pylori* as a carcinogen, screening for and treatment of infected individuals to prevent gastric cancer is not generally accepted. Yet, globally, gastric cancer is the second-leading cause of cancer deaths annually. Up to 80% of noncardia gastric adenocarcinomas are directly attributable to this bacterium, probably through the development of gastric atrophy followed by intestinal metaplasia. Although environmental and genetic exposures are important and 1% to 3% of cases are hereditary, *H pylori* is a necessary, albeit not sufficient, cause of most gastric adenocarcinoma. Once *H pylori* infection has led to gastric atrophy and intestinal metaplasia, it may be too late to eradicate the bacterium to reduce the later onset of cancer. Contrarily, if *H pylori* remains an important causal factor in gastric cancer, treating the infection—even in the setting of advanced gastric atrophy—could reduce subsequent risk of cancer.

What we see in the report of Fukase et al from Japan is an important randomized trial looking at whether eradication of *H pylori* does indeed reduce the risk of gastric cancer. The participants had early gastric carcinoma and were referred for endoscopic mucosal resection, and therefore were at very high risk for recurrent gastric cancer. Of nearly 550 patients, most had either intestinal metaplasia or moderate-to-severe gastric atrophy, yet the risk of subsequent cancer was reduced from 4 per 100 every year to just 1.4 per 100 every year in the group that received treatment for eradication of this bacterium. The results of this

Japanese study are clear. In a high-risk population, gastric cancer rates are substantially reduced, but not totally abolished, by *H pylori* eradication.

Compelling evidence now exists to show that *H pylori* eradication reduces risk of subsequent gastric adenocarcinoma irrespective of age, despite pre-existing severe gastric atrophy or intestinal metaplasia. While these conditions are not likely to occur in childhood, the start of the process certainly can begin on the pediatrician's watch. The benefits and risks of *H pylori* eradication still need to be tested in large randomized trials, most likely to occur in Asia, where the prevalence of gastric carcinoma is highest. Gastric cancer kills many more people than colon cancer, and we do screen adults with colonoscopy. Is it reasonable to screen adults for *H pylori* infection, or possibly even children? Only time and expensive further studies will give the answers.

J. A. Stockman III, MD

The changing epidemiology of infantile hypertrophic pyloric stenosis in Scotland

Sommerfield T, Chalmers J, Youngson G, et al (NHS National Services, Scotland, Edinburgh, UK; Univ of Aberdeen, UK)
Arch Dis Child 93:1007-1011, 2008

Background.—The aetiology of infantile hypertrophic pyloric stenosis (IHPS) has not been fully elucidated. Since the 1990s, a sharp decline in IHPS has been reported in various countries. Recent research from Sweden reported a correlation between falling rates of IHPS and of sudden infant death syndrome (SIDS). This was attributed to a reduction in the number of infants sleeping in the prone position following the "Back to Sleep" campaign.

Objectives.—To describe the changing epidemiology of IHPS in Scotland, to examine the relationship between IHPS and SIDS rates and to examine trends in other factors that may explain the observed reduction in IHPS incidence.

Design.—Incidence rates of IHPS and SIDS were derived from routine data and their relationship analysed. Trends in mean maternal age, maternal smoking, mean birth weight and breastfeeding rates were also examined.

Setting.—The whole of Scotland between 1981 and 2004.

Results.—IHPS incidence fell from 4.4 to 1.4 per 1000 live births in Scotland between 1981 and 2004. Rates were consistently higher in males, although the overall incidence patterns in males and females were similar. Rates showed a positive relationship with deprivation. The fall in the incidence of IHPS preceded the fall in SIDS by 2 years and the incidence of SIDS displayed less variability than that of IHPS. Significant temporal trends were also observed in other maternal and infant characteristics.

Conclusion.—There has been a marked reduction in Scotland's IHPS incidence, but this is unlikely to be a consequence of a change in infant sleeping position.

▶ It has been almost 125 years since infantile hypertrophic pyloric stenosis was first described; yet its cause or causes remain unclear.[1] Recent advances in understanding the control of gastrointestinal motility have provided a better basis for identification of the disease pathways underlying infantile hypertrophic stenosis. A decline in recent years in its incidence has been reported in a number of countries leading some to suggest that this decline is related somehow to the recent decrease in the incidence of sudden infant death syndrome as the result of the "Back To Sleep" campaign. For this reason, it has been suggested that a prone sleeping position in early infancy may also be an environmental risk factor for infantile hypertrophic pyloric stenosis. If one looks carefully, however, the decline in the incidence of pyloric stenosis appears to have preceded that of the sudden infant death syndrome. As we see in the report from Scotland, a parallel decline in the prevalence of these 2 disorders has not been noted in some places such as Scotland. We do know that there has been a several-fold increase in the incidence of pyloric stenosis among infants who have received erythromycin.

Many studies have attempted to identify the etiologic factors for pyloric stenosis. A better understanding of the pathophysiology of infantile hypertrophic pyloric stenosis will no doubt come from the elucidation of its molecular genetics. Pyloric stenosis is a disease in which genetics does play a role. Given the fact that boys outnumber girls with this disorder by 4 to 1, one can presume that there is some genetics involved with the etiology. Pyloric stenosis has been associated with several genetic syndromes such as Cornelia de Lange and Smith-Limli-Opitz syndromes and chromosomal abnormalities including translocation of chromosome 8 and 17 and partial trisomy of chromosome 9. Autosomal-dominant forms of pyloric stenosis have also been reported in several families.

Five specific idiopathic hypertrophic pyloric stenosis gene loci have been identified. One of these loci encodes for nitric oxide synthase, an enzyme critical for the production of nitric oxide, which mediates relaxation of the pyloric smooth muscle. Although the etiology of infantile hypertrophic pyloric stenosis remains unclear, we are seeing more and more epidemiological and genetic studies that are starting to provide glimpses of understandings that will unravel some of the genetic and environmental factors causing this fairly common problem.

J. A. Stockman III, MD

Reference

1. Rolins MD, Shields MD, Quinn RJN, et al. Pyloric stenosis: congenital or acquired? *Arch Dis Child.* 1989;64:138-147.

Recovery after open versus laparoscopic pyloromyotomy for pyloric stenosis: a double-blind multicentre randomised controlled trial

Hall NJ, Pacilli M, Eaton S, et al (UCL Inst of Child Health and Great Ormond Street Hosp, London, UK; et al)
Lancet 373:390-398, 2009

Background.—A laparoscopic approach to pyloromyotomy for infantile pyloric stenosis has gained popularity but its effectiveness remains unproven. We aimed to compare outcomes after open or laparoscopic pyloromyotomy for the treatment of pyloric stenosis.

Methods.—We did a multicentre international, double-blind, randomised, controlled trial between June, 2004, and May, 2007, across six tertiary paediatric surgical centres. 180 infants were randomly assigned to open (n=93) or laparoscopic pyloromyotomy (n=87) with minimisation for age, weight, gestational age at birth, bicarbonate at initial presentation, feeding type, preoperative duration of symptoms, and trial centre. Infants with a diagnosis of pyloric stenosis were eligible. Primary outcomes were time to achieve full enteral feed and duration of postoperative recovery. We aimed to recruit 200 infants (100 per group); however, the data monitoring and ethics committee recommended halting the trial before full recruitment because of significant treatment benefit in one group at interim analysis. Participants, parents, and nursing staff were unaware of treatment. Data were analysed on an intention-to-treat basis with regression analysis. The trial is registered with ClinicalTrials.gov, number NCT00144924.

Findings.—Time to achieve full enteral feeding in the open pyloromyotomy group was (median [IQR]) $23 \cdot 9$ h ($16 \cdot 0$–$41 \cdot 0$) versus $18 \cdot 5$ h ($12 \cdot 3$–$24 \cdot 0$; p=$0 \cdot 002$) in the laparoscopic group; postoperative length of stay was $43 \cdot 8$ h ($25 \cdot 3$–$55 \cdot 6$) versus $33 \cdot 6$ h ($22 \cdot 9$–$48 \cdot 1$; p=$0 \cdot 027$). Postoperative vomiting, and intra-operative and postoperative complications were similar between the two groups.

Interpretation.—Both open and laparoscopic pyloromyotomy are safe procedures for the management of pyloric stenosis. However, laparoscopy has advantages over open pyloromyotomy, and we recommend its use in centres with suitable laparoscopic experience.

▶ Pyloric stenosis has been with us a long time, as has its surgical correction technique. Back in 1912, Ramstedt first operated on a patient with pyloric stenosis showing how easy it was to perform a pyloromyotomy. This procedure is still considered a safe and effective one with an extremely low risk of complications. Nonetheless, individuals are continuously trying to improve on old surgical techniques. In 1991, the first laparoscopic pyloromyotomy was performed. This involves the introduction of small (3-5 mm) laparoscopic equipment to enable access into the abdomen of infants. A number of centers are now using this technique and the report of Hall et al describes the pros and cons of the use of laparoscopic pyloromyotomy in comparison with the traditional surgical incision technique.

Hall et al present the 3-year results of a multicenter, international comparison of laparoscopic versus open pyloromyotomy in 180 infants. The primary outcome measures were timed to achievement of full enteral feeds and the duration of postoperative hospital stay. The infants who had laparoscopic pyloromyotomy achieved full enteral feeds significantly more quickly and were discharged significantly earlier than infants who had open pyloromyotomy. These outcomes were achieved with no increase in intraoperative and postoperative complications. Parents or care providers also stated a significantly higher satisfaction score with cosmetic appearance of the surgical wounds. In fact, the trial was stopped early on the recommendations of the data monitoring and ethics committee in review of the statistically significant advantages of laparoscopic pyloromyotomy. The debate, however, about cosmetic outcomes will continue because some believe that circumumbilical pyloromyotomy in the performance of the Ramstedt procedure (where an incision is made around the umbilicus) is cosmetically better because the scar is almost totally hidden. With the laparoscopic technique, one will see 2 small puncture scars that are the accessory ports for the surgical technique.

If there is any downside to a laparoscopic pyloromyotomy and its use in children, it is the fact that it is a more difficult procedure to teach young physicians because only 1 set of hands can be the "driver." Thus, although a surgical attending may be in attendance, a resident in training will in essence be performing the procedure if allowed to because the attending will merely be able to observe. As of now, a higher proportion of laparoscopic than open procedures are being done by nontrainees because of lack of operative experience of trainees. This is true of laparoscopic techniques in general.

Overall, the data from this report do suggest that laparoscopy has several advantages over open pyloromyotomy without the occurrence of additional complications or negative cost implications. This large study, therefore, strongly recommends the use of this technique in centers that have suitable experience.

J. A. Stockman III, MD

Circumumbilical pyloromyotomy in the era of minimally invasive surgery
Cozzi DA, Ceccanti S, Mele E, et al (University of Rome "La Sapienza", Italy)
J Pediatr Surg 43:1802-1806, 2008

Purpose.—No studies have investigated the cosmetic outcome of current approaches to pyloromyotomy in infants with hypertrophic pyloric stenosis. The purpose of this study was to evaluate the final appearance of the scar in patients undergoing circumumbilical pyloromyotomy.

Methods.—During a 16-year period, 86 infants underwent circumumbilical pyloromyotomy at our institution. A detailed questionnaire was created to document the family members' perceptions of the esthetic appearance of the scar. Data were collected by telephone interview and at clinic visit. In addition, cosmesis was assessed by 5 staff members who scored blindly the esthetic outcome of the scars with comparative photographs, using a categorical scale.

Results.—Fifty-seven families were tracked by telephone contact. In the family questionnaire, 100% of families reported an excellent or good scar. Of these, forty-one (72%) were available for cosmetic assessment. Follow-up ranged between 5 months and 15 years (mean, 6 years). The panel members ranked the scar, on average, as excellent or good for 90% of the patients. No assessor stated that a scar was unacceptable. Intra- and interobserver agreement was 0.72 and 0.78, respectively.

Conclusions.—Overall satisfaction with the cosmetic outcome of circumumbilical pyloromyotomy is very high.

▶ This report shows that parents will go to some lengths to ensure that their offspring are cosmetically protected, even going so far as to request minimally invasive techniques for simple surgical procedures such as pyloromyotomy. The purpose of the report of Cozzi et al from Rome was to evaluate the final appearance of a scar in patients undergoing pyloromyotomy using an umbilical fold approach. This is a true surgical procedure, albeit minimally invasive, but does not require skill with an endoscope. Basically, a 180° circumlinear supraumbilical incision is made in the skin fold about the umbilicus. Through this incision, the pylorus can be delivered, obviating the need for the old-time vertical midline incision that has been used in years past. Among 57 youngsters who were followed up many years later, almost 100% of families reported a good or excellent scar. In fact, 72% of cases were available for cosmetic assessment by the surgical team who also rated the patients as having a good or excellent scar the majority of time (90%) (Fig 1). No scar was found to be unacceptable. In contrast to laparoscopic repair of pyloric stenosis, the circumumbilical pyloromyotomy has a significant cosmetic advantage in that it does not require the 2 stab incisions needed for port sites.

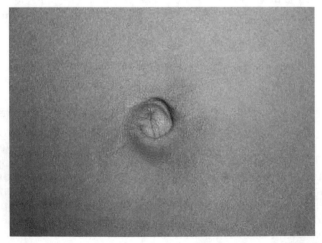

FIGURE 1.—Close-up view of an inconspicuous supraumbilical scar 7 years postoperatively. This scar was scored as an excellent result by the assessor team. (Reprinted from Cozzi DA, Ceccanti S, Mele E, et al. Circumumbilical pyloromyotomy in the era of minimally invasive surgery. *J Pediatr Surg.* 2008;43:1802-1806, with permission from Elsevier.)

The surgical technique reviewed in this report from Italy documents that there is one open surgical technique that produces better results, at least cosmetically, in comparison with more modern techniques such as laparoscopic surgery. The technique does appear to be safe, simple, and reproducible in a good surgeon's hands. It is also a procedure that can be performed essentially by any skilled personnel because it does not require specialized equipment or instrumentation. The authors conclude their report with the statement that while awaiting final answers from further randomized controlled trials with regard to safety, efficacy, cost-effectiveness, and long-term cosmesis of the laparoscopic approach, they feel that we should have second thoughts about laparoscopic techniques for pyloromyotomy because equally good and perhaps better cosmesis can be obtained with new variations of old techniques.

To read more about the laparoscopic pyloromyotomy and the perceived cosmetic benefits, see the recent report from Birmingham, Alabama.[1] In that report, 88% of parents said that they would pay an additional out-of-pocket amount for their daughter and 85% for their son to have the better cosmetic outcome after laparoscopic surgery in comparison with a vertical abdominal incision. One wonders if the money would be better spent on college tuition.

J. A. Stockman III, MD

Reference

1. Haricharan RN, Aprahamian CJ, Morgan TL, Harmon CM, Georgeson KE, Barnhart DC. Smaller scars–what is the big deal: a survey of perceived value of laparoscopic pyloromyotomy. *J Pediatr Surg.* 2008;43:92-96.

Minimally invasive closure of pediatric umbilical hernias
Feins NR, Dzakovic A, Papadakis K, (Children's Hosp Boston, MA)
J Pediatr Surg 43:127-130, 2008

Background.—Pediatric umbilical hernias may close spontaneously by concentric fibrosis and scar tissue formation. Some hernias do not close. This study was developed to assess this novel minimally invasive closure (MIC), using injectable material to close the umbilical defect.

Method.—Twenty-five children with umbilical hernias of 1.5 cm or less were included in the study. Deflux (Q Med, Uppsala, Sweden), a biodegradable compound of dextranomer microspheres in hyaluronic acid, was injected percutaneously in the border and preperitoneal space in 4 quadrants of the hernia defect, thereby occluding the lumen. Follow-up visits were obtained at approximately 1 week, 3 months, and 1 year.

Results.—Two to twenty-four months after surgery, 21 of the 25 umbilical hernias were closed (84%). To date, there have been no complications from the injected compound substance. The average age at the time of the MIC was 6 years and 7 months, ranging from 4 months to 17 years. The average defect was more than 6.4 mm, ranging from 4 to 14 mm.

Conclusion.—Minimally invasive closure procedure with injection of dextranomer hyaluronic acid copolymer can safely be used to close umbilical hernias. The procedure closed or reduced the size of hernias in our patients immediately after surgery; and within months, 21 (84%) of 25 were closed. One defect has not closed in 1 year and will need repair. The remaining 3 defects are small and may go on to close by ongoing fibroblast ingrowth and collagen deposit. The MIC procedure may be an alternative to open repair of umbilical hernias. Increased experience and long-term follow-up will determine the true efficacy of this new technique.

▶ Now we see another potential application of the agent known as Deflux, a compound of dextranomer microspheres in hyaluronic acid. This material has been used as part of the management of vesicoureteral reflux. The history behind this goes back to 1981 when the first reports appeared of the endoscopic treatment of vesicoureteral reflux as an alternative to surgery. Originally, polytetrafluoroethylene and silicone were used for subureteral injection, but concerns were raised about safety and migration of these substances. Then came along Deflux where an organic dextranomer hyaluronic acid compound was formulated with microspheres of 80µ to 250µ in size. This material is biodegradable and has no immunogenic properties nor has it been shown in extensive testing to have any malignant potential. As the material biodegrades, collagen fibers will ingrow between the microspheres. A mild granulomatous inflammatory reaction occurs as part of this process. Deflux is injected via a cystoscope into the subureteral meatal orifice. The ingrowth of fibroblasts

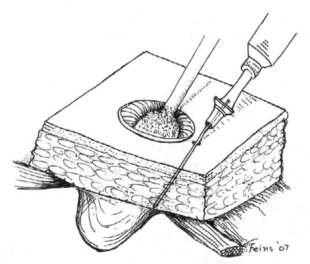

FIGURE 1.—The D/H is injected at the border of the umbilical ring in the preperitoneal space of all 4 quadrants obliterating the defect, using a 25-gauge needle with approximately 1 mL per injection. A Q-tip will define the borders, reduce the hernia contents, and facilitates the injection at the 12-o'clock and 3-o'clock positions. It is usually removed for the injections at the 6-o'clock and 9-o'clock positions. (Reprinted from Feins NR, Dzakovic A, Papadakis K, et al. Minimally invasive closure of pediatric umbilical hernias. *J Pediatr Surg.* 2008;43:127-130, with permission from Elsevier.)

and collagen corrects vesicoureteral reflux in up to 80% of patients without the need for surgery.

Now we see Deflux being used to treat umbilical hernias. The concept behind this actually goes back more than 60 years when attempts were first made to use sclerosing agents in an attempt to close inguinal hernias. More recently, Deflux has been used as part of the management of this problem. We see in this report that in the usual age group in which children are treated (4 to 5 years of age or older), successful closure of an umbilical hernia defect occurs in almost 85% of patients. Precise placement of the compound in the preperitoneal space surrounding the hernia to obliterate the defect is imperative for a successful closure (Fig 1). The procedure seems to be very well tolerated with no adverse side effects. Obviously the compound is substantially more expensive than conventional sutures, but the minimally invasive nature of the technique offsets most of the cost, and also there is no need for general anesthesia.

Sooner or later we will be seeing Super Glue used for the same purpose; you can count on it.

J. A. Stockman III, MD

Post-Infectious Functional Gastrointestinal Disorders in Children

Saps M, Pensabene L, Di Martino L, et al (Children's Memorial Hosp, Chicago, IL; Univ Magna Graecia, Catanzaro, Italy; Santo Bono Hosp, Naples, Italy; et al)
J Pediatr 152:812-816, 2008

Objective.—To investigate the development of functional gastrointestinal disorders (FGIDs) after an episode of acute bacterial gastroenteritis (AGE) in children.

Study Design.—A cohort study of children 3 to 19 years old with a positive result on a bacterial stool culture. 44 patients in each arm (unidirectional α of 0.05, power of 0.80). Children presenting at two pediatric hospitals (United States and Italy) for AGE who tested positive for bacteria on stool culture (2001-2005) were contacted at least 6 months after the episode. Exposed children were matched with control subjects of similar age and sex consulting to the same hospitals for trauma or well-child visit within 4 weeks of the index case. Symptoms were evaluated with a validated questionnaire for FGIDs assessing pain, diarrhea, and disability.

Results.—88 patients (46 boys; mean age, 8.1 years; age range, 3-19 years) were recruited. Bacteria included Salmonella (54%), Campylobacter (32%), and Shigella (14%). 36% of exposed patients and 11% of control subjects complained of abdominal pain ($P < .01$). 87% had irritable bowel syndrome and 24% had dyspepsia. 56% reported onset of pain following the AGE.

Conclusion.—There is a significant increase in cases of FGIDs after bacterial infections in children.

▶ This report documents that the effects of bacterial enteritis can linger on long after the acute infectious episode has ended. This report suggests that once one experiences an episode of bacterial enteritis, there is a high risk for the subsequent occurrence of a prolonged period of a functional gastrointestinal disorder (FGID). One of the most common FGID is the irritable bowel syndrome (IBS). Recent studies have shown that IBS can develop as a consequence of an acute gastrointestinal infection. Despite the high prevalence and morbidity of both acute gastroenteritis and FGID, the possible relation between these conditions in children has yet to have been investigated. Establishing a link between these conditions could lead to modifications of our current approach to the initial management of gastrointestinal infections.

These investigators have examined a large number of children in follow-up of an episode of acute bacterial gastroenteritis. Children presenting at 2 hospitals (Children's Memorial Hospital in Chicago and the Federico II School of Medicine in Naples, Italy) who had a bacterial enteritis documented by stool culture were followed up to see if they developed FGID, including IBS. The most common bacteria recovered included *Salmonella* (54%), *Campylobacter* (32%), and *Shigella* (14%). These data are totally consistent with preliminary data from other studies. Most importantly, it would appear that the FGID does not necessarily subside with time out from the occurrence of the bacterial enteritis.

If one recognizes that there are more than 200 million cases of diarrheal illness here in the United States each year, a significant proportion of which are occurring in children, and that many of these are due to *Salmonella*, *Shigella*, and *Campylobacter*, you can readily recognize the potential consequences on the occurrence of IBS. Giving someone a case of bacterial enteritis can therefore be the gift that lingers on. Indeed, this editor in his mid-30s contracted a case of *Salmonella* enteritis from 2 of his children who got this infection from contaminated commercially bottled milk. He has been left with the inability to tolerate any form of red or white wine, a rare but long-term consequence of bacterial enteritis. Adults all too frequently get bacterial enteritis from their kids. This is like insanity, also a disorder inheritable from your kids.

Needless to say, if one of the long-term consequences of bacterial enteritis is this high risk of functional gastrointestinal disorder, we need to rethink our early management of a bacterial enteritis. The pathophysiologic link between bacterial enteritis and long-term sequelae remains elusive, but the question does arise whether we should be more aggressive in eliminating pathogenic bacteria or perhaps starting to use probiotics early in the course of a bacterial enteritis. Obviously, we need to learn much more about the specific mechanism of this linkage.

This commentary closes with a *Clinical Fact/Curio* about a common GI problem, lactose intolerance. Are you aware of the consequence of thinking you are milk intolerant when you really are not? It appears that girls who think they are milk intolerant (and thus are more likely to cut dairy foods from their diet) actually consume on average 212 mg of calcium a day less than those who do not. A survey of 13-year-olds found that almost half of those who thought they were intolerant were proven, on hydrogen breath testing, not to be lactose intolerant.[1] Self-imposed restriction of dairy foods because of perceived milk intolerance occurred at ages as young as 10 years. This erroneous belief is without question associated with a greater risk of the development of diminished spinal bone mineral content and a later risk of osteoporosis.

J. A. Stockman III, MD

Reference

1. Matlik L, Savaiano D, McCabe G, VanLoan M, Blue CL, Boushey CJ. Perceived milk intolerance is related to bone mineral content in 10- to 13-year-old female adolescents. *Pediatrics.* 2007;120:e669-e677.

Increased Gastrointestinal Permeability and Gut Inflammation in Children with Functional Abdominal Pain and Irritable Bowel Syndrome

Shulman RJ, Eakin MN, Czyzewski DI, et al (Baylor College of Medicine, Houston, TX; The A.I. duPont Hosp for Children, Wilmington, DE; et al)
J Pediatr 153:646-650, 2008

Objectives.—To determine gastrointestinal (GI) permeability and fecal calprotectin concentration in children 7 to 10 years of age with functional abdominal pain and irritable bowel syndrome (FAP/IBS) versus control subjects and ascertain potential relationships with pain symptoms and stooling.

Study Design.—GI permeability and fecal calprotectin concentration were measured. Children kept a 2-week diary of pain episodes and stooling pattern.

Results.—Proximal GI permeability was greater in the FAP/IBS group (n = 93) compared with control subjects (n = 52) (0.59 ± 0.50 vs 0.36 ± 0.26, respectively; mean ± SD; $P < .001$) as was colonic permeability (1.01 ± 0.67 vs 0.81 ± 0.43, respectively; $P < .05$). Gastric and small intestinal permeability were similar. Fecal calprotectin concentration was greater in children with FAP/IBS compared with control children (65.5 ± 75.4 μg/g stool vs 43.2 ± 39.4, respectively; $P < .01$). Fecal calprotectin concentration correlated with pain interference with activities ($P = .01$, $r^2 = 0.36$). There was no correlation between GI permeability and pain related symptoms. Neither permeability nor fecal calprotectin correlated with stool form.

Conclusions.—Children with FAP/IBS have evidence of increased GI permeability and low-grade GI inflammation, with the latter relating to the degree to which pain interferes with activities.

▶ Many of us were trained at a time when the term "functional abdominal pain" implied that a child had a psychological cause for their abdominal pain. We have come a long way in our thinking, however, about both functional abdominal pain and the irritable bowel syndrome. The report of Shulman et al expands our knowledge of functional abdominal pain and irritable bowel syndrome by exploring the relationship of subclinical inflammation and its relationship to chronic pain in the GI tract. The investigators looked at 93 children with functional abdominal pain/irritable bowel syndrome, recruited from both general and subspecialty practices and compared these youngsters with several dozen healthy children recruited from the same pediatricians through a medical chart review. The investigators looked at differences in GI permeability and gut inflammation between these groups. Gastric permeability was measured by assessing the absorption of various sugars (sucrose, lactulose, mannitol, and sucralose). These sugars were given by mouth and the amount that appeared in the urine determined whether these sugars had leaked across the GI tract intact. The greater amount of these sugars that appeared in the urine, the more likely the gut had become permeable. With respect to gut inflammation, fecal calprotectin quantities were measured in stool. It is well known from studies of inflammatory bowel disease that fecal calprotectin adequately reflects the amount of bowel wall inflammation.

The findings from this report show that proximal GI permeability as well as colonic permeability, is significantly greater in youngsters with functional abdominal pain/irritable bowel syndrome compared with controls. Fecal calprotectin was also significantly higher in the functional abdominal pain/irritable bowel syndrome group. The fecal calprotectin concentration was shown to correlate with pain interference with normal activities.

If you are not familiar with the protein calprotectin, it is found in neutrophils and monocytes and in recent years has been shown to be a noninvasive marker of persistent gastrointestinal complaints. In pediatric patients with undiagnosed gastrointestinal symptoms, elevated fecal calprotectin is an accurate marker of colorectal inflammation and is helpful in selecting patients who require colonoscopy to exclude inflammatory bowel disease. With an upper reference limit of 50 μg/g, calprotectin stool testing has a sensitivity of 95%, a specificity of 93%, positive predictive value of 95%, and a negative predictive value of 93% in the assessment of whether a patient has bowel wall inflammation.

This report is important because it does increase our understanding about the presence of subclinical inflammation in a common pediatric practice disorder, functional abdominal pain/irritable bowel syndrome. As many as 20% of school-age children are thought to have this problem. Now we have better ways of thinking about the disorder and its pathophysiology. This should lead to improved diagnostic techniques, but more importantly, to more therapeutic options. For more on this topic, see the important and excellent editorial that accompanied the Shulman et al report, this by Roussef and Perez.[1]

J. A. Stockman III, MD

Reference

1. Roussef NN, Perez ME. When there is smoke, there may be fire: functional abdominal pain and the role of inflammation. *J Pediatr.* 2008;153:594-596.

Effect of fibre, antispasmodics, and peppermint oil in the treatment of irritable bowel syndrome: systematic review and meta-analysis
Ford AC, Talley NJ, Spiegel BMR, et al (McMaster Univ, Hamilton, Ontario, Canada; Mayo Clinic, Florida, Jacksonville; UCLA/VA Ctr for Outcomes Res and Education, CA; et al)
BMJ 337:a2313, 2008

Objective.—To determine the effect of fibre, antispasmodics, and peppermint oil in the treatment of irritable bowel syndrome.

Design.—Systematic review and meta-analysis of randomised controlled trials.

Data Sources.—Medline, Embase, and the Cochrane controlled trials register up to April 2008.

Review Methods.—Randomised controlled trials comparing fibre, antispasmodics, and peppermint oil with placebo or no treatment in adults with irritable bowel syndrome were eligible for inclusion. The minimum duration of therapy considered was one week, and studies had to report either a global assessment of cure or improvement in symptoms, or cure of or improvement in abdominal pain, after treatment. A random effects model was used to pool data on symptoms, and the effect of therapy compared with placebo or no treatment was reported as the relative risk (95% confidence interval) of symptoms persisting.

Results.—12 studies compared fibre with placebo or no treatment in 591 patients (relative risk of persistent symptoms 0.87, 95% confidence interval 0.76 to 1.00). This effect was limited to ispaghula (0.78, 0.63 to 0.96). Twenty two trials compared antispasmodics with placebo in 1778 patients (0.68, 0.57 to 0.81). Various antispasmodics were studied, but otilonium (four trials, 435 patients, relative risk of persistent symptoms 0.55, 0.31 to 0.97) and hyoscine (three trials, 426 patients, 0.63, 0.51 to 0.78) showed consistent evidence of efficacy. Four trials compared peppermint oil with placebo in 392 patients (0.43, 0.32 to 0.59).

Conclusion.—Fibre, antispasmodics, and peppermint oil were all more effective than placebo in the treatment of irritable bowel syndrome.

▶ We are seeing more and more use of complementary and alternative medicines related to the care of children. This report of Ford et al tells us about some interesting ways that one might attempt to manage the irritable bowel syndrome.

Irritable bowel syndrome is obviously a common condition with a community prevalence of 10% to 15% of the general population if one looks at both children and adults. The disorder is difficult to treat, hence the wide range of treatments used—dietary exclusion, fiber supplements, and probiotics; antispasmodic drugs, antidiarrheal agents, and laxatives; antidepressants, hypnotherapy, and cognitive behavioral therapy. The report of Ford et al summarizes data from the literature on the effects of 3 different agents—fiber, antispasmodic drugs, and peppermint oil. The report represents a systematic review and meta-analysis that includes data on more than 2500 subjects with irritable bowel syndrome.

The data from this report would appear to indicate there is good news for patients with irritable bowel who are treated with fiber, antispasmodics, and peppermint oil. However, as always, the devil is in the detail and if one scratches the surface, one can see that detail. Although trials of fiber do show an overall benefit, analysis of the effect of different kinds of fiber show that bran is not effective and that only ispaghula significantly reduces symptoms. Thus, insoluble fiber (such as bran) does not work well; soluble fiber possibly may. As far as antispasmodic agents are concerned, the best evidence for any benefit lies with the use of hyoscine. Hycosine butylbromide is an antimuscarinic agent extracted from the corkwood tree. In many places of the world it is available without prescription, including the United States. Peppermint oil is also available without a prescription and also seems to be a promising agent for the management of irritable bowel syndrome.

As you might suspect, the data from the Ford et al report relate to information obtained largely from adult studies. Many, however, will be tempted to apply the information to children. Unfortunately, the agents discussed in this report are by and large relatively safe if taken as directed. Thus, one might contemplate their use in the management of irritable bowel syndrome patients.

J. A. Stockman III, MD

Natural History of Paediatric Inflammatory Bowel Diseases Over a 5-Year Follow-up: A Retrospective Review of Data From the Register of Paediatric Inflammatory Bowel Diseases
Newby EA, Croft NM, Green M, et al (Countess of Chester Hosp, UK; St. Bartholomew's and the London Hosp, UK; Leicester Royal Infirmary, UK; et al)
J Pediatr Gastroenterol Nutr 46:539-545, 2008

Objectives.—The natural history of paediatric inflammatory bowel diseases (IBDs) is poorly understood. We aim to describe the disease course in this cohort and generate prognostic information for patients and clinicians.

Materials and Methods.—Patient records from 6 tertiary paediatric gastroenterology centres were reviewed to generate data concerning original diagnosis, change in diagnosis, family history, surgical interventions, growth, and presence of extragastrointestinal manifestations.

Results.—Data were collected on 116 children with Crohn disease (CD), 74 with ulcerative colitis (UC), and 20 with indeterminate colitis (IC), followed for a mean period of 3.42, 3.3, and 2.9 years from date of diagnosis, respectively. A male predominance is demonstrated in CD. Revision of diagnosis in patients with IC is mainly to UC, with most children receiving a definitive diagnosis within 2 years of initial presentation. Of the children with UC, 17.6% underwent 1 or more major operations with a median time to surgery of 1.92 years. Of children with CD, 11.6% underwent 1 or more major intraabdominal procedures with a median time to surgery of 1.83 years. We recorded a positive family history in 2.7%, 8.2%, and 10% of cases for CD, UC, and IC, respectively. For both boys and girls with CD, but only for boys with UC, height standard deviation score became more negative over time.

Conclusions.—This retrospective study quantifies certain distinctions between IBDs diagnosed in paediatric and adult populations. We document a trend toward male predominance in children with CD. We also note impaired linear growth in children with CD, whereas it appears maintained in girls with UC. We also have recorded a low incidence of IBDs in the families of this cohort and suggest that environmental influences may be of greater importance. We document that major intraabdominal surgery may be required in about 15% of patients with either UC or CD within 2 years of diagnosis, and that the majority of those diagnosed initially with IC will be reclassified as either UC or CD within 2 years.

► This report from Great Britain is a great one, outlining the natural history of pediatric inflammatory bowel disease (IBD). The investigators use this data from the register of pediatric IBD, which collects information from children at 50 hospitals throughout the United Kingdom. You might want to read this report in some detail to get a comprehensive update on the natural history of this disease in the context of modern therapies.

There are many new therapies to manage IBD, particularly Crohn's disease. In the past few years, antagonists of tumor necrosis factor have resulted in unforetold therapeutic benefits in Crohn's disease, but the magnitude and duration of responses have been variable in both children and adults. Thus the need for new agents. The traditional view of the pathogenesis of Crohn's disease is that intestinal inflammation is mediated by cells of the acquired immune system, with overly aggressive activity of effector lymphocytes and proinflammatory cytokines. Emerging evidence suggests that the disease process entails a dysregulated relationship between the intestinal microbiota and components of both the innate and adaptive immune systems. Investigators have long sought to identify a microorganism that causes IBD. Some have suggested that an imbalance between protective and harmful bacteria (dysbiosis) is the trigger. Recent studies have emphasized the potential importance of adherent invasive *Escherichia coli* in the initiation and maintenance of inflammation in Crohn's disease.

Treatment of IBD is now undergoing a transition from the era of tumor necrosis factor antagonists to an era of novel biological agents, including those that are able to stimulate the innate immune system. Clinicians are also working on new strategies aimed at modification of the natural history of Crohn's disease, by including an aggressive therapeutic approach. There is a lot going on, and patient safety concerns pop up frequently when it comes to IBD treatment. Most of us only recently learned about tumor necrosis factor antagonists, and now we are off and running with additional learnings about novel biological agents. To read more about this, see the extensive review by Peyrin-Viroulet et al.[1]

J. A. Stockman III, MD

Reference

1. Peyrin-Biroulet L, Desreumaux P, Sandborn WJ, et al. Crohn's disease: beyond antagonists of tumor necrosis factor. *Lancet.* 2008;372:67-81.

Use of complementary medicine in pediatric patients with inflammatory bowel disease: results from a multicenter survey
Wong AP, Clark AL, Garnett EA, et al (Univ of California, San Francisco)
J Pediatr Gastroenterol Nutr 48:55-60, 2009

Objectives.—We examined the use of complementary and alternative medicine (CAM) at 3 US pediatric medical centers, comparing a group of children with inflammatory bowel disease (IBD) with children presenting with chronic constipation.

Materials and Methods.—Surveys were administered by postal mail and at pediatric IBD centers in San Francisco, Houston, and Atlanta from 2001 to 2003. A comparison group consisting of pediatric patients with chronic constipation also was surveyed. Data were analyzed by t tests and by exact tests of contingency tables.

Results.—In all, 236 surveys were collected from the IBD group; 126 surveys were collected from the chronic constipation comparison group. CAM therapies were used by 50% in the IBD group and 23% in the chronic constipation group. The overall regional breakdown of CAM use in IBD revealed no differences, although the types of CAM therapy used varied by site. The most commonly used CAM therapies in the IBD group were spiritual interventions (25%) and nutritional supplements (25%). Positive predictors for CAM use in IBD include the patient's self-reported overall health, an increase in the number of side effects associated with allopathic medications, white ethnicity, and parental education beyond high school.

Conclusions.—This is the first US study to characterize CAM use in pediatric patients with IBD with another chronic gastrointestinal disorder. CAM use was twice as common with the IBD group compared with the chronic constipation group. Regional variations exist with the types of CAM therapy used. Practitioners should know that half of their pediatric patients with IBD may be using CAM in conjunction with or as an alternative to other treatments and that certain predictors can help identify those using CAM therapies.

▶ We are seeing more and more use of complementary and alternative medicine (CAM) in pediatric illnesses that are chronic. The National Institutes of Health defines CAM as a group of diverse medical and healthcare systems, practices, and products that are not presently considered to be part of conventional medicine. When prayer is included in the definition of CAM, some 62% of adults have used some form of CAM within the preceding 12 months.[1] This drops to 36% when prayer is excluded. When it come to adult inflammatory disease, there are numerous studies that have looked at the value of CAM, but data on its use in pediatrics has been quite limited, at least until this report of Wong et al appeared. Astoundingly, CAM therapies have been used in 50% of children with inflammatory bowel disease. The most common CAM intervention was spiritual therapy (25%) and almost as common was the use of unprescribed nutritional supplements. Unfortunately, in most instances these therapies were complementary to the traditional medicines that were being prescribed to treat the inflammatory bowel disease.

On a peripherally related topic, you might want to read the excellent invited review by Brent et al, which discusses psychological treatments for functional gastrointestinal disorders and children.[2] The number of psychological treatment outcome studies for pediatric functional gastrointestinal disorders has grown quite markedly in the last dozen or so years. These treatment outcomes are nicely summarized in the invited review and well worth your reading.

J. A. Stockman III, MD

References

1. Barnes PM, Powell-Griner E, McFann K, et al. Complementary and alternative medicine use among adults: United States, 2002. Advanced data report number 343 Centers for Disease Control and Prevention, http://nccam.nih.gov/news/report.pdf. Accessed January 30, 2009.
2. Brent M, Lobato E, Leiko N. Psychological treatments for pediatric functional gastrointestinal disorders. *J Pediatr Gastroenterol Nutr.* 2008;48:13-21.

Transition of adolescents with inflammatory bowel disease from pediatric to adult care: a survey of adult gastroenterologists

Hait EJ, Barendse RM, Arnold JH, et al (Children's Hosp Boston, MA)
J Pediatr Gastroenterol Nutr 48:61-65, 2009

Objectives.—Transition of patients with inflammatory bowel disease (IBD) from pediatric to adult providers requires preparation. Gastroenterologists for adult patients ("adult gastroenterologists") may have expectations of patients that are different from those of pediatric patients. We sought to explore the perspectives of adult gastroenterologists caring for adolescents and young adults with IBD, to improve preparation for transition.

Materials and Methods.—A survey sent to 1132 adult gastroenterologists caring for patients with IBD asked physicians to rank the importance of patient competencies thought necessary in successful transition to an adult practice. Providers reported which problems occurred in patients with IBD transitioning to their own practice. Adult gastroenterologists were asked about medical and developmental issues that are unique to adolescence.

Results.—A response rate of 34% was achieved. Adult gastroenterologists reported that young adults with IBD often demonstrated deficits in knowledge of their medical history (55%) and medication regimens

(69%). In addition, 51% of adult gastroenterologists reported receiving inadequate medical history from pediatric providers. Adult providers were less concerned about the ability of patients to identify previous and current health care providers (19%), or attend office visits by themselves (15%). Knowledge of adolescent medical and developmental issues was perceived as important by adult gastroenterologists; however, only 46% felt competent addressing the developmental aspects of adolescents.

Conclusions.—For successful transition, adolescents and young adults with IBD need improved education about their medical history and medications. Pediatric providers need to improve communication with the receiving physicians. In addition, adult providers may benefit from further training in adolescent issues. Formal transition checklists and programs may improve the transition of patients with IBD from pediatric to adult care.

▶ The transition of care for adolescents with chronic medical illnesses into the adult care system is fraught with many problems. All too often pediatric practitioners, both generalists and subspecialists, tend to "hang on to" these patients far beyond what otherwise might be appropriate age for provision of care. There are important differences between pediatric and adult systems of care. Pediatric care tends to be much more family focused, with parents involved in decision making. Although there is a lot of talk about the "medical home" now in the adult community of care providers, this is yet to have translated into anything as refined as what occurs in pediatrics. In contrast to pediatric providers, adult care providers often expect a patient to be autonomous and independent and may discourage input from family members, including parents, at the time of visits. Thus, internists and pediatricians often have different expectations of what might be required of the transitional age patient such as the adolescent with a chronic illness who is moving to the adult side of the health care system. Last, all too often the types of problems children have are of the sort that adult providers may not be familiar with. A good example of this is the young adult with cystic fibrosis. When it comes to inflammatory bowel disease, however, adult providers see this disease all the time and despite different styles of provision of care, should be able to provide quite adequate care to the transitional age patient.

What we learn from this report is that adult gastroenterologists when caring for a transitional age patient with inflammatory bowel disease often identify a deficiency in a young patient's knowledge about their disease, their medical history, and the medications they are taking. Internists also seem to believe that the pediatric care providers have not given adequate instruction on the risks posed by habits common to adults such as smoking and drinking, both of which can adversely affect one's general health and therefore the state of the patient's inflammatory bowel disease.

It is true that there is a tremendous variation in the intelligence and maturity of adolescents transitioning into adult care. Frankly, many such patients may not be able to recite their medical history in sufficient detail to allow good provision of care. This means that the pediatric care providers, in this case the gastroenterologist, must fill the gap with a detailed and informative medical summary, both to the patient and to the adult provider.

There is actually a fair paucity of information about transition of care of patients with inflammatory bowel disease. This is a circumstance that is very different than the literature on the related subject of transition of care of patients having congenital heart disease, type 1 diabetes mellitus, cystic fibrosis, sickle cell disease, and organ transplantation. Each of these diseases have common features regarding the difficulties associated with transition of care, but at the same time each of these diseases has unique differences that are substantial as well as subtle. Thus it is incumbent upon us to really refine our understanding about the transition of care of children with most every type of chronic illness. Clearly, more research is needed in this regard. Many in pediatrics do not recognize that there are more adults now with congenital heart disease than there are children given the survival status of the disease conditions associated with congenital heart disease. Also, given the fact that survivorship of patients with cystic fibrosis now approaches 50 years, there are almost as many adults with this disease as there are children. Given such facts, we cannot ignore this problem any longer. At the same time, our adult counterparts cannot either.

J. A. Stockman III, MD

Quality of life in adolescents with treated coeliac disease: influence of compliance and age at diagnosis

Wagner G, Berger G, Sinnreich U, et al (Med Univ of Vienna, Austria)
J Pediatr Gastroenterol Nutr 47:555-561, 2008

Objective.—To assess the influence of gluten-free diet (GFD) compliance on the quality of life (QOL) of adolescents with coeliac disease (CD), and the impact of patient's age at time of diagnosis.

Study Design.—Participants included 365 subjects: 283 adolescents (10-20 years old) with biopsy-proven CD and 82 adolescents without a chronic condition matched for age, sex, education, and social status. Their subjective QOL-comprising physical, mental, and social dimensions as defined by the World Health Organization-was measured and has been analyzed according to compliance status and age at CD diagnosis.

Results.—Adolescents noncompliant with GFD reported a lower general QOL, more physical problems, a higher burden of illness, more family problems, and more problems in leisure time than adolescents who are compliant with GFD. More frequent GFD transgressions were associated with poorer QOL. Higher problem anticipation and higher feelings of "ill-being" were found in the noncompliant group. No differences between compliant patients with CD and adolescents without any chronic condition were found in all QOL aspects. Adolescents with a late CD diagnosis showed more problems at school and in social contact with peers, as well as worse physical health and higher CD-associated burden.

Conclusions.—Compliance with GFD is an essential factor to obtain optimal QOL. Psychosocial and educational support should be provided for patients having difficulties strictly adhering to GFD. Early CD onset and diagnosis is associated with better physical health, lower CD-associated burden and fewer social problems, indicating the importance of the earliest CD diagnosis possible.

▶ Assessing quality of life in someone with coeliac disease is a complex process. Normally, quality of life is determined by how the disease in and of itself affects one's daily activities. When it comes to coeliac disease, there also needs to be an assessment of how the compliance with a gluten-free diet affects one's quality of life. The fact that someone with coeliac disease has a restricted variety of available foods, the fact that some of these gluten-free foods are often less palatable than comparable products in the normal diet (gluten is a crucial structure-forming component in baked products and is also important for taste and texture of other products containing flour), and that such food restrictions can make one's social life more restricted are parts of the quality of life formula. Also of concern is the fact that when compliance is good, nutrient intake is often not satisfactory because the affected patient may eat more fat (especially saturated) and sugar than might otherwise be desirable. In the long run, this type of gluten-free diet could increase the risk for other diet-related diseases. Add to this fact that vitamin and mineral content of foods is often lower in gluten-free varieties than in their gluten-containing counterparts, and you can see the wider scope of the problem. The upside, however, is the fact that while coeliac disease was once considered a rare disorder, it is fairly common now such that there have been many advances in the formulation of gluten-free cereal-based products that are both palatable and highly nutritious.

One can bet that quality of life issues in those with coeliac disease will be of increasing importance as more and more individuals are diagnosed. Screening studies show that there may be 3 to 7 undiagnosed cases for each diagnosed case of celiac disease, with as many as 2% of our population ultimately having the disorder.

The report of Wagner et al adds an enormous amount of understanding about quality of life in those affected with coeliac disease. The report represents the first time that quality of life, well-being and ill-being have been assessed in a well-defined adolescent population with coeliac disease. One of the conclusions of the report is that adolescents who are noncompliant with a gluten-free diet will experience a lower general quality of life, especially poorer physical health and a higher feeling of ill-being in general. In those who are compliant with their gluten-free diet, there was a self-perception of a good quality of life in all areas indicating that strictly adhering to a diet does not negatively affect quality of life during adolescence, a particularly vulnerable period of time for a youngster in terms of social connections. Regarding quality of life, social and psychological aspects absolutely must be taken into consideration. In doing so, lower quality of life in children with coeliac disease was observed mostly in those who were noncompliant. For those with coeliac disease who do experience problems in social contact with peers, these are mostly patients with a late diagnosis of coeliac disease. No differences between patients with an early diagnosis of coeliac disease and healthy controls and social contact with peers were observed in this report.

If there is a punch line here, it is that better physical, psychological, and social quality of life can be obtained by strict adherence to a gluten-free diet in those with coeliac disease. Also, the younger the age at diagnosis, the better the ultimate quality of life.

For more on the topic of coeliac disease and quality of life, see the excellent editorial by Hornell.[1]

J. A. Stockman III, MD

Reference

1. Hornell A. Living well with coeliac disease? *J Pediatr Gastroenterol Nutr.* 2008; 47:544-546.

Difference in Celiac Disease Risk Between Swedish Birth Cohorts Suggests an Opportunity for Primary Prevention

Olsson C, Hernell O, Hörnell A, et al (Umeå Univ, Sweden)
Pediatrics 122:528-534, 2008

Objectives.—Sweden experienced a unique epidemic of celiac disease in children <2 years of age. The epidemic was partly explained by changes in infant feeding over time and indicated a multifactorial pathogenesis. The main aim of this study was to analyze celiac disease risk in epidemic and postepidemic birth cohorts up to preschool age, to explore further the opportunity for primary prevention.

Methods.—A population-based incidence register of celiac disease in children covering the entire nation from 1998 to 2003 and part of the country back to 1973 was analyzed. European Society for Pediatric Gastroenterology, Hepatology, and Nutrition diagnostic criteria for celiac disease were used. The annual incidence rate for each age group and the cumulative incidence according to age for each birth cohort were calculated.

Results.—A considerable difference in cumulative incidences of celiac disease at comparable ages was demonstrated between birth cohorts from the epidemic and postepidemic periods. The difference persisted during the preschool years, although it decreased somewhat with age. During the last years of the follow-up period, there was again a successive increase in incidence rate among children <2 years of age.

Conclusions.—The difference in celiac disease risk between birth cohorts at comparable ages suggests an opportunity for primary prevention. This highlights the importance of further exploring the role of infant feeding and exogenous factors besides dietary gluten that might initiate or prevent disease development. Moreover, on the basis of postepidemic incidence trends, we speculate that the Swedish epidemic might not have been

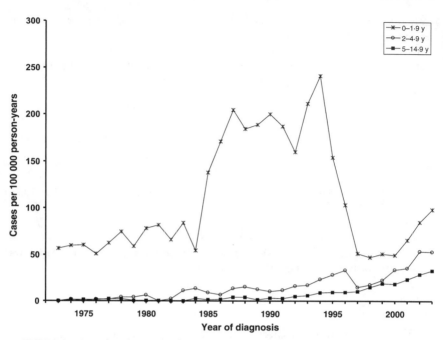

FIGURE 2.—Annual incidence rates of CD in children from 1973 to 2003. Calculations were based on retrospective data covering 15% of the Swedish childhood population during the period from 1973 to 1990, on prospective data covering 40% from 1991 to 1997, and on data with nationwide coverage from 1998 to 2003. (Reprinted from Olsson C, Hernell O, Hörnell A, et al. Difference in celiac disease risk between swedish birth cohorts suggests an opportunity for primary prevention. *Pediatrics*. 2008;122:528-534. Copyright © 2008 by the American Academy of Pediatrics.)

as unique as thought previously, although its magnitude was striking (Fig 2).

▶ It has only been in the last 20 years that we have learned just how common celiac disease is and how protean its manifestations can be. Most epidemiological studies now suggest that as many as 1 in 100 in a mixed population have celiac disease with the majority of affected individuals being unaware of the disorder they carry. The pathogenesis of celiac disease remains largely unknown, but both genetic and environmental factors seem to contribute to the problem and studies have suggested that in some cases the development of celiac disease is the result of an autoimmune problem. In any event, those with celiac disease must avoid wheat gluten and related proteins in rye and barley as these cause small-intestinal atrophy resulting in impaired nutrient absorption. The treatment of celiac disease includes life-long exclusion of all foods containing wheat, rye, and barley and adherence to a gluten-free diet will result in relief of symptoms and restore mucosal morphologic features. A recent report, however, suggests that as many as 50% of youngsters with celiac disease will not stay on a gluten-free diet.[1]

Sweden is an interesting country in which to study various patterns of prevalence of celiac disease over time. For example, unique to Sweden, the incidence of celiac disease in children less than 2 years of age showed an epidemic pattern during the period 1984 to 1996. The incidence rates in that country during that period reached levels higher than ever reported for any population. At that time, celiac disease was considered unavoidable when dietary gluten was given to genetically susceptible individuals. Therefore, both the abrupt 4-fold increase and the subsequent rapid decrease in the relatively genetically stable Swedish population was unexpected. The abrupt increase in the incidence of celiac disease in the middle 1980s resulted in a decision by the Swedish Pediatric Association to support initiation of a celiac disease epidemiological surveillance system that included a celiac disease registry It seemed as if the increase in the prevalence of celiac disease somehow related to recommendations to exclude gluten from the diet of infants. Subsequently, the decrease in celiac disease risk in infants seemed to occur when gluten was permitted to be introduced in small to medium amounts in the diet of babies who were still being breast-fed. This small/frequent introduction of gluten very early in life seemed to produce a 45% reduction in cases of celiac disease presenting symptomatically. The report of Olsson et al shows us that over time, this early protection fades and the annual incidence of celiac disease in the total childhood population ultimately reaches the same level as during the epidemic years, but with a shift toward older age at diagnosis If these data hold up, then a favorable exposure with regard to infant feeding might only delay the diagnosis because of milder symptoms, and/or individuals at risk might contract the disease at older ages anyway This would support the view that, given genetic susceptibility, celiac disease cannot be avoided in individuals exposed to gluten.

The authors of this report suggested Sweden might be facing a new epidemic of celiac disease, in as much as the incidence rate for the youngest age group increased fairly significantly in the last years studied. The bottom line is that if you are susceptible, celiac disease will catch up with you at some point.

This commentary closes with a *Clinical Fact/Curio* dealing with a disorder of the gastrointestinal tract, specifically celiac disease and its relationship to another problem. Social phobia is not yet fully accepted as a medical diagnosis, but it is creeping into academic parlance. A controlled study of social phobia in people with celiac disease reports that social phobia is significantly more prevalent in those with celiac disease in comparison with those control subjects who are healthy. Also, a higher proportion of the celiac disease population shows evidence of depression.[2]

J. A. Stockman III, MD

References

1. Jadresin O, Misak Z, Kolacek S, Sonicki Z, Zizić V. Compliance with gluten-free diet in children with celiac disease. *J Pediatr Gastroenterol Nutr.* 2008;47: 344-348.
2. Addolorato G, Mirijello A, D'Angelo C, et al. Social phobia in coeliac disease. *Scan J Gastroenterol.* 2008;43:410-415.

Fructose intolerance in children presenting with abdominal pain

Gomara RE, Halata MS, Newman LJ, et al (New York Med College, Valhalla)
J Pediatr Gastroenterol Nutr 47:303-308, 2008

Objectives.—We determined the occurrence of fructose malabsorption in pediatric patients with previous diagnoses of abdominal pain caused by a functional bowel disorder, whether the restriction of fructose intake changes the reporting of symptoms, the role of fructose dosage, and the severity of resultant symptoms.

Patients and Methods.—We administered a fructose breath test to children presenting with persistent unexplained abdominal pain. Patients randomly received 1, 15, or 45 g fructose, and breath hydrogen was measured for 3 hours after ingestion. Test results were positive when breath hydrogen was 20 ppm greater than baseline and was accompanied by gastrointestinal symptoms.

Results.—A total of 32 patients was enrolled, and none of the 9 who received 1 g had positive results. Three of 10 who received 15 g and 8 of 13 who received 45 g had positive results. All patients with positive test results restricted their fructose intake. Among the group with positive results, 9 of 11 had rapid improvement of their gastrointestinal symptoms. After 2 months, all 9 patients continued to report improvement.

Conclusions.—We concluded that fructose malabsorption may be a significant problem in children and that management of dietary intake can be effective in reducing gastrointestinal symptoms.

▶ When we think about carbohydrate intolerance as a cause of abdominal pain, lactose intolerance is what normally comes to mind. What we learn from this report, however, is that we might also be thinking about fructose intolerance. The role of fructose intolerance, though described in adults, has not been previously studied in the pediatric population.

We are seeing more and more fructose being used as a carbohydrate substitute in our diets. Fructose is a naturally occurring monosaccharide that has been increasingly used as a sweetener to process foods, particularly in the form of high-fructose corn syrups. These are a less expensive alternative to manufacture in comparison with table sugar and are being added with increasing frequency to sodas, fruit juices, and candy. Fructose, of course, is present in many naturally occurring fruits such as apples, peaches, melons, plums, cherries, pears, and oranges.

When fructose is not absorbed in the small intestine, colonic bacteria will ferment this sugar, producing hydrogen, methane, carbon dioxide, lactate, and short-chain fatty acids such as acetate, butyrate, and propionate. All this results in osmotic fluid shifts, the drawing of fluid into the bowel lumen, which causes distention of the small intestine resulting in abdominal pain and bloating. The hydrogen that is produced cannot be metabolized and is excreted in the breath or is passed as flatus. It can also be consumed by colonic bacteria. The hydrogen can be assayed in breath and is measured noninvasively in the same manner employed for the detection of lactose intolerance.

In the study of Gomara et al, 32 youngsters of both sexes with diagnoses of irritable bowel syndrome, functional dyspepsia, or functional abdominal pain syndrome were studied for fructose intolerance after being given fructose containing solutions. Breath hydrogen was examined. One-third of the patients had a definitively abnormal fructose breath hydrogen assay.

This report is important because it appears to be the first that has measured fructose malabsorption in children. Additionally, it documented that the ingestion of fructose reproduced many of the gastrointestinal symptoms these youngsters presented with. Fructose restriction also resulted in a significant decrease in the reporting of abdominal pain in subsequent weeks and months.

The authors of this report are not presuming to say that fructose intolerance is anywhere nearly as common as lactose intolerance, but they do warn us that fructose intolerance may not be a rare phenomenon. The treatment is obvious, avoidance of foods that contain excessive amounts of this sugar. Therefore, honey, dates, oranges, and drinks containing excess fructose should be avoided. Fruits that contain more glucose than fructose probably are alright (bananas and strawberries). These recommendations are made with some caution because we need more than one report warning us of the problem potentially associated with fructose ingestion to be totally convinced that another sugar must be added to the list of "intolerant" sweets.

This commentary closes with a *Clinical Fact/Curio* having to do with the consequences of too much fructose in your diet and the risk of gout. A recent cohort study by Choi and Curhan adds dietary fructose intake to the list of possible risk factors for gout.[1] Laboratory evidence that dietary fructose increases serum urate already exists and recent epidemiologic studies have found an association between dietary fructose and hyperuricemia in the United States. The analysis of Choi and Curhan has examined the role of nonalcoholic drinks and fruit on the first onset of gout. It finds a strong association between sugar-sweetened soft drinks, usually containing fructose, and gout. Consuming 2 servings a day of a sugar-sweetened soft drink increases the risk of developing gout by 85% (relative risk 1.85). This compares with an increased risk of 49% from drinking 15 g to 30 g per day of alcohol, 21% from eating an average serving of meat a day, and 95% from having a body mass index of 25.0 to 30.0 versus 21.0 to 22.9; consuming 240 ml of skim milk a day decreases the risk by 43%. A high intake of naturally occurring fructose also increases the risk of developing gout. Consuming 2 or more glasses of fruit juice each day increases the risk by 81% and eating an apple or orange a day increases the risk by 64%.

These new data suggest that dietary fructose is an important factor in the development of gout. However, the importance for public health is context specific. In the United States, soft drinks are usually sweetened with high-fructose corn syrup. In the rest of the world, soft drinks are usually sweetened with sucrose—a disaccharide consisting of fructose and glucose. High-fructose corn syrup is produced from corn syrups by enzymatic isomerization. The use of high-fructose corn syrup and thus dietary intake of free fructose has increased dramatically in the United States over the past 25 years. It is used in almost all soft drinks and in a variety of other manufactured goods. Concern exists that high-fructose corn syrup has a specific effect in promoting obesity as the rise in obesity corresponds directly with the use of such sugars. One reason may be that fructose may have less effect on satiety than other sugars. Thus far it is not entirely clear whether high-fructose corn syrup per se is a causal factor in the overweight and obesity problem as well as the high incidence of metabolic syndrome in the United States.

The reason high-fructose corn syrup is so widely used in the United States as opposed to sucrose is that the former is cheaper because of high tariffs on imported sugar and other measures used to support United States domestic sugar production. This is not true in Europe. While the United Kingdom produces only some 37 000 tons of high-fructose corn syrup, in the United States almost 8 million tons are produced annually.

Please note that the data emerging from the Choi and Curhan study should not be interpreted to mean that we should be eating less in the way of fresh fruits. Yes, it is possible that the fructose content of fresh fruit might increase the risk of gout, but the data are quite clear that fresh fruit independently reduces the risk of cardiovascular disease.

J. A. Stockman III, MD

Reference

1. Choi HK, Curhan G. Soft drinks, fructose consumption and the risk of gout in men: prospective cohort study. *BMJ.* 2008;336:309-312.

Health Utilization and Cost Impact of Childhood Constipation in the United States

Liem O, Harman J, Benninga M, et al (Nationwide Children's Hosp, Columbus, OH; Emma Children's Hosp, Amsterdam, The Netherlands; Management and Policy College of Public Health and Health Professions, Gainesville, FL)
J Pediatr 154:258-262, 2009

Objective.—To estimate the total health care utilization and costs for children with constipation in the United States.

Study Design.—We analyzed data from 2 consecutive years (2003 and 2004) of the Medical Expenditure Panel Survey (MEPS), a nationally representative household survey. We identified children who either had been reported as constipated by their parents or had received a prescription for laxatives in a given year. Outcome measures were service utilization and expenditures.

Results.—The MEPS database included a total of 21 778 children age 0 to 18 years, representing 158 million children nationally. An estimated 1.7 million US children (1.1%) reported constipation in the 2-year period. No differences with respect to age, sex, race, and socioeconomic status were found between the children with constipation and those without constipation. The children with constipation used more health services than children without constipation, resulting in significantly higher costs:

$3430/year vs $1099/year. This amounts to an additional cost for children with constipation of $3.9 billion/year.

Conclusions.—This study demonstrates that childhood constipation has a significant impact on the use and cost of medical care services. The estimated cost per year is 3 times than that in children without constipation, which likely is an underestimate of the actual burden of childhood constipation.

▶ Who would have thought that constipation would not only be a pain in the abdomen, but also a pain in the wallet? Recently, researchers evaluated the health care utilization of more than 75 000 patients with constipation enrolled in the California Medicaid program and estimated a total annual health care cost of close to $19 million for this problem.[1] In another study, Martin et al drew on 3 national surveys (the National Ambulatory Medical Care Survey, the National Hospital Ambulatory Medical Care Survey, and the 2001 National Hospital Discharge Survey) to estimate an annual cost of care of $235 million that can be directly attributed to constipation as the primary diagnosis or as the reason of health care visits.[2]

The report of Liem et al extends the knowledge we have of the cost implications of the diagnosis of constipation to the country as a whole by estimating health care utilization and cost for children with constipation using the Medical Expenditure Panel Survey (MEPS), a nationally representative survey that has been used previously to estimate health care utilization and costs in children with attention-deficit/hyperactivity disorder, influenza, and behavioral disorders.[3]

The findings from this report underscore that childhood constipation is not a laughing matter. One can extrapolate the data from this report to estimate that 1.1% of the childhood population has constipation resulting in an annual expenditure of $3362 per child, a figure that represents a $5.9 billion burden on the United States health care system. These costs are approximately 3 times that seen for the routine care of otherwise well children.

The United States government spent quite a few billion dollars getting our economy moving in 2009. At the same time, we could have saved almost $6 billion by getting something as simple as a bowel movement moving in kids at the national level. The money wasted is going down the toilet (no pun intended).

J. A. Stockman III, MD

References

1. Singh G, Lingala V, Wang H, et al. Use of healthcare resources and cost of care for adults with constipation. *Clin Gastroenterol Hepatol.* 2007;5:1053-1058.
2. Martin BC, Barghout V, Cerulli A. Direct medical cost of constipation in the United States. *Manag Care Interface.* 2006;19:43-49.
3. Guevara JP, Mandell DS, Rostain AL, et al. National estimates of health services expenditures for children with behavioral disorders: an analysis of the medical expenditure panel survey. *Pediatrics.* 2003;112:e440.

Waist circumference correlates with liver fibrosis in children with non-alcoholic steatohepatitis

Manco M, Bedogni G, Marcellini M, et al (Paediatric Hosp "Bambino Gesù", IRCCS, Rome, Italy; Liver Research Ctr Basovizza, Triesta, Italy; et al)
Gut 57:1283-1287, 2008

Objective.—Waist circumference is widely accepted as a risk factor for cardiovascular disease and metabolic syndrome. Non-alcoholic fatty liver disease (NAFLD) is a feature of the metabolic syndrome. A contribution of metabolic syndrome, and especially of waist circumference, to liver fibrosis in children with NAFLD is strongly suspected.

Design.—Cross-sectional study.

Setting.—Department of Hepatogastroenterology and Nutrition, Paediatric Hospital "Bambino Gesù", Rome, Italy.

Patients.—197 consecutive Caucasian children with NAFLD (136 males and 61 females) aged 3–19 years.

Main Outcome Measures.—Multivariale logistic regression models were used to examine the contribution of gender, age, body mass index (BMI) and metabolic syndrome components (waist circumference, high-density lipoprotein (HDL)-cholesterol, triglycerides, blood pressure and glucose) to the odds of liver fibrosis as detected by liver biopsy.

Results.—92% of the children had BMI $\geq 85^{th}$ percentile and 84% had a waist $\geq 90^{th}$ percentile for gender and age. Ten per cent of the children had metabolic syndrome and 67% had liver fibrosis, mostly of low degree. At multivariable analysis, waist was the only metabolic syndrome component to be associated with liver fibrosis. This was seen both when the components of the metabolic syndrome were coded as dichotomous (odds ratio (OR) = 2.40; 95% confidence interval (CI), 1.04 to 5.54) and continuous (OR = 2.07; 95% CI, 1.43 to 2.98 for a 5 cm increase). In the latter case, age was also associated with the outcome (OR = 0.70; 95% CI, 0.55 to 0.89 for a 1 year increase).

Conclusions.—Abdominal rather than generalised obesity contributes to liver fibrosis in children with NAFLD. Waist is also the only component of the metabolic syndrome to be associated with fibrosis in these children. Therefore, the presence of abdominal obesity is an additional criterion for the selection of children and adolescents who should undergo extensive investigation, including liver biopsy.

▶ Nonalcoholic fatty liver disease (NAFLD) is characterized by elevated intra-hepatic triglyceride content with varying degrees of inflammation and fibrosis. The prevalence of NAFLD is directly correlated with body mass index. The marked increase in the prevalence of obesity in recent years most likely is responsible for the current prevalence of NAFLD. In the United States, about 20% of adolescents are overweight (defined as BMI $\geq$ 95th percentile on the age-specific BMI-for-growth chart), and approximately one-third of these overweight children and adolescents have some degree of NAFLD. NAFLD in addition to damaging the liver is associated with insulin resistance in both children and adolescents. The intrahepatic triglyceride content is associated with dyslipidemia and insulin-resistant glucose metabolism in both the liver and skeletal muscle.[1]

One of the problems we have as pediatricians is attempting to determine just how bad the liver involvement is with NAFLD. Liver enzyme elevations provide a poor correlate with the degree of liver damage. Technically speaking, only a liver biopsy can really assess the degree of inflammation and fibrosis. For these reasons, it would be good to have a surrogate, noninvasive screening tool to tell which patients are at highest risk for serious NAFLD. The report of Manco et al helps us in this regard because it shows us that waist circumference, as one component of the metabolic syndrome, is the best indicator of liver fibrosis. The distribution of fat, both at the abdominal and dorso-cervical level appear to correlate well with liver inflammation and fibrosis. Other studies have confirmed that fat distribution particularly at the dorso-cervical level is among the most significant contributors to the severity of histological diagnosis of fibrosis of the liver.

Thus it is that while there are a number of components that define the metabolic syndrome, waist circumference among these parameters is the most diagnostic and predictive of liver disease. Why being fat in the tummy is such a predictor as opposed to generalized obesity is not clear, but the data in this regard are solid.

J. A. Stockman III, MD

Reference

1. Deivanayagam S, Mohammed BS, Vitola VE, et al. Non-alcoholic fatty liver disease is associated with hepatic and skeletal muscle insulin resistance in overweight adolescents. *Am J Clin Nutr*. 2008;88:257-262.

Wilson disease in children: analysis of 57 cases

Manolaki N, Nilkolopoulou G, Daikos GL, et al (Athens Univ, Greece)
J Pediatr Gastroenterol Nutr 48:72-77, 2009

Objectives.—Wilson disease (WD) has a wide spectrum of clinical manifestations. Affected children may be entirely asymptomatic and the diagnosis problematic. Herein we present the clinical and laboratory characteristics of 57 children with WD and point out the diagnostic difficulties in a pediatric population.

Patients and Methods.—Clinical and laboratory data were collected from 57 consecutive children with WD. Evaluation included detailed physical examination, conventional laboratory testing, genetic analysis, and liver biopsy.

Results.—The mean age at diagnosis was 9.27 ± 3.62 years (range 4 months-18 years). Twenty patients were symptomatic, 19 were referred because of abnormal liver function test results and/or hepatomegaly, and 18 received their diagnoses after family screening. Twenty-two patients had both Kayser-Fleischer ring and decreased serum ceruloplasmin levels, 13 had urinary copper excretion after penicillamine challenge >1600 microg/24 hours, and 3 had liver copper content >250 microg/g dry weight. Of the remaining 19 patients, 17 had both low serum ceruloplasmin ≤20 mg/dL and increased urinary copper excretion, >75 microg/24 hours before, or >1000 microg/24 hours after penicillamine challenge. In 2 patients with equivocal cases who had serum ceruloplasmin 26 mg/dL, the diagnosis was confirmed by genetic analysis. No correlation was found between specific mutations and the disease phenotypic expression. Chelating therapy was well tolerated, and the outcome was satisfactory.

Conclusions.—WD in children may be obscure and requires extensive investigation to establish the diagnosis. Genetic analysis is needed in equivocal cases.

▶ We should be grateful to our colleagues in Greece who have accumulated so many cases of Wilson disease in children. There is no single diagnostic test that can exclude or confirm Wilson disease with certainty; thus, the diagnosis tends to be thought of based on a combination of clinical features, laboratory findings, and the results of mutation analysis. Wilson disease is an autosomal recessive disorder, one which is characterized by a decreased biliary copper excretion and reduced incorporation into ceruloplasmin, leading to excessive copper accumulation in many organs, predominantly the liver, brain, and cornea. It is a rare inborn error of metabolism with a frequency of about 1 in 30 000 live births and a carrier frequency of 1 in 86. We do know the causative gene responsible, that having been identified in 1993. This gene consists of 21 exons and encodes a copper transporting *P*-type adenosine triphosphatase that has a high degree of similarity to the Menkes disease protein. More than 300 disease-causing mutations have been described that can cause Wilson disease.

Given the fact that the ability to make the diagnosis depends on a constellation of clinical and laboratory findings and the fact that there is no single diagnostic test for the disorder, it is incumbent upon us to be familiar with the clinical presentation. A number of investigators have suggested that a key finding is the presence of a Kayser-Fleischer ring and a low ceruloplasmin. Unfortunately for children, many of the traditional clinical symptoms seen in adults may be absent. Typical features such as the Kayser-Fleischer ring are rarely seen before 7 years of age, making the diagnosis of the disease quite a bit more difficult than in adults. This is why the report of Manolaki et al is so important because it describes the spectrum of findings in 57 pediatric patients with Wilson disease.

In this report, the mean age of the patients was 9.27 ± 3.6 years (range 4 months to 18 years) with a median age of 9 years. The presenting manifestations of the disease were as follows: jaundice in 14 of 57 patients (24.6%), epistaxis in 13 of 57 (23%), abdominal pain in 10 of 57 (17.5%), ankle edema in 7 of 57 (12.3%), ascites in 7 of 57 (12.3%), and acute Coombs-negative hemolytic anemia in 7 of 57 (12.3%). Two patients of the 57 were admitted to hospital with fulminant hepatic failure. Kayser-Fleischer rings were present in just 38% of the patients, all of whom were older than 8 years of age with the exception of a single 5-year-old asymptomatic child. The most common physical finding was hepatomegaly seen in 44 of 57 patients (77%), followed by splenomegaly in 21 of 57 (37%). A low serum ceruloplasmin was seen in 50 of 57 patients (88%). A similar percent of patients had a high urinary copper excretion. Mutation analysis showed the typical findings. Overall, just 38 of the 50 patients fulfilled the previously published traditional diagnostic criteria for Wilson disease.

This report reminds us that the presence of Kayser-Fleischer rings and a low serum ceruloplasmin constitute a sufficient set of findings to establish the diagnosis of Wilson disease. Unfortunately, this combination of findings is not always present and as we see in this report, it is actually fairly rare in young children. Only half of patients with Wilson disease who were 8 years of age or older had both Kayser-Fleischer rings and a low ceruloplasmin level. Genetic testing does not always provide the answer either since so many mutations can cause the problem. The detection of all the mutations is difficult in any one patient.

The bottom line here is that children with Wilson disease frequently go undiagnosed. The disease does require a high level of suspicion. While the average pediatrician is not likely to see very many patients with Wilson disease in her or his career, one does not want to miss this serious and life-threatening illness.

J. A. Stockman III, MD

8 Genitourinary Tract

Prevalence of Urinary Tract Infection in Childhood: A Meta-Analysis

Shaikh N, Morone NE, Bost JE, et al (Univ of Pittsburgh School of Med, PA; Univ of Pittsburgh, PA)
Pediatr Infect Dis J 27:302-308, 2008

Background.—Knowledge of baseline risk of urinary tract infection can help clinicians make informed diagnostic and therapeutic decisions. We conducted a meta-analysis to determine the pooled prevalence of urinary tract infection (UTI) in children by age, gender, race, and circumcision status.

Methods.—MEDLINE and EMBASE databases were searched for articles about pediatric urinary tract infection. Search terms included urinary tract infection, cystitis, pyelonephritis, prevalence and incidence. We included articles in our review if they contained data on the prevalence of UTI in children 0–19 years of age presenting with symptoms of UTI. Of the 51 articles with data on UTI prevalence, 18 met all inclusion criteria. Two evaluators independently reviewed, rated, and abstracted data from each article.

Results.—Among infants presenting with fever, the overall prevalence (and 95% confidence interval) of UTI was 7.0% (CI: 5.5–8.4). The pooled prevalence rates of febrile UTIs in females aged 0–3 months, 3–6 months, 6–12 months, and >12 months was 7.5%, 5.7%, 8.3%, and 2.1% respectively. Among febrile male infants less than 3 months of age, 2.4% (CI: 1.4–3.5) of circumcised males and 20.1% (CI: 16.8–23.4) of uncircumcised males had a UTI. For the 4 studies that reported UTI prevalence by race, UTI rates were higher among white infants 8.0% (CI: 5.1–11.0) than among black infants 4.7% (CI: 2.1–7.3). Among older children (<19 years) with urinary symptoms, the pooled prevalence of UTI (both febrile and afebrile) was 7.8% (CI: 6.6–8.9).

Conclusions.—Prevalence rates of UTI varied by age, gender, race, and circumcision status. Uncircumcised male infants less than 3 months of age and females less than 12 months of age had the highest baseline prevalence of UTI. Prevalence estimates can help clinicians make informed decisions regarding diagnostic testing in children presenting with signs and symptoms of urinary tract infection.

▶ Most of us tend to pursue laboratory testing when the likelihood of risk of a problem is high enough to warrant such testing. This is only common sense. More specifically, knowledge of the prevalence of urinary tract infection

155

(UTI) among different subgroups of children of various ages should guide us to determine whether further diagnostic testing is warranted, say in an infant or child presenting with fever. In children with a very low pretest probability of disease, routine diagnostic testing is not necessary. In fact, in such children an indiscriminate approach to diagnostic testing might lead to more harm than benefit as the result of false-positive laboratory results. In contrast, in children with a high pretest probability of disease, routine diagnostic testing would be appropriate. In a survey of 300 academic and community pediatricians regarding diagnostic testing in infants with unexplained fever, baseline risk was important in determining diagnostic decisions.[1] Specifically, only 10% of clinicians believe that a urine culture is indicated if the probability of UTI is >1%, whereas 80% to 90% would obtain a urine culture if the probability of disease were 3% to 5%, and all would do so if the probability exceeded 5%. To say this differently, baseline probability of a UTI makes a difference to the practicing clinician as to whether or not one should even obtain a culture of the urine in a febrile patient.

This report from Pittsburgh represents a meta-analysis of the world's literature in an attempt to integrate all the variables that would increase the risk of the likelihood of having a UTI. From a total of more than 4000 articles found through a search strategy, 330 underwent a full text review. Some 51 articles contained prevalence data, and of these, 18 articles met all the criteria for inclusion. The analysis allowed an estimate of the likelihood of UTI based on age, gender, and circumcision status. The findings were that female infants with fever have a relatively high prevalence rate of UTI, especially in the first year of life. Accordingly, it would be reasonable to consider obtaining a urine specimen from febrile girls younger than 1 year of age in virtually all circumstances. Among febrile boys, circumcision status was extremely important in determining the risk for a UTI. Uncircumcised male infants less than 3 months of age had the highest prevalence of UTI of any group, male or female, whereas circumcised males had one of the lowest rates. Among febrile male infants less than 3 months of age, just over 20% of uncircumcised males had a UTI. This finding suggests that clinicians need to carefully ascertain circumcision status in all male infants with unexplained fever. Among circumcised male infants less than 3 months of age who are febrile, the prevalence of UTI was just 2.4%. Accordingly, approximately 42 such infants will need to undergo catheterization to detect a single UTI. Although the prevalence of UTI is relatively low in this subgroup, the risk of a misdiagnosed UTI in the first few months of life (hematogenous dissemination, sepsis, and missed high-grade vesicoureteral reflux) is high. For this reason, the authors of this article recommend catheterization of all febrile male infants less than 3 months of age, at least as a consideration.

The data from this report also show that the overall prevalence of UTI among boys decreases rapidly with age. It is reasonable to assume that the prevalence of UTI among circumcised boys over 12 months of age is less than 1%.

This report from Pittsburgh is well worth reading. It may change your own approach to the management of fever in young children and infants. This commentary closes with a *Clinical Fact/Curio* having to do with the genitourinary tract. Wearing high heels might in fact enhance pelvic muscle tone, according to a small study. A urologist from the University of Verona, a self-professed lover of high heels, has found that 2 cm to 5 cm heels result in optimal pelvic floor muscle activity. If you want to tone those abs, walk on your tippy toes.[2]

J. A. Stockman III, MD

References

1. Roberts KB, Charney E, Sweren RJ, et al. Urinary tract infection in infants with unexplained fever: a collaborative study. *J Pediatr.* 1983;103:864-867.
2. Shoes and sex [editorial comment]. *BMJ.* 1999;353:27.

Delay in Diagnosis in Poststreptococcal Glomerulonephritis
Pais PJ, Kump T, Greenbaum LA (Children's Hosp of Wisconsin, Milwaukee; Emory Univ and Children's Healthcare of Atlanta, GA)
J Pediatr 153:560-564, 2008

Objective.—To determine the frequency and risk factors for diagnostic delays in children with poststreptococcal glomerulonephritis (PSGN).

Study Design.—We reviewed the charts of 52 children with PSGN, and identified children with a delay in diagnosis of more than 24 hours. We determined risk factors for delay in diagnosis using univariate and multivariate logistic regression.

Results.—17 children (33%) with PSGN had a delay in diagnosis. Delay in diagnosis occurred in 14% of children with gross hematuria as a presenting complaint and in 54% of children without gross hematuria as a presenting complaint (3.8 increased relative risk, 95% CI = 1.4 to 10; $P = .02$). A delay in diagnosis was more common in children with a negative infection history ($P = .04$). In multiple logistic regression, only the absence of gross hematuria as a presenting complaint was associated with a delay in diagnosis ($P = .01$). All children with a delay in diagnosis had microscopic hematuria on their initial urinalysis.

Conclusions.—Delay in diagnosis is common in children with PSGN, especially if visible hematuria is not a presenting complaint. Physicians should consider the possibility of PSGN in children with symptoms that may be secondary to volume overload. A urinalysis is a helpful initial diagnostic test.

▶ It sometimes can be difficult to think of a diagnosis of poststreptococcal glomerulonephritis (PSGN) in a patient presenting without hematuria, but with other signs and symptoms suggestive of PSGN. This report from the Children's Hospital of Wisconsin and Children's Healthcare of Atlanta attempts to assist us in finding out why some patients have a delay in diagnosis (the latter defined as greater than 1 day past presentation to hospital). The absence of visible hematuria as a presenting complaint is the single greatest risk factor for a delay in diagnosis even though many of the patients had other classical features of PSGN (Table 1).

Other findings from this report indicate that more than 80% of patients with PSGN had a positive ASO titer. Other studies have shown that ASO titer in patients with PSGN may be negative despite other serologic evidence of a recent streptococcal infection. Also, despite the classic textbook description that PSGN follows an episode of impetigo or streptococcal pharyngitis, the investigators in Wisconsin and Georgia found that very few patients had a history of a documented infection with group A beta-hemolytic streptococci. Even when the investigators broadened their criteria to include all patients with a history of impetigo, sore throat, or documented streptococcal infection, most patients still did not have a clinical history that was consistent with the classic description. These findings should be a strong reminder to all of us that a documented preceding streptococcal infection should not be considered an absolute criterion for the diagnosis of PSGN.

In the last couple of decades, there has been a decrease in the incidence of PSGN in children such that many newly trained pediatricians have not seen a lot of this problem and therefore tend not to think of it. The association of a delay in diagnosis associated with the absence of gross hematuria as a presenting complaint therefore is not surprising. The absence of visible hematuria makes it difficult to suspect the diagnosis of PSGN without performing additional laboratory tests. This absence of visible hematuria decreases the probability that a patient will be placed in the correct category of kidney disease, even when the presenting sign is hypertension. The authors of this report remind us that physicians tend to arrive at a provisional diagnosis based on history and that there is "tendency to look for evidence that supports an early

TABLE 1.—Children with a Delay in Diagnosis

Chief Complaint(s)	Initial Diagnosis
Altered mental status, seizures	Acute disseminated encephalomyelitis
Shortness of breath, edema	Allergies
Shortness of breath, edema	Allergies/asthma
Shortness of breath, edema	CHF due to myocarditis
Unresponsive	Encephalopathy and seizures
Hematuria	Hemolytic anemia
Headaches, blurry vision	Hypertension
Shortness of breath	Hypertension
Shortness of breath	Hypertension/pulmonary edema
Seizures	Hypertensive encephalopathy
Shortness of breath	Pneumonia
Seizures	Seizure disorder
Shortness of breath	Tonsillar hypertrophy
Hematuria	UTI
Hematuria	UTI
Hematuria	UTI
Headaches, disorientation	Viral syndrome

CHF, Congestive heart failure; URI, upper respiratory infection.
(Reprinted from Pais PJ, Kump T, Greenbaum LA. Delay in diagnosis in poststreptococcal glomerulonephritis. *J Pediatr.* 2008;153:560-564.)

working hypothesis and to ignore data that contradicts it." In the case of patients presenting with what appears to be hypertension and neurologic signs and symptoms, the hypertension is often ascribed to the central nervous system, rather than to a problem with the kidneys.

When in doubt, in those presenting with altered mental status, shortness of breath, edema, blurry vision, and headaches, even in the absence of hematuria, think renal disease as the cause.

J. A. Stockman III, MD

Risk Factors for End Stage Renal Disease in Children With Posterior Urethral Valves

DeFoor W, Clark C, Jackson E, et al (Cincinnati Children's Hosp, OH)
J Urol 180:1705-1708, 2008

Purpose.—Obstructive uropathy secondary to posterior urethral valves is an important cause of end stage renal disease in children. Early diagnosis and intervention to decrease bladder pressure and stabilize the upper urinary tract are important to delay or prevent the progression of renal insufficiency. We analyzed the records of patients with posterior urethral valves to determine risk factors that might be predictive of ultimate renal failure.

Materials and Methods.—A retrospective cohort study was performed of children presenting to our institution with a diagnosis of posterior urethral valves from 1975 to 2005. Patient demographics, clinical background, laboratory and radiographic data, and renal outcomes were abstracted from the medical record. Potential risk factors were analyzed, such as high grade vesicoureteral reflux at diagnosis, nadir serum creatinine greater than 1.0 mg/dl, urinary tract infection and severe bladder dysfunction requiring clean intermittent catheterization. Risk factors were analyzed by univariate analysis with Fisher's exact test. Those achieving significance were placed in a multivariate logistic regression model and an OR was generated.

Results.—A total of 142 patients were identified, of whom half presented in the neonatal period. Of the patients 119 had sufficient records for evaluation and mean followup was 7.2 years. A total of 15 patients progressed to end stage renal disease. The mean interval from diagnosis to end stage renal disease was 8.1 years. Of these patients 93% initially presented with vesicoureteral reflux and 87% ultimately required clean intermittent catheterization. Increased nadir creatinine was seen in 80% of cases. Multivariate analysis revealed that increased nadir creatinine and bladder dysfunction were independent risk factors for end stage renal disease (OR 71 and 8.9, respectively). Vesicoureteral reflux was also associated with an increased risk of end stage renal disease (OR 2.0), although this was not statistically significant. Urinary tract infections were not associated with end stage renal disease.

Conclusions.—Patients with posterior urethral valves and severe bladder dysfunction in whom nadir creatinine remains increased are at risk for upper urinary tract deterioration, requiring renal replacement therapy. It is unclear whether high grade vesicoureteral reflux at diagnosis may also be a poor prognostic sign. Further analysis is necessary to evaluate the effects of early aggressive bladder management on renal outcomes.

▶ The message of this report is quite clear and readily understandable. In boys with posterior urethral valves who have the latter corrected, if the serum creatinine does not promptly fall into a normal range, trouble is brewing. Specifically, if the nadir of serum creatinine is greater than 1.0 mg/dL, the likelihood of developing end-stage renal disease approaches 80% at some point in later childhood.

While the cutoff for the nadir for serum creatinine, set at 1.0 mg/dL in this report, could be construed as arbitrary, it does seem to discriminate very nicely in determining who is or is not likely to get into trouble with chronic renal failure. Please note that the serum creatinine may return totally to normal if there is unilateral reflux and severe damage to one kidney. Thus serum creatinine alone cannot give a clean bill of health in terms of preservation of bilateral renal function. When it comes to all boys presenting with posterior urethral valves, the statistics show that just 13% will progress to end-stage renal disease. The median age at this progression in this report was 8.2 years.

This commentary closes with a *Clinical Fact/Curio* having loosely to do with the genitourinary tract. A 3-cents-a-day incentive is enough to get people to do what in India? The answer is that residents in the town of Tamil Nadu, India are being paid to relieve themselves in public urinals rather than out in the open in a bid to promote good hygiene. Apparently most everyone is a taker. Town folk are earning close to $1.00 (US) per month by complying. By the way, the urine is also being collected and tested for its effectiveness as a crop fertilizer, given the nitrogen content of the liquid.[1]

J. A. Stockman III, MD

Reference

1. Penny for your... [editorial comment]. *Lancet.* 2008;372:804.

Long-Term Consequences of Kidney Donation
Ibrahim HN, Foley R, Tan L, et al (Univ of Minnesota, Minneapolis; Chronic Disease Research Group, Minneapolis)
N Engl J Med 360:459-469, 2009

Background.—The long-term renal consequences of kidney donation by a living donor are attracting increased appropriate interest. The overall evidence suggests that living kidney donors have survival similar to that of nondonors and that their risk of end-stage renal disease (ESRD) is not increased. Previous studies have included relatively small numbers of donors and a brief follow-up period.

Methods.—We ascertained the vital status and lifetime risk of ESRD in 3698 kidney donors who donated kidneys during the period from 1963 through 2007; from 2003 through 2007, we also measured the glomerular filtration rate (GFR) and urinary albumin excretion and assessed the prevalence of hypertension, general health status, and quality of life in 255 donors.

Results.—The survival of kidney donors was similar to that of controls who were matched for age, sex, and race or ethnic group. ESRD developed in 11 donors, a rate of 180 cases per million persons per year, as compared with a rate of 268 per million per year in the general population. At a mean ($\pm$ SD) of 12.2 ± 9.2 years after donation, 85.5% of the subgroup of 255 donors had a GFR of 60 ml per minute per 1.73 m² of body- surface area or higher, 32.1% had hypertension, and 12.7% had albuminuria. Older age and higher body-mass index, but not a longer time since donation, were associated with both a GFR that was lower than 60 ml per minute per 1.73 m² and hypertension. A longer time since donation, however, was independently associated with albuminuria. Most donors had quality-of-life scores that were better than population norms, and the prevalence of coexisting conditions was similar to that among controls from the National Health and Nutrition Examination Survey (NHANES) who were matched for age, sex, race or ethnic group, and body-mass index.

Conclusions.—Survival and the risk of ESRD in carefully screened kidney donors appear to be similar to those in the general population. Most donors who were studied had a preserved GFR, normal albumin excretion, and an excellent quality of life.

▶ While children are rarely kidney donors, they are not infrequently recipients of kidneys from adults, including the youngster's adult relatives. This report tells us exactly what happens on the long haul to adult kidney donors. The life expectancy of kidney donors based on early studies appears to be similar to that of nondonors or perhaps even longer. There have been concerns, however, about the longterm effects of kidney donation. The present study was undertaken to ascertain vital status and the risk of end-stage renal disease (ESRD) in a large number of kidney donors and compared these donors' health with that of controls. These donors had donated kidneys as long as 45 years before the study began. The results indicate that the lifespan of kidney donors is indeed similar to that of persons who have not donated a kidney, and that the risk of ESRD does not appear to be increased among donors and their current health seems to be similar to that of the general population. In addition, these donors' quality of life appears to be excellent.

All of us learned in medical school that uninephrectomy is followed by a compensatory increase in glomerular filtration rate in the remaining kidney of about 70% of prenephrectomy values. In the report abstracted, it was observed that this compensatory increase was higher in donors who were younger at the time of donation. There has been concern that kidney donors, who undergo a 50% reduction in renal mass with donation, might have hyper-filtration damage in addition to the normal loss of kidney function with age. This does not appear to happen based on the information from this report.

All in all, this study underscores the fact that kidney donors can be expected to have a normal life span, a normal health status that is similar to that of the general population, and an excellent quality of life with no excessive risk of ESRD. This is some of the best news that we could possibly learn since it allows us, with a high degree of confidence, to inform prospective donors who pass the initial screening for donation that they will not be harmed, on the long haul, by their generous offer of a kidney.

This commentary closes with a query related to a *Clinical Fact/Curio* about the genitourinary tract. From time to time, you cross-cover at nights and week-ends for a family physician. You are asked to see a young adult who appears in quite a state of distress with renal colic. On reviewing his chart you note that he has had oxalate stones in the past. The patient tells you that this episode and one previous one seemed to be related in time to the ingestion of a liberal amount of a specific spice. What might that spice be?

Lovers of tumeric beware. Tumeric can predispose one to the development of renal stones because of high urinary oxalate levels. Cinnamon, another spice being consumed in high supplemental doses by many these days because of its purported health benefits, does not lead to the problem. It turns out that tumeric contains a highly water soluble form of oxalate. Water solubility of this crystal seems to be the main cause of the greater urinary oxalate excretion resulting from tumeric ingestion.[1]

J. A. Stockman III, MD

Reference

1. Tang M, Larson-Meyer DE, Liebman M. Effect of cinnamon and turmeric on urinary oxalate excretion, plasma lipids, and plasma glucose in healthy subjects. *Am J Clin Nutr.* 2008;87:1262-1267.

Genetic Alterations Associated With Cryptorchidism
Ferlin A, Zuccarello D, Zuccarello B, et al (Univ of Padova, Italy; Univ of Messina, Italy)
JAMA 300:2271-2276, 2008

Context.—Cryptorchidism is the most frequent congenital birth defect in male children and represents an important risk factor for infertility and testicular cancer. Major regulators of testicular descent are the hormones insulin-like factor 3 (INSL3) and testosterone, and disruption of these pathways might cause cryptorchidism.

Objective.—To determine the frequency of genetic alterations in cryptorchidism.

Design and Setting.—Case-control study in 2 departments of pediatric surgery in Italy between January 2003 and March 2005.

Patients.—Six hundred male infants with cryptorchidism. Boys were followed up for 2 to 3 years (through January 2008) and orchidopexy was performed in those who were persistently cryptorchid. We analyzed 300 noncryptorchid male children aged 1 to 4 years as controls.

Main Outcome Measures.—Karyotype anomalies and *INSL3*, INSL3 receptor, and androgen receptor gene mutations.

Results.—The frequency of genetic alterations in boys with cryptorchidism was low (17/600 [2.8%; 95% confidence interval {CI}, 1.7%-4.5%]) and was significantly higher in participants with persistent cryptorchidism (16/303 [5.3%; 95% CI, 3.0%-8.4%]; $P = .001$) and those with bilateral cryptorchidism (10/120 [8.3%; 95% CI, 4.1%-14.8%]; $P - .001$) than in controls (1/300 [0.3%; 95% CI, 0.1%- 0.8%]). Boys with persistent cryptorchidism had a 17-fold greater odds of having a genetic alteration (odds ratio, 16.7; 95% CI, 2.2-126.5). The most common genetic findings in those with cryptorchidism were 8 cases of Klinefelter syndrome and 5 cases of mutations in the INSL3 receptor gene. Genetic alterations were not found in boys with low birth weight or low gestational age, who had frequent spontaneous descent of the testes.

Conclusion.—In a small percentage of the study population, there was a statistically significant association between bilateral and persistent cryptorchidism and genetic alterations, including Klinefelter syndrome and INSL3 receptor gene mutations.

▶ This report adds an enormous amount of new information to the knowledge base of most of us who are somewhat intellectually deprived when it comes to knowing the latest about hormone receptors, particularly how the knowledge of these interrelates to our understanding of common problems such as cryptorchidism. Recent studies have documented that major regulators of testicular descent are the Leydig cell-derived hormones insulin-like factor 3 (INSL3) and testosterone. As we have learned more about testicular descent and the identification of animal models of cryptorchidism, this knowledge has facilitated research on the possible genetic contribution to cryptorchidism. Specifically, we are learning about the links between cryptorchidism and chromosomal aberrations including mutations in INSL3/RXFP2 and in androgen receptor genes. The study of Ferlin et al screened and then followed up on a large number of boys with cryptorchidism for these gene mutations to see if there were any linkages between these mutations and the clinical expression of cryptorchidism.

The findings from this report are quite fascinating. While the overall frequency of genetic alterations in boys with cryptorchidism was found to be low (just 2.8%), boys with persistent cryptorchidism had 17-fold greater odds of having a genetic abnormality. The most common genetic findings in those with cryptorchidism included 8 cases of Klinefelter syndrome (out of some 300 cases of persistent cryptorchidism) and 5 cases of mutations in the INSL3 receptor gene. Genetic alterations were not found in those who had low birth weight or low gestational age, conditions frequently associated with cryptorchidism.

The conclusion of this report is that chromosomal aberrations do occur in some with isolated cryptorchidism, particularly in those with persistent cryptorchidism (1.6% in unilateral forms and 4.2% in bilateral forms) and that chromosomal alterations if found are largely represented by Klinefelter syndrome. It is known that the prevalence of Klinefelter syndrome in the general population runs 1 in 500 and therefore is much higher in boys who have cryptorchidism. Studies of boys with Klinefelter syndrome suggest that almost 30% will have a history of an undescended testis. It is also recognized that Klinefelter syndrome is an under-diagnosed condition, with the majority of cases not being diagnosed before puberty. Diagnosis of Klinefelter syndrome early in childhood would allow better management of these patients during puberty, preservation of fertility, and initiation of androgen replacement therapy before signs and symptoms of hypogonadism develop. Needless to say, the earliest sign of Klinefelter syndrome, therefore, may be cryptorchidism and one should be alert to the small but real chance that a boy with cryptorchidism might in fact have Klinefelter syndrome.

J. A. Stockman III, MD

Transient Asynchronous Testicular Growth in Adolescent Males With a Varicocele
Kolon TF, Clement MR, Cartwright L, et al (Univ of Pennsylvania School of Medicine, Philadelphia)
J Urol 180:1111-1115, 2008

Purpose.—We assessed the testicular growth of adolescent males followed nonsurgically for the presence of left varicocele.

Materials and Methods.—We retrospectively reviewed the charts of adolescent males with a diagnosis of unilateral left varicocele and ultrasound testis volume measurements seen during a 10-year period. A total of 161 boys underwent at least 2 testicular ultrasounds as part of the evaluation for left varicocele. Patients were excluded from study for a history of inguinal/scrotal pathology or endocrinopathy that could affect testicular size. Sonographic testicular volume was calculated using the Lambert volume (length × width × height × 0.71). The resulting volumes were compared to previously published criteria for surgical repair (15%, 20% and 2 cc size differentials).

Results.—Of the 71 boys with 3 followup ultrasounds 38 (54%) initially had a 15% or greater volume differential. After nonsurgical followup with ultrasounds for 2 years 60 boys (85%) had testicular volume differentials in the normal range (less than 15%). Of the patients 71% were spared potential surgery by size criteria and 50% were spared surgery by the same 15% volume differential criteria.

Conclusions.—Adolescent males with unilateral left varicocele often demonstrate asynchronous testicular growth that usually equalizes in time. Therefore, sonographic testicular size measurement at a single point during adolescence is insufficient to determine the need for varicocelectomy. When contemplating varicocelectomy we recommend at least 2, and preferably 3, testicular volume measurements 1 year apart to establish accurately decreased left testicular volume compared to a normal right testis.

▶ This is a quite interesting report of some significant clinical relevance. Adult men with varicocele commonly have problems with infertility and decreased testicular volume. In fact, discrepancy in size of the testes has been used as an indication for varicocele repair. In adolescents, testicular size has been used by many authors as a gauge of developing spermatogenic potential in boys with varicocele. Unfortunately, testicular size is an imperfect measure of testicular function and fertility potential. The actual measurement of testicular size is quite subjective when done solely clinically. While semen analysis can be undertaken, normal ranges are not established for this age group.

What we learn from this report by Kolon et al is that a single measurement of testicular size demonstrating a discrepancy between the testes is not a good indicator of the need for surgery in boys with varicocele. The investigators document that just as female breast development frequently occurs asynchronously, testes may also normally grow asynchronously during puberty. Of 71 patients in this report who were followed with 3 ultrasound examinations, each at lest 6 months apart, 38 exhibited a 15% or more size differential at some point during evaluation. This in tact historically has been used as the volume differential threshold for varicocele repair in the surgical literature. Two-thirds of these boys with discrepant testicular size eventually exhibited "catch-up growth" of the testes without any surgical intervention. Given these data, the authors propose that adolescent males with asymptomatic varicocele be followed with at least 2, but preferably 3, serial scrotal ultrasounds 1 year apart with testicular volumes calculated using ultrasound examination, not clinical examination alone as usually performed with Prader and Rochester orchidometers. Needless to say, if the data from this report hold up, two-thirds of boys with varicocele might be spared surgery using the criteria presented.

There are other good data now to suggest that if you really need to know testicular volume, you should do it with ultrasound, not with the clinical use of an orchidometer. This was documented in a report by Paltiel et al.[1] Dogs who were being neutered under anesthesia had their testicular volumes measured using an orchidometer followed then by ultrasound in vivo. The testes, once removed, had their volumes definitively measured by water displacement. Paltiel et al found that ultrasound measurement of testicular volume was far more accurate and precise than orchidometry. For us clinicians, orchidometers will remain the logical instrument of choice for determining testicular size, but if careful measurement is needed, there is nothing better than the use of ultrasound.

The lesson learned from this report is that testicular growth in adolescents may be similar to female breast development in that it can occur asynchronously and a single measurement of a discrepancy and size of the 2 testes should not be of great alarm. This commentary closes with another *Clinical Fact/Curio*, this having to do with the testes. In a very interesting article titled "Dissent of the Testes," investigators remind us of an earlier report about 2 chocolates, Teasers and Truffles (available largely in Great Britain), that were strikingly similar to the 8 ml bead of the orchidometer used to assess testicular volume.[2] The 8 ml bead is used by many generalists as well as endocrinologists as a hallmark of the onset of puberty in the male, since at puberty, the testes measure in volume approximately 8 ml. It was suggested, therefore, that Teasers and Truffles could be used to stage puberty in males, because of their wide availability and low cost, and needless to say are edible after the fact. Unfortunately, the manufacturer of these chocolates has changed the shape of both of these. They are now flat bottomed and even nonspecialists will note that they bare little resemblance to the human testes and are no longer of much use for assessing testicular volume. Only 1 of 6 pediatric endocrinologists felt confident that they could use the new Teasers or Truffles to gauge testicular volume relative to the 8 ml cut-off, which indicates that puberty is proceeding satisfactorily.[3]

In decrying the shift to nontesticular-like chocolates, Williams and Dharmar comment that the change in appearance is a major setback for pediatric endocrinology given the fact that both Teasers and Truffles tasted better than wooden orchidometer beads and, "we speculate, better than testes."[4] As of this writing, British physicians were encouraged to sign a petition asking the manufacturer of Teasers and Truffles to restore their former aesthetic and functional glory (a petition that could be found at chocnuts@vris.ac.uk). Nothing quite like British humor.

J. A. Stockman III, MD

References

1. Paltiel HJ, Diamond DA, DiCanzio J, Zurakowski D, Borer JG, Atala A. Testicular volume: comparison of orchidometer and US measurements in dogs. *Radiol.* 2002; 222:114-119.
2. Bhalla P, Sally P, Williams G. An inexpensive and edible aid for the diagnosis of puberty in the male: multispecies evaluation of an alternative orchidometer. *BMJ.* 2001;323:1486.
3. Tanner JM, Whitehouse RH. Clinical longitudinal standards for height, weight, height velocity, weight velocity, and stages of puberty. *Arch Dis Child.* 1976;51: 170-179.
4. Williams G, Dharmar P. Descent of the testes. *BMJ.* 2007;335:1287.

9 Heart and Blood Vessels

Prevalence of Congenital Heart Defects in Metropolitan Atlanta, 1998-2005
Reller MD, Strickland MJ, Riehle-Colarusso T, et al (Oregon Health and Science Univ, Portland; Natl Ctr on Birth Defects and Developmental Disabilities, Atlanta, GA; et al)
J Pediatr 153:807-813, 2008

Objective.—To determine an accurate estimate of the prevalence of congenital heart defects (CHD) using current standard diagnostic modalities.

Study Design.—We obtained data on infants with CHD delivered during 1998 to 2005 identified by the Metropolitan Atlanta Congenital Defects Program, an active, population-based, birth defects surveillance system. Physiologic shunts in infancy and shunts associated with prematurity were excluded. Selected infant and maternal characteristics of the cases were compared with those of the overall birth cohort.

Results.—From 1998 to 2005 there were 398 140 births, of which 3240 infants had CHD, for an overall prevalence of 81.4/10 000 births. The most common CHD were muscular ventricular septal defect, perimembranous ventricular septal defect, and secundum atrial septal defect, with prevalence of 27.5, 10.6, and 10.3/10 000 births, respectively. The prevalence of tetralogy of Fallot, the most common cyanotic CHD, was twice that of transposition of the great arteries (4.7 vs 2.3/10 000 births). Many common CHD were associated with older maternal age and multiple-gestation pregnancy; several were found to vary by sex.

Conclusions.—This study, using a standardized cardiac nomenclature and classification, provides current prevalence estimates of the various CHD subtypes. These estimates can be used to assess variations in prevalence across populations, time, or space.

▶ Most congenital heart defect (CHD) prevalence estimates are based on data from population-based birth defects surveillance systems that were established quite some time ago. If one takes all types of CHD combined, the range of CHDs seems to be 60 to 105 CHDs per 10 000 births. Obviously, routine utilization of echocardiography has significantly enhanced the ability to diagnose CHD, particularly when it comes to minor abnormalities such as small VSDs in asymptomatic infants. Much of the variation that exists in the prevalence

TABLE 1.—Definitions of Congenital Heart Defects with Inclusion and Exclusion Criteria

Defect Group	Definition
Left-to-right shunts	
Ventricular septal defect (VSD)	Includes type 2 (perimembranous), type 4 (muscular), type 1 (subarterial, conoseptal, infundibular, supracristal), and unspecified types of VSD. Excludes VSD with interrupted aortic arch type B or cyanotic defects.
Atrial septal defect (ASD)	Includes secundum, sinus venosus, and unspecified types of ASD >4 mm in size. Excludes patent foramen ovale and obligatory shunts.
Atrioventricular septal defect (AVSD)	Includes complete, intermediate, and unbalanced AVSD and those associated with tetralogy of Fallot, ostium primum atrial septal defect, and type 3 (inlet) ventricular septal defect.
Complete atrioventricular septal defect	Includes complete atrioventricular septal defect.
Patent ductus arteriosus (PDA)	Includes term infants (≥36 weeks' gestation) with patent ductus arteriosus persisting for ≥6 weeks after delivery. Excludes obligatory shunt lesions or if maintained by prostaglandin infusion.
Cyanotic congenital heart defects	
Tetralogy of Fallot (TOF)	Includes typical TOF, TOF with absent pulmonary valve, pulmonary atresia with ventricular septal defect, pulmonary atresia with major aortopulmonary collateral arteries, and TOF-type double-outlet right ventricle.
Transposition of the great arteries (TGA)	Includes concordant atrioventricular connections and discordant ventricular arterial connections, with or without ventricular septal defect or left ventricular outflow tract obstruction. Also includes double-outlet right ventricle with malpositioned great arteries.
Discordant atrioventricular connections	Includes discordant atrioventricular and ventriculo-arterial connections (congenitally corrected transposition of the great arteries), with or without ventricular septal defect or outflow tract obstruction; and discordant atrioventricular with concordant ventriculo-arterial connections.
Truncus arteriosus	Includes all truncus arteriosus subtypes. Excludes hemitruncus and pseudotruncus
Total anomalous pulmonary venous return	Includes all types of total anomalous pulmonary venous return.
Tricuspid atresia	Includes tricuspid valve atresia with normally related great arteries.
Ebstein's anomaly	Includes Ebstein's anomaly of the right heart with atrioventricular concordance.
Single ventricle complex	Includes double-inlet left or right ventricle, mitral or tricuspid valve atresia with aortic malposition, or other specified or unspecified types of single ventricle.
Heterotaxy syndrome	Includes atrial situs abnormalities, situs inversus with or without dextrocardia, situs ambiguous, isolated dextrocardia, and unspecified heterotaxy. Cases with other heart defects and heterotaxy syndrome are only considered in the heterotaxy group, and excluded from the other heart defect groups.
Left heart obstructive defects	
Coarctation of the aorta	Includes coarctation of the aorta with or without aortic valve stenosis, aortic arch hypoplasia, and interrupted aortic arch type A.
Valvar aortic stenosis	Includes valvar or unspecified aortic valve stenosis, dysplasia, or atresia. Excludes isolated bicuspid aortic valve and aortic stenosis with coarctation.

(Continued)

TABLE 1. *(continued)*

Defect Group	Definition
Interrupted aortic arch type B	Includes type B and unspecified type of interrupted aortic arch.
Hypoplastic left heart syndrome (HLHS)	Includes HLHS with or without ventricular septal defect.
Right heart obstructive defects	
Valvar pulmonic stenosis	Includes valvar and unspecified pulmonary stenosis or valvar dysplasia.
Pulmonary atresia	Includes pulmonary atresia with intact ventricular septum.

(Reprinted from Reller MD, Strickland MJ, Riehle-Colarusso T, et al. Prevalence of congenital heart defects in metropolitan Atlanta, 1998-2005. *J Pediatr.* 2008;153:807-813.)

of CHD is a reflection of this ascertainment of minor forms of CHD in recent years. Another important source of variation, however, is the nomenclature and classification systems used in previous prevalence studies, including the International Classification of Disease, Ninth Revision (ICD-9), the modified version of the British Pediatric Association system, and the International Society of Cardiology. More recently there has been developed an even more standard CHD nomenclature, the International Pediatric and Congenital Cardiac Code. Table 1 reflects the contemporary definition of congenital heart defects using this classification. The report from Emory University is one of the first to document the current prevalence of congenital heart defects using modern coding based on the International Pediatric and Congenital Cardiac Code system. Using this system in the past decade, in Metropolitan Atlanta, it was determined that the overall prevalence of congenital heart defects runs 81.4 per 10 000 births, with the most common forms of CHD being muscular ventricular septal defect, followed by perimembranous ventricular septal defect and secundum atrial septal defect with prevalence of 27.5, 10.6, and 10.3 per 10 000 births, respectively. Serious heart defects such as tetralogy of Fallot, the most common cyanotic CHD, was found to be twice that of transposition of the great arteries (4.7 versus 2.2 per 10 000 births).

The detection of a heart murmur may be the initial presentation of CHD in a newborn. The problem is that murmurs are common in newborns with a reported prevalence as high as 77%. Given the fact that the actual prevalence of CHD is a tiny fraction of this, this implies that many neonates with murmurs have structurally normal hearts. Distinguishing innocent from pathologic murmurs is a common clinical scenario for general pediatricians, neonatologists, and pediatric cardiologists. While echocardiography is the gold standard for distinguishing innocent from pathologic murmurs in children, given the high prevalence of murmurs in the newborn period, were one to use an echocardiogram to distinguish every murmur, one would find this to be not only time consuming, but inordinately expensive and impractical. For this reason, we must rely on our physical examination. Unfortunately, neonates have high heart rates, which only increases the difficulty of auscultation. All too commonly, innocent murmurs may be mistaken for heart disease and vice versa. This is where having someone who knows what they are listening to is helpful in making the initial assessment. A recent report of Mackie et al showed that when a pediatric cardiologist listened to the heart of a newborn potentially suspected of having congenital heart disease, clinical assessment alone identified patients with CHD with a sensitivity of 80.5%, a specificity of 90.9%, a positive predictive value of 91.9%, and a negative predictive value of 78.4%.[1] Unfortunately, all too often, the cardiologist will still wind up deferring to the echocardiogram in uncertain cases.

One wonders if it is time to think about the possibility of the echocardiogram being simply an extension of the physical examination. Sure we cannot do an echocardiogram on every newly minted baby, but maybe we are shortchanging ourselves if we are too restrictive in the application of such a "simple" technique.

J. A. Stockman III, MD

Reference

1. Mackie AS, Jutras LC, Dancea AB, Rohlicek CV, Platt R, Béland MJ. Can cardiologists distinguish innocent from pathologic murmurs in neonates? *J Pediatr.* 2009;154:50-54.

Effectiveness of teaching cardiac auscultation to residents during an elective pediatric cardiology rotation

Mattioli LF, Belmont JM, Davis AM (Univ of Kansas Med Ctr)
Pediatr Cardiol 29:1095-1100, 2008

This study aimed to assess the effectiveness of randomized tracks of prerecorded cardiac sounds as a teaching tool for cardiac auscultation. The study focused on recognizing murmurs when present, distinguishing functional from organic murmurs, and detecting heart disease by auscultation. At both pre- and posttesting, 26 residents listened to 15 randomized tracks of live-recorded cardiac sounds and identified key features. The results indicate that the residents improved at detecting any murmur (66% vs 76%, $p = 0.007$) and functional murmur (37% vs 54%, $p = 0.048$), and marginally improved at detecting organic murmur (75% vs 84%, $p = 0.129$). Detection of absence of murmur declined slightly (69% vs 62%, $p = 0.723$). The posttest difference in identifying organic versus functional murmurs was striking (84% vs 54%, $p < 0.001$). Detection of heart disease (sensitivity) improved significantly (76% to 86%, $p = 0.016$), but there was scant improvement in detecting no disease (specificity) (55% vs 59%, $p = 0.601$). The residents increased in their ability to detect heart disease when present. However, the false-positive rate for a diagnosis of heart disease remained quite high. To ensure that appropriate referrals will be made, teaching should specifically target the confident recognition of functional murmurs.

▶ There has been a great deal written about whether the training we currently provide adequately prepares a resident for general pediatric practice when it comes to listening for potential heart murmurs. A study performed not that long ago among more than 500 medical students and residents in training showed that they correctly recognized only 20% of recorded sounds and murmurs.[1] This study involved internal medicine and family practice trainees. When it comes to pediatric residents, one study suggests that those listening to simulated sounds and murmurs have an overall diagnostic accuracy of just 33%.[2] In the report of Mattioli et al, a concerted effort was made to train residents during a cardiology rotation to detect and sort out potential murmurs in children. The decision was made to do this based on the Accreditation Council for Graduate Medical Education (ACGME) requirements that all residencies have written detailed goals and standards for each rotation, including a standardized test of performance. During the cardiology rotation, residents were given careful definitions of what murmurs are and are not. The residents were also given scoring sheets that they could use to check off certain characteristics of possible murmurs. Prerecorded murmurs were used as part of the assessment. At the completion of the rotation, the resident was able 86% of the time to make a satisfactory diagnosis of a recorded murmur. Obviously, this is not quite the same as listening to the chest of a youngster in an environment with a fair amount of background noise, but the results were quite compelling in the sense that it was clear that one could teach the required skill.

It would behoove those who are exiting training to maintain their skills in auscultation by periodically listening to prerecorded murmurs. Pathologic murmurs are not all that common in pediatric practice and it is possible for one to lose skills fairly quickly.

This commentary closes with another *Clinical Fact/Curio*, this having to do with cardiopulmonary fitness. Investigators in Canada have done a study that mathematically calculates the number of lives saved or lost as a direct consequence of a runner's participation in a marathon.[3] The authors hypothesized that even though people occasionally die from running a marathon, in the aggregate, not only is such exercise safe, but it in fact may well save lives at the time the marathon is run. The specific speculation is that the closure of roads at the time of a marathon run prevents more deaths from concurrent road accidents than might be occasioned by loss of life from a runner participating in the marathon. The investigators designed a very unique analysis to address this. They screened some 328 marathons listed in the "Runners' World Registry" and randomly selected 26 marathons to provide a diverse sample that covered a period of 30 years. All the marathons that were included in the analysis were run in the United States. They obtained data on sudden cardiac deaths from local newspapers on the days after each marathon. Because such deaths tend to be quite high profile, the assumption was that all deaths were captured in the analysis. Also retrieved was information from the National Highway Traffic Safety Administration, which provided population-based data for all fatal crashes on public roads on the days of the marathon run. The authors distinguished counties in the state that were inside and outside the marathon course and hours that were inside and outside the general interval of marathon-related road closures. For comparative reasons, they looked at deaths for the same specific geography for the same hours 1 week before and 1 week after for the counties involved in the marathon route.

The analysis performed amounted to 3 329 268 participants each running 42 km (26.2 miles). Over the 30-year period studied among these more than 3 million participants, there were 26 sudden cardiac deaths. Fifteen of the 26 marathons studied in more detail had no deaths, 6 had 1, 5 had more than 1 (Boston, New York, Chicago, Honolulu, Washington, DC/Marine Corp). One marathon had more than 1 death in a single year, this being New York with 2 deaths in 1994. The typical participant with sudden cardiac death was a middle-aged man (average age 41 years, 81% men). Five deaths occurred in individuals who had previously completed a marathon. Autopsy results were available for 24, the most common finding being coronary atherosclerosis ($n = 21$). Other contributory factors in scattered cases included electrolyte abnormalities ($n = 4$), coronary anomalies ($n = 2$), and heat stroke ($n = 1$). The most common course location of cardiac death was at or within 1.6 km (one mile) of the finish line. Approximately one-half of all deaths occurred that close to the end of the run.

From these data, one can extrapolate that the overall risk of sudden death from participation in a marathon is equal to 0.8 per 1000 participants. This is the equivalent of about 2 deaths per million hours of vigorous exercise. A total of 85 individuals died in fatal car crashes on marathon days in counties inside the course during hours when roads were closed. In contrast, 262 individuals died in fatal crashes on the control days in the corresponding county road. Given that each marathon was paired with 2 control days, the discrepancy between observed and expected crash deaths on marathon days corresponded to a marked relative decrease in risk meaning that it was significantly safer to be running a marathon than driving a comparable distance. The ratio of crash deaths prevented was about 1.8 for each case of sudden cardiac death attributed to a marathon. The data, interestingly, were consistent across different regions of the United States, decades of the century, seasons of the year, days of the week, degree of competition (as measured by prize money), and course difficulty (as measured by winning race time).

This report also highlights the fact that we tend to pay attention to "high profile" deaths such as the passing of a young adult male voluntarily participating in a marathon, but pay little attention to a motor vehicle crash resulting in a death. The bottom line here is that it is not all that risky to run a marathon assuming that you are not born with a fixed number of heartbeats that are being wasted on the exercise (this author's theory). Given the fact that the final 1.6 km (1 mile) of the marathon represents less than 5% of the total distance and yet accounts for almost 50% of sudden cardiac deaths, one can see that simply by shortening a marathon a very modest amount, one could decrease the mortality rate related running to a marathon by almost half. Obviously, this is not going to happen anymore than one could have altered the distance between Marathon and Athens by 1.6 km.

J. A. Stockman III, MD

References

1. Mangione S, Nieman LZ. Cardiac auscultatory skills of internal medicine and family practice trainees: a comparison of diagnostic proficiency. *JAMA*. 2007; 278:1717-1722.

2. Gaskin PR, Owens SE, Talner NS, Sanders SP, Li JS. Clinical auscultation skills and pediatric residents. *Pediatrics.* 2000;105:1184-1187.

3. Redelmeier DA, Greenwald A. Competing risk of mortality with marathons: retrospective analysis. *BMJ.* 2007;335:1275-1277.

First Day of Life Pulse Oximetry Screening to Detect Congenital Heart Defects

Meberg A, Brügmann-Pieper S, Due R Jr, et al (Vestfold Hosp, Tønsberg, Norway; Buskerud Hosp, Drammen, Norway; Bærum Hosp, Sandvika, Norway; et al)
J Pediatr 152:761-765, 2008

Objective.—To evaluate the efficacy of first day of life pulse oximetry screening to detect congenital heart defects (CHDs).

Study Design.—We performed a population-based prospective multicenter study of postductal (foot) arterial oxygen saturation (SpO_2) in apparently healthy newborns after transfer from the delivery suite to the nursery. $SpO_2 < 95\%$ led to further diagnostic evaluations. Of 57,959 live births, 50,008 (86%) were screened. CHDs were prospectively registered and diagnosed in 658 newborns (1.1%), of whom 35 (5%) were classified as critical (ductus dependent, cyanotic).

Results.—Of the infants screened, 324 (0.6%) failed the test. Of these, 43 (13%) had CHDs (27 critical), and 134 (41%) had pulmonary diseases or other disorders. The remaining 147 infants (45%) were healthy with transitional circulation. The median age for babies with CHDs at failing the test was 6 hours (range, 1-21 hours). For identifying critical CHDs, the pulse oximetry screening had a sensitivity rate of 77.1% (95% CI, 59.4-89.0), specificity rate of 99.4% (95% CI, 99.3-99.5), and a false-positive rate of 0.6% (95% CI, 0.5-0.7).

Conclusions.—Early pulse oximetry screening promotes early detection of critical CHDs and other potentially severe diseases. The sensitivity rate for detecting critical CHDs is high, and the false-positive rate is low.

▶ Unfortunately, newborn physical findings in infants afflicted with congenital heart disease are frequently inconsistent. One study in fact suggests that the routine examination of a newborn will fail to detect critical congenital heart disease in almost 70% of cases.[1] Part of the problem here is that some babies with cyanotic forms of congenital heart disease may not have sufficient amounts of unoxygenated hemoglobin to produce findings on physical examination. In general, 4 g/dL of deoxygenated hemoglobin is needed to produce visible cyanosis, and those children with mild hypoxemia (arterial oxygen saturations of 80%-95%) might not be obviously cyanotic. Add to that the difficulty of detecting cyanosis in babies with darkly pigmented skin and you see the problem.

Some have suggested that neonatal pulse oximetry should be used to identify congenital heart disease cases, or some other cases. Studies to date have reported that pulse oximetry can identify many newborn infants with critical congenital heart disease who are otherwise asymptomatic and hence might elude clinical detection before discharge from the newborn nursery. Given the small numbers of babies included in previous studies, there has been insufficient data to convince many that pulse oximetry screening should be incorporated into routine newborn nursery care. This is where the report of Meberg et al comes into play.

Meberg et al report the outcomes of a screening strategy to detect congenital heart disease using pulse oximetry in 14 centers in Norway—accounting for approximately 50% of all deliveries in this country. The investigators identified 40 asymptomatic newborns with congenital heart defects out of a group of 50 000 children. The majority of infants with congenital heart disease (some 94%) were identified by methods other than screening pulse oximetry. These methods included prenatal diagnosis, newborn nursery physical examination, or identification after discharge from the newborn nursery. Thus, the detection rate of newborn oximetry for all forms of congenital heart disease would be considered to be quite poor. However, if one considers only those infants with critical congenital heart disease, and those lesions that require intervention and that can result in hemodynamic compromise, screening oximetry faired much better. Only 8 newborn infants with critical congenital heart disease were not detected by pulse oximetry screening.

The naysayers for using pulse oximetry complain about the false-positive rates of the technique. In the study from Norway, false positives were seen in 0.6% of newborns. While this percentage seems fairly modest, in absolute numbers it is high. One of the reasons that the false-positive rate was high in this report is that the authors chose to screen soon after birth. It is known that the oxygen saturations of newborns are lower in the first few hours after birth. By a day of life, however, the average oxygen saturation of a newborn is about 97%. The false-positive rate seen in the Meberg et al study could be lessened by screening after 24 hours of age but before hospital discharge. Studies have suggested that the false-positive rate when testing is done after a day of age is less than 0.1%.

Another limitation of using newborn pulse oximetry screening is the false-negative rate associated with it. Obviously, not all babies with critical congenital heart disease will have desaturation. Examples of such babes are those with coarctation of the aorta and to a much lesser extent, hypoplastic left heart syndrome. Many of these babies will have oxygen saturations in excess of 95% at least for the first few days of life. Interestingly, in the present study, screening oximetry did identify several newborn infants with coarctation of the aorta. These findings are consistent with other reports that suggest that about half of babies with coarctation will have some level of desaturation.

This editor has been a strong proponent of the routine screening of all newborns with pulse oximetry. As this report suggests, such screening is best done before discharge but after 1 day of age. Yes, it is true that pulse oximetry will have a small false-positive rate and will miss perhaps as many as half of all infants with noncyanotic forms of congenital heart disease, but importantly it clearly will detect some babies who would otherwise be missed with critical congenital heart disease who may ultimately present in dire straits. Studies here in the United States suggest that for every 1000 live births, there are approximately 1 to 3 deaths directly attributable to the delayed diagnosis of critical congenital heart disease.[2]

This commentary closes with another miscellaneous *Clinical Fact/Curio*, this having to do with cell phones and hospitals. For too long the myth has been perpetuated that the use of cell phones in hospitals is dangerous. A recent report tells us that mobile phone use may in fact be safe within the confines of hospitals. An online search found no cases of death caused by the use of a mobile phone in any medical facility worldwide. Less serious incidents, including false alarms on monitors, malfunctions of infusion pumps, and incorrect readings on cardiac monitors, have occasionally been reported. Although no reference or dates are given, one government web site published an anecdote in 2002 saying that use of a mobile phone in an intensive care unit resulted in an unintended bolus of epinephrine from an infusion pump. After a journal cited more than 100 reports of suspected electromagnetic interference with medical devices before 1993, the *Wall Street Journal* highlighted this danger on its front page. That was the point at which many hospitals banned the use of mobile phones, further perpetuating the belief.

Studies have been performed to show that mobile phones interfere with fewer than 4% of devices and then only at a distance of < 1 m. Fewer than 0.1% of events showed serious effects. At the Mayo Clinic in 2005, in 510 tests with 16 medical devices and 6 mobile phones, the incidence of clinically important interference was 1.2%. Rigorous testing in Europe found minimal interference and only at distances < 1 m. Recent technological improvements may be lessening even this minimal interference. A 2007 study found no interference in 300 tests in 75 treatment rooms. Interestingly, a large survey of anesthetists found that the use of mobile phones by doctors was associated with reduced risk of medical error or injury resulting from delays in communication (relative risk 0.78; 95% confidence interval 0.62 to 0.96).

To read more about whether mobile phones are dangerous in hospitals as well as many other medical myths, see the interesting article by Vreeman and Carroll.[3]

J. A. Stockman III, MD

References

1. Richmond S, Wren C. Early diagnosis of congential heart disease. *Semin Neonatal.* 2001;6:27-35.
2. Chang RK. How many infants with critical congenital heart disease are missed? *Circulation.* 2007;116:612-614.
3. Vreeman RC, Carroll AE. Medical myths. Sometimes even doctors are duped. *BMJ.* 2007;335:1288-1289.

Impact of pulse oximetry screening on the detection of duct dependent congenital heart disease: a Swedish prospective screening study in 39 821 newborns
de-Wahl Granelli A, Wennergren M, Sandberg K, et al (Queen Silvia Children's Hosp, Göteborg, Sweden; Sahlgrenska Univ Hosp, Göteborg, Sweden; et al)
BMJ 338:a3037, 2009

Objective.—To evaluate the use of pulse oximetry to screen for early detection of life threatening congenital heart disease.

Design.—Prospective screening study with a new generation pulse oximeter before discharge from well baby nurseries in West Götaland. Cohort study comparing the detection rate of duct dependent circulation in West Götaland with that in other regions not using pulse oximetry screening. Deaths at home with undetected duct dependent circulation were included.

Setting.—All 5 maternity units in West Götaland and the supraregional referral centre for neonatal cardiac surgery.

Participants.—39 821 screened babies born between 1 July 2004 and 31 March 2007. Total duct dependent circulation cohorts: West Götaland n = 60, other referring regions n = 100.

Main Outcome Measures.—Sensitivity, specificity, positive and negative predictive values, and likelihood ratio for pulse oximetry screening and for neonatal physical examination alone.

Results.—In West Götaland 29 babies in well baby nurseries had duct dependent circulation undetected before neonatal discharge examination. In 13 cases, pulse oximetry showed oxygen saturations $\leq 90\%$, and (in accordance with protocol) clinical staff were immediately told of the results. Of the remaining 16 cases, physical examination alone detected 10 (63%). Combining physical examination with pulse oximetry screening had a sensitivity of 24/29 (82.8%(95% CI 64.2% to 95.2%)) and detected 100% of the babies with duct dependent lung circulation. Five cases were missed (all with aortic arch obstruction). False positive rate with pulse oximetry was substantially lower than that with physical examination alone (69/39 821 (0.17%) v 729/38 413 (1.90%), P<0.0001), and 31/69 of the "false positive" cases with pulse oximetry had other pathology. Thus, referral of all cases with positive oximetry results for echocardiography resulted in only 2.3 echocardiograms with normal cardiac findings for every true positive case of duct dependent circulation. In the cohort study, the risk of leaving hospital with undiagnosed duct dependent circulation was 28/100 (28%) in other referring regions versus 5/60 (8%) in West Götaland (P=0.0025, relative risk 3.36 (95% CI 1.37 to 8.24)). In the other referring regions 11/25 (44%) of babies with transposition of the great arteries left hospital undiagnosed versus 0/18 in West Götaland (P=0.0010), and severe acidosis at diagnosis was more common (33/100 (33%) v 7/60 (12%), P=0.0025, relative risk 2.8 (1.3 to 6.0)). Excluding premature babies and Norwood surgery, babies discharged without diagnosis had higher mortality than those diagnosed in hospital (4/27 (18%) v

1/110 (0.9%), P=0.0054). No baby died from undiagnosed duct dependent circulation in West Götaland versus five babies from the other referring regions.

Conclusion.—Introducing pulse oximetry screening before discharge improved total detection rate of duct dependent circulation to 92%. Such screening seems cost neutral in the short term, but the probable prevention of neurological morbidity and reduced need for preoperative neonatal intensive care suggest that such screening will be cost effective long term.

▶ We have written previously about the use of neonatal pulse oximetry. The study by de-Wahl Granelli et al addresses the contribution of neonatal pulse oximetry saturation screening to early detection of life-threatening congenital heart disease. Critical congenital heart disease—cardiac malformations that are either ductal dependent or need surgery in the first month of life—occurs in about 170 per 100 000 live births. One would possibly think that clinical examination would be capable of detecting most of these cases. Unfortunately, it is not. Clinical cyanosis, for example, is poorly identified even when severe. As many as 15% of babies with cyanotic congenital heart disease are discharged from their hospital of birth without being diagnosed. Infants with critical congenital heart disease as a result of obstructive left heart lesions, such as coarctation of the aorta, interrupted aortic arch, and hypoplastic left heart syndrome are even more difficult to diagnose and generally present only when postnatal closure of the ductus arteriosus leads to acute and life-threatening deterioration. When a late diagnosis is made, there is a higher mortality rate before and postsurgery, so early detection theoretically would improve outcomes. The study of de-Wahl Granelli et al assesses the introduction of universal oximetry screening in one region of Sweden.

This Swedish study found a low false-positive rate (0.17%) after the introduction of postoximetry screening. All infants with cyanotic critical congenital heart disease in the screened population were able to be identified. Detection of left-sided disease was more difficult, and as in earlier studies, some infants were missed. Nonetheless, fewer infants with the latter type lesions were missed in the screening region. Even the "false-positive" babies frequently turned out to have diagnoses such as high pulmonary artery pressure, perhaps at one end of a spectrum of normal.

Please recognize that a study performed in the United States has suggested that no additional infants are detected with pulse oximetry screening compared with usual care in hospital.[1] It should be noted that the latter report emanated from a single hospital that looked at all babies with close observation for a minimum of 4 hours after birth before the pulse oximetry screening was performed. Other evaluations in the United States have shown that up to 30% of affected infants with congenital heart disease are being discharged with no diagnosis.

Please note that the best criterion for adequately diagnosing critical congenital heart disease seems to be a lower limb saturation of less than 96% with a measurement obtained with a new generation motion artifact resistant oximeter more than 20 hours after birth. Adequately trained screening technicians are needed and the oximetry should last for at least 360 seconds. A saturation gradient of more than 3% between the infant's right hand and foot may be a useful indicator of left-sided critical congenital heart disease.

One of the reasons why neonatal screening with pulse oximetry has not caught on like wildfire is the concern about an unacceptably high false-positive rate that might lead to high cost to exclude disease in infants with positive screens. The data suggest that if the false-positive rate can be driven down to as low as that found in the Swedish report, the benefit-cost analysis would suggest that screening is indeed cost-effective.

Needless to say, the debate about universal pulse oximetry screening for all newborns will continue in the United States. One suspects that with time that the tide will trend toward such screening. Chances are this will occur within the next few years in most centers.

J. A. Stockman III, MD

Reference

1. Sendelbach DM, Jackson GL, Lai SS, Fixler DE, Stehel EK, Engle WD. Pulse oximetry screening at four hours of age to detect critical congenital heart disease. *Pediatrics.* 2008;122:e815-e820.

Screening newborns for congenital heart disease with pulse oximetry: survey of pediatric cardiologists
Chang RK, Rodriguez S, Klitzner TS (Harbor-UCLA Med Ctr, CA)
Pediatr Cardiol 30:20-25, 2008

Background.—Controversies exist regarding the use of pulse oximetry for routine screening of newborns. This study aimed to evaluate current practices and opinions of pediatric cardiologists in relation to newborn screening for congenital heart disease (CHD) using pulse oximetry.

Methods.—Email invitations were sent to 1,045 pediatric cardiologists in North America. The survey was Internet based and included multiple-choice questions. Two repeat email reminders were sent after the initial invitation.

Results.—A total of 363 responses (35%) were returned. In terms of experience, 40% of the respondents had more than 20 years, 32% had 10 to 20 years, 21% had 5 to 10 years, and 6% had less than 5 years of experience. More than 90% agreed that an early diagnosis of CHD for newborns prevents morbidity and mortality. In terms of practice, 96% reported that all newborns are examined by a clinician before discharge, 29% reported that newborns get a pulse oximetry reading, and 1.4% (n = 5) reported the use of electrocardiogram. Only 58% of respondents thought that current practice is adequate for detecting significant CHD. With regard to their experience with pulse oximetry, 26% reported "too many false-positives," 21% described it as "prone to noise and artifact," and 30% viewed it as "very operator dependent." The overall support for mandated pulse oximetry screening was 55%. The support for mandate decreased with years of experience, with 76% of the supporters having less than 5 years, 58% of those having 5 to 10 years, 53% of those having 10 to 20 years, and 51% of those having more than 20 years of experience.

Conclusions.—Pediatric cardiologists recognize that current practice is inadequate for detecting significant CHD. Slightly more than half of the pediatric cardiologists in this study supported a mandate for pulse oximetry screening, but there were many concerns, and the support decreased with increasing years of clinical experience.

▶ Another report dealing with screening newborns for congenital heart disease with the use of pulse oximetry. This topic has proven to be a highly controversial one. Sometimes when controversies exist in terms of optional treatments, it is wise to test the waters by doing a survey of those currently in practice to see what the "experts" are recommending. This is exactly what Chang et al did. In recent years there have been a number of studies that have looked at the possibility that pulse oximetry in the immediate newborn period would be an aid to clinical examination for detecting some forms of congenital heart disease. A systematic review of 8 clinical studies on pulse oximetry concluded, however, that pulse oximetry screening is not sufficiently sensitive to serve as an independent screen.[1] Others have interpreted the literature differently, however. Little is known regarding the collective opinions of pediatric cardiovascular specialists on this highly debated topic. For this reason, current practices and opinions were evaluated on this subject by a survey that was undertaken of pediatric cardiologists in North America. Some 1086 pediatric cardiologists were polled.

It was clear from the survey that the importance of an early detection of cyanotic congenital heart disease was understood. Only 58% of respondents thought that the current practice of clinical examination was adequate for detecting significant congenital heart disease. At the same time, 1 in 4 pediatric cardiologists indicated that based on their experience with pulse oximetry, adding this technique produced too many false positives. About the same percentage viewed it as very operator dependent. In the aggregate, only about half indicated support for mandated pulse oximetry screening. Support for pulse oximetry screening was inversely related to years out of training.

Given the fact that there have been no earlier surveys of this type performed, it is hard to tell whether there is an increasing trend toward the acceptance of newborn pulse oximetry screening as a complement to physical diagnosis. At least at the present time, just over half of all pediatric cardiologists seem to believe that there is some merit in such screening.

J. A. Stockman III, MD

Reference

1. Valmar IP. Should pulse oximetry be used to screen for congenital heart disease? *Arch Dis Child Fetal Neonatal Ed.* 2007;92:F219-F224.

Cardiac surgery in adults performed at children's hospitals: Trends and outcomes

Mahle WT, Kirshbom PM, Kanter KR, et al (Emory Univ School of Medicine, Atlanta, GA)

J Thorac Cardiovasc Surg 136:307-311, 2008

Objective.—The number of adults with congenital heart disease who require cardiac surgery is projected to increase dramatically. Controversy exists as to whether such procedures should be performed in pediatric centers, which generally have the greatest experience with operations for congenital heart disease. We sought to report the outcomes for cardiac surgery performed in adults (≥21 years of age) at children's hospitals and determine how these practices varied among institutions.

Methods.—Data from July 2005 to June 2007 from the Child Health Corporation of America, a consortium of 37 free-standing children's hospitals, were analyzed to determine the institutional volume, type of cardiac procedure, outcome, and hospital charges. Individual institutional variables were analyzed to determine which factors might be associated with the practice of performing adult cardiac surgery in children's hospitals.

Results.—During the study period, there were 719 admissions for cardiac surgery in adults at Child Health Corporation of America institutions. The median age at the time of operation was 26 years (range, 21–86 years). The most common surgical procedures were implantation or revision of a pacemaker or defibrillator (n = 207 [29.2%]), pulmonary valve replacement (n = 119 [16.8%]), aortic valve replacement (n = 59 [8.3%]), and Fontan revision (n = 37 [5.2%]). The median hospital length of stay was 6 days (range, 1–175 days). The hospital mortality was 1.9%. Comorbid conditions likely to require other subspecialty care were present in more than 30% of patients. Among the Child Health Corporation of America centers, adult operations as a proportion of overall cardiac operations varied from 0% to 10.9%. There was no relationship between overall cardiac surgical volume and proportion of adult cases performed in Child Health Corporation of America centers.

Conclusions.—A significant number of adult cardiac surgical procedures are being performed at children's hospitals with excellent results. The majority of procedures are not related to complex shunt lesions but rather pacemaker/defibrillator implantation and semilunar valve surgery. Whether adult patients with congenital heart disease should continue to undergo most cardiac surgery in children's hospitals is worthy of discussion (Tables 2 and 4).

▶ The number of adult survivors of congenital heart disease now exceeds the number of children with these disorders. Since the number of adult patients with congenital heart disease has been increasing, there has been interest in creating regional adult congenital heart disease centers. This seems to make good sense given that adults can have comorbid conditions that are uncommon in children, such as deep venous thrombosis, atherosclerotic coronary artery

TABLE 2.—Most Common Principal Cardiac Surgical Procedures and Hospital Mortality

	No. (%)
Pulmonary valve replacement	119 (16.6)
Revision of pacemaker/defibrillator	75 (10.4)
Defibrillator implantation	68 (9.5)
Pacemaker implantation	64 (8.9)
Aortic valve replacement	59 (8.2)
Fontan procedure revision	37 (5.1)
Atrioventricular valve repair	35 (4.9)
ASD closure	28 (3.9)
Atrioventricular valve replacement	27 (3.8)
RV to PA conduit replacement	18 (2.5)
Aortic valve repair	13 (1.8)
Heart transplantation	12 (1.7)
Coarctation of the aorta	10 (1.4)
VSD closure	9 (1.3)
Other procedures	145 (20.1)

ASD, Atrial septal defect; RV, right ventricle; PA, pulmonary artery; VSD, ventricular septal defect.
(Reprinted from Mahle WT, Kirshbom PM, Kanter KR, et al. Cardiac surgery in adults performed at children's hospitals: trends and outcomes. *J Thorac Cardiovasc Surg.* 2008;136:307-311.)

disease, or peripheral vascular disease and emphysema. At least theoretically, it would be better that adult patients with congenital heart disease are treated in adult hospitals with specialized congenital heart cardiologists and surgeons. Unfortunately, the numbers of the latter are insufficient to handle the clinical case burden. Thus the alternative is to perform adult congenital heart disease surgery in children's hospitals that are familiar with the cardiac physiology of

TABLE 4.—Associated medical conditions among adults (n = 719) at children's hospitals

	No. (%)
Renal	
Acute renal failure	27 (3.8)
Chronic renal failure	7 (1.0)
Gastrointestinal	
Cirrhosis of liver	8 (1.1)
Acute pancreatitis	4 (0.6)
Viral hepatitis	7 (1.0)
Psychiatric	
Depression	19 (2.6)
Anxiety state/panic disorder	24 (3.3)
Manic–depression	3 (0.4)
Substance abuse	21 (2.9)
Hematologic	
Blood disorder other than anemia	46 (6.5)
Endocrinologic	
Hypothyroidism	48 (6.4)
Diabetes	18 (2.5)
Gout	6 (0.8)
Obstructive sleep apnea	14 (1.9)
Alzheimer's dementia	3 (0.4)

(Reprinted from Mahle WT, Kirshbom PM, Kanter KR, et al. Cardiac surgery in adults performed at children's hospitals: trends and outcomes. *J Thorac Cardiovasc Surg.* 2008;136:307-311.)

these patients. This report, using data from 37 children's hospitals, examines the outcomes of adults who are operated on in a children's hospital. Apparently, adults fair very well when operated on in a children's hospital.

You can debate whether it is good or bad for adults, especially those who have complex comorbid conditions, to be operated on in a children's hospital. An argument in favor of this is that adult patients with congenital heart disease are best served by those facilities that have personnel familiar with the physiology, and complications that are unique to congenital heart disease such as might occur in those with a functional single ventricle or in those who have had unique procedures designed for pediatric patients. Please note, however, that such complex physiology is not a major issue for most adults who require some type of surgical procedure who have a diagnosis of congenital heart disease. Implantation of pacemakers or defibrillators, placement of pulmonary valves, aortic valve repair or replacement, etc, are the type of operations that account for more than 70% of all adult congenital heart disease procedures performed in children's hospitals in this study. Although the technical expertise of a surgeon trained in congenital heart disease lesions would seem crucial for some lesions, the postoperative physiology for many of the subjects in this report would not require management of complex intracardiac shunts. This does not mean that adults should not be operated on in children's hospitals, rather, that there might be better solutions some time in the future with greater attention paid on the part of adult specialists to the problems that survivors of congenital heart disease have. This is a hot topic under debate right now within the house of medicine.

For more on the topic of congenital heart defects and their associated developmental and functional outcomes, see the report of Majnemer et al.[1] You will learn that mean IQ scores tend to be in the low average range (90 to 94) and that behavioral difficulties are quite common (27.1%). Predictors of developmental and functional limitations were observed and included abnormal postoperative neurologic examination, microcephaly, deep hypothermic circulatory arrest time, acyanotic heart lesions, age at surgery, and maternal education.

J. A. Stockman III, MD

Reference

1. Majnemer A, Limperopoulos C, Shevell M, et al. Developmental and functional outcomes at school entry in children with congenital heart defects. *J Pediatr.* 2008;153:55-60.

Hospital mortality for Norwood and arterial switch operations as a function of institutional volume
Hirsch JC, Gurney JG, Donohue JE, et al (Univ of Michigan Med Ctr, Ann Arbor, MI)
Pediatr Cardiol 29:713-717, 2008

Regionalization of complex surgical procedures to high-volume centers is a model for improving hospital survival. We analyzed the effect of institutional volume on hospital mortality for the Norwood and arterial switch operations (ASO) as representative high-complexity neonatal cardiac procedures. Analysis of discharge data from the 2003 Kids' Inpatient Database (KID) was conducted. Association between institutional volume and in-hospital mortality was examined for the ASO or Norwood procedure. Logistic regression analysis was performed to calculate the probability of hospital mortality for both procedures. Significant inverse associations between institutional volume and in-hospital mortality for the Norwood procedure ($p \leq 0.001$) and the ASO ($p = 0.006$) were demonstrated. In-hospital mortality decreased for the ASO as institutional volume increased, with mortality rates of 9.4% for institutions performing two ASOs/year, 3.2% for 10 ASOs/year, and 0.8% for 20 ASOs/year. Similarly, in-hospital mortality rates for hypoplastic left heart syndrome were 34.8% for two Norwood procedures/year, 25.7% for 10 Norwood procedures/year, and 16.7% for 20 Norwood procedures/year. An inverse relation was observed between in-hospital mortality and institutional volume for ASO and the Norwood procedure. These results suggest that selective regionalization of complex neonatal cardiac procedures might result in significant improvement in hospital survival nationally.

▶ This report represents a complex analysis aimed at defining the relationship between institutional volume and hospital mortality for congenital heart surgery, and, not surprisingly, the report suggests that a high-volume institution will have lower hospital mortality in comparison with a low-volume institution. Although the data presented are restricted to 2 specific procedures, the conclusions are consistent with the majority of reports examining this issue using a wider range of procedures. It should be noted that others have not always found a consistent relationship between hospital volume and outcome, perhaps suggesting the possibility that hospital volume is merely a proxy for other aspects of care that are important predictors of survival. This concern is supported by the observation that in most published analyses there are some low-volume centers that have risk-adjusted mortality that is equivalent, or in fact superior, to that of large-volume centers. Also, an institution with superb performance in the management of one cardiac lesion may have mediocre performance with another lesion. In fact, if you look at some of the studies showing an inverse relationship between volume and outcome and simply remove just one large center with highly superior outcomes, you often see no difference in the other institutional outcomes.

The recognition that some low-volume centers can deliver performance that is equivalent to that of high-volume centers suggests that there is more afoot than simply the number of procedures performed. Other factors than "practice makes perfect" may be at play. For example, rapid transfer, known to improve survival, may be independent of this. If there is a bottom line here, it is that there is a little good and a little bad in any group of large or small hospitals when it comes to outcomes. To learn more about this, see the excellent discussion of this topic by Caldarone and Al-Radi.[1] In this day and age, there should be complete transparency for both providers and the public about outcomes (risk adjusted, of course) of all types of procedures.

J. A. Stockman III, MD

Reference

1. Caldarone CA, Al-Radi O. The limits of confidence: at what price a baby's life? *Pediatr Cardiol.* 2008;29:704-705.

Developmental and Functional Outcomes at School Entry in Children with Congenital Heart Defects

Majnemer A, Limperopoulos C, Shevell M, et al (McGill Univ, Montreal, Quebec, Canada)

J Pediatr 153:55-60, 2008

Objective.—To describe developmental and functional outcomes of children with congenital heart defects (CHDs) at school entry after open heart surgery.

Study Design.—Infants with CHDs who underwent surgical repair in infancy were recruited and assessed prospectively for developmental progress. At 5 years of age (64.2 ± 11.3 months), 94 subjects were evaluated in a blind fashion by using a variety of standardized measures.

Results.—Mean IQ scores were in the low average range (90-94). Receptive language was in the average range (103.6 ± 14.4). Behavioral difficulties were common (27.1%), with internalizing problems being more frequent. Functional limitations in socialization (93.0 ± 17.1), daily living skills (94.6 ± 16.4), communication (90.0 ± 14.1), and adaptive behavior (92.1 ± 15.8) were noted in 11% to 17% of children. With the Functional Independence Measure for Children, 20% to 22% of subjects were more dependent than their peers in self-care and social cognition, although few (4.5%) had mobility restrictions. Predictors of developmental and functional limitations included: abnormal postoperative neurologic examination, microcephaly, deep hypothermic circulatory arrest time, palliation, acyanotic heart lesion, age at surgery, and maternal education.

Conclusions.—After infant open-heart surgery, children with CHDs may exhibit a range of developmental difficulties at school entry that enhances risk for learning challenges and decreased social participation.

▶ Until this report appeared, this editor was not aware of the full magnitude of the developmental and functional deficits that children with congenital heart defects may have. The study from Montreal Children's Hospital involved a prospective evaluation of a consecutive sample of newborns and infants who underwent open-heart surgery during the period of 1994 through early 1998, employing a wide range of outcome measures. These youngsters were followed with developmental assessments that included: (1) the Wechsler

Preschool and Primary Scale of Intelligence, (2) the Peabody Picture Vocabulary Test for receptive language skills, and (3) the Child Behavior Checklist for identification of behavior problems. Functional performance was also evaluated by using the Vineland Adaptive Behavior Scale, which measures a child's typical performance in everyday activities (ie, socialization, communication, daily living skills, and adaptive behavior). Last, the Functional Independence Measure for Children was also assessed. This evaluates the level of assistance required to carry out everyday activities independently.

The study from Montreal confirms earlier studies that have demonstrated that children undergoing early open heart surgery when evaluated at preschool age, school age, and adolescence have a mean IQ score in the low normal range (90-99, generally). Socioeconomic status and prolonged deep hypothermic circulatory arrest were found to be associated with lower IQ. The study also found that children who had surgery delayed well into infancy had lower IQ scores than children who had surgery in the first days of life. Subjects with acyanotic lesions had lower IQ scores than in subjects with cyanotic lesions. This may reflect the fact that these types of heart lesions are more likely to be associated with poor cerebral blood flow because of poor systemic profusion, often beginning in the fetal period and extending until surgical correction.

Needless to say, congenital heart disease, even when adequately corrected through surgery, can have long-term sequelae. Families need to be aware of this so that proper interventions, including those related to schooling can be in place, if needed.

J. A. Stockman III, MD

Outcomes in Adults With Bicuspid Aortic Valves

Tzemos N, Therrien J, Yip J, et al (Univ of Toronto, Ontario, Canada; McGill Univ, Montreal, Quebec, Canada; Natl Univ Hosp, Singapore; et al)
JAMA 300:1317-1325, 2008

Context.—Bicuspid aortic valve is the most common congenital cardiac anomaly in the adult population. Cardiac outcomes in a contemporary population of adults with bicuspid aortic valve have not been systematically determined.

Objective.—To determine the frequency and predictors of cardiac outcomes in a large consecutive series of adults with bicuspid aortic valve.

Design, Setting, and Participants.—Cohort study examining cardiac outcomes in 642 consecutive ambulatory adults (mean [SD] age, 35 [16] years; 68% male) with bicuspid aortic valve presenting to a Canadian congenital cardiac center from 1994 through 2001 and followed up for a mean (SD) period of 9 (5) years. Frequency and predictors of major cardiac events were determined by multivariate analysis. Mortality rate in the study group was compared with age- and sex-matched population estimates.

Main Outcome Measures.—Mortality and cause of death were determined. Primary cardiac events were defined as the occurrence of any of the following complications: cardiac death, intervention on the aortic valve or ascending aorta, aortic dissection or aneurysm, or congestive heart failure requiring hospital admission during the follow-up period.

Results.—During the follow-up period, there were 28 deaths (mean [SD], 4% [1%]). One or more primary cardiac events occurred in 161 patients (mean [SD], 25% [2%]), which included cardiac death in 17 patients (mean [SD], 3% [1%]), intervention on aortic valve or ascending aorta in 142 patients (mean [SD], 22% [2%]), aortic dissection or aneurysm in 11 patients (mean [SD], 2% [1%]), or congestive heart failure requiring hospital admission in 16 patients (mean [SD], 2% [1%]). Independent predictors of primary cardiac events were age older than 30 years (hazard ratio [HR], 3.01; 95% confidence interval [CI], 2.15-4.19; $P<.001$), moderate or severe aortic stenosis (HR, 5.67; 95% CI, 4.16-7.80; $P<.001$), and moderate or severe aortic regurgitation (HR, 2.68; 95% CI, 1.93-3.76; $P<.001$). The 10-year survival rate of the study group (mean [SD], 96% [1%]) was not significantly different from population estimates (mean [SD], 97% [1%]; $P=.71$). At last follow-up, 280 patients (mean [SD], 45% [2%]) had dilated aortic sinus and/or ascending aorta.

Conclusions.—In this study population of young adults with bicuspid aortic valve, age, severity of aortic stenosis, and severity of aortic regurgitation were independently associated with primary cardiac events. Over the mean follow-up duration of 9 years, survival rates were not lower than for the general population (Table 4).

▶ Obviously, this report deals with adults with bicuspid aortic valves. Needless to say, however, every adult with a bicuspid aortic valve was born in infancy

TABLE 4.—Predictors of Primary Cardiac Events

Candidate Variables	Univariate Analysis		Multivariate Analysis	
	HR (95% CI)	*P* Value	HR (95% CI)	*P* Value
Baseline age >30 y	2.11 (1.56-2.87)	<.001	3.01 (2.15-4.19)	<.001
Male sex	1.82 (1.27-2.62)	.002		
Hypertension	1.65 (1.24-2.20)	.002		
Hyperlipidemia	2.66 (1.70-4.18)	<.001		
Diabetes mellitus	1.00 (0.35-2.84)	.95		
Smoking	5.36 (1.89-15.24)	.004		
Family history of coronary artery disease	0.52 (0.21-1.29)	.20		
Body mass index[a]	1.00 (0.97-1.04)	.91		
Prior diagnosis of aortic coarctation	0.30 (0.19-0.48)	<.001		
Prior aortic valvuloplasty or valvotomy	1.92 (1.29-2.85)	.004		
Prior pregnancy	0.38 (0.13-1.08)	.10		
Right-left leaflet orientation	1.57 (1.11-2.21)	.02		
Moderate or severe aortic stenosis	5.31 (3.98-7.09)	<.001	5.67 (4.16-7.80)	<.001
Moderate or severe aortic regurgitation	2.61 (1.96-3.48)	<.001	2.68 (1.93-3.76)	<.001
Left ventricular ejection fraction <55%	3.22 (1.98-5.24)	<.001		
Aortic sinus >35 mm	1.93 (1.45-2.58)	<.001		

Abbreviations: CI, confidence interval; HR, hazard ratio.
[a]Calculated as weight in kilograms divided by height in meters squared.

with this defect, thus its relevance to pediatrics. In fact, one of the co-authoring institutions on this report was the Congenital Heart Center at the Children's Hospital of Philadelphia. Bicuspid aortic valves are quite common and in adults are reported to be the most common congenital cardiac anomaly. Despite its prevalence, the exact morbidity and mortality associated with the defect have remained somewhat elusive, at least until this large cohort study examining cardiac outcomes in more than 600 adults with bicuspid aortic valve was published. The subjects reported on were ambulatory and asymptomatic and had an average (mean) age of 35 years (standard deviation 16 years). Thus, pediatric age patients were included in this report.

So what do we learn? Reassuringly, the overall mortality rate of this ambulatory cohort with bicuspid aortic valves was not significantly different from population estimates of peers. Nonetheless, 25% of patients experienced a primary cardiac event during a mean follow-up of 9 years. A noninvasive or invasive workup or therapeutic procedure on the aortic valve and/or the aorta comprised the vast majority of these primary cardiac events. At follow-up, almost half of the population had dilatation of either the aortic root or ascending aorta. The relatively high frequency of cardiac events in association with extraordinarily little serious cardiac morbidity and mortality is a testimony to the quality of care that is able to be given these days to prevent significant adverse outcomes.

Given the fact that the average age of entry into this longitudinal study was just 35 years (±16 years) and 25% of the population had already required some type of intervention within the subsequent 9 years, one could cautiously project that many adults with bicuspid aortic valve will eventually need intervention for aortic valve disease or aortic dilatation. Even in the absence of symptoms, moderate or severe aortic stenosis is likely to eventually cause problems. This report confirms this statement.

The association between orientation of bicuspid aortic valve leaflets, aortic valve dysfunction, and subsequent intervention has been reported in children and adolescents.[1] This association may be mediated by the influence of bicuspid aortic valve leaflet spacial orientation on the elastic properties of the aorta.

Often there is a bit of good news mixed with not so good news in longitudinal studies. The good news in this report is that at least over a period of 9 years, survival rates in subjects with bicuspid aortic valves are not lower than for the general population. The not so good news is that there is a high likelihood that such individuals will at some point in time require interventions on their aortic valve and/or their aorta. Age, severity of aortic stenosis, and severity of aortic regurgitation all independently predict the need for intervention. In most instances, a pediatric diagnosis is made following the detection of a systolic murmur with the confirmation of diagnosis made by echocardiography. This is not an uncommon circumstance on our watch. This report allows us pediatricians and pediatric cardiologists to better inform our patients with this condition about their long-term prognosis.

This commentary closes with a *Clinical Fact/Curio* posed in the form of a query having to do with a cardiac defect. What common congenital heart defect, one that most of us consider to be relatively benign, actually causes more morbidity than all other congenital heart defects combined? The answer is that the most common congenital heart defect, present in 1% to 2% of the population, is a bicuspid aortic valve. If one considers the span of a lifetime, over that span, about one-third of affected people will have a serious complication—valvular stenosis, regurgitation, infective endocarditis, or aortic dissection. If one runs the math on this, the bicuspid valve may be responsible for more deaths and morbidity than all other congenital heart defects combined.[2]

J. A. Stockman III, MD

References

1. Fernandes SM, Khairy P, Sanders SP, et al. Bicuspid aortic valve morphology and interventions in the young. *J Am Coll Cardiol.* 2007;49:2211-2214.
2. De Mozzi P, Longo UG, Galanti G, et al. Bicuspid aortic valve: a literature review and its impact on sport activity. *Br Med Bull.* 2008;85:63-65.

Shared Genetic Causes of Cardiac Hypertrophy in Children and Adults

Morita H, Rehm HL, Menesses A, et al (Harvard Med School, Boston, MA; Harvard Med School–Partners HealthCare Ctr for Genetics and Genomics, Boston, MA; Baylor College of Med, Houston, TX; et al)

N Engl J Med 358:1899-1908, 2008

Background.—The childhood onset of idiopathic cardiac hypertrophy that occurs without a family history of cardiomyopathy can portend a poor prognosis. Despite morphologic similarities to genetic cardiomyopathies of adulthood, the contribution of genetics to childhood-onset hypertrophy is unknown.

Methods.—We assessed the family and medical histories of 84 children (63 boys and 21 girls) with idiopathic cardiac hypertrophy diagnosed before 15 years of age (mean [± SD] age, 6.99 ± 6.12 years). We sequenced eight genes: *MYH7, MYBPC3, TNNT2, TNNI3, TPM1, MYL3, MYL2,* and *ACTC.* These genes encode sarcomere proteins that, when mutated, cause adult-onset cardiomyopathies. We also sequenced *PRKAG2* and *LAMP2,* which encode metabolic proteins; mutations in these genes can cause early-onset ventricular hypertrophy.

Results.—We identified mutations in 25 of 51 affected children without family histories of cardiomyopathy and in 21 of 33 affected children with familial cardiomyopathy. Among 11 of the 25 children with presumed sporadic disease, 4 carried new mutations and 7 inherited the mutations. Mutations occurred predominantly (in >75% of the children) in *MYH7* and *MYBPC3;* significantly more *MYBPC3* missense mutations were detected than occur in adult-onset cardiomyopathy (P<0.005). Neither hypertrophic severity nor contractile function correlated with familial or genetic status. Cardiac transplantation and sudden death were more prevalent among mutation-positive than among mutation-negative children; implantable cardioverter–defibrillators were more frequent (P=0.007) in children with family histories that were positive for the mutation.

Conclusions.—Genetic causes account for about half of presumed sporadic cases and nearly two thirds of familial cases of childhood-onset hypertrophy. Childhood-onset hypertrophy should prompt genetic analyses and family evaluations.

▶ It is quite amazing how much we have learned about the relationship between cardiac hypertrophy in children in particular and related genetic influences. This report is important because it gives us solid information about the genetic causes of cardiac hypertrophy, which unfortunately can first present with a life-threatening event. Despite sophisticated medical management, rates of death and cardiac transplantation among children with symptomatic childhood-onset cardiomyopathy approach 10%. The early age of diagnosis and the striking differences in morbidity and mortality that distinguish childhood cardiomyopathies from adult-onset cardiomyopathies have been interpreted to indicate distinct causes of these conditions. We do know that adult-onset hypertrophic cardiomyopathy is a fairly prevalent genetic condition caused by inherited or new mutations in genes that encode sarcomere proteins. There is a whole list of these genes that have been elucidated. Less commonly, hypertrophic cardiomyopathy can be caused by mutation in other genes, but manifestations before 14 years of age are atypical, even in children with an inherited gene mutation.

The study reported from Boston was undertaken to determine whether some childhood-onset left ventricular hypertrophies share a genetic cause with hypertrophic cardiomyopathy. These genetic studies of childhood-onset cardiomyopathy presenting as unexplained left ventricular hypertrophy in the absence of systemic disease reveal a gene mutation in 46 of 84 patients (55%). The rates of mutation detection are similar among children with familial cardiomyopathy (64%) and among children with presumed sporadic cardiomyopathy (49%). This suggests that unexplained hypertrophy that presents during childhood should prompt evaluation for a potential genetic cause of the cardiac findings. It should also be noted that all but one of the 46 mutations identified occurred in a sarcomere-protein gene. Thus, despite considerable clinical differences between childhood-onset hypertrophy and hypertrophic cardiomyopathy in the adult, the data from this study do seem to define an etiologic relationship between these 2 pathologic conditions.

For whatever reason, children affected with cardiomyopathy who have a documented genetic cause or a strong family history seem to be the ones who receive the most aggressive therapy in the form of placement of an implantable cardioverter-defibrillator. These devices can and do prevent sudden death in children with familial diseases, whereas sudden deaths still have been reported in children with presumed sporadic disease. Perhaps, cardiologists will be more aggressive not only in finding out whether there is a genetic cause but also, in fact, using implantable cardioverter-defibrillators, because approximately half of all cases of childhood-onset isolated cardiac hypertrophy are in fact now known to be caused by gene mutations.

There is a great push these days to screen all young athletes for existing cardiac disease with tools such as an electrocardiogram (ECG), an echocardiogram, and/or an exercise test. The value of this remains controversial. Basavarajaiah et al assess the prevalence of hypertrophic cardiomyopathy in 3500 elite British athletes by use of the clinical history, physical examination, screening ECG, and echocardiogram.[1] One percent had deep T-wave inversion and 1.5% had echocardiographic evidence of left ventricular hypertrophy. Physiological adaptation to training explained the findings in 50 subjects. Just 0.08% had left ventricular hypertrophy with nondilated left ventricles and associated T-wave inversion. All had normal cardiac MRI, normal right-ventricular and left-ventricular structure and function, and normal 48-hour ambulatory ECG monitoring. The results of this study suggest that routine noninvasive testing with an echocardiogram appears to be a cost inefficient way to prospectively screen highly trained athletes, particularly those competing at the Olympic level. Also, the role of the resting ECG, a much less expensive modality as a pre-screening requirement, seems to remain controversial. Needless to say, all of us will be hearing more on this topic as time goes by.

This commentary closes with a *Clinical Fact/Curio* about preventive cardiology. For some time, it has been thought that the ingestion of garlic might be protective of one's heart. Indeed, recent animal studies have suggested that one mechanism of garlic's protection may have to do with its ability to decrease pulmonary hypertension. This potentially lethal condition increases the work of the right side of the heart leading to heart failure. This particular form of high blood pressure might be prevented by a daily downing of 2 cloves of fresh garlic or its powered equivalent, a recent study shows. A pharmacologist at the University of Alabama in Birmingham has reported experiments showing that constituents of some garlic tablets could relax constricted blood vessels, just what is needed to alleviate pulmonary hypertension. The tablets that were most effective had been prepared from fresh garlic or were labeled as likely to contain allicin. The latter is a highly reactive compound, responsible for garlic's characteristic pungent aroma. It is normally formed only when raw garlic is crushed. The recent experiment consisted of giving pure allicin or over-the-counter garlic supplements containing allicin to rats for 3 weeks before administering a drug that causes pulmonary hypertension. Control animals were given a placebo. Only animals receiving allicin were protected from progressive injury to the walls of blood vessels and elevated blood pressure in their lungs.

While an apple a day may keep the doctor away, a garlic clove, or two, surely will.[2]

J. A. Stockman III, MD

References

1. Basavarajaiah S, Wilson M, Whyte G, et al. Prevalence of hypertrophic cardiomyopathy in highly trained athletes. *J Am Coll Cardiol.* 2008;51:1033-1039.
2. Fallon MB, Abrams GA, Abdel-Razek TT, et al. Garlic prevents hypoxic pulmonary hypertension in rats. *Am J Physiol Lung Cell Mol Physiol.* 1998;275: L283-L287.

Angiotensin II Blockade and Aortic-Root Dilation in Marfan's Syndrome

Brooke BS, Habashi JP, Judge DP, et al (Johns Hopkins Univ School of Medicine, Baltimore, MD)

N Engl J Med 358:2787-2795, 2008

Background.—Progressive enlargement of the aortic root, leading to dissection, is the main cause of premature death in patients with Marfan's syndrome. Recent data from mouse models of Marfan's syndrome suggest that aortic-root enlargement is caused by excessive signaling by transforming growth factor β (TGF-β) that can be mitigated by treatment with TGF-β antagonists, including angiotensin II–receptor blockers (ARBs). We evaluated the clinical response to ARBs in pediatric patients with Marfan's syndrome who had severe aortic-root enlargement.

Methods.—We identified 18 pediatric patients with Marfan's syndrome who had been followed during 12 to 47 months of therapy with ARBs after other medical therapy had failed to prevent progressive aortic-root enlargement. The ARB was losartan in 17 patients and irbesartan in 1 patient. We evaluated the efficacy of ARB therapy by comparing the rates of change in aortic-root diameter before and after the initiation of treatment with ARBs.

Results.—The mean ($\pm$SD) rate of change in aortic-root diameter decreased significantly from 3.54 ± 2.87 mm per year during previous medical therapy to 0.46 ± 0.62 mm per year during ARB therapy ($P<0.001$). The deviation of aortic-root enlargement from normal, as expressed by the rate of change in z scores, was reduced by a mean difference of 1.47 z scores per year (95% confidence interval, 0.70 to 2.24; $P<0.001$) after the initiation of ARB therapy. The sinotubular junction, which is prone to dilation in Marfan's syndrome as well, also showed a reduced rate of change in diameter during ARB therapy ($P<0.05$), whereas the distal ascending aorta, which does not normally become dilated in Marfan's syndrome, was not affected by ARB therapy.

Conclusions.—In a small cohort study, the use of ARB therapy in patients with Marfan's syndrome significantly slowed the rate of progressive aortic-root dilation. These findings require confirmation in a randomized trial.

▶ All too frequently, pediatricians tend not to think Marfan's syndrome causes that much difficulty during childhood. Indeed, it can. This is an autosomal dominant connective tissue disorder affecting about 1 in 5000 people. In the last 10 years, we have learned the genetic and molecular basis for the problem. Marfan's syndrome is caused by mutations in the gene encoding fibrillin-1 (FBN1). These FBN1 mutations cause defects in a variety of different organs, but the most life threatening are those defects causing progressive enlargement and dissection of the aortic root.

Both pediatric and adult patients with Marfan's syndrome should be followed serially with cardiac imaging studies to determine whether anatomical changes due to the gene mutation are occurring. The management of the syndrome usually involves the use of beta-blockers and other agents such as angiotensin-converting-enzyme (ACE) inhibitors and calcium-channel blockers.

The authors of this report decided to see if angiotensin II blockade might halt or at least slow down the rate of vascular problems in patients with Marfan's syndrome. They decided to study this in a model of Marfan's syndrome in mice shown to have a deficiency of fibrillin-1 leading to excessive signaling by transforming growth factor β (TGF-β), the underlying mechanism that leads to progressive enlargement of the aortic root in the human. Interestingly, these genetically engineered mice that have been developed to have a deficiency of fibrillin-1 and who have pathologic changes in their aortic root closely mimicking those in humans will benefit from treatment with TGF-β antagonists. A drug currently on the market, the angiotensin II-receptor blocker, losartan, will attenuate or prevent changes in the aortic wall and halt the progressive dilation of the aortic root in these Marfan-ized mice. Losartan (trade name Cozaar) is a commonly used antihypertensive medication.

The report of Brooke et al represents a retrospective review of all pediatric patients treated in the medical genetics clinic of Johns Hopkins Hospital with a diagnosis of Marfan's syndrome. Patients had echocardiograms performed to measure the aortic-root diameter. The effects of losartan therapy were evaluated to determine whether this drug was capable of preventing or slowing down aortic-root enlargement. The age of initiation of therapy ranged from just 14 months to 16 years. The study does provide preliminary evidence suggesting that the addition of losartan to traditional treatment regimens used to manage aortic aneurysm in patients with Marfan's syndrome indeed may be beneficial. The initiation of losartan therapy resulted in a significant reduction in the rate of change in aortic-root diameter, for example, when compared with the effects of beta-blocker therapy alone. The use of angiotensin II blockade did not totally arrest aortic growth, but did reduce the pathologic rate of increase in the diameter of the aortic segments.

Before jumping on the angiotensin II blockade bandwagon, recognize that the study out of Johns Hopkins did have some limitations. The study represented a nonrandomized, retrospective, observational study that evaluated only a small subset of pediatric patients with Marfan's syndrome who had existing evidence of severe aortic-root enlargement or rapid increase in aortic diameter. Selection bias may have resulted in the identification of patients who were more adherent to and therefore more likely to have a response to angiotensin II blockade therapy. The bottom line is that the findings from this report must be confirmed by a prospective, randomized trial. A trial coordinated by the Pediatric Heart Network of the National Heart, Lung and Blood Institute, comparing losartan with atenolol (the most commonly used beta-blocker) in patients with Marfan's syndrome, began enrolling patients in the winter of 2007. Any patient with Marfan's syndrome who might be eligible to be part of this study should be enrolled.

The authors of this report conclude that until the NIH trial begins to produce data that may show evidence for the potential efficacy of angiotensin II blockade in subjects with Marfan's syndrome, patients should not be put on this therapy willy-nilly. This will be a hard recommendation to accept, largely because therapy with a simple antihypertensive is so seductively easy to use and may in fact turn out to be of great benefit during the waiting period until this trial ends. Obviously, clinicians will have to use their own judgment in this regard. The bottom line, however, is that if the data from this report hold up, we finally have found something that can either stop or slow down the progression of a highly lethal component of Marfan's syndrome.

This commentary closes with a *Clinical Fact/Curio* regarding the cardiovascular system. It is in the form of a question. Is an aortic aneurysm more likely to rupture on a day with a high or a low barometric pressure? Specifically, are periods of low atmospheric pressure associated with an increased risk of rupture of an abdominal aortic aneurysm? The answer is probably yes, as reported in the *Annals of the Royal College of Surgeons of England.*[1] When 182 cases of aortic aneurysm rupture were examined retrospectively, the days on which these patients presented exhibited a significantly lower mean atmospheric pressure than days when no rupture occurred. Regression analysis showed an association between low daily atmospheric pressure and the incidence of rupture. This finding was independent of temperature.

Perhaps those with a high risk of rupture of an abdominal aortic aneurysm should purchase a Speedo LZR racer suit, which debuted in March 2008. At the time of the Olympics, the new Speedos were all the buzz. Swimmers donning the suit have broken 46 world records so far. The suit contains polyurethane panels that strategically are placed around parts of the torso, abdomen, and lower back. It is sort of an expensive corset that keeps the body in a streamlined position. If your aorta is a little larger than normal and you wish to avoid the vicissitudes of a low barometric pressure day, don your Speedo LZR!

J. A. Stockman III, MD

Reference

1. Smith RA, Edwards PR, Da Silva AF. Are periods of low atmospheric pressure associated with an increased risk of abdominal aortic aneurysm rupture? *Ann R Coll Surg Engl.* 2008;90:389-393.

Left Ventricular Mass Index in Children with White Coat Hypertension

Lande MB, Meagher CC, Fisher SG, et al (Univ of Rochester Med Ctr, NY)
J Pediatr 153:50-54, 2008

Objectives.—To determine whether children with white coat hypertension (WCH) have evidence of target-organ damage by comparing the left ventricular mass index (LVMI) of subjects with WCH with that of matched normotensive and hypertensive controls.

Study Design.—Each subject in the WCH group was matched by body mass index (BMI; ± 10%), age (± 1 year), and sex to a normotensive control and a hypertensive control. Echocardiograms were reviewed to determine the LVMI for each subject. These triple matches were analyzed using repeated-measures analysis of variance to detect differences in LVMI among the 3 groups.

Results.—A total of 27 matched triplets were established. The groups were comparable for sex, age, and BMI. Mean LVMI was 29.2 g/m$^{2.7}$ for the normotensive group, 32.3 g/m$^{2.7}$ for the WCH group, and 35.1 g/m$^{2.7}$ for the sustained hypertensive group (normotensive vs WCH, $P = .028$; WCH vs sustained hypertension, $P = .07$). Left ventricular hypertrophy was not present in any subject in the normotensive or WCH groups, but was found in 26% of the sustained hypertensive subjects ($P < .001$).

Conclusions.—After controlling closely for BMI, the LVMI in the subjects with WCH was between that of the normotensives and sustained hypertensives, suggesting that WCH may be associated with hypertensive end-organ effects.

▶ When this editor went to medical school, we were taught that white coat hypertension was nothing to worry about. Lots of patients were afraid of doctors. As it turns out, white coat hypertension in many ways is a misnomer because the problem really relates to an excessive variability in blood pressure, often triggered by certain stimulants, only one of which is the sight of a white coat. Studies in recent years in adults do suggest that white coat hypertension is not a benign condition. A significant proportion of adults with this entity progress to sustained hypertension. To date, there have been relatively few studies of the cardiovascular implications of white coat hypertension in children, but the studies do suggest that children may be prone to progress to sustained hypertension as well.

The study of Lande et al from Rochester, New York goes one step further in its design by comparing left ventricular mass in children with white coat hypertension in comparison to children with normotension and sustained hypertension. The study was unique in that it had close matching of subjects for body mass index (BMI), itself an independent determinant of left ventricular mass. The results of the study demonstrated that subjects with white coat hypertension have a mean ventricular mass between that of normotensive and sustained hypertensive children. The results also provided evidence that white coat hypertension has an effect on the cardiovascular system of youngsters that is independent of BMI, supporting the theory that white coat hypertension in children may represent a prehypertensive state.

So what should we do with this information? If you see a child in your office who you suspect might have white coat hypertension, the way of confirming the diagnosis is with ambulatory blood pressure monitoring. Criteria do exist not only to define the presence of true hypertension, but also white coat hypertension. Once a diagnosis is made of white coat hypertension, youngsters with it should be counseled in lifestyle modifications and monitored for the development of sustained hypertension. As of now, there is no evidence that one can do anything to prevent the occurrence of sustained hypertension, but there certainly is value in picking it up earlier than otherwise might happen. The lesson learned, most importantly, is that white coat hypertension is not likely to be a benign condition.

This commentary closes with a *Clinical Fact/Curio* related to the diagnosis of hypertension. Just how important is it to fully remove an outer garment before taking a blood pressure? Is such a determination really that much less accurate than with taking the blood pressure over bare skin? The answer is, contrary to popular opinion, that taking a blood pressure reading over a sleeved arm may be just as good as taking it over bare skin, at least in adults.[1] Over a 2-year period, 376 patients aged 18 to 85 had their blood pressure taken in a family practice clinic with the same automatic device. Everyone had a first reading obtained on bare skin. Patients then were randomly assigned to the sleeved arm group or bare arm group for the second reading. There was no statistical difference between the 2 methods of blood pressure taking. Whether or not patients rolled up their sleeves appeared to be clinically irrelevant.

It would be interesting for someone to do this same study on youngsters. Needless to say, when talking about a "sleeved" arm, one is talking about a simple garment such as a shirt, not a parka.

J. A. Stockman III, MD

Reference

1. Ma G, Sabin N, Dawes M. A comparison of blood pressure measurement over a sleeved arm versus a bare arm. *CMAJ.* 2008;178:585-589.

Effect of Domperidone on QT Interval in Neonates

Djeddi D, Kongolo G, Lefaix C, et al (School Hosp of Amiens, France)
J Pediatr 153:663-666, 2008

Objectives.—To determine whether oral domperidone is associated with QT interval prolongation and ventricular arrhythmia and to identify factors that can influence these effects.

Study Design.—An electrocardiogram was performed before and after oral administration of domperidone in 31 neonates or infants classified into 3 groups according to gestational age.

Results.—Oral domperidone is associated with QTc prolongation except in infants with a gestational age less than 32 weeks of amenorrhea ($P < .005$). Mean QTc prolongation was 14 msec. On univariate analysis, oral domperidone-induced QTc prolongation was correlated with gestational age, birth weight, and elevated serum potassium. On multivariate analysis, after adjustment for gestational age, serum potassium was the only factor independently associated with interval QT prolongation during treatment. No ventricular arrhythmias were observed.

Conclusions.—This study shows a significant association between oral domperidone therapy and QTc prolongation. Two risk factors were identified: advanced gestational age and serum potassium at the upper limit of normal. It is recommended that measurement of the QT interval be done before and after oral domperidone therapy.

▶ The story linking the use of gastrointestinal prokinetics and induction of QT prolongation is getting longer and longer. For some time it has been known that certain drugs are likely to produce excessive prolongation of the QT interval and that when these drugs are stopped, the QT interval reverts back to normal. QT prolongation places a subject at risk for torsades de pointes, a potentially fatal arrhythmia. The number of drugs with the potential to cause QT prolongation has grown with time. If you want to look this list up, it can be found at http://www.torsades.org. The report of Djeddi et al adds one more agent to this list of drugs, that drug being domperidone, a drug used to help manage gastroesophageal reflux.

Most pediatric practitioners learned about the interaction between drugs and the QT interval when cisapride was recognized to cause this problem. Cisapride is a prokinetic agent that was widely used in the 1980s and 1990s for gastrointestinal disorders, especially gastrointestinal reflux. Although initially considered safe, marketing of the drug was stopped in 2000 after the publication of multiple reports of QT prolongation, ventricular arrhythmia and cardiac arrest in adults and children. In studies of children, cisapride was associated with a QTc prolongation of 10 to 15 msec. Like cisapride, domperidone is a prokinetic agent, but one that is chemically distinct. As cisapride was being withdrawn from the market due to its malignant side effect profile, domperidone was becoming the preferred prokinetic agent in Europe. The drug was never approved for use by the United States Food and Drug Administration, however. Domperidone's effect on cardiac repolarization involves the same mechanism as for cisapride and other medications known to prolong the QT interval. In the current study, Djeddi et al report QT prolongation in 31 infants taking oral domperidone. The mean QTc prolongation was 14 msec, similar to that seen for cisapride. Only one infant developed a QTc of longer than 450 msec, which did return to normal on discontinuation of the drug. None of the patients studied had a malignant arrhythmia.

Fortunately, in the United States, the use of prokinetic medications to manage gastroesophageal reflux has diminished quite significantly and not just due to the known side effects of drugs like cisapride. Prokinetic medications have been shown to be not all that effective at controlling symptoms, despite the fact they improve test results for reflux disease such as esophageal pH, esophageal sphincter pressure, and gastric emptying time. While there are certainly legitimate indications for using prokinetic agents in some disorders of gastrointestinal motility, when it comes to gastroesophageal reflux, prokinetics may not be worth their risk. In a summary of randomized trials using prokinetics, none provided any robust evidence of domperidone's efficacy for the management of reflux.[1]

For more on the topic of prokinetics and QT prolongation, see the superb editorial by Collins and Sondheimar.[2] This commentary closes with a *Clinical Fact/Curio* about a cardiac condition. You should be aware of a disorder known as Brugada syndrome. Brugada syndrome (right bundle branch block,

ST segment elevation in electrocardiography leads V_1 to V_3, and a high inci-dence of ventricular fibrillation) is an important, although uncommon, cause of sudden cardiac death in young, asymptomatic men from Southeast Asia. Many genetic mutations affecting a sodium channel gene have been identified in the 15 years since the syndrome was first described.[3]

J. A. Stockman III, MD

References

1. Pritchard DS, Baber N, Stephenson T. Should domperidone be used for the treat-ment of gastroesophageal reflux in children? Systematic review of randomized control trials in children age one month to 11 years. *Br J Clin Pharmacol.* 2005; 59:725-729.
2. Collins KK, Sondheimar JM. Domperidone-induced QT prolongation: another drug added to the list. *J Pediatr.* 2008;153:596-598.
3. Chen PS, Priori SG. The Brugada syndrome. *J Am Coll Cardiol.* 2008;51: 1176-1180.

Cardiovascular evaluation, including resting and exercise electrocardiography, before participation in competitive sports: cross sectional study

Sofi F, Capablo A, Pucci N, et al (Univ of Florence, Italy; et al)
BMJ 337:a346, 2008

Objective.—To evaluate the clinical usefulness of complete preparti-cipation cardiovascular screening in a large cohort of sports participants.

Design.—Cross sectional study of data over a five year period.

Setting.—Institute of Sports Medicine in Florence, Italy.

Participants.—30 065 (23 570 men) people seeking to obtain clinical eligibility for competitive sports.

Main Outcome Measures.—Results of resting and exercise 12 lead elec-trocardiography.

Results.—Resting 12 lead ECG patterns showed abnormalities in 1812 (6%) participants, with the most common abnormalities (>80%) concerning innocent ECG changes. Exercise ECG showed an abnormal pattern in 1459 (4.9%) participants. Exercise ECG showed cardiac anomalies in 1227 athletes with normal findings on resting ECG. At the end of screening, 196 (0.6%) participants were considered ineligible for competitive sports. Among the 159 participants who were disqualified at the end of the screening for cardiac reasons, a consistent proportion (n=126, 79.2%) had shown innocent or negative findings on resting 12 lead ECG but clear pathological alterations during the exercise test. After adjustment for possible confounders, logistic regres-sion analysis showed that age >30 years was significantly associated with an increased risk of being disqualified for cardiac findings during exercise testing.

Conclusions.—Among people seeking to take part in competitive sports, exercise ECG can identify those with cardiac abnormalities. Follow-up studies would show if disqualification of such people would reduce the incidence of CV events among athletes.

▶ Few among us have been immune to the controversy about how thoroughly we should be evaluating young athletes before their participation in sporting activities. Indeed, the screening strategy that should be used to identify young athletes at risk for sudden cardiac death is a highly controversial matter. For many years, the medical community has disputed the cost effectiveness, feasibility, and accuracy of including 12-lead electrocardiography in the cardiovascular screening of athletes. Sudden cardiac death in young athletes is caused by a diverse set of structural diseases of the heart (such as cardiomyopathies) and electrical defects (such as ion channelopathies). In the United States alone, one competitive athlete dies every 3 days from an unrecognized cardiovascular disorder. American and European authorities have recommended a comprehensive preparticipation evaluation, which includes a detailed patient and family history and a physical examination, for all athletes of 12 years or more. Warning symptoms of an underlying cardiovascular disease—exertional chest pain, syncope or near syncope, palpitations, excessive dyspnea, and unexplained seizures—warrant cessation of sports activity pending the results of diagnostic tests. A family history of unexplained death or sudden death before the age of 50 as the result of cardiac problems may also indicate the presence of a genetic cardiovascular disorder. A substantial challenge to screening is that apparently healthy asymptomatic athletes may have unsuspected cardiovascular disease—death is the first clinical manifestation of cardiac disease in somewhere between 60% and 80% of athletes with sudden cardiac death. To date, no study monitoring sudden cardiac death has shown that a preparticipation evaluation based on history and physical examination alone can prevent or detect athletes at risk for sudden death.

The value of adding noninvasive cardiovascular tests such as ECG to the screening process in athletes has been widely debated. In 2007, the American Heart Association reaffirmed its recommendations against universal ECG screening in athletes, citing a low prevalence of disease, poor sensitivity, high false-positive rate, poor cost-effectiveness, and lack of clinicians to interpret the results. In contrast, the European Society of Cardiology, the International Olympic Committee, and the governing associations of several United States and international professional sports leagues endorse the use of ECG in preparticipation screening of athletes. These recommendations are supported by studies showing that ECG is more sensitive than history and physical examination alone in identifying athletes with underlying cardiovascular disease. In 2006, a study of more than 40 000 athletes in Italy over a 25-year period found that disqualification on the basis of a standardized history, physical examination, and electrocardiography produced a 10-fold reduction in the incidence of sudden cardiac death in young competitive athletes and an 89% reduction of sudden death as the result of a cardiomyopathy, in comparison to preparticipation screening that did not include an ECG.[1]

The report of Sofi et al seems to confirm that among people seeking to take part in competitive sports, an exercise ECG is better at identifying those with cardiac abnormalities. An important element of the Sofi et al study is that only a small proportion (1.2%) of athletes had distinct abnormalities identified on resting ECG. The issue is whether exercise ECG should be a substitute for a resting ECG. If this were to be the recommendation, it severely ups the ante in terms of the logistics of doing a preparticipation screening in a young athlete. Needless to say, the controversy regarding what is practical and what is ideal in this regard will continue for some time. To read more about this, see the excellent editorial by Drezner and Kahn.[2]

This commentary closes with a *Clinical Fact/Curio* about cardiovascular fitness of women over the years as evidenced by age of participation in Olympic Games. 2008 was a pretty significant year for the Olympics, with a 41-year-old woman swimmer garnering a silver medal. The following shows the age spectrum, over the years, of those competing and winning in the Olympics[3]:

- Age 11: Italy's Lugina Giavotti won silver in gymnastics in 1928.
- Age 13: Marjorie Gestring of the US won gold in diving in 1936 the youngest gold medalist ever.
- Age 14: Hungarian swimmer Krisztine Egerszegi won gold in 1988.
- Age 15: US runner Pearl Jones won gold in the 4 x 100 m relay in 1952.
- Age 33: US swimmer Dara Torres won 2 gold and 3 bronze medals in 2000. Dara was the winner of a silver medal in Beijing, 2008.
- Age 34: UK sprinter Kelly Holmes won gold in the 800 and 1500 m events in 2004.
- Age 46: Ethel Seymour won a bronze medal with Great Britain's gymnastics team in 1928.
- Age 59: Bill Northam of Australia won gold in yachting in 1964.
- Age 72: Swedish shooter Oscar Swahn won silver in the team double-shot running deer event in 1920.

J. A. Stockman III, MD

References

1. Corrado D, Basso C, Pavei A, Michieli P, Schiavon M, Thiene G. Trends in sudden cardiovascular death in young competitive athletes after implementation of a pre-participation screening program. *JAMA*. 2006;296:1593-1601.
2. Drezner JA, Kahn K. Sudden cardiac death in young athletes. Evidence supports a systematic screening program before participation. *BMJ*. 2008; 337:61-62.
3. Stokstad E. What's age got to do with it: medalists span the decades. *Science*. 2008;321:625.

Mandarin juice improves the antioxidant status of hypercholesterolemic children

Codoñer-Franch P, López-Jaén AB, Muñiz P, et al (Univ of Valencia, Spain)
J Pediatr Gastroenterol Nutr 47:349-355, 2008

Background.—Oxidative stress has been linked to such degenerative diseases as atherosclerosis, and it has been suggested that increased dietary intake of antioxidants may reduce its progression.

Objective.—To determine the effect of mandarin juice consumption on biomarkers related to oxidative stress in hypercholesterolemic children.

Materials and Methods.—The diet of 48 children with plasma cholesterol >200 mg/dL and low-density lipoprotein cholesterol >130 mg/dL was supplemented for 28 days with 500 mL/day of pure (100%) mandarin juice (Citrus clementina Hort. ex Tan.). The composition of the mandarin juice was analyzed, and its antioxidant antiradical activity was evaluated in vitro. Malondialdehyde, carbonyl groups, vitamins E and C, erythrocyte-reduced glutathione, and plasma lipids were measured at the onset and at the end of the supplementation period. The paired Student t test was used to compare values before and after supplementation.

Results.—Mandarin juice exerted a strong antioxidant effect mainly due to its high hydroxyl activity and, to a lesser extent, to its superoxide scavenger activity. At the end of the study, levels of the plasma biomarkers of oxidative stress were significantly decreased (malondialdehyde -7.4%, carbonyl groups -29.1%, P < 0.01), whereas the plasma antioxidants vitamin E and C (13.5%, P < 0.001 and 68.2%, P < 0.00001, respectively) and intraerythrocyte glutathione level (36.7%, P < 0.00001) were significantly increased. Plasma lipids and antibodies to oxidized low-density lipoproteins remained unchanged.

Conclusions.—Regular ingestion of mandarin juice significantly reduces plasma biomarkers of lipid and protein oxidation and enhances the antioxidant status of consumers.

▶ Who would have thought that mandarin juice would be truly good for us and serve as a strong antioxidant! Natural citrus juices contain vitamin C, folate, and carotenoids, as well as some flavonoids that are almost exclusively found in the citrus species. Flavonoids exert antioxidant effects. Sweet orange juice has been reported to exert a beneficial effect in animals and humans and is, by far, the most frequently studied citrus fruit juice. However, despite the high consumption of mandarin worldwide, there are no data available about the potential antioxidant effect of mandarin juice in vivo. As far as kids are concerned, if there is some therapeutic benefit to the ingestion of mandarin juice, the latter has the added value of its sweet taste, attractive color, and aroma. Other citrus fruits and their juices can be a bit sour tasting, a turn off for some kids.

The report of Codoñer-Franch et al studied the effects of regular consumption of mandarin juice on the oxidant status of children with high cholesterol levels. Measured were plasma levels of biomarkers derived from the oxidation of lipids as well as the antioxidants vitamin C and E, cellular reduced gluta-thione, and the blood lipid profile before and after daily consumption of half a liter of commercial mandarin juice for a period of 28 days. It was clear that mandarin juice exerted a strong antioxidant effect producing a positive influ-ence on most of the biomarkers measured. As would be expected, the ingestion of half a liter of mandarin juice daily for 1 month did not significantly affect total cholesterol, high-density lipoprotein (HDL), or low-density lipoprotein (LDL) levels. The antioxidant properties, however, theoretically should protect against the oxidation of LDL, a known risk factor for coronary heart disease.

No one would argue that fruit juices are better than fresh fruits. However, kids seem to preferentially enjoy drinking juices. It is conceivable that drinking 100% pure mandarin juice could reduce the intake of other beverages and snacks, increasing the antioxidant status of those who consume this juice. It goes without saying that while mandarin juice most likely is an excellent source of antioxidants and could theoretically protect against atherosclerotic disease, further studies are necessary to be sure about this and in the meantime, if one is to imbibe of the mandarin, this dietary maneuver should be combined with other dietary and life-style factors to lower the risk of coronary heart disease. The Florida Citrus Growers Association should take due note of this report and its implications.

This commentary closes with a *Clinical Fact/Curio* describing one way to enhance cardiovascular performance. At the 2004 Olympic Games, 30 minutes before the women's marathon, Deena Kastor of the United States began her "warm-up." Instead of jogging in the 35°C heat, she donned an ice-filled vest, sat down and waited for the start of the 42.2-kilometer run. More than 2 hours later, staying cool seemed to pay off. A kilometer from the finish, Kastor pulled into third place to secure a bronze medal. The logic of using an ice vest seemed somewhat unimpeachable: as body temperature climbs to 40°C, strength and endurance evaporate. So cooling off before the competition should enable an athlete to push harder and longer. Runners, rowers, cyclists, and others are already using ice vests. Since the 1970s, numerous studies have shown that precooling dramatically affects some measures of athletic output. A 1995 study of 14 male runners found that if they were first chilled for 30 minutes in a chamber at 5°C, they could run on a treadmill at a certain level of exertion for an average of 26.4 minutes, 4 minutes longer than they averaged otherwise. A study in 2005 involving 18 female cross-country runners who had ingested encapsulated thermometers showed that those who wore ice vests an hour before their 4- to 5-kilometer race, on average, had a core body temperature half a degree lower than those who did not, even at the end of the race. This same study found only an insignificant difference of a few seconds between the times of those who wore the ice vests and those who did not. A subsequent study looking at participants in a 5-kilometer race did show that the wearing of an ice vest during a 38-minute warm-up of jogging and stretching provided a 13-second advantage, on average.

How chilling out helps one's competitiveness is a mystery. When the skin is cool, less blood flows to carry heat away, leaving more to course through the muscles. Precooling may also change the input from the body's heat sensors to the brain, which regulates pacing, enabling the athlete to push harder. This much is certain: using an ice vest will not make an athlete unbeatable. Paula

Radcliffe of the United Kingdom, the world's record holder for the women's marathon, wore one before the Athens race. She overheated and dropped out 6 kilometers from the finish.[1]

J. A. Stockman III, MD

Reference

1. Cho A. Can ice vests provide a competitive chill? *Science.* 2008;321:625.

Spectrum and Management of Hypertriglyceridemia Among Children in Clinical Practice
Manlhiot C, Larsson P, Gurofsky RC, et al (Univ of Toronto, Ontario, Canada)
Pediatrics 123:458-465, 2009

Objectives.—The prevalence and identification of hypertriglyceridemia in youths will likely will increase in the future as a consequence of childhood obesity and increased screening for dyslipidemias. We sought to review our clinical experience with hypertriglyceridemia, evaluate factors associated with increased triglyceride levels, and review treatment options to provide guidance for management.

Methods.—Clinical review of data for all patients who had ≥1 elevated triglyceride level (>4 mmol/L [>350 mg/dL]) while being monitored in a specialized lipid disorders clinic was performed.

Results.—The study population consisted of 76 patients with 761 clinic visits. Hypertriglyceridemia was secondary to lifestyle factors for 13 patients. The rest had primary hypertriglyceridemia, with 32 patients having familial combined hypertriglyceridemia and hypercholesterolemia (type II), 25 patients having primary hypertriglyceridemia (type IV), 4 patients having familial lipase deficiency (type I), and 2 patients having hyperlipoproteinemia E2/E2 phenotype (type III). Triglyceride levels were highest in type I and III hypertriglyceridemia (>10 mmol/L [>900 mg/dL]), followed by type IV and adiposity-related hypertriglyceridemia (>4 mmol/L [>350 mg/dL]) and finally type II familial combined hypertriglyceridemia and hypercholesterolemia (>2 mmol/L [>180 mg/dL]). A total of 34 patients received 37 trials of drug therapy as part of triglyceride level management (bile acid–binding resins, n = 12; fibrates, *n* = 19; statins, *n* = 6). Triglyceride levels were found to decrease over time with the use of fibrates, to increase with the use of bile acid–binding resins, and not to change with the use of statins.

Conclusions.—Lifestyle modifications remain the primary therapeutic avenue for the management of pediatric hypertriglyceridemia. We propose an algorithm for the management of this heterogeneous population to guide clinicians in their treatment decisions.

▶ So much has been written about hypercholesterolemia that little in the way of light has been shown on the problem of hypertriglyceridemia. Few studies have explored hypertriglyceridemia in children despite the massive volume of literature that exists referable to adults. The condition tends to be under-recognized in children and adolescents, and we have paid modest attention to the many causes of hypertriglyceridemia in the pediatric age group. That is why this report from the Hospital for Sick Children in Toronto is so important.

This study reviews the clinical data for all patients being followed at the Hospital for Sick Children who have elevated triglyceride levels (> 350 mg/dL). One of the most important things we learn from this report is that while hypertriglyceridemia in childhood is a rare disorder, it has many different causes. Whatever the many causes are, hypertriglyceridemia is an independent risk factor for coronary artery disease. It has been suggested that there is more than an 11-fold increase in coronary artery disease risk for patients with triglyceride levels in the range of 500 mg/dL to 800 mg/dL and even values greater than 80 mg/dL carry a 3-fold increased risk of coronary artery disease.[1]

The authors of this report remind us that the classification of pediatric hypertriglyceridemia into etiologic groups can be quite challenging, mainly because hypertriglyceridemia can be multifactorial with both genetic and lifestyle related factors contributing to elevated triglyceride levels. While not perfect, the classification system used in the study of Manlhiot et al is quite helpful for better understanding the phenotypic distribution of dyslipidemias in the pediatric population. The authors divide hypertriglyceridemia into the following groups: adiposity related; type II combined familial hypertriglyceridemia and hypercholesterolemia; and type IV hypertriglyceridemia (characterized by increased triglyceride levels but normal or nearly normal cholesterol levels). They also include the rare type I (familial lipase deficiency) and type III (hyperlipoproteinemia). Triglyceride levels are highest in type I and type III hypertriglyceridemia followed by type IV and adiposity-related hypertriglyceridemia and finally type II familial combined hypertriglyceridemia and hypercholesterolemia.

So what should be done with those who have hypertriglyceridemia? If you are a child, current guidelines suggest that these types of lipid disorders are initially best managed by lifestyle changes as the primary therapeutic intervention. This includes a diet with reduced saturated fat, cholesterol, long-chain fatty acids, refined sugar, sucrose intake, limited alcohol intake, and increased dietary polyunsaturated fat, complex carbohydrate, and soluble protein intake, along with an increase in physical activity. Lifestyle changes should be prioritized over pharmacologic treatment for all types of dyslipidemia except for the most severe forms. If appropriate lifestyle changes fail to lower triglyceride levels sufficiently, then drug therapy should be considered. Because of the scarcity of data on the safety and efficacy of lipid-lowering medications for children and adolescents, pediatric lipid disorder specialists probably should be consulted before medication is prescribed. There are a variety of pharmaceuticals available to manage hypertriglyceridemia, but no one is a silver bullet. Figure 3 in the original article shows a suggested approach. There is a great deal of wisdom contained in the thinking behind this figure, but again it might be wise to use a consultant to help guide one along the way.

The bottom line here is that one should be screening for triglyceride levels and for cholesterol levels in the pediatric age population. Lifestyle changes are the first thing to try to manage either of these problems, but failing that, drug therapy is available. This commentary closes with a *Clinical Fact/Curio* about a dietary risk factor for heart disease. A Physicians' Health Study has found that eating 7 or more eggs a week is associated with a statistical greater probability of the development of heart failure. However, eating up to 6 eggs a week is not associated with such an increased risk.[2] This association has been found to be independent of obesity, smoking, alcohol, atrial fibrillation, and previous myocardial infarction. It will be interesting to see what the Egg Council does with this data from the Physicians' Health Study. One interpretation can be that one can eat 0.85 eggs a day to your heart's delight with sheer abandon.

J. A. Stockman III, MD

References

1. Hopkins PN, Wu LL, Hunt SC, Brinton EA. Plasma triglycerides and type III hyperlipidemia are independently associated with premature familial coronary artery disease. *J Am Coll Cardiol.* 2005;45:1003-1012.
2. Djoussé L, Gaziano JM. Egg consumption and risk of heart failure in the Physicians' Health Study. *Circulation.* 2008;117:512-516.

10 Infectious Diseases and Immunology

The stethoscope as a vector of infectious diseases in the paediatric division
Youngster I, Berkovitch M, Heyman E, et al (Assaf Harofeh Med Ctr, Zerifin, Israel; et al)
Acta Paediatr 97:1253-1255, 2008

Aim.—Nosocomial infections are of great concern in hospital settings, and even more so in the paediatric ward. Health professionals and their medical equipment have long been known to act as vectors of infectious diseases. This study aimed at evaluating the presence of bacterial pathogens on the stethoscopes of medical personnel in the paediatric division.

Methods.—Forty-three stethoscopes belonging to senior physicians, residents, interns and medical students at the paediatric ward were sampled. Bacterial cultures and antibiotic sensitivity testing were carried out.

Results.—All but six bacterial cultures were positive (85.7%). Staphylococcal species were the most common contaminants (47.5%). One case of methicillin-resistant *Staphylococcus aureus* was encountered. Gram-negative organisms were isolated in nine different samples (21%) including one case of *Acinetobacter baumannii* in the neonatal intensive care unit.

Conclusion.—Most stethoscopes harbour potential pathogens. The isolation of Gram-negative organisms pose a real risk of spreading potentially serious infections, especially in the setting of intensive care departments. Apparently, the current recommendations of regular disinfection of stethoscopes are not carried out by health personnel that participated in the study.

▶ One wonders why a report like this would appear in the literature when it is so intuitively obvious that the stethoscope is hardly a sterile instrument. It is good, however, to see reports such as this because they do remind us how dirty we and the equipment we carry around are. In the report of Youngster et al, a total of 43 stethoscopes belonging to attending physicians, residents, interns, and medical students were sampled by swabbing the surface of the diaphragm with a sterile cotton-tip applicator moistened with a physiological solution. Routine bacterial cultures were performed on the swabs. Eight-six percent of the cultures were positive for organisms, some of these not exactly benign organisms. Methicillin-resistant *Staphylococcus aureus* was cultured along with other gram-positive bacilli and some gram-negative organisms including *Escherichia coli, Pseudomonas aeruginosa*, and *Burkholderia cepacia*. Gram-negative organisms were cultured in 21% of the samples.

The solution to this problem is obvious. When it comes to inpatients, it would seem wise to have a stethoscope assigned to each patient and that it be left in the room. Obviously this will not work all that terribly well because such stethoscopes will frequently be deposited around other rooms by care providers. The other solution is also obvious and that is to wipe the stethoscope head with alcohol before and/or after each use. It has been shown that cleaning a stethoscope's diaphragm in this manner results in an immediate reduction in bacterial count by 94% if alcohol swabs are used, 90% with a nonionic detergent, and 75% with soap.[1]

There are only a few studies in the literature that document how frequently we clean our stethoscopes. Those studies suggest that fewer than half of physicians do this just once a day. If you are moving around a hospital and fail to keep your stethoscope clean, please recognize that you are at high risk of spreading nosocomial infections. Carry some alcohol wipes with you in your pocket and use them.

This commentary closes with a *Clinical Fact/Curio* about transmission of infection by things we wear. In Great Britain, the government is trying to ban physicians from wearing white coats in hospitals.[2] Britain is the only country in the world where this has happened so far. A consulting gynecologist at the Royal Free Hospital in London, Dr Adam Magos, has made a proposal for what to do with all the discarded white coats.[3] Dr Magos notes that there will be many thousands of white coats lying idle in hospital laundries and that rather than throwing them away, these are his thoughts of how they might be recycled:

1. Use it as a projector screen.
2. Donate it to developing countries.
3. Give it to any developed country apart from the UK.
4. Give it to the butcher.
5. Give it to the dentist.
6. Cut it up into handkerchiefs.
7. Turn it into nappies.
8. Make sails out of it.
9. Make it into dusters or dishcloths.
10. Give it to a pharmacist.
11. Turn it into napkins.
12. Use it for a shadow theatre screen.
13. Give it to your child for a school play.
14. Donate it to a science museum.
15. Give it to the Catholic Church for priest collars.
16. Give it to the Catholic Church for nuns' head covers.
17. Turn it into hair ribbons.

18. Turn it into curtains.
19. Turn it into a demonstration banner.
20. Wave it as a white flag in case of surrender.
21. Use as a dust sheet when you are painting the house.
22. Give it to your child to play doctors and nurses.
23. Cut it into bandages.
24. Donate it to the local abattoir.
25. Use for white balance for endoscopy camera.
26. Make it into a scarecrow.
27. Make it into a windshield for the summer holidays.
28. Wear it at a fancy dress party.
29. Give it to the local school dinner lady.
30. Donate it to the local laboratory.
31. Give it to your vet.

J. A. Stockman III, MD

References

1. Jones JS, Hoerle D, Riekse R. Stethoscopes: a potential vector of infection? *Ann Emerg Med*. 1995;26:296-299.
2. Department of Health. *Uniforms and workwear: an evidence-base for developing local policy*. London, http://www.dh.gov.uk/en/Publicationsandstatistics/Publications/PublicationsPolicyAndGuidance/DH_078433; 2007. Accessed July 23, 2009.
3. Magos A. 31 uses for a white coat. *BMJ*. 2008;336:346.

Influenza-Associated Pediatric Mortality in the United States: Increase of *Staphylococcus aureus* Coinfection

Finelli L, Fiore A, Dhara R, et al (Natl Ctr for Immunization and Respiratory Diseases, Atlanta, GA)
Pediatrics 122:805-811, 2008

Objective.—Pediatric influenza-associated death became a nationally notifiable condition in the United States during 2004. We describe influenza-associated pediatric mortality from 2004 to 2007, including an increase of *Staphylococcus aureus* coinfections.

Methods.—Influenza-associated pediatric death is defined as a death of a child who is younger than 18 years and has laboratory-confirmed influenza. State and local health departments report to the Centers for Disease Control and Prevention demographic, clinical, and laboratory data on influenza-associated pediatric deaths.

Results.—During the 2004–2007 influenza seasons, 166 influenza-associated pediatric deaths were reported ($n = 47$, 46, and 73, respectively). Median age of the children was 5 years. Children often progressed rapidly to death; 45% died within 72 hours of onset, including 43% who died at home or in an emergency department. Of 90 children who were recommended for influenza vaccination, only 5 (6%) were fully vaccinated. Reports of bacterial coinfection increased substantially from 2004–2005 to 2006–2007 (6%, 15%, and 34%, respectively). *S aureus* was isolated from a sterile site or endotracheal tube culture in 1 case in 2004–2005, 3 cases in 2005–2006, and 22 cases in 2006–2007; 64% were methicillin-resistant *S aureus*. Children with *S aureus* coinfection were significantly older and more likely to have pneumonia and acute respiratory distress syndrome than those who were not coinfected.

Conclusions.—Influenza-associated pediatric mortality is rare, but the proportion of *S aureus* coinfection identified increased fivefold over the past 3 seasons. Research is needed to identify risk factors for influenza coinfection with invasive bacteria and to determine the impact of influenza vaccination and antiviral agents in preventing pediatric mortality.

▶ It is the youngest in our population and the oldest who tend to have the greatest morbidity and mortality associated with influenza infection. Although the influenza virus infection itself can lead to death, most influenza-related deaths are the result of either exacerbation of underlying medical conditions or invasive coinfection with another infectious pathogen, particularly a bacterium. A common problem, sometimes fatal, is a secondary bacterial pneumonia after influenza has been established in a patient. For this reason, it is important not only to attempt to immunize against influenza virus, but also certain strains of bacteria, including the pneumococcis. Most data telling us about the morbidity and mortality associated with secondary bacterial infections derive from adult studies. This report, however, investigates influenza-associated pediatric deaths related to secondary *Staphylococcus aureus* coinfection.

This report describes 166 cases of laboratory-confirmed influenza-associated deaths that occurred in children over a 3-year series of influenza seasons. We learned that influenza was rapidly fatal with almost half of infected children dying within 72 hours of the onset of symptoms and 75% dying within 75 days. Almost half died at home or in the emergency department before ever being admitted to hospital. The number of bacterial infections increased substantially in the 2006-2007 influenza season with most infections resulting in death caused by *S aureus*, primarily methicillin-resistant *S aureus*. Many of these deaths occurred among children without a prior condition or at a young age that would make them unusually susceptible to influenza infection. Unfortunately, among the children who died, just 21% had been vaccinated during the season in which they died.

There are a number of hypotheses that have been suggested to explain why bacterial coinfection frequently occurs with influenza virus infection. Certainly the virus damages the tracheobronchial tree, enhancing staphylococcal adherence. Influenza virus also suppresses the respiratory burst response and the phagocytic function of neutrophils and macrophages. Given the fact that up to 40% of children are colonized with *S aureus*, it is not too surprising that this bacterium can take over quite readily and cause significant morbidity and mortality. In this report, the proportion of children with bacterial coinfection increased more than 5-fold between the 2004 and 2005 and 2006 and 2007 influenza seasons, when nearly all the increase was attributable to *S aureus* coinfections. During this period, about one-quarter of the children who had data able to be analyzed in fact died from influenza-associated complications most probably related to bacterial coinfection. Methicillin-resistant *S aureus* was the principal culprit in these cases. Obviously, prevention by following the recommendation that all children who are age 6 to 59 months and those with underlying chronic conditions receive the vaccine is part of the solution as is the use of influenza antiviral treatment, which studies have shown to be effective in preventing secondary complications. We should consider treating children with suspected *S aureus* pneumonia during influenza season with vancomycin or other antibiotics to treat methicillin-resistant *S aureus*, particularly when they reside in areas where this organism is highly prevalent.

J. A. Stockman III, MD

Effectiveness of Maternal Influenza Immunization in Mothers and Infants
Zaman K, Roy E, Arifeen SF, et al (International Ctr for Diarrheal Disease Res, Dhaka, Bangladesh; et al)
N Engl J Med 359:1555-1564, 2008

Background.—Young infants and pregnant women are at increased risk for serious consequences of influenza infection. Inactivated influenza vaccine is recommended for pregnant women but is not licensed for infants younger than 6 months of age. We assessed the clinical effectiveness of inactivated influenza vaccine administered during pregnancy in Bangladesh.

Methods.—In this randomized study, we assigned 340 mothers to receive either inactivated influenza vaccine (influenza-vaccine group) or the 23-valent pneumococcal polysaccharide vaccine (control group). Mothers were interviewed weekly to assess illnesses until 24 weeks after birth. Subjects with febrile respiratory illness were assessed clinically, and ill infants were tested for influenza antigens. We estimated the incidence of illness, incidence rate ratios, and vaccine effectiveness.

Results.—Mothers and infants were observed from August 2004 through December 2005. Among infants of mothers who received influenza vaccine, there were fewer cases of laboratory-confirmed influenza than among infants in the control group (6 cases and 16 cases, respectively), with a vaccine effectiveness of 63% (95% confidence interval [CI], 5 to 85). Respiratory illness with fever occurred in 110 infants in the influenza-vaccine group and 153 infants in the control group, with a vaccine effectiveness of 29% (95% CI, 7 to 46). Among the mothers, there was a reduction in the rate of respiratory illness with fever of 36% (95% CI, 4 to 57).

Conclusions.—Inactivated influenza vaccine reduced proven influenza illness by 63% in infants up to 6 months of age and averted approximately a third of all febrile respiratory illnesses in mothers and young infants. Maternal influenza immunization is a strategy with substantial benefits for both mothers and infants. (ClinicalTrials.gov number, NCT00142389.)

▶ For half a dozen years now, in the United States, influenza immunization has been recommended for infants between the ages of 6 months and 24 months, although vaccine immunogenicity may be reduced in children under the age of 2 years. Influenza vaccines are not licensed in the United States for use in infants less than 6 months, and antiviral drugs for influenza therapy are not licensed for infants under the age of 1 year. Studies from the United States and elsewhere have shown high rates of hospitalization among infants with influenza, especially those less than 6 months of age. Indeed, the rate of hospitalization for such infants is higher than for other high-risk groups and a national survey in the United States has shown that childhood deaths associated with influenza are most frequent in infants under 6 months of age.[1] For these reasons, anything that can be done to help protect infants under 6 months of age from contracting influenza would be most helpful.

It is well known that maternal influenza antibodies are capable of protecting infants in the first few months of life. Influenza immunization of pregnant women will produce antibodies that can be actively transported in utero via the umbilical cord. What is not known is whether active immunization of women during pregnancy might in fact be of true benefit to their infants, thus the purpose of this report from Bangladesh. The report summarizes a prospective, controlled, blinded, randomized trial to assess the safety and immunogenicity of pneumococcal vaccines and the clinical effectiveness of influenza vaccine given during pregnancy. A total of 340 women in the third trimester of pregnancy who met the inclusion criteria agreed to participate in the study. Data from the study show that maternal immunization with influenza vaccine had significant clinical effectiveness, resulting in a 63% reduction in laboratory-proven influenza illness in offspring of these pregnancies up to 6 months of age. Needless to say, the women who received the influenza vaccine also were significantly protected. Specifically, the absolute reduction data in the rate of illness show that every 100 influenza immunizations in pregnancy prevented respiratory illness with fever of more than 38°C in 14 infants and 4 mothers. In other words, 5 pregnant women would need to be vaccinated to prevent a single case of respiratory illness with fever in a mother or infant, thus demonstrating reasonable and expected value for such an approach.

Sooner or later we are going to see another pandemic of influenza. When that comes, everything possible to protect the youngest in our population will be needed, including vaccines that effectively produce high-titer antibody in pregnant women. It has been estimated that if we have an influenza pandemic similar to the Spanish flu that started in 1918 (H1N1 virus), one could anticipate close to 10 million hospitalizations and 2 million deaths in the United States and somewhere between 50 and 80 million deaths worldwide, the significant majority of which would occur in developing countries. The economic cost associated with this in the United States has been estimated to potentially approach $200 billion.[2] It has been now more than a decade since highly pathogenic avian influenza viruses of the H5N1 subtype were first found to infect humans. Although time has passed, the fear that these strains will cause the next pandemic has increased rather than subsided. There is only limited evidence so far to support the idea that H5N1 strains are evolving toward a human-adapted strain that can transmit efficiently, but recently H5N1 strains have acquired several mutations thought to be important for generation of a pandemic strain. Sooner or later, many believe, we will face a serious pandemic and the most we can do to understand how to protect all of our population, but importantly also the very young, should be undertaken now.

J. A. Stockman III, MD

References

1. Bhat N, Wright JG, Broder KR, et al. Influenza-associated deaths among children in the United States, 2003-2004. *N Engl J Med.* 2005;353:2559-2567.
2. McCullers JA. Preparing for the next influenza pandemic. *Pediatr Infect Dis J.* 2008;10:S57-S60.

Influenza Vaccine Effectiveness Among Children 6 to 59 Months of Age During 2 Influenza Seasons: A Case-Cohort Study

Szilagyi PG, for the New Vaccine Surveillance Network (Univ of Rochester School of Medicine and Dentistry, NY; et al)
Arch Pediatr Adolesc Med 162:943-951, 2008

Objective.—To measure vaccine effectiveness (VE) in preventing influenza-related health care visits among children aged 6 to 59 months during 2 consecutive influenza seasons.

Design.—Case-cohort study estimating effectiveness of inactivated influenza vaccine in preventing inpatient/outpatient visits (emergency department [ED] and outpatient clinic). We compared vaccination status of laboratory-confirmed influenza cases with a cluster sample of children from a random sample of practices in 3 counties (subcohort) during the 2003-2004 and 2004-2005 seasons.

Setting.—Counties encompassing Rochester, New York, Nashville, Tennessee, and Cincinnati, Ohio.

Participants.—Children aged 6 to 59 months seen in inpatient/ED or outpatient clinic settings for acute respiratory illnesses and community-based subcohort comparison.

Main Exposure.—Influenza vaccination.

Main Outcome Measures.—Influenza vaccination status of cases vs subcohort using time-dependent Cox proportional hazards models to estimate VE in preventing inpatient/ED and outpatient visits.

Results.—During the 2003-2004 and 2004-2005 seasons, 165 and 80 inpatient/ED and 74 and 95 outpatient influenza cases were enrolled, while more than 4500 inpatient/ED and more than 600 outpatient subcohorts were evaluated, respectively. In bivariate analyses, cases had lower vaccination rates than subcohorts. However, significant influenza VE could not be demonstrated for any season, age, or setting after adjusting for county, sex, insurance, chronic conditions recommended for influenza vaccination, and timing of influenza vaccination (VE estimates ranged from 7%-52% across settings and seasons for fully vaccinated 6- to 59-month-olds).

Conclusion.—In 2 seasons with suboptimal antigenic match between vaccines and circulating strains, we could not demonstrate VE in preventing influenza-related inpatient/ED or outpatient visits in children younger than 5 years. Further study is needed during years with good vaccine match.

▶ We tend to rely on seasonal use of influenza vaccine to mitigate the spread of influenza to the most vulnerable in the pediatric population. Included in that population are those 6 to 59 months of age, the age group in which the influenza vaccination is recommended. Unfortunately, and surprisingly, there is relatively little information regarding the effectiveness of the influenza vaccine in this age group, most probably because it is only been recently that the vaccine has been used routinely for children other than those with chronic conditions. We are grateful to the New Vaccine Surveillance Network for designing a study that was capable of estimating the effectiveness of the inactivated influenza vaccine in preventing inpatient/outpatient visits during the 2003-2004 and 2004-2005 influenza seasons. It is unfortunate, but it appears that the vaccine did not work very well, most likely because of suboptimal antigenic match between the vaccines in each of those years and the circulating strains of influenza. Thus, in youngsters younger than 5 years of age who received the vaccines, there was no significant reduction in influenza-related inpatient, emergency room, or outpatient visits. To say this differently, the vaccines are only as good as their match with what is circulating in the community at that particular point in time. It should be noted, though, that this report analyzes data using the inactivated influenza vaccine only. Most information suggests that the live vaccine is somewhat more antigenic and possibly more protective...another study waiting to be done.

On a different topic, there have been some new and important insights derived into the basis upon which the influenza vaccine causes so much damage to the respiratory tract. Recent work suggests that epithelial cells in the respiratory tract contribute to the inflammatory milieu during influenza H5N1 infection. In vitro studies among tissue specimens from autopsies of patients who died from H5N1 infection indicate that these activated epithelial cells produce tumor necrosis factor alpha and cyclooxygenase-2 (COX-2). Zheng et al have described the specific inhibition of COX-2 expression in mice infected with H5N1 influenza virus and then treated these with COX inhibitors.[1] This key finding suggests that the coadministration of COX inhibitors such as celecoxib and antiviral therapy might significantly improve outcomes, a finding that has been now documented in influenza-infected mice. COX inhibitors, of course, are frequently used in clinical practice to treat noninfectious, inflammatory disorders, and wouldn't it be wonderful if something as simple as this class of drug would help minimize the morbidity and mortality associated with influenza infection? Needless to say, randomized, controlled clinical trials in this regard in humans are badly needed, but should be undertaken as soon as possible. To learn more about COX inhibitors, inflammation and influenza, see the excellent editorial on this topic by Simmons and Farrar.[2]

J. A. Stockman III, MD

References

1. Zheng BJ, Chan KW, Lin YP, et al. Delayed antiviral plus immunomodulator treatment still reduces mortality in mice infected by high inoculum of influenza A/H5N1 virus. *Proc Natl Acad Sci.* 2008;105:8091-8096.
2. Simmons C, Farrar J. Insights into inflammation and influenza. *N Engl J Med.* 2008;359:1621-1623.

Prognostic Factors in Influenza-associated Encephalopathy

Nagao T, Morishima T, Kimura H, et al (Okayama Univ; Nagoya Univ Graduate School of Medcinie, Japan; et al)
Pediatr Infect Dis J 27:384-389, 2008

Background.—Recently, reports of influenza-associated encephalopathy have increased worldwide. Given the high mortality and morbidity rates attributable to this severe neurologic complication of influenza, we conducted a nationwide study in Japan to identify the prognostic factors.

Methods.—We retrospectively evaluated 442 cases of influenza-associated encephalopathy that were reported to the Collaborative Study Group on Influenza-Associated Encephalopathy, which was organized by the Japanese Ministry of Health, Labor, and Welfare in collaboration with hospitals, clinics, and local pediatric practices in Japan between 1998 and 2002. The outcome for each patient was classified as either survival or death. Predictors of death were identified using logistic regression analysis.

Results.—Four major prognostic factors for death were found to be significant by multivariate analysis ($P < 0.05$) in the 184 patients for whom we had complete data: elevation of aspartate aminotransferase, hyperglycemia, the presence of hematuria or proteinuria, and use of diclofenac sodium.

Conclusions.—We identified patients who had factors associated with a poor prognosis, and these findings might be clinically useful for the management of this illness.

▶ This report from Japan reminds us that although there is a great deal of emphasis being placed on the potential for a pandemic of the avian flu virus H5N1, we should not take our eyes off the more common influenza viruses that run through countries seasonally. One of the most devastating complications of influenza is not the respiratory problem it can cause, but rather the neurologic disorders this virus can cause. Influenza-associated encephalopathy represents a severe complication of influenza and is characterized by an abrupt onset of seizure and coma within just a few days of developing a high fever. This report of Nagao et al from Japan, where influenza-associated encephalopathy has increased in recent years, with more than 100 youngsters under 6 years of age dying annually as a result of this complication. The issue that has come up is whether the encephalopathy might in fact result from the treatment of the fever these youngsters have. For example, it is well known that cyclooxygenase inhibitors, particularly aspirin, are known to cause Reye syndrome. In Japan, cyclooxygenase inhibitors such as diclofenac sodium and mefenamic acid (but not aspirin) are widely used as antipyretic drugs in children. It has been suggested that these nonsalicylate antipyretic drugs may be associated with the development of influenza-associated encephalopathy. Thus far, the relationship between antipyretics and influenza-associated encephalopathy remains tenuous.

The authors of this report attempt to provide us with information about prognostic factors influencing the outcome of influenza infection, particularly the complication of influenza-associated encephalopathy. The information provided is important because the mortality of this complication is as high as 30% without treatment. It was observed that a markedly elevated transaminase level, thrombocytopenia, and hematuria or proteinuria are associated with a nonfavorable influenza-associated encephalopathy. It has been suggested that activation of cytokines and other inflammatory mediators triggers this complication of influenza infection. It has also been shown that hyperglycemia is an additional factor leading to a poor prognosis. These should be added high fever, particularly a fever of over 41 °C, as adverse prognostic factors. Also, if there is any antipyretic that seems to be most problematic in causing the neurologic problem, it is diclofenac sodium.

J. A. Stockman III, MD

Acute Childhood Encephalitis and Encephalopathy Associated With Influenza: A Prospective 11-Year Review

Amin R, Ford-Jones E, Richardson SE, et al (The Hosp for Sick Children, Toronto, Ontario, Canada; Univ of Toronto, Ontario, Canada; et al)
Pediatr Infect Dis J 27:390-395, 2008

Background.—Influenza virus infection has been associated with a variety of neurologic complications. The objective of this study was to evaluate prospectively the role of influenza viruses in acute childhood encephalitis/encephalopathy (ACE).

Methods.—All children admitted to the Hospital for Sick Children, Toronto, during an 11-year period with ACE and evidence of acute influenza virus infection were included. Acute influenza virus infection was defined by detection of the organism in the nasopharynx by direct immunofluorescence microscopy or viral culture and/or by a 4-fold or greater rise in complement fixation titer.

Results.—A total of 311 children with ACE were evaluated; evidence of influenza infection was detected in 7% (22 of 311). Eight were excluded from the main analysis because of evidence implicating other potential pathogens. Eleven of the 14 included subjects were <5 years of age. A respiratory prodrome was documented in 93% of subjects. In 64% neurologic manifestations developed within 5 days of onset of respiratory symptoms. Neuroimaging abnormalities were more common in children <2 years of age. Neurologic sequelae occurred in more than one-half of subjects.

Conclusions.—In this prospective registry, influenza virus infection was associated with 5% of ACE cases. The majority of children were <5 years of age and the prevalence of neuroimaging abnormalities was higher in children <2 years of age suggesting that younger children are predisposed to the neurologic complications of influenza. An acute rather than a post-infectious process was suggested by the briefness of the respiratory prodrome in most cases.

▶ The previous report showed us how common and problematic encephalop athy is in association with influenza infection in Japan. This report of Amin et al comes from North America, Toronto in particular. The same problem exists on our continent as well. Since January 1994, the Hospital for Sick Children in Toronto has maintained a prospective encephalitis registry. Any child admitted to the hospital with acute encephalitis undergoes extensive neurologic and microbiologic investigation. This database has allowed the investigators from the Hospital for Sick Children to examine the relationship between influenza A and B infection, and the occurrence of childhood encephalitis/encephal-opathy.

What we learn from this report is that of a 311 children admitted to the hospital with acute childhood encephalitis, 22 had evidence of acute infection with influenza A or B. Of these, 14 fulfilled the study criteria for acute influenza-associated encephalopathy/encephalitis. Other patients were excluded because of the possibility of at least 1 additional potential pathogen as a possible cause of the neurologic problem. In affected children, fever occurred in all and a respiratory component was seen in 13 of the 14 patients. The interval between the onset of respiratory symptoms and the development of neurologic symptoms varied from 1 to 14 days with an average of 3 days. The interval was less than 5 days in the significant majority of patients. None of the patients in this series, unlike Japan, had multisystem organ failure or disseminated intravascular coagulation. Neurologic manifestations included seizures, cranial nerve abnormalities, focal motor deficits, gait abnormalities, as well as nonspecific abnormalities such as persistent irritability, meningismus, torticollis, hyperreflexia or hyporeflexia, and opisthotonus. Seizures occurred in 10 of the 14 children. Eight had generalized tonic clonic seizures alone, 1 had focal seizures alone, and 1 had both focal and generalized seizures. Two of the children presented in status epilepticus, one of whom was diagnosed with acute myelinating encephalomyelitis. Hemiparesis was observed in 2 cases.

As far as laboratory findings were concerned, leukocytosis was unusual, but half of the patients were anemic. Thrombocytopenia was not observed, again unlike what was seen in Japan. CSF pleocytosis was unusual, being observed in just 3 patients. An elevated protein was seen in 4.

Fortunately, among the 14 youngsters infected with influenza encephalitis (they ranged in age from 14 months to 10 years) there were no deaths. Eight of the 14, however, had neurologic sequelae at follow-up. These included seizure disorders, developmental delay, hemiparesis, and speech disorders.

In children admitted to hospital with a diagnosis of encephalitis, one should think about the possibility of influenza A or B being the cause. In this series from the Hospital for Sick Children, some 5% of acute childhood encephalitis was the result of infection with this group of viruses. The report from Canada also speculated that the cause of the neurologic problem is the systemic immune response observed to influenza virus resulting in high levels of proinflammatory cytokines interleukin (IL)-6 and tumor necrosis factor-alpha and the anti-inflammatory cytokine IL-10. These inflammatory cytokines have been found at elevated levels in the CSF of children infected with influenza A and B viruses.

It is only by improving our understanding of the pathogenesis of influenza-associated encephalitis that we will advance our ability to prevent and treat this devastating illness. There are no data on the use of antiviral agents with respect to their effectiveness in improving clinical outcomes. Also, if we learn anything from the experience in Toronto, it is that registries add valuable and important information to our knowledge of unusual or infrequent events.

J. A. Stockman III, MD

Probable limited person-to-person transmission of highly pathogenic avian influenza A (H5N1) virus in China

Wang H, Feng Z, Shu Y, et al (Jiangsu Provincial Centre for Disease Control and Prevention, Nanjing, China; Chinese Centre for Disease Control and Prevention (China CDC), Beijing; Natl Inst for Viral Disease Control and Prevention, China CDC, Beijing; et al)

Lancet 371:1427-1434, 2008

Background.—In December, 2007, a family cluster of two individuals infected with highly pathogenic avian influenza A (H5N1) virus was identified in Jiangsu Province, China. Field and laboratory investigations were implemented immediately by public-health authorities.

Methods.—Epidemiological, clinical, and virological data were collected and analysed. Respiratory specimens from the patients were tested by reverse transcriptase (RT) PCR and by viral culture for the presence of H5N1 virus. Contacts of cases were monitored for symptoms of illness for 10 days. Any contacts who became ill had respiratory specimens collected for H5N1 testing by RT PCR. Sera were obtained from contacts for H5N1 serological testing by microneutralisation and horse red-blood-cell haemagglutinin inhibition assays.

Findings.—The 24-year-old index case died, and the second case, his 52-year-old father, survived after receiving early antiviral treatment and post-vaccination plasma from a participant in an H5N1 vaccine trial. The index case's only plausible exposure to H5N1 virus was a poultry market visit 6 days before the onset of illness. The second case had substantial unprotected close exposure to his ill son. 91 contacts with close exposure to one or both cases without adequate protective equipment provided consent for serological investigation. Of these individuals, 78 (86%) received oseltamivir chemoprophylaxis and two had mild illness. Both ill contacts tested negative for H5N1 by RT PCR. All 91 close contacts tested negative for H5N1 antibodies. H5N1 viruses isolated from the two cases were genetically identical except for one non-synonymous nucleotide substitution.

Interpretation.—Limited, non-sustained person-to-person transmission of H5N1 virus probably occurred in this family cluster.

Funding.—Chinese Ministry of Science and Technology; US National Institute of Allergy and Infectious Diseases, National Institutes of Health; China-US Collaborative Program on Emerging and Re-emerging Infectious Diseases.

▶ By the end of 2007, there had been 346 confirmed human cases of A/H5N1 infection reported to the World Health Organization from 14 countries, although 5 countries where the infection seems to be endemic in poultry (China, Egypt, Indonesia, Thailand, and Vietnam) account for nearly 90% of these cases. A total of 213 were known to have died by the end of 2007, a case fatality rate of about 60%. Serologic studies suggest that there are only a few asymptomatic or mild cases. Fortunately, person-to-person transmission has been uncommon and very limited, the subject of the report of Wang et al. Children, adolescents, and young women are disproportionately represented among the cases of human disease probably because almost all infections come from close contact with sick chickens and ducks and the care of domestic poultry is traditionally a task for younger members of families and women in endemic countries.

Clinically, the children and adults present with a febrile respiratory illness and sometimes also with diarrhea, which can progress to multiorgan involvement. Treatment with antivirals and other agents has not been conclusively shown to end in a positive outcome. Most cases come to the attention of healthcare providers only at a later stage of illness, so experience with early use of antivirals is limited in this regard. The experience with A/H5N1 is very different from the influenza viruses previously causing pandemics. For example, the previous highest recorded all age case fatality rate during a pandemic was 2% to 3% in the 1918-1919 influenza epidemic. Children with other underlying medical conditions fare much worse. Although respiratory system problems are often the major cause of morbidity, there are a plethora of other occasional complications, including Reye's syndrome, encephalitis, neuritis, Guillain-Barré syndrome, transverse myelitis, and cardiac problems (myocarditis and pericarditis).

What we learn from the report of Wang et al is quite troublesome. As recently as February 2004, the Prime Minister of Thailand said that the "possibility of person-to-person transmission of H5N1 is 0.00001%."[1] In fact, person-to-person transmission of H5N1 was first noted after the 1997 Hong Kong outbreak in which family members and at least 2 healthcare workers might have been infected by contact with patients. Since then, one report of a family cluster concluded that person-to-person transmission was probable and an additional 4 reports stated that it could not be ruled out in at least 6 families. The report of Wang et al gives another convincing analysis of probable person-to-person transmission by researchers from China and here in the United States.

Transmission of avian flu virus between mammals is not restricted to H5N1 in human beings: H7N7 can also be transmitted from person-to-person and there is evidence of transmission of H5N1 among other mammalian species. Given that species barriers can be breached, the intriguing issue so far is why transmissibility of H5N1 among people remains so low. This is the subject of an interesting commentary that appeared in the *Lancet*.[2]

With the exception of occasional infection in healthcare workers, all published incidents of possible or probable person-to-person transmission have been between genetically related individuals. Although this finding could be related to the intensity and intimacy of contact between family members, postgenetic factors may also play a part in susceptibility to H5N1. Whatever the underlying determinants, if we continue to experience widespread, uncontrolled outbreaks of H5N1 in poultry, the appearance of strains well adapted to human beings might just well be a matter of time. In the meantime, all family contacts of a patient with probable or confirmed H5N1 should be given chemoprophylaxis and placed under surveillance. Personal protection from infected individuals should be undertaken.

The study of Wang et al is an excellent example of epidemiologic work showing the benefit of a long-standing and trusting international collaboration that began during the acute respiratory syndrome epidemic. Only by such cooperation will we see the earliest signs of a greater spread of human-to-human transmission, at which point we better be prepared to deal with it.

For more on the topic of preparing for the next epidemic, possibly of avian flu H5N1, and the implications for pediatric care providers, see the excellent review by Nocholl.[3]

As this commentary closes, a *Clinical Fact/Curio*, this having to do with avian flu. We all know that the risk of avian flu and contagion to humans persists. We also know that the type of birds that cause this, at least as of now, do not fly. Were they to fly, an interesting question arises, however. That question is, how far can a bird actually fly? Is it theoretically possible for a bird, for example, to fly from China to the United States and make it there alive? The answer to this question actually is not known, but recently a female bartailed godwit was documented to have flown nonstop from Alaska to New Zealand, the longest documented direct bird flight ever.[4]

J. A. Stockman III, MD

References

1. Times Online. Bird flu death reaches 12 in Asia. http://www.timesonline.co.uk/tol/news/uk/health/article1009480.ece; February 2, 2004. Accessed May 8, 2008.
2. Tran Hien EN, Farrar J, Horby P. Person-to-person transmission of influenza A (H5N1). *Lancet.* 2008;371:1392-1394.
3. Nocholl A. Children, avian influenza H5N1 and preparing for the next pandemic. *Arch Dis Child.* 2008;93:433-438.
4. Avian airlines [editorial comment]. *Sci News.* November 22, 2008;14.

A Clinical Trial of a Whole-Virus H5N1 Vaccine Derived from Cell Culture

Ehrlich HJ, Müller M, Oh HML, et al (Baxter BioScience, Vienna; Med Univ of Vienna; Changi General Hosp, Singapore; et al)
N Engl J Med 358:2573-2584, 2008

Background.—Widespread infections of avian species with avian influenza H5N1 virus and its limited spread to humans suggest that the virus has the potential to cause a human influenza pandemic. An urgent need exists for an H5N1 vaccine that is effective against divergent strains of H5N1 virus.

Methods.—In a randomized, dose-escalation, phase 1 and 2 study involving six subgroups, we investigated the safety of an H5N1 whole-virus vaccine produced on Vero cell cultures and determined its ability to induce antibodies capable of neutralizing various H5N1 strains. In two visits 21 days apart, 275 volunteers between the ages of 18 and 45 years received two doses of vaccine that each contained 3.75 µg, 7.5 µg, 15 µg, or 30 µg of hemagglutinin antigen with alum adjuvant or 7.5 µg or 15 µg of hemagglutinin antigen without adjuvant. Serologic analysis was performed at baseline and on days 21 and 42.

Results.—The vaccine induced a neutralizing immune response not only against the clade 1 (A/Vietnam/1203/2004) virus strain but also against the clade 2 and 3 strains. The use of adjuvants did not improve the antibody response. Maximum responses to the vaccine strain were obtained with formulations containing 7.5 µg and 15 µg of hemagglutinin antigen without adjuvant. Mild pain at the injection site (in 9 to 27% of subjects) and headache (in 6 to 31% of subjects) were the most common adverse events identified for all vaccine formulations.

Conclusions.—A two-dose vaccine regimen of either 7.5 µg or 15 µg of hemagglutinin antigen without adjuvant induced neutralizing antibodies against diverse H5N1 virus strains in a high percentage of subjects, suggesting that this may be a useful H5N1 vaccine. (ClinicalTrials.gov number, NCT00349141.)

▶ There are few who are not worried about the emergence of a pandemic caused by the avian virus strain H5N1. The quest for a fully immunogenic vaccine against influenza H5N1 virus has gone on for more than a decade ever since this family of potentially pandemic viruses emerged as a cause of human disease in Hong Kong in 1997. By 2008, H5N1 had caused almost 400 human cases of influenza, with a mortality rate exceeding 60%. H5 strains had been found in birds throughout much of the world (though not yet in the Americas) by 2008. At that point in time, human illness had occurred in 14 countries throughout Asia and Northern Africa. For whatever reasons, the much-feared rapid spread through and between communities, however, had not occurred. Aside from small clusters of cases within families, each human case has been associated with close contact with poultry. The culling of poultry in the face of recognized bird disease has been a major defense strategy since the very first outbreak. The fact that no epidemic has occurred during the first decade of the virus infection has prompted questions about whether H5 viruses face some insurmountable barrier of viral fitness that renders them incapable of causing widespread illness in humans. Nonetheless, there is not a person who would not agree that history is a powerful teacher, and that future influenza pandemics caused by novel strains are highly probable.

The history of vaccine development against influenza virus goes back some time. During the pandemics of Asian influenza in 1957 and Hong Kong influenza in 1968, there were efforts to explore possible vaccines, but the first systematic attempt to develop vaccines against an influenza virus representing a pandemic threat was made in the face of the swine influenza of 1976. Vaccine trials were carried out in both children and adults and showed that whole-virus vaccine was not only more immunogenic, but also more reactogenic than subvirion vaccine. It was also suggested that 2 doses of vaccine were needed. These lessons, coupled with other data on the seasonal impact of influenza, have formed the basis for the broadening use of influenza here in the United States for yearly epidemic influenza.

The first attempts to develop an H5 vaccine involved the testing of a subvirion vaccine. Limited benefit was seen with this vaccine. The next vaccine trials increased the dose of the subvirion vaccine substantially and it was given in 2 doses. Only with this higher amount did it appear that the vaccine might potentially be effective in more than 50% of those vaccinated. This vaccine was approved by the Food and Drug Administration and is indeed being stockpiled. It is now the benchmark against which new vaccines will be judged. The article by Ehrlich et al extends our understanding of influenza vaccines in several ways. Perhaps most importantly, it introduces the concept that influenza vaccines may be produced in substrates rather than embryonated eggs. The idea that a vaccine might be grown in tissue culture under controlled conditions has excited investigators for a number of years. Embryonated eggs are available only seasonally, creating a time constraint in the manufacturing of yearly vaccine that is a serious impediment for any preparedness for a pandemic. As of now, decisions have to be made by February each year about what the best bet is for the following winter's vaccine strains. With tissue culture methodologies, this decision could be delayed until it is more apparent what strains will be needed. The vaccine used in the Ehrlich et al trial was also not a subvirion vaccine, harkening back to the 1976 trial in which it was shown that whole virus type vaccine is of greater effectiveness.

As of this writing, it is fairly clear that we are at least on the right trajectory to develop an adequate vaccine against avian influenza. The report of Ehrlich et al demonstrates significant progress. Fortunately, vaccine can now be grown in tissue culture so we don't have to put all of our eggs in 1 basket. For more on vaccine preparedness, see the superb editorial on this topic by Wright.[1]

J. A. Stockman III, MD

Reference

1. Wright PF. Vaccine preparedness – are we ready for the next influenza pandemic? *N Engl J Med*. 2008;358:2540-2543.

The Burden of Respiratory Syncytial Virus Infection in Young Children

Hall CB, Weinberg GA, Iwane MK, et al (The Univ of Rochester School of Medicine and Dentistry, NY; Ctrs for Disease Control and Prevention, Atlanta; et al)
N Engl J Med 360:588-598, 2009

Background.—The primary role of respiratory syncytial virus (RSV) in causing infant hospitalizations is well recognized, but the total burden of RSV infection among young children remains poorly defined.

Methods.—We conducted prospective, population-based surveillance of acute respiratory infections among children under 5 years of age in three U.S. counties. We enrolled hospitalized children from 2000 through 2004 and children presenting as outpatients in emergency departments and pediatric offices from 2002 through 2004. RSV was detected by culture and reverse-transcriptase polymerase chain reaction. Clinical information was obtained from parents and medical records. We calculated population-based rates of hospitalization associated with RSV infection and estimated the rates of RSV-associated outpatient visits.

Results.—Among 5067 children enrolled in the study, 919 (18%) had RSV infections. Overall, RSV was associated with 20% of hospitalizations, 18% of emergency department visits, and 15% of office visits for acute respiratory infections from November through April. Average annual hospitalization rates were 17 per 1000 children under 6 months of age and 3 per 1000 children under 5 years of age. Most of the children had no coexisting illnesses. Only prematurity and a young age were independent risk factors for hospitalization. Estimated rates of RSV-associated office visits among children under 5 years of age were three times those in emergency departments. Outpatients had moderately severe RSV-associated illness, but few of the illnesses (3%) were diagnosed as being caused by RSV.

Conclusions.—RSV infection is associated with substantial morbidity in U.S. children in both inpatient and outpatient settings. Most children with RSV infection were previously healthy, suggesting that control strategies targeting only high-risk children will have a limited effect on the total disease burden of RSV infection.

▶ This report is an absolute read for anyone involved in the care of children. The report outlines the population-based burden of respiratory syncytial virus (RSV) infection among hospitalized children and outpatients in emergency departments and primary care settings. Eligible children were under 5 years of age and had received a diagnosis of acute respiratory infection, which was defined as an illness presenting with one or more of the following symptoms: fever, cough, earache, nasal congestion, rhinorrhea, sore throat, vomiting after coughing, wheezing, and labored, rapid, or shallow breathing. RSV was detected by culture and reverse-transcriptase polymerase chain reaction. With this information, it was possible to calculate population-based rates of hospitalization associated with RSV infection and rates of RSV-associated outpatient visits. One sees that rates of hospitalization for RSV-associated illness are 3 times as high as those associated with influenza or parainfluenza viruses, and the proportion of children receiving influenza vaccine was low (18%). The estimated rates of outpatient visits associated with RSV infection were similar to those associated with influenza for all children under 5 years of age, but were markedly greater for children under the age of 6 months.

One can take the data generated from this report out of Rochester, New York and extrapolate the information to the nation as a whole. If one did this, one could estimate that there are 2.1 million children under the age of 5 years with RSV infection requiring medical attention in the United States every year. Of these children, approximately 3% will be hospitalized and 25% will be treated in emergency departments. The remainder will be treated in the office setting. Of these outpatients, 61% are between the ages of 2 and 5 years of age. These numbers may in fact be underestimates because many with RSV infection do not have the cause of the illness diagnosed specifically.

The rates of RSV infection requiring medical attention are high not only during infancy, but throughout the whole first 5 years of life, underscoring the need for an effective vaccine. When 2 million children a year under the age of 5 experience an RSV infection and 80% are over the age of 1, you see the magnitude of the problem. The authors of this report estimate that among children under the age of 5 years, RSV infection results in approximately 1 of 334 hospitalizations, 1 of 38 visits to emergency departments, and 1 of 13 visits to primary care offices each year here in the United States.

Before leaving the topic of wheezing in children associated with viral illness, a recent report documented that rhinoviruses are in fact a major cause of wheezing and hospitalization in children less than 2 years of age.[1] The human rhinoviruses are the cause of 80% of cases of common colds in adults who have self-diagnosed colds. These viruses belong to the picornavirus family that includes polio virus, enterovirus, and hepatitis A virus, among others. We generally think of rhinoviruses as causing mainly mild upper respiratory tract infections. We now see that they can, along with RSV, cause significant wheezing associated illness in children.

J. A. Stockman III, MD

Reference

1. Piotrowska Z, Vazquez M, Shapiro ED, et al. Rhinoviruses are a major cause of wheezing and hospitalization in children less than two years. *Pediatr Infect Dis J.* 2009;28:25-29.

Lack of antibody affinity maturation due to poor Toll-like receptor stimulation leads to enhanced respiratory syncytial virus disease

Delgado MF, Coviello S, Monsalvo AC, et al (INFANT Found, Buenos Aires, Argentina)
Nat Med 15:34-41, 2009

Respiratory syncytial virus (RSV) is a leading cause of hospitalization in infants. A formalin-inactivated RSV vaccine was used to immunize children and elicited nonprotective, pathogenic antibody. Immunized infants experienced increased morbidity after subsequent RSV exposure. No vaccine has been licensed since that time. A widely accepted hypothesis attributed the vaccine failure to formalin disruption of protective antigens. Here we show that the lack of protection was not due to alterations caused by formalin but instead to low antibody avidity for protective epitopes. Lack of antibody affinity maturation followed poor Toll-like receptor (TLR) stimulation. This study explains why the inactivated RSV vaccine did not protect the children and consequently led to severe disease, hampering vaccine development for 42 years. It also suggests that inactivated RSV vaccines may be rendered safe and effective by inclusion of TLR agonists in their formulation, and it identifies affinity maturation as a key factor for the safe immunization of infants.

▶ This report reminds us that about half of infants are infected with respiratory syncytial virus (RSV) during their first year of life. For reasons that have yet to be explained, we are actually seeing more and more RSV infection as time passes. Hospital rates, for example, related to RSV in the United States have risen by almost 240% in recent decades, and there still is no vaccine licensed against the virus.[1] During the 1960s, researchers thought they had a vaccine, but the experimental, formalin-inactivated vaccine administered to children, not only failed to protect, but also exacerbated illness in response to natural RSV infection. Many of the children developed bronchiolitis and pneumonia so severe that it required hospitalization, and unfortunately, 2 of the vaccinated children died. The formalin-inactivated RSV vaccine did elicit antibodies—but these were not neutralizing, meaning that they did not inactivate the virus. High titers of RSV were recovered from the lungs of the 2 children that died, demonstrating the ineffectiveness of the vaccine in producing a protective response.

The report of Delgado et al provides insight into the failure of the formalin-inactivated RSV vaccine. The investigators tell us that inactivated forms of RSV do not sufficiently activate pattern recognition receptors, molecules important for the recognition of pathogens by immune cells and expressed by several cell types including B-cells, the cells that produce antibodies. As a result of this poor activation, B-cells produce only low-avidity antibodies that poorly recognize the virus. Because the vaccine elicited such poor antibodies, it failed to inhibit virus replication and resulted in enhanced disease, probably caused by the host immune response. It has taken more than 40 years to figure out why the 1960s vaccine did not work, but thanks to Delgado et al, we now know why.

What is also interesting about the Delgado report is that it shows that the vaccine-enhanced disease exhibited by children during the 1960s can be recapitulated in mice. As in people, immunization with formalin-inactivated RSV results in the production of non-neutralizing RSV-specific antibodies. After RSV challenge, these non-neutralizing antibodies cause the formation of immune complexes consisting of antibodies bound to the surface of the RSV virion. One hypothesis is that formalin treatment disrupts the folding of proteins on the surface of the RSV virion that harbors protective antibody epitopes – accounting for the inability to induce a neutralizing antibody response. Delgado et al suggest that the situation is somewhat more complicated than this. They compared the antibody response after immunization with either live RSV or inactivated forms of the virus. As expected, inactivated forms of the virus elicited only low-avidity antibodies, whereas live RSV induced neutralizing antibodies of high avidity. Immunization with the inactivated forms of RSV resulted in increased airway hyperresponsiveness and increased virus titers in the lung after RSV challenge as compared to mice previously vaccinated with live virus. Delgado et al hypothesize that the inability of the inactivated forms of RSV to replicate compromised their ability to activate pattern recognition receptors, resulting in less efficient B-cell stimulation. At the same time, the formalin inactivated RSV vaccine triggers a robust RSV-specific CD4 T-cell response, but no cytotoxic CD8 T-cell response. The exacerbated disease in children observed in the 1960s was probably due to these unique circumstances that together created the perfect storm. Thus the vaccine not only failed to inhibit the RSV infection itself, but produced an exuberant T-cell response that did nothing to clear the virus, while raising the level of inflammation, the latter causing the excess morbidity.

The findings from this report could possibly have broader implications for vaccine development given the fact that a number of formalin-inactivated virus vaccines are being used these days. It is important to figure out why some vaccines cause more harm than good as we introduce additional new vaccines into the marketplace. Obviously not everything that looks good on paper works all that well in vivo.

J. A. Stockman III, MD

Reference

1. Shay DK, Holman RC, Roosevelt GE, Liu LL, Stout JW, Anderson LJ. Bronchio-litis-associated hospitalization among US children 1980-1996. *JAMA.* 1999;282: 1414-1446.

Human bocavirus infection in children with respiratory tract disease

Brieu N, Guyon G, Rodière M, et al (Montpellier Univ Hosp, France)

Pediatr Infect Dis J 27:969-973, 2008

Background.—Human bocavirus (HBoV) is a ubiquitous, newly described member of the Parvoviridae family frequently detected in the respiratory tract of children, but only few reports provide data proving the link between HBoV and respiratory tract disease (RTD).

Objectives.—To evaluate the incidence of HBoV infection in children with RTD; to analyze the clinical features of HBoV infection; and to clinically compare HBoV, respiratory syncytial virus (RSV), and human metapneumovirus (HMPV) infections.

Study Design.—A prospective 1-year study was conducted in children <5 years of age hospitalized with RTD and in asymptomatic control children.

Results.—Human bocavirus was detected in 55 (10.8%) of the 507 children tested and in none of the 68 asymptomatic control children (P = 0.01). About 80% of these infections occurred between November and March. Coinfection with another virus was observed in 22 (40%) of the HBoV-positive children. HBoV viral load was significantly higher in samples from children with HBoV monoinfection than in those with coinfection. Subsequent detection of HBoV more than 2 months after the initial detection could be documented in 3 children. Clinical features associated with HBoV infection were similar to those observed with either RSV or HMPV infections, but HBoV infections were less severe than RSV infections.

Conclusions.—The difference observed in HBoV prevalence between children with RTD and controls provides support for a role of this virus in RTD. The frequent associations of HBoV with other respiratory viruses might be explained by the persistence of HBoV in the respiratory tract. The significance of HBoV viral load in nasopharyngeal secretions as a marker of pathogenicity merits further investigation.

▶ We all know about respiratory syncytial virus (RSV), influenza viruses, parainfluenza viruses, adenoviruses, and coronaviruses as causes of respiratory tract disease in children. Many, however, have not heard of the bocavirus. Recently, a new virus, a member of the Parvoviridae family, has been identified in respiratory tract secretions in children with respiratory tract disease. This virus has been classified in the *Bocavirus* genus and named the human bocavirus (HBoV). This virus is now been found worldwide, but we have known relatively little about its impact in the United States. The report of Brieu et al has examined the clinical features of children under the age of 5 years who have been hospitalized with respiratory tract disease and who were found to be positive for HBoV.

What we learn from this report is that approximately 10% of children hospitalized with respiratory tract disease who are less than 5 years of age will be infected with HBoV. In fact, the median age of HBoV-infected children is less than 2 years of age. A study undertaken in Japan has shown that nearly all individuals over the age of 5 years have serologic evidence of a previous HBoV infection.[1] Thus, HBoV infection is a disease of young children. In the report of Brieu et al, HBoV turned out to be second only to RSV in terms of prevalence in this young population as a cause of respiratory tract illness. The virus was not able to be detected in children free of respiratory symptoms, clearly arguing for a role of HBoV in causing respiratory tract illness. Another interesting finding from this report is that persistent shedding of HBoV was observed in 3 children. By persistent is meant several months of shedding.

As far as clinical illness is concerned, the findings of this report indicate that the clinical signs associated with HBoV infection cannot be distinguished from those related to other respiratory viruses, including RSV. HBoV infection, however, appears to be less severe than RSV infection. In most instances, the infection with HBoV presents with what looks like atypical RSV-negative bronchiolitis. Thus, the next time you see a child with what appears to be bronchiolitis who is RSV negative, think bocavirus.

J. A. Stockman III, MD

Reference

1. Endo R, Ishiguro N, Kikuta H, et al. Seroepidemiology of human bocavirus in Hokkaido prefecture, Japan. *J Clin Microbiol.* 2007;45:3218-3223.

Measles in Europe: an epidemiological assessment
Muscat M, for the EUVAC.NET group (Statens Serum Institut, Copenhagen, Denmark)
Lancet 373:383-389, 2009

Background.—Measles persists in Europe despite the incorporation of the measles vaccine into routine childhood vaccination programmes more than 20 years ago. Our aim was therefore to review the epidemiology of measles in relation to the goal of elimination by 2010.

Methods.—National surveillance institutions from 32 European countries submitted data for 2006–07. Data for age-group, diagnosis confirmation, vaccination, hospital treatment, the presence of acute encephalitis as a complication of disease, and death were obtained. 30 countries also supplied data about importation of disease. Clinical, laboratory-confirmed, and epidemiologically linked cases that met the requirements for national surveillance were analysed. Cases were separated by age: younger than 1 year, 1–4 years, 5–9 years, 10–14 years, 15–19 years, and older than 20 years. Countries with indigenous measles incidence per 100 000 inhabitants per year of 0, less than 0·1, 0·1–1, and more than 1 were grouped into categories of zero, low, moderate, and high incidence, respectively.

Findings.—For the 2 years of the study, 12 132 cases of measles were recorded with most cases (n=10 329; 85%) from five countries: Romania,

Germany, UK, Switzerland, and Italy. Most cases were unvaccinated or incompletely vaccinated children; however, almost a fifth were aged 20 years or older. For the same 2 years, seven measles-related deaths were recorded. High measles incidence in some European countries revealed suboptimum vaccination coverage. Of the 210 cases that were reported as being imported, 117 (56%) came from another country within Europe and 43 (20%) from Asia.

Interpretation.—The suboptimum vaccination coverage raises serious doubts that the goal of elimination by 2010 can be attained. Achievement and maintenance of optimum vaccination coverage and improved surveillance are the cornerstones of the measles elimination plan for Europe.

▶ There is a lot to be learned from the measles situation in Europe. There, a measles surveillance data system exists for vaccine-preventable diseases (EUVAC.NET). EUVAC.NET includes the 27 European Union (EU) member states together with Croatia, Iceland, Norway, Switzerland, and Turkey. The EUVAC.NET group was formed in 2006. The intent was to record data on measles outbreaks with the intention of eliminating measles in the World Health Organization European region by 2010. The good news is that only half as many (3909) measles cases occurred in 2007 as in 2006. However, preliminary data suggest that measles incidence was about 3 times higher during the first half of 2008 than in the same period of 2007, suggesting that the earlier decline was just a waning of a natural cycle of measles that is seen from time to time. Such periodicity of measles outbreaks more likely than not accounts for these changes rather than any sudden progress in vaccination. What is encouraging, however, is that most of the cases reported are occurring in unvaccinated individuals, confirming vaccine efficacy in diverse socioeconomic settings of participating countries.

The situation in vaccinated individuals in the EUVAC.NET study, however, seems more complex. Some 10% to 17% of cases occurred in people vaccinated with 1 vaccine dose. Some 9% to 15% of cases occurred in infants who were infected before they could be vaccinated. Such infants can only be protected by high population immunity, which normally cannot be reached without the opportunity for a second vaccine dose.

The obstacles to measles vaccination in Europe are not dissimilar to what we see here in the United States. The United Kingdom, for example, is only slowly recovering from an unsubstantiated scare that the measles, mumps, and rubella vaccination was linked to an increased risk of autism.[1] For a period of time in the Ukraine, the measles and rubella vaccination campaign had to be stopped because of unfounded reports of side effects. Although Germany has its anthroposophic communities and measles parties, the Netherlands struggles with religious objectors in their Bible belt, which, after an outbreak in 1999 and 2000, is again moving toward critical numbers of susceptible individuals sufficient to sustain a large outbreak of measles. Disruption of vaccine supplies after the disintegration of the Soviet Union and political unrest in the Balkans has also caused problems with measles control in Eastern Europe. More than 50 000 cases were recorded in 2005 and 2006 in the Ukraine, which is not part of the EUVAC.NET. Many of the cases occurred in 15- to 29-year-olds. In 2006, a very large outbreak in Romania was reported. Strains of the measles virus that caused this outbreak crept into parts of Europe.

So why are the data from the EU important to us? As long as measles is endemic on other continents, the risk of virus importation into susceptible communities anywhere remains. Many of the strains of measles virus that came into the EU in 2006 and 2007 originated from regions with high measles lethality, confirmed by molecular epidemiology. The only way for the EU (and us) to avoid this problem of importation measles is to maintain high vaccination coverage within our own borders. Thus, identification of final hurdles to measles elimination is essential. The harm done by the bogus reports of autism cannot be underestimated in this regard.

J. A. Stockman III, MD

Reference

1. Friederichs V, Cameron JC, Robertson C. Impact of adverse publicity on MMR vaccine update: population-based analysis of vaccine uptake records for one million children, born 1987-2004. *Arch Dis Child.* 2006;91:465-468.

Factors associated with uptake of measles, mumps, and rubella vaccine (MMR) and use of single antigen vaccines in a contemporary UK cohort: prospective cohort study
Pearce A, Law C, Elliman D, et al (UCL Inst of Child Health, London; Hospital for Children NHS Trust, London)
BMJ 336:754-757, 2008

Objectives.—To estimate uptake of the combined measles, mumps, and rubella vaccine (MMR) and single antigen vaccines and explore factors associated with uptake and reasons for not using MMR.

Design.—Nationally representative cohort study.

Setting.—Children born in the UK, 2000-2.

Participants.—14 578 children for whom data on immunisation were available.

Main Outcome Measures.—Immunisation status at 3 years defined as "immunised with MMR," "immunised with at least one single antigen vaccine," and "unimmunised."

Results.—88.6% (13 013) were immunised with MMR and 5.2% (634) had received at least one single antigen vaccine. Children were more likely to be unimmunised if they lived in a household with other children (risk ratio 1.74, 95% confidence interval 1.35 to 2.25, for those living with three or more) or a lone parent (1.31, 1.07 to 1.60) or if their mother was under 20 (1.41, 1.08 to 1.85) or over 34 at cohort child's birth (reaching 2.34, 1.20 to 3.23, for ≥40), more highly educated (1.41, 1.05 to 1.89, for a degree), not employed (1.43, 1.12 to 1.82), or self employed (1.71, 1.18 to 2.47). Use of single vaccines increased with household income (reaching 2.98, 2.05 to 4.32, for incomes of ≥£52 000 (€69 750, $102 190)), maternal age (reaching 3.04, 2.05 to 4.50, for ≥40), and education (reaching 3.15, 1.78 to 5.58, for a degree). Children were less likely to have received single vaccines if they lived with other children (reaching 0.14, 0.07 to 0.29, for three or more), had mothers who were Indian (0.50, 0.25 to 0.99), Pakistani or Bangladeshi (0.13, 0.04 to 0.39), or black (0.31, 0.14 to 0.64), or aged under 25 (reaching 0.14, 0.05 to 0.36, for 14-19). Nearly three quarters (74.4%, 1110) of parents who did not immunise with MMR made a 'conscious decision' not to immunise.

Conclusions.—Although MMR uptake in this cohort is high, a substantial proportion of children remain susceptible to avoidable infection, largely because parents consciously decide not to immunise. Social differentials in uptake could be used to inform targeted interventions to promote uptake.

▶ Even though this report emanates from Great Britain, there are quite a few analogies to the situation here in the United States when it comes to acceptance of the measles, mumps, and rubella (MMR) vaccine. The use of the MMR vaccine in the United Kingdom reached its peak in the mid-1990s when well over 90% of toddlers were getting the vaccine. Unfortunately, 1998 saw the publication of a report suggesting a link between the administration of the vaccine and the development of autism, and possibly certain forms of bowel disease. This report shot like a rocket around Great Britain, and also here in the United States. Within the British Isles, the receptivity to using the vaccine declined to less than 80% by 2003. It has made a slow comeback on the Isles, reaching a penetration of about 85% in the last couple of years. Despite subsequent research showing no link between MMR and autism and bowel disorders, some parents still seem to be hesitant about allowing their children to receive the vaccine.

What we have learned from this experience is quite interesting. Before the report of Wakefield et al, suggesting a link with autism, it was largely lower income single-parent families in socially deprived areas that comprised the largest population with under immunized children when it came to MMR.[1] Since 1998, however, the decline in uptake has been mostly among parents living in affluent situations.

What we see in this report is that many parents make a conscious decision not to have their child immunized with MMR, with a substantial proportion of parents, in Great Britain, opting to use single antigen vaccines or no vaccines at all. There is significant variation among socioeconomic, cultural, demographic, and ethnic groups. Although economic deprivation is still a risk factor for underimmunization, one sees that among the highest household income families there is the greatest risk for an unwillingness to be immunized with MMR. If there is any value to this report, it is that it informs us of who the target population should be to receive the greatest attention with educational programs to demystify the pros and the cons of MMR vaccination.

At the time this report appeared, Dr Wakefield, the author of the now infamous article attempting to link MMR vaccine to autism, was under review for misconduct in Great Britain by the General Medical Counsel. Years after the publication of his study, it has emerged that 10 of 12 patients involved in the research had legal aid backing to sue vaccine manufacturers and that the Legal Services Commission had funded his research. Dr Wakefield also received some $860 000 from the Legal Services Commission in fees to investigate and write reports on the safety of MMR vaccine—fees that were not disclosed at the time of the publication of the *Lancet* report. The Legal Services Commission is the equivalent of an entity that sues for malpractice recovery. When the payments to Dr Wakefield became apparent in 2004, the *Lancet* repudiated the article citing support of Dr Wakefield's research by this group of attorneys as a "fatal conflict of interest." Dr Wakefield has disputed allegations that while at the Royal Free Hospital, London, he conducted invasive tests on the study subjects, including colonoscopies and lumbar punctures, not approved by the hospital's Research Ethics Committee.

Clearly, the purported link between MMR and autism has been debunked. Also debunked appears to be the senior author of the report that started all the hubbub. The unfortunate consequence has been the thousands of children worldwide who have been put at risk for serious disease by not having received the MMR vaccine. This commentary closes with a *Clinical Fact/Curio* about vaccines. German scientists have found a novel way of delivering therapeutic vaccines—a rapidly vibrating tattoo needle. In studies with mice, tattooing a vaccine produced 16 times more antibodies than did conventional methods. Unfortunately, such preventative vaccine delivery systems would likely be too painful for humans. The heck with the mice.[2]

J. A. Stockman III, MD

References

1. Wakefield A, Murch S, Anthony A, et al. Ileal-lymphoid-nodular hyperplasia, nonspecific colitis and pervasive developmental disorder in children. *Lancet.* 1998;351:637-641.
2. Vaccine tattoos [editorial comment]. *Lancet.* 1999;354:21.

Human Papillomavirus Vaccination Coverage on YouTube
Ache KA, Wallace LS (Univ of Tennessee, Knoxville)
Am J Prev Med 35:389-392, 2008

Background.—A large percentage of Internet users regularly search for health-related information. In recent years, participatory Internet sites such as YouTube have become increasingly popular, in part because individuals are able to both retrieve and post information. This study analyzed how human papillomavirus (HPV) vaccination was portrayed in video-clips and viewer-posted comments available on YouTube.

Methods.—YouTube (www.youtube.com) was queried on February 8, 2008, using the search terms *Gardasil, cervical cancer vaccination*, and

HPV vaccination to identify and download relevant videoclips. Videoclips were classified as either positively or negatively portraying HPV vaccination, and viewer-posted comments were enumerated. Data analyses were conducted immediately following videoclip retrieval.

Results.—A total of 146 unique YouTube videoclips were located, using the three search keywords combined. Three quarters ($n=109$; 74.7%) of the videoclips portrayed HPV vaccination in a positive manner. One third ($n=47$; 32.2%) of the videoclips had generated at least one posted comment.

Conclusions.—These results demonstrate that there is a wide variety of information on YouTube regarding HPV vaccination and cervical cancer. As a result, public health and medical professionals need to be cognizant of the nature of the HPV-related information available, so that they are better equipped to respond to patients who acquire information posted on YouTube and other Internet sources.

► Who would have thought that YouTube would turn out to be a rich source of health information? Although YouTube seems to have been around forever, it was launched only in 2005. YouTube, of course, is a site where users can broadcast themselves by uploading and sharing videos. Worldwide, YouTube is one of the most frequently visited Internet sites. It has been estimated that the average Internet user watches at least 2 YouTube videos daily.[1] It has been shown that information gathered on YouTube can be influential in health-care decision making. Studies have reported the quality of immunization and tobacco information available on YouTube. The report of Ache et al looks at the quality of health care information related to human papillomavirus (HPV) vaccination.

So what will YouTube yield if you plug in the search words "HPV vaccination"? What you will see is that 75% of the clips portray HPV vaccination in a quite positive manner. This is actually quite remarkable because YouTube has a reputation for dissing things in general. It is clear that these YouTube postings are being looked at because the number of searches is listed. Unfortunately, we do not know who is doing the searching.

Care providers should take note of this report and pay some attention to it. There is no reason why accurate information on a variety of health subjects cannot be posted by health care providers. YouTube is one really good place to do this.

J. A. Stockman III, MD

Reference

1. Meiners J, Marketing Pilgrim Web Site. Average internet user watches two You-Tube videos a day. www.marketingpilgrim.com/2007/10/average-internet-user-watches-two-youtube-videos-a-day.html. Accessed July 30, 2009.

Monovalent Type 1 Oral Poliovirus Vaccine in Newborns

El-Sayed N, El-Gamal Y, Abbassy AA, et al (Ministry of Health and Population, Cairo, Egypt; Ain Shams Univ, Cairo, Egypt; Alexandria Univ, Egypt; et al)
N Engl J Med 359:1655-1665, 2008

Background.—In 1988, the World Health Assembly resolved to eradicate poliomyelitis. Although substantial progress toward this goal has been made, eradication remains elusive. In 2004, the World Health Organization called for the development of a potentially more immunogenic monovalent type 1 oral poliovirus vaccine.

Methods.—We conducted a trial in Egypt to compare the immunogenicity of a newly licensed monovalent type 1 oral poliovirus vaccine with that of a trivalent oral poliovirus vaccine. Subjects were randomly assigned to receive one dose of monovalent type 1 oral poliovirus vaccine or trivalent oral poliovirus vaccine at birth. Thirty days after birth, a single challenge dose of monovalent type 1 oral poliovirus vaccine was administered in all subjects. Shedding of serotype 1 poliovirus was assessed through day 60.

Results.—A total of 530 subjects were enrolled, and 421 fulfilled the study requirements. Thirty days after the study vaccines were administered, the rate of seroconversion to type 1 poliovirus was 55.4% in the monovalent-vaccine group, as compared with 32.1% in the trivalent-vaccine group (P<0.001). Among those with a high reciprocal titer of maternally derived antibodies against type 1 poliovirus (>64), 46.0% of the subjects in the monovalent-vaccine group underwent seroconversion, as compared with 21.3% in the trivalent-vaccine group (P<0.001). Seven days after administration of the challenge dose of monovalent type 1 vaccine, a significantly lower proportion of subjects in the monovalent-vaccine group than in the trivalent-vaccine group excreted type 1 poliovirus (25.9% vs. 41.5%, P = 0.001). None of the serious adverse events reported were attributed to the trial interventions.

Conclusions.—When given at birth, monovalent type 1 oral poliovirus vaccine is superior to trivalent oral poliovirus vaccine in inducing humoral antibodies against type 1 poliovirus, overcoming high preexisting levels of maternally derived antibodies, and increasing the resistance to excretion of type 1 poliovirus after administration of a challenge dose. (Current Controlled Trials number, ISRCTN76316509.)

▶ A lot has happened since 1963 when the trivalent oral polio vaccine developed by Albert Sabin was first licensed in the United States. It was this vaccine that was the one that was part of the polio eradication campaign initiated in 1988 by the World Health Organization, a campaign that has led to an impressive decline in cases of paralytic poliomyelitis around the world. In fact, monovalent versions of oral polio vaccine had been licensed earlier but were abandoned in favor of trivalent combination of oral polio vaccine to simplify immunization schedules. Differences between monovalent and trivalent vaccines were never formally addressed. However, by the turn of the century, global transmission of wild-type poliovirus type 2, one of the 3 serotypes of the virus, had been successfully interrupted. Elimination of this particular serotype represented a major milestone for the eradication initiative. Further progress, however, toward eradication has stalled somewhat with a continuation of circulation of endemic virus in several geographic pockets of the world such as northern Nigeria, northern India, and the Pakistan-Afghanistan border. It has been suspected that the trivalent oral polio vaccine is not sufficiently immunogenic to eliminate the circulation of wild-type virus, and new vaccine products have been sought to achieve the final goal of eradication. A few studies done a while back have suggested that monovalent oral poliovirus vaccine, in particular that containing monovalent type 1 virus, was 2 to 3 times as immunogenic as trivalent oral polio virus vaccine because it eliminated interference from the other 2 polio virus serotypes. The Global Polio Eradication Initiative encouraged the development of a new monovalent type 1 oral poliovirus vaccine, which was licensed and put into use in 2005.

Two studies simultaneously appeared in the *New England Journal of Medicine* that tell us about how well the monovalent type 1 poliovirus vaccine actually works. The report of El-Sayed et al was designed to directly measure immunogenicity and took place in Egypt. Seroconversion rates were determined after the administration of a dose of either trivalent vaccine or monovalent vaccine given at birth, and virus excretion was measured after subsequent challenge with monovalent type 1 oral poliovirus vaccine. The results show that when given at birth, monovalent type 1 oral poliovirus vaccine was more effective in inducing production of humoral antibodies and at reducing virus excretion after challenge.

The report of Jenkins et al tells us more about the monovalent type 1 oral poliovirus vaccine and summarizes a study performed in northern Nigeria.[1] This commentary closes with an infectious disease *Clinical Fact/Curio*. If you are traveling to Uganda, beware of bats and for reasons that go well beyond rabies. The World Health Organization has warned Ugandans and tourists to avoid caves with bats after a Dutch tourist, exposed to fruit bats, was infected and died from Marburg hemorrhagic fever. Marburg infection is caused by a virulent filovirus of the family also responsible for Ebola hemorrhagic fever. It is fatal and death is usually preceded by severe blood loss. No vaccine or treatment has been identified.[2]

J. A. Stockman III, MD

References

1. Jenkins HE, Aylward RB, Gasasira A, et al. Effectiveness of immunization against paralytic poliomyelitis in Nigeria. *N Engl J Med.* 2008;359:1666-1674.
2. Deadly bats [editorial comment]. *Lancet.* 2008;372:821.

Effectiveness of Immunization against Paralytic Poliomyelitis in Nigeria
Jenkins HE, Aylward RB, Gasasira A, et al (Imperial College London, UK; World Health Organization (WHO), Geneva; WHO–Nigeria, Abuja)
N Engl J Med 359:1666-1674, 2008

Background.—The number of cases of paralytic poliomyelitis has declined in Nigeria since the introduction of newly licensed monovalent oral poliovirus vaccines and new techniques of vaccine delivery. Understanding the relative contribution of these vaccines and the improved coverage to the decline in incident cases is essential for future planning.

Methods.—We estimated the field efficacies of monovalent type 1 oral poliovirus vaccine and trivalent oral poliovirus vaccine, using the reported number of doses received by people with poliomyelitis and by matched controls as identified in Nigeria's national surveillance database, in which 27,379 cases of acute flaccid paralysis were recorded between 2001 and 2007. Our estimates of vaccine coverage and vaccine-induced immunity were based on the number of doses received by children listed in the database who had paralysis that was not caused by poliovirus.

Results.—The estimated efficacies per dose of monovalent type 1 oral poliovirus vaccine and trivalent oral poliovirus vaccine against type 1 paralytic poliomyelitis were 67% (95% confidence interval [CI], 39 to 82) and 16% (95% CI, 10 to 21), respectively, and the estimated efficacy per dose of trivalent oral poliovirus vaccine against type 3 paralytic poliomyelitis was 18% (95% CI, 9 to 26). In the northwestern region of Nigeria, which reported the majority of cases during the study period, coverage with at least one dose of vaccine increased from 59 to 78%. Between 2005 and 2007, vaccine-induced immunity levels among children under the age of 5 years more than doubled, to 56%.

Conclusions.—The higher efficacy of monovalent type 1 oral poliovirus vaccine (four times as effective as trivalent oral poliovirus vaccine) and the moderate gains in coverage dramatically increased vaccine-induced immunity against serotype 1 in northern Nigeria. Further increases in coverage in Nigerian states with infected populations are required to achieve the levels of vaccine-induced immunity associated with the sustained elimination achieved in other parts of the country.

▶ This report represents the second of 2 studies appearing in the same issue of the *New England Journal of Medicine*. This study was conducted in northern Nigeria, where temporary suspension of all poliovirus immunization in one state in 2003 contributed to a national epidemic of poliomyelitis and reinfection in more than 20 countries that had been poliomyelitis-free. Even after the reversal of the suspension, vaccine coverage remained low in northern Nigeria. According to field studies of the reported number of doses of polio vaccine received by case patients and matched controls, the estimated efficacy of monovalent type 1 oral poliovirus vaccine per dose against type 1 poliomyelitis was 4 times as great as that of the trivalent oral poliovirus vaccine. At the same time, a new strategy of vaccine delivery, in which oral poliovirus vaccine was offered together with a range of additional pediatric vaccinations and other health services, resulted in moderate gains in coverage. Taken together, these 2 interventions significantly increased vaccine-induced immunity in this region.

Based on all the information we have now, one can say that the monovalent oral poliovirus vaccine is an effective tool for interrupting persistent chains of wild-type virus transmission, particularly now that serotype 2 polio seems to have been eradicated throughout the world. Although reducing vaccine failure does not compensate for failure to vaccinate, the newly formulated monovalent type 1 oral poliovirus vaccine, and by extrapolation, monovalent type 3 oral poliovirus vaccine, are now welcome additions to the toolbox we need to eliminate transmission of wild-type polioviruses.

One final comment having to do with poliovirus vaccines. Most now consider it critical that we eliminate polio from the face of the earth, not just because this can be a devastating infection, but also because of the dangers of the live oral poliovirus vaccine itself, whether trivalent or monovalent. It has now been documented that the oral poliovirus vaccine contains virus that is genetically unstable and that there has been some emergence of circulating neurovirulent vaccine-derived polioviruses. In addition, long-term excretion of virus by immunodeficient vaccines is a well-known phenomenon and just as worrisome is the fact that vaccine-related polioviruses can recombine with non-poliovirus enteroviruses, and theoretically these recombined viruses can cause problems. Even if we are able to eradicate wild-type virus, chances are that it will be necessary to maintain high levels of immunity throughout the world, but this can be safely done with inactivated poliovirus vaccine. While not as immunogenic as a live-virus vaccine, inactivated poliovirus vaccine is capable of maintaining levels of immunity to achieve this goal.

To read more about monovalent oral poliovirus vaccines, see the excellent editorial on this topic by Ehrenfeld and Chumakov.[1]

J. A. Stockman III, MD

Reference

1. Ehrenfeld E, Chumakov K. Monovalent oral poliovirus vaccines – a good tool, but not a total solution. *N Engl J Med*. 2008;359:1726-1727.

Hepatitis B Virus Screening for Internationally Adopted Children

Stadler LP, Mezoff AG, Staat MA (Cincinnati Children's Hosp Med Ctr, OH; Children's Med Ctr, Dayton, OH)
Pediatrics 122:1223-1228, 2008

Objectives.—The objectives of this study were to estimate the prevalence of hepatitis B virus protection, infection, and recovery among internationally adopted children and to examine the need for repeat testing 6 months after arrival in the United States.

Methods.—From November 1999 through October 2006, 1282 international adoptees were screened for hepatitis B virus, and results were examined with regard to age, gender, and birth country. The prevalence of hepatitis B virus protection, infection, and recovery was determined.

Results.—The prevalence of hepatitis B virus in internationally adopted children at our large international adoption center was 4%, including 1.1% with acute or chronic infection and 2.9% with resolved infection. Overall, 64% of internationally adopted children had evidence of hepatitis B virus immunization, with protective antibodies. We also report a case that highlights the need for repeat serological testing to detect hepatitis B virus infection or immunization in internationally adopted children who might have been infected or vaccinated just before adoption and thus not have serological evidence in initial testing.

Conclusions.—These data reinforce the American Academy of Pediatrics recommendations regarding hepatitis B virus screening and infection control measures for international adoptees.

▶ The *Red Book* recommends that all children being adopted from overseas should be screened for a variety of infectious diseases. Among these is hepatitis related to the hepatitis B virus (HBV). The report of Stadler et al provides us with information about how frequently HBV is picked up as part of this screening. We learn that 4% of internationally adopted children either have or have had HBV infections (1.1% with acute or chronic disease and 2.9% with resolved infection). The highest prevalence of infection was found in children being adopted from Africa, Southeast Asia (including China), Korea, Indonesia, the Philippines, Haiti, and the Dominican Republic. High prevalence countries were defined as having an ≥8% likelihood of children being internationally adopted having evidence of HBV. Intermediate prevalence (2%-7%) countries and regions include South Central and Southwest Asia, Israel, Japan, Eastern and Southern Europe, Russia, most areas surrounding the Amazon river basin, Honduras, and Guatemala. One hundred percent of the children infected with HBV came from these countries and regions.

It should be recognized that HBV has a long incubation period, and negative serologic results need to be followed up on at 6 months with repeat testing. It would be wise to recommend to families adopting children from disease-endemic areas to receive the HBV vaccine before the adoption process proceeds because horizontal transmission from undetected internationally adopted children to household members has been described.

Recognize that HBV causes chronic infection worldwide to the tune of about 400 million people. Most carriers of chronic HBV, including Asians, Africans, and a proportion of persons in the Mediterranean countries, acquire infection at birth or within the first 1 to 2 years after birth. It is estimated that 50% of male carriers and 14% of female carriers will eventually die of complications of cirrhosis and hepatocellular carcinoma. To say this differently, HBV is no laughing matter. It is very important to follow the American Academy of Pediatrics *Red Book* recommendation religiously and to screen for this infection in internationally adopted children.

J. A. Stockman III, MD

Tenofovir Disoproxil Fumarate versus Adefovir Dipivoxil for Chronic Hepatitis B

Marcellin P, Heathcote EJ, Buti M, et al (Univ of Paris 7 and INSERM Unité 773, France; Univ of Toronto, Canada; Hebron Hosp, Barcelona; et al)
N Engl J Med 359:2442-2455, 2008

Background.—Tenofovir disoproxil fumarate (DF) is a nucleotide analogue and a potent inhibitor of human immunodeficiency virus type 1 reverse transcriptase and hepatitis B virus (HBV) polymerase.

Methods.—In two double-blind, phase 3 studies, we randomly assigned patients with hepatitis B e antigen (HBeAg)–negative or HBeAg-positive chronic HBV infection to receive tenofovir DF or adefovir dipivoxil (ratio, 2:1) once daily for 48 weeks. The primary efficacy end point was a plasma HBV DNA level of less than 400 copies per milliliter (69 IU per milliliter) and histologic improvement (i.e., a reduction in the Knodell necroinflammation score of 2 or more points without worsening fibrosis) at week 48. Secondary end points included viral suppression (i.e., an HBV DNA level of <400 copies per milliliter), histologic improvement, serologic response, normalization of alanine aminotransferase levels, and development of resistance mutations.

Results.—At week 48, in both studies, a significantly higher proportion of patients receiving tenofovir DF than of those receiving adefovir dipivoxil had reached the primary end point (P<0.001). Viral suppression occurred in more HBeAg-negative patients receiving tenofovir DF than patients receiving adefovir dipivoxil (93% vs. 63%, P<0.001) and in more HBeAg-positive patients receiving tenofovir DF than patients receiving adefovir dipivoxil (76% vs. 13%, P<0.001). Significantly more HBeAg-positive patients treated with tenofovir DF than those treated with adefovir dipivoxil had normalized alanine aminotransferase levels (68% vs. 54%, P = 0.03) and loss of hepatitis B surface antigen (3% vs. 0%, P = 0.02). At week 48, amino acid substitutions within HBV DNA polymerase associated with phenotypic resistance to tenofovir DF or other drugs to treat HBV infection had not developed in any of the patients. Tenofovir DF produced a similar HBV DNA response in patients who had previously received lamivudine and in those who had not. The safety profile was similar for the two treatments in both studies.

Conclusions.—Among patients with chronic HBV infection, tenofovir DF at a daily dose of 300 mg had superior antiviral efficacy with a similar safety profile as compared with adefovir dipivoxil at a daily dose of 10 mg through week 48. (ClinicalTrials.gov numbers, NCT00116805 and NCT00117676.)

▶ There is a relatively high prevalence of hepatitis B virus (HBV) infection in internationally adopted children. Children and adults who have active and/or chronic HBV infection now need to be treated. An elevated HBV DNA level of more than 2000 IU/milliliter is a strong predictor of the risk of complications of cirrhosis and hepatocellular carcinoma. Prolonged, effective suppression of

HBV DNA has been shown to decrease the risk of the development of cirrhosis and of hepatocellular carcinoma. The goal for the treatment of chronic HBV infection is sustained suppression of HBV DNA to very low levels, preferably to below the detection limit of sensitive polymerase chain-reaction (PCR) assays. The liver enzyme alanine aminotransferase level should also ideally be lower than half the upper limit of the normal range.

The first licensed agent for the treatment of chronic HBV infection was the conventional form of interferon alfa, which acts mainly through immunomodulation and has the advantage of being given over a fixed period of time, although this is partly because of its often severe side effects. Unfortunately, most patients treated with interferon alfa will still have levels of HBV DNA that are detectable by PCR assay and most studies show no decrease in the occurrence of hepatocellular carcinoma on long-term follow-up. The short-term efficacy of pegylated interferon (Pegterferon), licensed in 2005, is almost identical to that of conventional interferon. Data on its long-term effects with respect to the development of cirrhosis and hepatocellular carcinoma have not been published.

There is another form of treatment available. This is with lamivudine, a nucleoside analogue. The drug was licensed in 1998. Nucleoside and nucleotide analogues suppress HBV replication through inhibition of the reverse transcriptase and DNA polymerase activities. In the past decade, 4 other nucleoside and nucleotide analogues have been licensed: adefovir (2002), entecavir (2005), telbivudine (2006), and most recently, tenofovir disoproxil fumarate (2008). Marcellin reported on 2 studies comparing the antiviral efficacy of tenofovir with that of adefovir dipivoxil in both HBeAg-negative and HBeAg-positive patients. After 48 weeks of treatment, tenofovir was superior to adefovir dipivoxil in suppressing levels of HBV DNA to less than 400 copies per milliliter. Many of the patients who responded had been previously treated with lamivudine and were resistant to the latter drug. The most obvious niche for tenofovir therefore is in the treatment of patients with lamivudine resistance. It is to be expected that resistance to tenofovir will be lower because of its greater efficacy in viral suppression.

For more on the moderate management of chronic hepatitis B infection, see the excellent editorial on this topic by Lai and Lyuen.[1] This commentary closes with a *Clinical Fact/Curio* of profound significance. Once and for all, did Christopher Columbus bring epidemic typhus to the New World upon his arrival? The answer is that it is entirely likely that Christopher Columbus actually was not the source of epidemic typhus in the western hemisphere. Typhus, a potentially deadly flu-like illness, is spread by body lice. A biologist at the Florida Museum of Natural History in Gainesville has sequenced DNA from ancient life preserved in the scalps and braids of 1000-year-old Peruvian mummies. Surprisingly, it was discovered that the lice belonged to a common subtype that is found all over the world. This subtype typically infests the head, but it also includes body lice that thrive in clothing and spread diseases, including epidemic typhus. Thus it is reasonable to believe that body lice were in the New World well before Columbus and that the typhus the lice carried was around many centuries if not millennia before the arrival of those from Spain.

The studies from Gainesville are unique in their own right even though studies of ancient DNA are not new. The DNA in lice tends to degrade quite quickly, and the oldest lice genetic material sequenced to date comes only from Napoleonic soldiers—bodies buried 200 years ago. The feat of being able to sequence lice that is over a millennium old is quite remarkable and does give insights into how pristine, or not, the western hemisphere was, or was not, before contamination from those visiting its shores from Europe.[2]

J. A. Stockman III, MD

References

1. Lai C-L, Lyuen M-F. Chronic hepatitis B – new goals in treatment. *N Engl J Med.* 2008;359:2488-2491.
2. Molecular nit picking [editorial comment]. *Science.* 2008;319:1019.

Estimation of HIV incidence in the United States

Hall III, Song R, Rhodes P, et al (Ctrs for Disease Control and Prevention, Atlanta, GA; et al)
JAMA 300:520-529, 2008

Context.—Incidence of human immunodeficiency virus (HIV) in the United States has not been directly measured. New assays that differentiate recent vs long-standing HIV infections allow improved estimation of HIV incidence.

Objective.—To estimate HIV incidence in the United States.

Design, Setting, and Patients.—Remnant diagnostic serum specimens from patients 13 years or older and newly diagnosed with HIV during 2006 in 22 states were tested with the BED HIV-1 capture enzyme immunoassay to classify infections as recent or long-standing. Information on HIV cases was reported to the Centers for Disease Control and Prevention through June 2007. Incidence of HIV in the 22 states during 2006 was estimated using a statistical approach with adjustment for testing frequency and extrapolated to the United States. Results were corroborated with back-calculation of HIV incidence for 1977-2006 based on HIV diagnoses from 40 states and AIDS incidence from 50 states and the District of Columbia.

Main Outcome Measure.—Estimated HIV incidence.

Results.—An estimated 39 400 persons were diagnosed with HIV in 2006 in the 22 states. Of 6864 diagnostic specimens tested using the BED assay, 2133 (31%) were classified as recent infections. Based on extrapolations from these data, the estimated number of new infections for the United States in 2006 was 56 300 (95% confidence interval [CI], 48 200-64 500); the estimated incidence rate was 22.8 per 100 000 population (95% CI, 19.5-26.1). Forty-five percent of infections were among black individuals and 53% among men who have sex with men. The back-calculation (n = 1.230 million HIV/AIDS cases reported by the end of 2006) yielded an estimate of 55 400 (95% CI, 50 000-60 800) new infections per year for 2003-2006 and indicated that HIV incidence increased in the mid-1990s, then slightly declined after 1999 and has been stable thereafter.

Conclusions.—This study provides the first direct estimates of HIV incidence in the United States using laboratory technologies previously implemented only in clinic-based settings. New HIV infections in the United States remain concentrated among men who have sex with men and among black individuals.

▶ The report showing the estimate of HIV incidence in the United States was viewed by some as a sign of success in the battle against the transmission of HIV infection and by others as an indication that we have a long way to go. It is now almost 30 years since HIV infection and its consequence, AIDS, have mingled within our societies throughout the world. While millions of lives have been lost to this illness, it is quite amazing, actually, how much progress has been made. What was once a quickly lethal disease has now been converted in those who are able to receive adequate treatment regimens to a chronic illness, albeit still likely a fatal one.

Progress against HIV infection has come on many fronts, one of which has been the development of new drug therapies. It was in 1987 that the drug known as azidothymidine became available and was welcomed for the brief reprieve it gave to severely immunocompromised patients with AIDS. Unfortunately, the drug is extraordinarily toxic. By the mid-1990s, a wide variety of drugs of several classes collectively known as HAART entered our therapeutic armamentarium. Once again, not all patients could tolerate combination therapy and even more unfortunate was the extraordinary cost of these drugs. We quickly learned that in order for drug resistance not to occur, these drugs had to be given in combination. It was HAART that converted HIV infection and AIDS from what was clearly a universal death sentence to a survivable chronic disease. If one could get these drugs and could afford them, there was finally hope for a reasonably normal existence for most patients with HIV infection. All during this period, we learned much about the public health aspects of HIV infection and the behaviors that predispose to the acquiring of the infection.

So where are we with HIV/AIDS today? It is estimated that more than 25 million individuals worldwide have already died of AIDS and that somewhat more than this number are currently infected. Vast populations are at risk, particularly emerging parts of the world such as Asia. HIV infection struck with a fury in South Africa with an estimated 2.5 million individuals newly infected in recent years. For more than a decade, however, in the United States, a "steady state" of about 40 000 new HIV infection cases have been reported, although in the study abstracted, it does appear that about 50 000 incident cases may be occurring if one accounts for both reported and likely cases.

It is hard to say exactly where we are in the battle against HIV infection and AIDS. Virologic concerns remain. The HIV genome has been mutating continuously from the outset of the description of the disease. It is clear also that HIV-1 has multiple subtypes, and while a number of them can be traced back to the beginning of the epidemic, others have unquestionably arisen since then. Most believe that these subtypes represent hybrid viruses that arise when a single individual is coinfected with 2 subtypes of virus and then the viral offspring express recombined genomic content. The fact that this occurs changes our whole concept of virus transmission. Early in the AIDS epidemic it was assumed that individuals once infected posed no additional risk to another infected individual. Actually, once infected, individuals can pass around many different virus subtypes.

Well worth reading is the commentary on the current and future status of AIDS by June Osborn.[1] Dr Osborn reminds us that like the day after Hiroshima, it is now evident that a new primal force has unequivocally altered the world and its future. HIV infection hopefully will be able to be managed, dealt with, and confronted in a number of ways, but it never will be likely gone from the face of the earth. Most of us, as adults, can remember a world without AIDS. Many of our children do not. The unfortunate fact is there never will again be a world without AIDS.

As this commentary closes, another *Clinical Fact/Curio*, this having to do with infectious diseases. Were you aware of which institutions were getting the most money to support HIV/AIDS research? The following table shows the so-called fat cats as published in *Science* recently.[2] The University of Washington in Seattle leads the pack by a significant margin. The R01 Top Dogs had 28 grants among them and received $1.95 million to $2.6 million each—4 to 5 times as much as the average age researcher. Many of these top dogs ran expensive clinical or epidemiological studies outside of established networks funded by the NIH. These networks account for $300 million annually. The 10 best funded universities in the table run many of these networks, which helps explain why they rake in about one-fourth of the NIH's entire HIV/AIDS research budget which annually runs in the $3 billion-a-year range.

Best HIV/AIDS-Funded Institutions (FY '07)

Institution	Amount ($M)
University of Washington	138.1
Harvard University	103.0
Johns Hopkins University	98.3
University of California, San Francisco	70.8
Duke University	68.6
University of California, Los Angeles	62.6
University of Pittsburgh	55.2
University of Minnesota	51.5
University of Pennsylvania	39.0
University of California, San Diego	32.6
Total	719.7

J. A. Stockman III, MD

References

1. Osborn JE. The past, present and future of AIDS. *JAMA.* 2008;300:581-583.
2. Cohen J. Where have all the dollars gone? *Science.* 2008;321:519-520.

CD4+/CD8+ T Cell Ratio for Diagnosis of HIV-1 Infection in Infants: Women and Infants Transmission Study

Pahwa S, Read JS, Yin W, et al (Univ of Miami, FL; Eunice Kennedy Shriver Natl Inst of Child Health and Human Development, Bethesda, MD; Clinical Trials & Surveys Corp, Baltimore, MD; et al)

Pediatrics 122:311-339, 2008

Objective.—In this study, we tested the hypothesis that the CD4+/CD8+ T cell ratio could predict HIV infection status in HIV-exposed infants.

Methods.—CD4+/CD8+ T cell ratios were determined from data for live-born singleton infants who had been prospectively enrolled in the Women and Infants Transmission Study. Data for 2208 infants with known HIV infection status (179 HIV-infected and 2029 uninfected infants) were analyzed.

Results.—Receiver operating characteristic curves indicated that the CD4+/CD8+ T cell ratio performed better than the proportion of CD4+ T cells for diagnosis of HIV infection as early as 2 months of age, and this relationship was unaffected by adjustment for maternal race/ethnicity, infant birth weight, gestational age, and gender. At 4 months of age, 90% specificity for HIV diagnosis was associated with 60% sensitivity. For ease of use, graphical estimates based on cubic splines for the time-dependent parameters in a Box-Cox transformation (L), the median (M), and the coefficient of variation (S) were used to create LMS centile curves to show the sensitivity and specificity of CD4+/CD8+ T cell ratios in HIV-infected and uninfected infants until 12 months of age. At 6 months of age, a simplified equation that incorporated sequential CD4+/CD8+ T cell ratios and hematocrit values resulted in improved receiver operating characteristic curves, with 94% positive predictive value and 98% negative predictive value. The positive and negative predictive values remained above 90% in simulated infant populations over a wide range of HIV infection prevalence values.

Conclusions.—In the absence of virological diagnosis, a presumptive diagnosis of HIV infection status can be made on the basis of CD4+/CD8+ T cell ratios in HIV-1- exposed infants after 2 months of age; sensitivity and specificity can be improved at 6 months by using a discriminant analysis equation.

▶ The determination of the HIV status of infants born to HIV-infected women is key for proper care of both infected and uninfected infants. No one argues that HIV nucleic acid amplification assays, including DNA polymerase chain reaction (PCR) assays, are the standards for the diagnosis of HIV infection among HIV-exposed infants. HIV-DNA PCR assays are almost 100% sensitive and specific at 6 weeks of age. Unfortunately, HIV nucleic acid testing is not available in many areas of the world that are resource poor and where the burden of HIV infection is the greatest. In such settings serological testing may be the only type of testing available, resulting in delays in the diagnosis of HIV-exposed infants. The delay is due to the fact that infection status cannot be established until a seroreversion after decay of passively transferred maternal antibodies occurs in the case of uninfected children or until the development of HIV-associated clinical symptoms or documented persistence of anti-HIV antibodies beyond 18 months is documented in the case of HIV-infected children. Until appropriate HIV serological assays for the diagnosis of HIV infection become universally available, it is critical to develop alternative diagnostic methods for perinatally HIV-exposed infants, in order to make a diagnosis as soon after birth as possible. Several approaches are currently being examined in this regard. The report of Pahwa et al looks at this conundrum by evaluating whether CD4$^+$/CD8$^+$ T-cell ratio might be useful as a diagnostic tool for identifying HIV-exposed infants. Such an approach, if successful, would prove quite useful because in many parts of the world where HIV nucleic acid testing is impossible, access to T-cell subset analysis does exist.

For some time now, CD4$^+$ T-cells have been used to monitor the degree of immunosuppression in HIV-infected infants, children, and adults. Concurrent with the loss of CD4$^+$ T-cells, a predominant consequence of HIV infection is expansion of CD8$^+$ T-cells, a component of the immune activation that is a pathogenic feature of HIV infection. The authors of this report hypothesize that an inverse CD4$^+$/CD8$^+$ T-cell ratio would likely be a more sensitive discriminator of HIV infection status than depilation of CD4$^+$ T-lymphocytes alone. In this study, they analyze CD4$^+$/CD8$^+$ T-cell ratios in infants born of HIV-infected mothers. At 16 weeks of age, the CD4$^+$/CD8$^+$ T-cell ratio turns out to be 90% specific for HIV infection with a sensitivity of approximately 60%. By 6 months of age, these assays have a 94% positive predictive value and a 98% predictive value. In other words, a presumptive diagnosis of HIV infection can be made on the basis of CD4$^+$/CD8$^+$ T-cell ratios in HIV-1-exposed infants as early as 2 months of age and certainly by 4 months later. The predictive value can be further improved by adding a few other simple tests, including hematocrit levels, a simple laboratory marker that is relatively easy to measure in low-resource areas.

Thus it may be that in resource-poor areas of the world lacking the routine availability of virological assays for infant diagnosis, a presumptive diagnosis of HIV infection can be made with alternative laboratory studies such as measurement of CD4$^+$/CD8$^+$ T-cell ratios early in life.

J. A. Stockman III, MD

Early Antiretroviral Therapy and Mortality among HIV-Infected Infants

Violari A, Cotton MF, Gibb DM, et al (Univ of the Witwatersrand, Johannesburg; Stellenbosch Univ, Tygerberg; Med Research Council Clinical Trials Unit, London; et al)

N Engl J Med 359:2233-2244, 2008

Background.—In countries with a high seroprevalence of human immunodeficiency virus type 1 (HIV-1), HIV infection contributes significantly to infant mortality. We investigated antiretroviral-treatment strategies in the Children with HIV Early Antiretroviral Therapy (CHER) trial.

Methods.—HIV-infected infants 6 to 12 weeks of age with a CD4 lymphocyte percentage (the CD4 percentage) of 25% or more were randomly assigned to receive antiretroviral therapy (lopinavir–ritonavir, zidovudine, and lamivudine) when the CD4 percentage decreased to less than 20% (or 25% if the child was younger than 1 year) or clinical criteria were met (the deferred antiretroviral-therapy group) or to immediate initiation of limited antiretroviral therapy until 1 year of age or 2 years of age (the early antiretroviral-therapy groups). We report the early outcomes for infants who received deferred antiretroviral therapy as compared with early antiretroviral therapy.

Results.—At a median age of 7.4 weeks (interquartile range, 6.6 to 8.9) and a CD4 percentage of 35.2% (interquartile range, 29.1 to 41.2), 125 infants were randomly assigned to receive deferred therapy, and 252 infants were randomly assigned to receive early therapy. After a median follow-up of 40 weeks (interquartile range, 24 to 58), antiretroviral therapy was initiated in 66% of infants in the deferred-therapy group. Twenty infants in the deferred-therapy group (16%) died versus 10 infants in the early-therapy groups (4%) (hazard ratio for death, 0.24; 95% confidence interval [CI], 0.11 to 0.51; P<0.001). In 32 infants in the deferred-therapy group (26%) versus 16 infants in the early-therapy groups (6%), disease progressed to Centers for Disease Control and Prevention stage C or severe stage B (hazard ratio for disease progression, 0.25; 95% CI, 0.15 to 0.41; P<0.001). Stavudine was substituted for zidovudine in four infants in the early-therapy groups because of neutropenia in three infants and anemia in one infant; no drugs were permanently discontinued. After a review by the data and safety monitoring board, the deferred-therapy group was modified, and infants in this group were all reassessed for initiation of antiretroviral therapy.

Conclusions.—Early HIV diagnosis and early antiretroviral therapy reduced early infant mortality by 76% and HIV progression by 75%. (ClinicalTrials.gov number, NCT00102960.)

▶ This report is one more example of why infants and children are not just "little adults." While highly active antiretroviral therapy (HAART) has changed the face of HIV infection in children and has turned a deadly disease into a chronic one by reducing mortality, it is clear that infants, in particular, cannot be considered little adults in how the task of therapy is administered. Infants with HIV infection tend to progress more rapidly and have higher mortality rates than older children even when CD4 cell counts are taken into account. Given the limitations of the available drugs, the long-term toxicity of antiretroviral therapy, adherence issues, the risk of resistance to antiretroviral therapy, and limited resources, administering a treatment throughout an entire lifespan for these infants is obviously problematic. This is where the report of Violari becomes important because it represents a study that addresses the optimal time of initiation and duration of antiretroviral therapy in infants with in utero or intrapartum HIV infection. The investigators hypothesize that early initiation of limited antiretroviral therapy soon after primary infection, when the immune system is most immature, would be ideally beneficial and would delay the time to initiation of continuous antiretroviral therapy. The study represents a randomized trial where some infants received deferred therapy and others received early antiretroviral treatment. The deferred antiretroviral therapy group included HIV-infected infants 6 to 12 weeks of age with 25% or more CD4 cells who received antiretroviral therapy only when the CD4 percentage decreased to less than 20% (or 25% if the child was younger than 1 year) or clinical criteria were otherwise met. The remainder of the infants were given HAART immediately until 1 year of age or 2 years of age (the early antiretroviral-therapy groups). Outcomes then were looked at over time. On follow-up, it was absolutely clear that the early introduction of antiretroviral therapy (median age 7 weeks) reduced mortality by almost 75% (actual mortality 4% versus 16%). A rapid decrease in CD4 values, rapid disease progression, and sudden death were all evident among infants in the deferred-therapy group despite very close follow-up and regular CD4 monitoring. Although the large majority of infants in this group in fact did receive antiretroviral therapy, mainly because of decreasing CD4 percentage, excess deaths could not be prevented. To say this differently, once the manifestations of this infection take hold, it becomes very difficult to reverse the clinical course even with aggressive antiretroviral therapy.

The conclusion here is very straightforward. The data from this report provide extraordinarily strong support for the early initiation of antiretroviral therapy in all infants developing HIV infection in utero or during the birthing process. Early diagnosis is obviously fundamental to the success of this program.

It should be noted that the results of the report abstracted are consistent with those of the pediatric AIDS clinical trials group, which recently reported that in a treatment-experienced population with a low percentage of T-cells, a sustainable suppression of HIV virus can be achieved with early initiation of HAART. The latter trial has looked at the optimal time to challenge HIV-infected infants and young children with vaccines.[1]

J. A. Stockman III, MD

Reference

1. Rigaud M, Borkowsky W, Muresan P, et al. Impaired immunity to recall antigens and neoantigens in severely immunocompromised children and adolescents during the first year of effective highly active antiretroviral therapy. *J Infect Dis*. 2008; 198:1123-1130.

Extended Antiretroviral Prophylaxis to Reduce Breast-Milk HIV-1 Transmission

Kumwenda NI, Hoover DR, Mofenson LM, et al (Johns Hopkins Univ, Baltimore, MD; Rutgers Univ, Piscataway, NJ; Natl Insts of Health, Bethesda, MD; et al)
N Engl J Med 359:119-129, 2008

Background.—Effective strategies are urgently needed to reduce mother-to-child transmission of human immunodeficiency virus type 1 (HIV-1) through breast-feeding in resource-limited settings.

Methods.—Women with HIV-1 infection who were breast-feeding infants were enrolled in a randomized, phase 3 trial in Blantyre, Malawi. At birth, the infants were randomly assigned to one of three regimens: single-dose nevirapine plus 1 week of zidovudine (control regimen) or the control regimen plus daily extended prophylaxis either with nevirapine (extended nevirapine) or with nevirapine plus zidovudine (extended dual prophylaxis) until the age of 14 weeks. Using Kaplan–Meier analyses, we assessed the risk of HIV-1 infection among infants who were HIV-1–negative on DNA polymerase-chain-reaction assay at birth.

Results.—Among 3016 infants in the study, the control group had consistently higher rates of HIV-1 infection from the age of 6 weeks through 18 months. At 9 months, the estimated rate of HIV-1 infection (the primary end point) was 10.6% in the control group, as compared with 5.2% in the extended-nevirapine group (P<0.001) and 6.4% in the extended-dual-prophylaxis group (P = 0.002). There were no significant differences between the two extended-prophylaxis groups. The frequency of breastfeeding did not differ significantly among the study groups. Infants receiving extended dual prophylaxis had a significant increase in the number of adverse events (primarily neutropenia) that were deemed to be possibly related to a study drug.

Conclusions.—Extended prophylaxis with nevirapine or with nevirapine and zidovudine for the first 14 weeks of life significantly reduced postnatal HIV-1 infection in 9-month-old infants. (ClinicalTrials.gov number, NCT00115648.)

▶ Although peripartum prophylaxis with a single dose or a short course of antiretroviral agents effectively reduces intrapartum HIV transmission, its effect does not extend much beyond 4 to 6 weeks in breast-feeding populations. In many parts of Africa where breast-feeding is critical for infant survival, postnatal transmission of HIV occurs in up to 16% of uninfected infants when breast-feeding continues into the second year of life.

In an effort to reduce the risk of transmission of HIV through breast milk but still maintain the benefits of breast-feeding, Kumwenda et al compared the efficacy of 3 antiretroviral prophylaxis regimens for infants that were begun on prophylaxis at birth. An extended 14-week course of nevirapine, with or without zidovudine, was 40% to 51% better in preventing HIV transmission at 9 months than a one-week standard regimen (single-dose nevirapine combined with one week of zidovudine). Unfortunately, rates of HIV transmission more than doubled in both of the extended-prophylaxis groups in the period between 9 and 24 months, time periods during which many of the mothers continued breast-feeding (eg, breast-feeding rates of 14% to 19% at 15 months). In contrast to HIV-infection rates, mortality rates did not differ according to treatment group. Although HIV-free survival was slightly better in both extended-prophylaxis groups at 9 months of age, this advantage was lost by 12 months in the group that received extended prophylaxis with nevirapine plus zidovudine and by 15 months in the group that received extended prophylaxis with nevirapine only. Continued breast-feeding beyond the period of antiretroviral prophylaxis clearly affected the durability of the extended regimens, making it difficult to recommend widespread implementation of the study strategies in populations that favor prolonged breast-feeding.

Thus, it stands to reason that in settings where breast-feeding must be the practice for socioeconomic reasons, antiretroviral prophylaxis for infants for the duration of breast-feeding may be the logical approach. However we need to learn more about the potential toxic effect of prolonged antiviral prophylaxis at such a young age on the developing infant.

J. A. Stockman III, MD

Effects of Early, Abrupt Weaning on HIV-free Survival of Children in Zambia
Kuhn L, for the Zambia Exclusive Breastfeeding Study (Columbia Univ, NY; et al)
N Engl J Med 359:130-141, 2008

Background.—In low-resource settings, many programs recommend that women who are infected with the human immunodeficiency virus (HIV) stop breast-feeding early. We conducted a randomized trial to evaluate whether abrupt weaning at 4 months as compared with the standard practice has a net benefit for HIV-free survival of children.

Methods.—We enrolled 958 HIV-infected women and their infants in Lusaka, Zambia. All the women planned to breast-feed exclusively to 4 months; 481 were randomly assigned to a counseling program that encouraged abrupt weaning at 4 months, and 477 to a program that encouraged continued breast-feeding for as long as the women chose. The primary outcome was either HIV infection or death of the child by 24 months.

Results.—In the intervention group, 69.0% of the mothers stopped breast-feeding at 5 months or earlier; 68.8% of these women reported the completion of weaning in less than 2 days. In the control group, the median duration of breast-feeding was 16 months. In the overall cohort, there was no significant difference between the groups in the rate of HIV-free survival among the children; 68.4% and 64.0% survived to 24 months without HIV infection in the intervention and control groups, respectively ($P = 0.13$). Among infants who were still being breast-fed and were not infected with HIV at 4 months, there was no significant difference between the groups in HIV-free survival at 24 months (83.9% and 80.7% in the intervention and control groups, respectively; $P = 0.27$). Children who were infected with HIV by 4 months had a higher mortality by 24 months if they had been assigned to the intervention group than if they had been assigned to the control group (73.6% vs. 54.8%, $P = 0.007$).

Conclusions.—Early, abrupt cessation of breast-feeding by HIV-infected women in a low-resource setting, such as Lusaka, Zambia, does not improve the rate of HIV-free survival among children born to HIV-infected mothers and is harmful to HIV-infected infants. (ClinicalTrials.gov number, NCT00310726.)

▶ The report of Kumwenda et al documents that babies who must be breast-fed for long periods of time and whose mothers have HIV infection most likely will need to be treated with antiviral prophylaxis during the entire period of breast-feeding.[1] An alternative, if possible, is to abruptly cease breast-feeding as soon as reasonably possible to potentially lessen the transmission of HIV from breast milk. Kuhn et al report the results of a randomized trial looking at HIV-infected women in Zambia to evaluate whether exclusive breast-feeding to 4 months of age, followed by an abrupt weaning, would reduce postnatal transmission of HIV and mortality in the first 2 years of life. Four months was selected as the weaning time because this was the minimal duration of exclusive breast-feeding that was recommended at the time the study was designed and was considered to be a reasonable period for exclusive breast-feeding to be maintained. The study found no significant difference in HIV-survival at 24 months between children whose mothers were randomly assigned to a 2-month counseling program that encouraged abrupt weaning at 4 months and those whose mothers were encouraged to continue breast-feeding for a duration of their own choice (a median of 16 months). Among children who were infected with HIV by 4 months of age, being assigned to abrupt weaning significantly increased their risk of death. The authors conclude that early abrupt cessation of breast-feeding by HIV-infected women in a low-resource setting is unwarranted for children who are exposed to HIV, but who are uninfected, and is harmful for infants who are known to be infected with HIV.

It is estimated that about half a million new HIV infections occur each year in children and that 40% of these are the result of transmission of the virus through a mother's breast milk, with the remainder occurring during pregnancy. In resource-constrained environments, it is important to promote breast-feeding, which is known to increase survivorship related to infectious diarrheal diseases. In resource-constrained settings, current policies with respect to breast-feeding by mothers who are infected with HIV are guided by observational evidence that exclusive breast feeding for the first 4 to 6 months of life reduces the risk of transmission of HIV as compared with mixed breast-feeding (ie, feeding both breast milk and formula) and may have survival benefits at 18 to 24 months that are similar to those for exclusive breast feeding. Although peripartum prophylaxis with a single dose or a short course of antiretroviral agents effectively reduces intrapartum HIV transmission, its effect does not extend much beyond 4 to 6 weeks in breast-feeding populations. From the data of Kuhn et al, it would seem that early, abrupt cessation of breast-feeding for HIV-infected women in low resource settings should be avoided. The benefit of diminishing the time exposure to HIV for uninfected babies is offset by the consequences of no longer having the benefits of being breast-fed.

J. A. Stockman III, MD

Reference

1. Kumwenda NI, Hoover DR, Mofenson LM, et al. Extended antiretroviral prophylaxis to reduce breast-milk HIV-1 transmission. *N Engl J Med*. 2008;359:119-129.

Circumcision Status and Risk of HIV and Sexually Transmitted Infections Among Men Who Have Sex With Men: A Meta-analysis

Millett GA, Flores SA, Marks G, et al (Ctrs for Disease Control and Prevention, Atlanta, GA)
JAMA 300:1674-1684, 2008

Context.—Randomized controlled trials and meta-analyses have demonstrated that male circumcision reduces men's risk of contracting human immunodeficiency virus (HIV) infection during heterosexual intercourse. Less is known about whether male circumcision provides protection against HIV infection among men who have sex with men (MSM).

Objectives.—To quantitatively summarize the strength of the association between male circumcision and HIV infection and other sexually transmitted infections (STIs) across observational studies of MSM.

Data Sources.—Comprehensive search of databases, including MEDLINE, EMBASE, ERIC, Sociofile, PsycINFO, Web of Science, and Google Scholar, and correspondence with researchers, to find published articles, conference proceedings, and unpublished reports through February 2008.

Study Selection.—Of 18 studies that quantitatively examined the association between male circumcision and HIV/STI among MSM, 15 (83%) met the selection criteria for the meta-analysis.

Data Extraction.—Independent abstraction was conducted by pairs of reviewers using a standardized abstraction form. Study quality was assessed using the Newcastle-Ottawa Scale.

Data Synthesis.—A total of 53 567 MSM participants (52% circumcised) were included in the meta-analysis. The odds of being HIV-positive were nonsignificantly lower among MSM who were circumcised than uncircumcised (odds ratio, 0.86; 95% confidence interval, 0.65-1.13; number of independent effect sizes [k] = 15). Higher study quality was associated with a reduced odds of HIV infection among circumcised MSM (β, -0.415; $P = .01$). Among MSM who primarily engaged in insertive anal sex, the association between male circumcision and HIV was protective but not statistically significant (odds ratio, 0.71; 95% confidence interval, 0.23-2.22; $k = 4$). Male circumcision had a protective association with HIV in studies of MSM conducted before the introduction of highly active antiretroviral therapy (odds ratio, 0.47; 95% confidence interval, 0.32-0.69; $k = 3$). Neither the association between male circumcision and other STIs (odds ratio, 1.02; 95% confidence interval, 0.83-1.26; $k = 8$), nor its relationship with study quality was statistically significant (β, 0.265; $P = .47$).

Conclusions.—Pooled analyses of available observational studies of MSM revealed insufficient evidence that male circumcision protects against HIV infection or other STIs. However, the comparable protective effect of male circumcision in MSM studies conducted before the era of highly active antiretroviral therapy, as in the recent male circumcision trials of heterosexual African men, supports further investigation of male circumcision for HIV prevention among MSM.

▶ Arguments for and against male circumcision have raged for years. Clearly the pendulum has swung toward circumcision when it comes to the reduction and risk of sexually transmitted infections including HIV, at least among men who have sex with women. A number of studies, mostly conducted in Africa, have illustrated that male circumcision does reduce the likelihood of female-to-male transmission of HIV infection by as much as 60%. Other studies have documented protection against acquisition of other sexually transmitted infections such as syphilis, chlamydial infection, and genital ulcer disease. Still outstanding is the question of whether circumcision might protect men who have sex with men against HIV infection, the purpose of this report, which is a comprehensive search of many databases that have looked at this subject. The biological plausibility of HIV protection resulting from male circumcision has been supported by immunohistological and histopathological studies indicating the susceptibility of the inner foreskin for virus-target cell contact.

Millett et al report the results of a meta-analysis evaluating the evidence for male circumcision in reducing risk of HIV and other sexually transmitted infections in a group of men who were not well represented in 3 African clinical trials of heterosexual men, that is, men who have sex with men. The bottom line is that the analyses of available studies of men who have sex with men reveal insufficient evidence that male circumcision does in fact protect against HIV infection or other sexually transmitted diseases. In many respects, this is not at all surprising. Men who have sex with men practice receptive anal sex, a circumstance in which that male's circumcision status is largely irrelevant. Also, in the United States, men have high circumcision rates already and no one has shown that this circumcision status in any way diminishes the seroprevalence rates of HIV infection in men who have sex with men in comparison with other parts of the world where circumcision rates are much lower.

The meta-analysis by Millett et al is likely to be used by both advocates and detractors of clinical trial investment. Some will argue the benefit is likely to be too modest to justify a multimillion-dollar clinical trial, while others will argue that further trials are necessary to be absolutely sure that circumcision is not of some benefit.

Circumcisions do occur more often than not on our watch as pediatricians, and the data from these adult studies should influence, at least to some small extent, decisions about infant circumcision. Infant and adult circumcision is clearly recommended in regions with high HIV prevalence such as sub-Saharan Africa. The question, however, as to whether men who have sex with men should be circumcised to reduce their HIV risk largely remains an outstanding issue and one very worthy of further investigation.

As this commentary closes, another *Clinical Fact/Curio*, this having to do with another infectious disease transmission. Would you believe there is a correlation between the recent mortgage crisis and West Nile virus!? In 2007 and into 2008, there was a tripling of cases of West Nile virus infection in Bakersfield, California, corresponding to a 300% increase in mortgage delinquency. Some .

smart investigator in the public health department there recognized that those with delinquent mortgages rarely took care of their swimming pools, allowing swarms of mosquitoes carrying the West Nile virus to overpopulate. The public health department got smart later in 2008 and sprayed all abandoned pools periodically. This essentially eliminated the problem![1]

J. A. Stockman III, MD

Reference

1. The mortgage crisis and West Nile virus [editorial comment]. *Pediatr Infect Dis.* January, 2009;3.

Extensively Drug-Resistant Tuberculosis in the United States, 1993-2007
Shah NS, Pratt R, Armstrong L, et al (Ctrs for Disease Control and Prevention, Atlanta, GA)
JAMA 300:2153-2160, 2008

Context.—Worldwide emergence of extensively drug-resistant tuberculosis (XDR-TB) has raised global public health concern, given the limited therapy options and high mortality.

Objectives.—To describe the epidemiology of XDR-TB in the United States and to identify unique characteristics of XDR-TB cases compared with multidrug-resistant TB (MDRTB) and drug-susceptible TB cases.

Design, Setting, and Patients.—Descriptive analysis of US TB cases reported from 1993 to 2007. Extensively drug-resistant TB was defined as resistance to isoniazid, a rifamycin, a fluoroquinolone, and at least 1 of amikacin, kanamycin, or capreomycin based on drug susceptibility test results from initial and follow-up specimens.

Main Outcome Measures.—Extensively drug-resistant TB case counts and trends, risk factors for XDR-TB, and overall survival.

Results.—A total of 83 cases of XDR-TB were reported in the United States from 1993to 2007. The number of XDR-TB cases declined from 18 (0.07% of 25 107 TB cases) in 1993 to 2 (0.02% of 13 293 TB cases) in 2007, reported to date. Among those with known human immunodeficiency virus (HIV) test results, 31 (53%) were HIV-positive. Compared with MDR-TB cases, XDR-TB cases were more likely to have disseminated TB disease (prevalence ratio [PR], 2.06; 95% confidence interval [CI], 1.19-3.58), less likely to convert to a negative sputum culture (PR, 0.55; 95% CI, 0.33- 0.94), and had a prolonged infectious period (median time to culture conversion, 183 days vs 93 days for MDR-TB; $P < .001$). Twenty-six XDR-TB cases (35%) died during treatment, of whom 21 (81%) were known to be HIV-infected. Mortality was higher among XDR-TB cases than among MDR-TB cases (PR, 1.82; 95% CI, 1.10-3.02) and drug-susceptible TB cases (PR, 6.10; 95% CI, 3.65-10.20).

Conclusion.—Although the number of US XDR-TB cases has declined since 1993, coinciding with improved TB and HIV/AIDS control, cases continue to be reported each year.

▶ While not exactly true in the United States, tuberculosis remains the leading cause of infectious disease-related death among adults worldwide. Complicating this fact is that drug-resistant tuberculosis has emerged as an expanding threat throughout the world, including in the United States in recent years. Multidrug-resistant tuberculosis (MDR-TB) not only represents a threat to survivorship, it is 100 times as costly to treat as drug-susceptible TB. Treatment successes in those with MDR-TB range only from 40% to 80%, much lower than the 85% to 99% cure rates achievable for drug-susceptible TB. The report of Shah et al outlines the nature of MDR-TB in the United States. The report is important to pediatric practitioners because the data from this report include individuals of all ages. The report provides detailed information on those 0 to 14 years as well as those 15 to 24 years of age.

It is clear throughout the world that greater and greater drug resistance has occurred in those with tuberculosis. In 2005, a global survey of reference laboratories defined a new TB disease category termed "extensively drug-resistant TB" (XDR-TB), and also determined that XDR-TB cases had emerged in every region of the world.[1] This problem was even more serious in terms of excess morbidity and mortality in those who are HIV-infected.

The report of Shah et al describes the epidemiology of XDR-TB in the United States and identifies the unique characteristics of those with this form of infection, compared with MDR-TB and drug-susceptible TB cases. The data from this report enable us to think about earlier diagnosis, implementation for appropriate infection control measures, and initiation of early, aggressive treatment to improve clinical outcomes and to curb transmission of this increasingly problematic variety of TB. The report does give us the first comprehensive assessment of the burden of XDR-TB in the United States based on surveillance data going back a decade and a half. From 1993 through 2007, there have been 83 cases of XDR-TB, accounting for 0.04% of all culture-confirmed TB cases. The outcomes for these cases compared with MDR-TB and drug susceptible TB cases were much poorer. Death rates were nearly 2 times greater than among MDR-TB cases and more than 6 times greater than among drug-susceptible TB cases. Infection with HIV plays an important role in both the occurrence and outcomes of XDR-TB cases consistent with prior reports. HIV-infected patients not only have a higher death rate, but also account for most but not all XDR-TB deaths.

This report also provides us with some other new insights about XDR-TB. XDR-TB cases are more likely to be infectious, with three-quarters of cases having positive sputum smear results for acid-fast bacilli. In addition, the higher prevalence of disseminated disease among XDR-TB cases may indicate delays in diagnosis, longer duration of disease, greater virulence of XDR-TB strains, and a more immunocompromised state, not just limited to those with HIV infection.

No physician likes to face the reality that some patients under their care cannot be cured. While TB was once a quite curable disease, there are now among us those with TB who may actually be declared to be incurable given the level of drug resistance they may possess. The management of tuberculosis in both children and adults is a very sophisticated process, one that is probably well beyond the competency of most of us. Thank goodness for our colleagues in pediatric infectious disease with whom we can hold hands in the eradication of this infection.

J. A. Stockman III, MD

Reference

1. Shah NS, Wright A, Bai GH, et al. Worldwide emergence of extensively drug-resistant tuberculosis. *Emerg Infect Dis.* 2007;13:380-387.

Latent Tuberculosis Diagnosis in Children by Using the QuantiFERON-TB Gold In-Tube Test

Lighter J, Rigaud M, Eduardo R, et al (New York Univ School of Medicine)
Pediatrics 123:30-37, 2009

Background.—The QuantiFERON-TB Gold test was the first blood test to be approved for the diagnosis of latent tuberculosis infection. Although it has been shown to be sensitive and specific in adults, limited data on its performance in children are available.

Methods.—This was a prospective study of children receiving health care in New York, New York. Each child was assessed for risk factors for *Mycobacterium tuberculosis* infection, underwent tuberculin skin testing, and had a QuantiFERON-TB Gold In-Tube test performed. The concordance between tuberculin skin test and QuantiFERON-TB Gold In-Tube test results was calculated, and the results were analyzed according to the likelihood of exposure to *M tuberculosis*.

Results.—Data for 207 children with valid tuberculin skin test and QuantiFERON-TB Gold In-Tube test results were analyzed. There was excellent correlation between negative tuberculin skin test results and negative QuantiFERON-TB Gold In-Tube test results; however, only 23% of children with positive tuberculin skin test results had positive QuantiFERON-TB Gold In-Tube test results. Positive QuantiFERON-TB Gold In-Tube test results were associated with increased likelihood of *M tuberculosis* exposure, and interferon γ levels were higher in children with known recent exposure to *M tuberculosis*, compared with children with older exposure histories. Younger children produced lower interferon γ levels in response to the mitogen (phytohemagglutinin) control used in the QuantiFERON-TB Gold In-Tube test, but indeterminant results were low for children of all ages. Performance characteristics were similar across all age groups.

Conclusion.—The QuantiFERON-TB Gold In-Tube test is a specific test for *M tuberculosis* exposure in children, with performance characteristics similar to those for adults residing in regions with low levels of endemic disease. Concerns about test sensitivity, especially for children <2 years of age, will require additional prospective long-term evaluation.

▶ This article reminds us how common tuberculosis remains. *Mycobacterium tuberculosis* is estimated to infect one-third of the world's population at any one point in time. A good bit of this infection exists as what we now call latent tuberculosis infection (LTBI). To decrease the incidence of active tuberculosis, we need better and better tools to detect LTBI. For more than a century, the methodology used to do this has been the tuberculin skin test, a test that is neither particularly sensitive nor specific. False-positive rates with the tuberculin skin test are well known to us and largely occur because of cross-reactivity to environmental mycobacteria and the BCG vaccination, which is given in many parts of the world. The result is that many children who do not have *M tuberculosis* infection are overtreated for it. Another problem with the tuberculin skin test, of course, is the need to have 2 encounters with the patient. All too often patients do not return to have the skin test read. For these reasons, a good deal of effort has been expended on the development of new techniques for diagnosing LTBI in both adults and children. The most widely studied technique to date involves the detection of interferon gamma released by T-cells after in vitro exposure to antigens from *M tuberculosis*.

In 2005, the United States Food and Drug Administration approved the QuantiFERON-TB Gold assay and the Centers for Disease Control and Prevention recommended its usage for diagnosing LTBI in "all circumstances in which the tuberculin skin test (TST) is currently used" including testing of children, with the caveat that the sensitivity for young children had not yet been determined. The CDC also said that treatment decisions could be entertained solely on the results of the assay results. Despite these recommendations, as of this writing the American Academy of Pediatrics has withheld recommending the use of the QuantiFERON assay until more data from children had become available, thus the importance of this report from the New York City Department of Health and Mental Hygiene, which has been using only the QuantiFERON-TB gold test for the diagnosis of latent tuberculosis in adults and children.

Because there is no gold standard method to determine LTBI, the applicability of any new test for LTBI can only be based on its assessing the likelihood of *M tuberculosis* exposure and correlating it with the TST. The data from New York City do show that the QuantiFERON-TB Gold test is more specific than the TST. The strongest concordance between the TST and the QuantiFERON-TB Gold test was found in children with a skin test result of 15 mm of induration in those who had not received BCG vaccination. Another finding from this report was that 77% of children with a positive skin test turned out to have a negative QuantiFERON-TB Gold test. The authors of this report did not feel that this was because of a lower sensitivity of the newer test, rather a lack of specificity of the tuberculin skin test. Also, discordant QuantiFERON-TB Gold test-positive/tuberculin skin test-negative results were much less common, occurring in only 4 children out of many tested in New York City. One of those children had active tuberculosis and the other 3 children had moderate risk factors for *M tuberculosis* exposure. The study did show that the assay cutoff value for the QuantiFERON-TB Gold test might need to be lowered for the younger children who do not seem to produce quite the same level of production of interferon gamma. Establishing better cutoffs and increasing the assay incubation time for children may significantly improve the sensitivity of the new test in the identification of children exposed to *Mycobacterium tuberculosis*.

So what is the bottom line from the New York City experience? If the QuantiFERON-TB Gold test were to be used as the diagnostic test for latent tuberculosis in children and treatment decisions were based on its results alone, as is now the case for adults, and also the practice for children in some health departments, including that in New York City, many fewer children would require isoniazid prophylaxis. On the basis of the results of this study, up to three-fourths of children with positive TST would not have required treatment. The bottom line is that the new test is highly specific, easy to perform, and requires only 1 visit. It may ultimately be the recommended way to go for all children who are being screened for latent tuberculosis. It will be interesting to see how our Academy recommendations reflect the findings observed in New York City.

It would be worthwhile reading an article by Nicol that looked at another type of interferon gamma release assay for the diagnosis of active and latent tuberculosis infection in children.[1] In this report, children with a history of exposure to tuberculosis and children presenting to a local clinic or hospital with symptoms suggesting tuberculosis were tested with the T-SPOT.TB assay. It was observed that for young children presenting in this way, the T-SPOT.TB cannot be used to exclude active disease. The sensitivity of this assay seems to be impaired for very young children.

J. A. Stockman III, MD

Reference

1. Nicol MP, Davies M-A, Wood K, et al. Comparison of T-spot TB assay and tuberculin skin test for the evaluation of young children at high risk for tuberculosis in a community setting. *Pediatrics.* 2009;123:38-43.

Effect of Pneumococcal Conjugate Vaccine on Pneumococcal Meningitis
Hsu HE, Shutt KA, Moore MR, et al (Univ of Pittsburgh, PA; Natl Ctr for Immunization and Respiratory Diseases, Ctrs for Disease Control and Prevention, Atlanta, GA; et al)
N Engl J Med 360:244-256, 2009

Background.—Invasive pneumococcal disease declined among children and adults after the introduction of the pediatric heptavalent pneumococcal conjugate vaccine (PCV7) in 2000, but its effect on pneumococcal meningitis is unclear.

Methods.—We examined trends in pneumococcal meningitis from 1998 through 2005 using active, population-based surveillance data from eight sites in the United States. Isolates were grouped into PCV7 serotypes (4, 6B, 9V, 14, 18C, 19F, and 23F), PCV7-related serotypes (6A, 9A, 9L, 9N, 18A, 18B, 18F, 19B, 19C, 23A, and 23B), and non-PCV7 serotypes (all others). Changes in the incidence of pneumococcal meningitis were assessed against baseline values from 1998–1999.

Results.—We identified 1379 cases of pneumococcal meningitis. The incidence declined from 1.13 cases to 0.79 case per 100,000 persons between 1998–1999 and 2004–2005 (a 30.1% decline, P<0.001). Among persons younger than 2 years of age and those 65 years of age or older, the incidence decreased during the study period by 64.0% and 54.0%, respectively (P<0.001 for both groups). Rates of PCV7-serotype meningitis declined from 0.66 case to 0.18 case (a 73.3% decline, P<0.001) among patients of all ages. Although rates of PCV7-related–serotype disease decreased by 32.1% (P = 0.08), rates of non-PCV7–serotype disease increased from 0.32 to 0.51 (an increase of 60.5%, P<0.001). The percentages of cases from non-PCV7 serotypes 19A, 22F, and 35B each increased significantly during the study period. On average, 27.8% of isolates were nonsusceptible to penicillin, but fewer isolates were nonsusceptible to chloramphenicol (5.7%), meropenem (16.6%), and cefotaxime (11.8%). The proportion of penicillin-nonsusceptible isolates decreased between 1998 and 2003 (from 32.0% to 19.4%, P = 0.01) but increased between 2003 and 2005 (from 19.4% to 30.1%, P = 0.03).

Conclusions.—Rates of pneumococcal meningitis have decreased among children and adults since PCV7 was introduced. Although the overall effect of the vaccine remains substantial, a recent increase in meningitis caused by non-PCV7 serotypes, including strains non-susceptible to antibiotics, is a concern.

▶ The pediatric heptavalent pneumococcal conjugate vaccine (PCV7; Prevnar, Wyeth) has had a major effect on the incidence of pneumococcal disease in the United States. Licensed in 2000, PCV7 is recommended by the Advisory Committee on Immunization Practices for all children 2 to 23 months of age and for children 24 to 59 months of age who are at increased risk for pneumococcal disease. In 2000, coverage by PCV7 among children 19 to 35 months of age was estimated to exceed 68% for the full vaccine series of 4 or more doses and to exceed 87% with 3 or more doses. PCV7 not only protects immunized children from pneumococcal disease, but also provides protection to nonimmunized children and adults through herd immunity, resulting from reduced transmission of *Streptococcus pneumoniae* from immunized children.

The potential unwanted effect of decreasing vaccine serotypes in circulation is the emergence of non-PCV7 pneumococcal serotypes. The absence of substantial increases in the rates of non-PCV7-serotype invasive disease, despite increased nasopharyngeal colonization with non-PCV7 serotypes, is presumably because of reduced invasive potential of most non-PCV7 serotypes. Non-PCV7 serotypes can result in invasive disease in immunocompromised individuals such as has been noted with HIV-infected patients.

The report of Hsu et al tells us about current trends in pneumococcal meningitis among children and adults for the period 1998 through 2005. Overall, rates of pneumococcal meningitis in the population at large declined by slightly over 30% between the 1998–1999 baseline period and 2004–2005, from 1.1 cases to 0.79 case per 100 000 persons. Among patients younger than 2 years of age, however, rates of meningitis decreased by some 64%. Similar rates of decrease were seen in those over 65 years of age. Much more modest declines were noted in the age group 18 to 39 years. In children younger than 2 years of age, there was a very modest increase in the frequency of non-PCV7 serotypes causing meningitis.

The data from this report provide extraordinarily strong evidence of the benefit of PCV7 in reducing the rate of pneumococcal meningitis, including cases caused by strains nonsusceptible to commonly used antimicrobial agents. These decreases reflect the direct effect of the vaccine and herd effect. Despite these successes, all of us know that there has been an increase in strains non-susceptible to antibiotics in recent years. To achieve better effects in the future, we will need to develop more broadly protective vaccines that go beyond the 7 serotypes we are currently using. We also must remind ourselves that pneumococcal meningitis is still a problem despite the presence of the PCV7 vaccine. One in 12 children developing pneumococcal meningitis will die as a result of this infection.

This commentary closes with an infectious disease *Clinical Fact/Curio*. Many naively suppose that Lyme disease, first reported out of Lyme, Connecticut, most likely started somewhere in the New England area of the United States. A genetic study has now examined the evolutionary history of *Borrelia burgdorferi* by sequencing 8 of its "housekeeping" genes. Analysis of 64 samples of bacterial DNA taken from infected individuals in Europe and the United States points to Europe as the mostly likely source of the evolution of this bacterium. What is surprising is that *B. burgdorferi* is likely to have reached the United States before humans did.[1]

J. A. Stockman III, MD

Reference

1. Margo G, Gatewood AG, Aanensen DM, et al. MLST of housekeeping genes captures geographic population structure and suggests a European origin of *Borrelia burgdorferi*. *Proc Natl Acad Sci U S A*. 2008;105:8730-8735.

Performance of a Rapid Antigen-Detection Test and Throat Culture in Community Pediatric Offices: Implications for Management of Pharyngitis

Tanz RR, Gerber MA, Kabat W, et al (Children's Memorial Hosp and Northwestern Univ Feinberg School of Medicine, Chicago, IL; Univ of Cincinnati College of Medicine, OH; Children's Memorial Hosp, Chicago, IL; et al)

Pediatrics 123:437-444, 2009

Objectives.—The goals were to establish performance characteristics of a rapid antigen-detection test and blood agar plate culture performed and interpreted in community pediatric offices and to assess the effect of the pretest likelihood of group A streptococcus pharyngitis on test performance (spectrum bias).

Methods.—Two throat swabs were collected from 1848 children 3 to 18 years of age who were evaluated for acute pharyngitis between November 15, 2004, and May 15, 2005, in 6 community pediatric offices. One swab was used to perform the rapid antigen-detection test and a blood agar plate culture in the office and the other was sent to our laboratory for blood agar plate culture. Clinical findings were used to calculate the McIsaac score for each patient. The sensitivities of the office tests were calculated, with the hospital laboratory culture results as the criterion standard.

Results.—Thirty percent of laboratory blood agar plate cultures yielded group A streptococcus (range among sites: 21%–36%). Rapid antigen-detection test sensitivity was 70% (range: 61%–80%). Office culture sensitivity was significantly greater, 81% (range: 71%–91%). Rapid antigen-detection test specificity was 98% (range: 98%–99.5%), and office culture specificity was 97% (range: 94%–99%), a difference that was not statistically significant. The sensitivity of a combined approach using the rapid antigen-detection test and back-up office culture was 85%. Among patients with McIsaac scores of >2, rapid antigen-detection test sensitivity was 78%, office culture sensitivity was 87%, and combined approach sensitivity was 91%. Positive diagnostic test results were significantly associated with McIsaac scores of >2.

Conclusions.—The sensitivity of the office culture was significantly greater than the sensitivity of the rapid antigen-detection test, but neither test was highly sensitive. The sensitivities of each diagnostic modality and the recommended combined approach were best among patients with greater pretest likelihood of group A streptococcus pharyngitis.

▶ The pediatrician has, in general, 2 options for the diagnosis of a group A streptococcal pharyngitis. One is to do a throat culture on a blood agar plate (BAP). The other option is one of the available rapid antigen-detection tests (RADTs). The latter have been around now for almost 20 years. Compared with BAP cultures, however, the specificity of these RADTs is considered to be excellent (at least 90%-95%), but the sensitivity is a bit lower (often 75%-85%). For this reason, the current recommendation emanating from the Infectious Diseases Society of America, the American Heart Association, and the

American Academy of Pediatrics is that if the RADT is negative, one should do a BAP. If the RADT is positive, one can feel confident that one has appropriately made a diagnosis of a group A streptococcal infection.

The study emanating from Chicago was designed to tell us the performance characteristics of RADTs and BAPs performed and interpreted in community pediatric offices. The study confirmed that the sensitivity of the office BAP culture was significantly greater than sensitivity of the RADT when the 2 tests were compared with a simultaneously collected swab that was plated and processed in the hospital laboratory. Both office-based tests perform better among patients with symptoms characteristic of acute streptococcal pharyngitis. Spectrum bias of RADTs has been noted previously. Based on the information from this report, pretest likelihood of group A streptococcal pharyngitis should now be added to the list of factors that affect office BAP culture sensitivity. If the diagnostic goal is to maximize identification of patients infected with this organism, then the data from this report indicate that negative office test results, including throat culture results, should be confirmed with BAP cultures processed in a hospital or commercial laboratory. While this theoretically sounds appropriate, given the logistics and cost implications it is reasonable not to follow this recommendation.

The currently recommended diagnostic approach to detect group A streptococcal pharyngitis is intended to identify patients as accurately as possible so that they can be treated with antibiotics. The philosophy has been driven for more than half a century by the desire to prevent acute rheumatic fever. Surveys of clinicians show that 95% signify this as the most important reason to identify and treat children as opposed to a lower percentage of pediatricians indicating that this approach should be used to prevent suppurative complications, for symptom relief, or for reduction of contagiousness. It should be recognized, however, that rates of acute rheumatic fever, suppurative complications of group A streptococcal pharyngitis, and invasive disease are quite low in the United States, and the significant decrease in the prevalence of acute rheumatic fever within our boarders began before effective antibiotics were available.

The RADT, office BAP culture, and office BAP culture confirmation of negative RADT results all exhibit spectrum bias supporting the selective testing of patients with pharyngitis. Specifically, the yields become much better when patients who are quite unlikely to have group A streptococcal pharyngitis are excluded from having cultures. In other words, in a viral season think twice about the need for looking for group A streptococcal pharyngitis. If you are not familiar with the term "spectrum effect" or "spectrum bias," this phenomenon occurs when test performance is affected by variations in disease presentation or population subgroups. For example, tests may have low sensitivity for young children and much higher sensitivity for teenagers (eg, heterophile test for infectious mononucleosis), or sensitivity may vary according to the course of a disease (eg, chest x-rays early or later in the course of pneumonia). In the case of pharyngitis, RADT results may be affected by clinical disease severity or presentation.

This commentary closes with a *Clinical Fact/Curio* about wearing a mask to prevent the spread of infection, this by an operating surgeon. Sneezing and the efficacy of mask wearing while operating has been a matter of some debate.

Standard teaching dictates that while operating with a face mask on, one must face the wound when sneezing, so that droplets escape backwards via the sides of the mask. The hypothesis behind this had never been studied until a recent report appeared. In a carefully constructed study, a surgeon wearing a surgical mask was encouraged to sneeze by inhaling finely ground pepper. A small reservoir of water was held in the floor of the mouth to improve the appearance of the droplets on photographs that were taken during the episode of sneezing. Photographs were taken from the back of the surgeon as well as from the side. All photographs were taken by highly skilled medical photographers in a dark room with a dark background using a quick flash gun that was strobed. It was clear from the photographs that very little if any spray droplets escaped from the sides of the mask. What did escape fell inferiorly from the mask onto the surgeon's upper chest. None of the photographs showed substantial numbers of droplets passing behind the head of the operating surgeon.

The doctrine of facing the wound when sneezing seems logical. The study, however, does not necessarily support this hypothesis. Few, if any, droplets of spray escaped sideways and none passed behind the surgeon's head. The photographs showed only that the most important visible escape of spray comes from below the mask onto a surgeon's chest. Therefore, theoretically, a surgeon can sneeze in any direction he or she wishes following their native instincts when sneezing during operations.[1]

J. A. Stockman III, MD

Reference

1. Granville-Chapman J, Dunne RL. Mixed messages: excuse me! *BMJ.* 2007;335: 1293.

Streptococcal Infection and Exacerbations of Childhood Tics and Obsessive-Compulsive Symptoms: A Prospective Blinded Cohort Study
Kurlan R, the Tourette Syndrome Study Group (Univ of Rochester School of Medicine, NY; et al)
Pediatrics 121:1188-1197, 2008

Objective.—If pediatric autoimmune neuropsychiatric disorders associated with streptococcal infections is a unique clinical entity, we hypothesized that children meeting diagnostic criteria would have more clinical exacerbations temporally linked to bona fide group A β-hemolytic streptococcus infection than matched control subjects (chronic tic and/or obsessive-compulsive disorder with no known temporal relationship to group A β-hemolytic streptococcus infection).

Patients and Methods.—Subjects included 40 matched pediatric autoimmune neuropsychiatric disorders associated with streptococcal infections case-control pairs who were prospectively evaluated with intensive laboratory testing for group A β-hemolytic streptococcus and clinical measures for an average of 2 years. Additional testing occurred at the time of any clinical exacerbations or illness. Laboratory personnel were blinded to case or control status and clinical (exacerbation or not) condition. Clinical raters were blinded to the results of laboratory tests.

Results.—The cases had a higher clinical exacerbation rate and a higher bona fide group A β-hemolytic streptococcus infection rate than the control group. Only 5 of 64 exacerbations were temporally associated (within 4 weeks) with a group A β-hemolytic streptococcus infection, and all occurred in cases. The number (5.0) was significantly higher than the number that would be expected by chance alone (1.6). Yet, ≥75% of the clinical exacerbations in cases had no observable temporal relationship to group A β-hemolytic streptococcus infection.

Conclusions.—Patients who fit published criteria for pediatric autoimmune neuropsy-chiatric disorders associated with streptococcal infections seem to represent a subgroup of those with chronic tic disorders and obsessive-compulsive disorder who may be vulnerable to group A β-hemolytic streptococcus infection as a precipitant of neuropsychiatric symptom exacerbations. Group A β-hemolytic streptococcus infection is not the only or even the most common antecedent event associated with exacerbations for these patients. Additional intensive studies are needed to determine whether there is clinical or scientific evidence to support separating out subgroups of tic disorder and/or obsessive-compulsive disorder patients based on specific symptom precipitants.

▶ By now everyone has heard about PANDAS, the abbreviation for Pediatric Autoimmune Neuropsychiatric Disorders Associated with Streptococcal infections. PANDAS are characterized by recurrent, acute fulminate tics and/or obsessive compulsive behaviors that are temporarily associated with a streptococcal infection. The disorder is proposed to be an autoimmune entity similar in pathophysiology to Sydenham chorea. It is hypothesized that tics and obsessive-compulsive symptomatology result from group A beta-hemolytic streptococcal activation of the immune system, either by the induction of antibodies that cross react against neuronal tissue (molecular mimicry) or by the production of proteins that mediate and regulate immunity and inflammation (cytokines and chemokines).

It is now 12 years since the first description of PANDAS. In the interim, support for the PANDAS hypothesis has come from studies reporting the presence of circulating antineuronal antibodies and from an increased prevalence of a B-cell surface marker, which has been reported to be associated with the onset of rheumatic fever in patients who previously had a streptococcal infection. Anyone who has followed the PANDAS story knows how controversial it has been, particularly given the absence of accurate and intensive prospective data confirming a temporal relationship between antecedent group A beta-hemolytic streptococcal infection and the onset or exacerbation of clinical manifestations. Given the frequency of such infections in children, many have questioned whether chance alone is the basis for the purported relationship with the neurologic findings.

Kurlan et al undertook an interesting study to address some of the outstanding issues with PANDAS. To accurately determine whether there is a specific temporal relation between bona fide antecedent group A beta hemolytic streptococcal infection and exacerbations of symptoms in children meeting published diagnostic criteria for PANDAS, a study was conducted involving an intensive, blinded clinical and laboratory prospective cohort study that included non-PANDAS control subjects. The theory was that if PANDAS were a unique clinical entity, then children meeting the diagnostic criteria would have more clinical exacerbations temporally linked to antecedent infections than control subjects without PANDAS. The data showed that PANDAS cases did have a higher clinical exacerbation rate in association with a higher bona fide group A beta hemolytic *streptococcus* infection in comparison with the control group. When one looked carefully at the data, however, only 5 of 64 exacerbations were temporally associated within a 4-week period with a group A beta hemolytic *streptococcus* infection. The 5 cases, nonetheless, were statistically higher than the number that would have been expected by chance alone, yet more than 75% of clinical exacerbations in PANDAS cases had no observable temporal relationship to group A beta hemolytic *streptococcus* infection.

One can interpret these data to indicate that children with PANDAS may represent a subgroup of patients with tics or obsessive-compulsive disorder who may be susceptible to group A beta hemolytic *streptococcus* infection as a precipitant of their symptoms. Further research on disease mechanisms and therapy are needed to determine for sure what these relationships are. Given the greater likelihood of a family history of rheumatic fever in subjects with PANDAS, there is a suggestion that the disorder may have a genetic vulnerability to streptococcal infection in general or infection with certain strains of *streptococcus* that might induce autoimmunity.

J. A. Stockman III, MD

Impact of rapid screening tests on acquisition of meticillin resistant *Staphylococcus aureus*: cluster randomised crossover trial

Jeyaratnam D, Whitty CJM, Phillips K, et al (Guys and St. Thomas' NHS Foundation Trust, London; London School of Hygiene and Tropical Med; et al)
BMJ 336:927-930, 2008

Objective.—To determine whether introducing a rapid test for meticillin resistant *Staphylococcus aureus* (MRSA) screening leads to a reduction in MRSA acquisition on hospital general wards.

Design.—Cluster randomised crossover trial.

Setting.—Medical, surgical, elderly care, and oncology wards of a London teaching hospital on two sites.

Main Outcome Measure.—MRSA acquisition rate (proportion of patients negative for MRSA who became MRSA positive).

Participants.—All patients admitted to the study wards who were MRSA negative on admission and screened for MRSA on discharge.

Intervention.—Rapid polymerase chain reaction based screening test for MRSA compared with conventional culture.

Results.—Of 9608 patients admitted to study wards, 8374 met entry criteria and 6888 had full data (82.3%); 3335 in the control arm and 3553 in the rapid test arm. The overall MRSA carriage rate on admission was 6.7%. Rapid tests led to a reduction in median reporting time from admission, from 46 to 22 hours (P<0.001). Rapid testing also reduced the number of inappropriate pre-emptive isolation days between the control and intervention arms (399 *v* 277, P<0.001). This was not seen in other measurements of resource use. MRSA was acquired by 108 (3.2%) patients in the control arm and 99 (2.8%) in the intervention arm. When predefined confounding factors were taken into account the adjusted odds ratio was 0.91 (95% confidence interval 0.61 to 1.234). Rates of MRSA transmission, wound infection, and bacteraemia were not statistically different between the two arms.

Conclusion.—A rapid test for MRSA led to the quick receipt of results and had an impact on bed usage. No evidence was found of a significant reduction in MRSA acquisition and on these data it is unlikely that the increased costs of rapid tests can be justified compared with alternative control measures against MRSA.

Trial registration.—Clinical controlled trials ISRCTN75590122.

▶ Some have suggested that the rate of hospital-acquired methicillin-resistant *Staphylococcus aureus* (MRSA) can be partially dealt with by screening patients as they are hospitalized and cohorting these patients while they are in the hospital. Indeed, a number of countries have taken this approach. A valid criticism, however, of most MRSA screening studies has been that the delay in obtaining a result following admission screening means that transmission of MRSA from colonized patients may have already occurred before the carrier has been able to be detected.

There are 2 approaches to laboratory screening for MRSA—conventional culture-based testing which can give a provisional result in 24 hours (but more usually 48 hours), and the newer "rapid" nucleic acid amplification methods. Obviously, there is significant cost difference between these 2 methods. The cost for routine culturing in most laboratories is just $2 to $3, whereas molecular triage runs well over $20. Using "rapid" nucleic acid amplification methods to screen hospitalized patients for MRSA and then cohorting positive patients, Jeyaratnam et al found no benefit of rapid versus conventional screening in terms of rates of MRSA acquisition by contacts of positive patients on 10 wards of a London teaching hospital. The authors concluded that the additional expense associated with rapid screening is unlikely to be justifiable. Laboratory costs associated with rapid screening as noted are somewhere between 3 and 4 times higher than for conventional testing. Please note that the findings do not preclude a benefit of rapid screening for admission to specialized units such as intensive care units, which were not studied. Such units generally have the most robust infection control measures already in place, which would limit any added value of rapid screening.

We here in the United States generally use no screening of hospitalized patients at the time of admission. If there is a lesson to be learned from our European colleagues, it is that current evidence does not support routine rapid screening as opposed to conventional MRSA screening. All too often, we fail to use rapid detection tools when time is truly of the essence such as in someone who is actually clinically infected with an organism that could be MRSA. In such instances, being penny wise is indeed being dollar foolish. It is time to have molecular techniques available for such purposes.

This commentary closes with a *Clinical Fact/Curio* about transmission of infection. Ron Rivera was a Nicaraguan potter whose ingenuity brought clean drinking water to many people. He developed a water filter made from clay mixed with finely milled sawdust. The sawdust burned away during firing, leaving a network of pores that were then coated with colloidal silver, a bactericide. The filters halved the incidence of diarrheal disease among the families that used them. Working through Potters for Peace and funded by the Red Cross and other organizations, he hoped to establish 100 locally owned pottery factories around the world. He was working on his 30th factory in Nigeria when he contracted falciparum malaria, from which he died.[1]

J. A. Stockman III, MD

Reference

1. The Guardian Web site, www.guardian.co.uk/science/208/Oct/16/1. Accessed March 5, 2009.

Methicillin-Resistant *Staphylococcus aureus* Central Line–Associated Bloodstream Infections in US Intensive Care Units, 1997-2007
Burton DC, Edwards JR, Horan TC, et al (Ctrs for Disease Control and Prevention, Atlanta, GA)
JAMA 301:727-736, 2009

Context.—Concerns about rates of methicillin-resistant *Staphylococcus aureus* (MRSA) health care–associated infections have prompted calls for mandatory screening or reporting in efforts to reduce MRSA infections.

Objective.—To examine trends in the incidence of MRSA central line–associated bloodstream infections (BSIs) in US intensive care units (ICUs).

Design, Setting, and Participants.—Data reported by hospitals to the Centers for Disease Control and Prevention (CDC) from 1997-2007 were used to calculate pooled mean annual central line–associated BSI incidence rates for 7 types of adult and non-neonatal pediatric ICUs. Percent MRSA was defined as the proportion of *S aureus* central line–associated BSIs that were MRSA. We used regression modeling to estimate percent changes in central line–associated BSI metrics over the analysis period.

Main Outcome Measures.—Incidence rate of central line–associated BSIs per 1000 central line days; percent MRSA among *S aureus* central line–associated BSIs.

Results.—Overall, 33 587 central line–associated BSIs were reported from 1684 ICUs representing 16 225 498 patient-days of surveillance; 2498 reported central line–associated BSIs (7.4%) were MRSA and 1590 (4.7%) were methicillin-susceptible *S aureus* (MSSA). Of evaluated ICU types, surgical, nonteaching-affiliated medical-surgical, cardiothoracic, and coronary units experienced increases in MRSA central line–associated BSI incidence in the 1997-2001 period; however, medical, teaching-affiliated medical-surgical, and pediatric units experienced no significant changes. From 2001 through 2007, MRSA central line–associated BSI incidence declined significantly in all ICU types except in pediatric units, for which incidence rates remained static. Declines in MRSA central line–associated BSI incidence ranged from −51.5% (95% CI, −33.7% to −64.6%; *P* < .001) in nonteaching-affiliated medical-surgical ICUs (0.31 vs 0.15 per 1000 central line days) to −69.2% (95% CI, −57.9% to −77.7%; *P* < .001) in surgical ICUs (0.58 vs 0.18 per 1000 central line days). In all ICU types, MSSA central line–associated BSI incidence declined from 1997 through 2007, with changes in incidence ranging from −60.1% (95% CI, −41.2% to −73.1%; *P* < .001) in surgical ICUs (0.24 vs 0.10 per 1000 central line days) to −77.7% (95% CI, −68.2% to −84.4%; *P* < .001) in medical ICUs (0.40 vs 0.09 per 1000 central line days). Although the overall proportion of *S aureus* central line–associated BSIs due to MRSA increased 25.8% (*P* = .02) in the 1997-2007 period, overall MRSA central line–associated BSI incidence decreased 49.6% (*P* < .001) over this period.

Conclusions.—The incidence of MRSA central line–associated BSI has been decreasing in recent years in most ICU types reporting to the CDC. These trends are not apparent when only percent MRSA is monitored.

▶ Methicillin-resistant *Staphylococcus aureus* (MRSA) continues to plague us. Infections with this organism have become a focus of national attention over the past several years. Over the last decade, the number of hospitalizations with infections due to MRSA have nearly doubled in a number of areas in this country. Klevens et al have estimated that up to 18 000 deaths in the United States are the result of invasive MRSA infection.[1] These statistics coupled with the increasing number of outbreaks of MRSA infections in the community setting have helped to ignite a contentious public debate about the best means of control, including calls for increased surveillance for MRSA infections, new prevention activities such as screening of all patients admitted to hospitals to detect colonization with MRSA (universal screening), and public reporting of hospital-acquired MRSA infection.

What we learn from the report of Burton et al is that the incidence of MRSA central line-associated bloodstream infections has been decreasing in recent years in most ICUs reporting to the Centers for Disease Control. The data are emanating from adult ICUs, but similar outcomes seem to be accruing in pediatric ICUs as well. Specifically, overall MRSA central line-associated bloodstream infection incidence decreased by just under 50% over the period 1997 through 2007.

In pediatrics, the decreasing prevalence of catheter-associated bloodstream infections appears to in part be the result of a national collaboration undertaken and sponsored by the National Association of Children's Hospitals and Related Institutions. Almost 5 dozen large pediatric facilities have entered a quality improvement collaboration to determine the best ways to reduce line infections. This collaboration has been a fabulous success, saving over 20 children's lives and millions of dollars in the first year of the collaboration's activity.

We need more of such collaborations in pediatrics. This commentary closes with a *Clinical Fact/Curio* about a source of an infectious disease. Beware of moisturizing body milk creams! Moisturizing body milk has caused a severe outbreak of *Burkholderia cepacia* in an intensive care unit in Spain. This outbreak occurred over an 18-day period. Biological samples of the moisturizing body milk available in treatment carts were collected and cultured. The organism, which matched strains cultured from the patients, was readily isolated from open containers of the body milk and from 2 hermetically sealed ones. While this outbreak occurred across "the pond," there is little reason to think that similar quality control issues might not occur on our shores.[2]

J. A. Stockman III, MD

References

1. Klevens RM, Morrison MA, Nadle J, et al. Invasive methicillin-resistant Staphylococcus aureus infections in the United States. *JAMA*. 2007;298:1763-1771.
2. Alvarez-Lerma F, Maull E, Terradas R, et al. Moisturizing body milk as a reservoir of *Burkholderia cepacia*: outbreak of nosocomial infection in a multidisciplinary intensive care unit. *Crit Care*. 2008;12:R10.

Prevalence of and Risk Factors for Community-Acquired Methicillin-Resistant and Methicillin-Sensitive *Staphylococcus aureus* Colonization in Children Seen in a Practice-Based Research Network

Fritz SA, Garbutt J, Elward A, et al (Washington Univ School of Medicine, St Louis, MO)
Pediatrics 121:1090-1098, 2008

Objective.—We sought to define the prevalence of and risk factors for methicillin-resistant *Staphylococcus aureus* nasal colonization in the St Louis pediatric population.

Methods.—Children from birth to 18 years of age presenting for sick and well visits were recruited from pediatric practices affiliated with a practice-based research network. Nasal swabs were obtained, and a questionnaire was administered.

Results.—We enrolled 1300 participants from 11 practices. The prevalence of methicillin-resistant *S aureus* nasal colonization varied according to practice, from 0% to 9% (mean: 2.6%). The estimated population prevalence of methicillin-resistant *S aureus* nasal colonization for the 2 main counties of the St Louis metropolitan area was 2.4%. Of the 32 methicillin-resistant *S aureus* isolates, 9 (28%) were health care-associated types and 21 (66%) were community-acquired types. A significantly greater number of children with community-acquired methicillin-resistant *S aureus* were black and were enrolled in Medicaid, in comparison with children colonized with health care-associated methicillin-resistant *S aureus*. Children with both types of methicillin-resistant *S aureus* colonization had increased contact with health care, compared with children without colonization. Methicillin-sensitive *S aureus* nasal colonization ranged from 9% to 31% among practices (mean: 21%). The estimated population prevalence of methicillin-sensitive *S aureus* was 24.6%. Risk factors associated with methicillin-sensitive *S aureus* colonization included pet ownership, fingernail biting, and sports participation.

Conclusions.—Methicillin-resistant *S aureus* colonization is widespread among children in our community and includes strains associated with health care-associated and community-acquired infections.

▶ To date, there have been few studies assessing the community rates of methicillin-resistant *Staphylococcus aureus* (MRSA) colonization. The studies that have been done have looked at the colonization rates of MRSA in the anterior nares, which is the most consistent colonization site for *S aureus*. The report of Fritz et al is the largest community-based pediatric MRSA nasal colonization prevalence study to date. The study was undertaken in the St. Louis, Missouri community. Of some 1300 children cultured in 11 general pediatric practices, 32 were colonized with MRSA. Within each practice, the colonization rate varied from 0% to 9% (mean 2.6%). This corresponded to approximately 8400 children in the St. Louis metropolitan area being likely to be colonized with MRSA. It should be noted that the rates of MRSA colonization were similar in all age groups, but the rate of colonization in black children was roughly quadruple that seen in white children. Children with chronic health problems, those taking daily medications, those having visited an emergency department, or those having been hospitalized in the past year had somewhere between a 2- and 3-fold increased risk of carrying MRSA. Interestingly, the highest risk for having MRSA colonization was seen in adolescents who either shaved and/or waxed (or 5.0 and 11.5, respectively). Unexpectedly, daycare attendance (for children 5 and under) was a significant protective factor (or: 0.10). Several risk factors associated previously with MRSA infections were not associated with colonization in this study population.

Suggestions for limiting transmission of MRSA within family members and teammates include not sharing personal hygiene items such as towels and washcloths. In this study, however, children sharing bath towels or face cloths were not at increased risk for MRSA colonization. Although outbreaks of MRSA infections have been reported among athletes and within prisons, sports participation, contact with a recent inmate, and a household member working in the corrections system were not significant risk factors for MRSA colonization in this study. The finding that shaving and waxing of body hair are each associated with higher MRSA colonization rates suggests that MRSA may be transmitted through depilatory wax, or related equipment, or that these practices create microscopic damage or other changes in the skin that favor colonization.

As of now, the data from this report are most useful if they are considered to be "baseline" for future studies, because there is not much we can actually do with the data right now. Strains of MRSA associated with community-acquired infection have distinct features in contrast with those associated with healthcare-associated infection. Methicillin resistance is conferred by the *mecA* gene, which is located in the staphylococcal cassette chromosome *mec* (SCC*mec*). The SCC*mec* elements are different in hospital-acquired and community-acquired MRSA strains. Community-acquired MRSA is often resistant to fewer classes of non-β-lactam antibiotics. Knowing the rates of colonization in a community should help us to follow over time trends in the rates of colonization and should alert us to the emergence of even greater problems than we currently have.

This commentary closes with a *Clinical Fact/Curio* about an infectious disease that causes enteritis. History records that the Crusaders invading the Holy Land during the 12th and 13th centuries were frequently devastated and decimated with debilitating and at times lethal cases of dysentery. Whole armies of Crusaders were wiped out. Paleopathologists have nailed the cause of dysentery that devastated these Crusaders. It is not possible to detect dysentery-causing parasites, the presumed etiology of the problem, by microscopic study of archeological samples because parasitic cysts tend to degrade in soil. Investigators from London studied the problem using an ELISA assay employing antibodies specific to proteins produced by parasites. Samples were taken from 2 locations in Israel: a cesspool used by the citizens of Acre and the Hospital of St. John, whose latrines were used by knights, soldiers, and pilgrims. The researchers unveiled traces of 2 dysentery-causing parasites, *Entamoeba histolytica* and *Giardia duodenalis*, at the St. John Hospital latrine. No parasites were found in samples from the public cesspool that was not frequented by the Crusaders, suggesting that locals did not suffer from the problem.

The latrine as St. John Hospital still exists, although it has not been used since the medieval period. Despite its being out of commission, it still harbors evidence of organisms in the doo-doo of the Crusaders.[1]

J. A. Stockman III, MD

Reference

1. Crusaders' bug [editorial comment]. *Science*. 2008;320:1139.

Methods of Investigation and Management of Infections Causing Febrile Seizures

Millichap JJ, Millichap JG (Northwestern Univ Med School, Chicago, IL)
Pediat Neurol 39:381-386, 2008

The management of febrile seizures is reviewed, with emphasis on methods of investigation and treatment of associated infections. Records of 100 consecutive febrile seizure patient-visits were examined retrospectively at an East Carolina University-affiliated hospital. Causes of fever and infection, viral and bacterial studies, antipyretic, antibiotic, and antiviral treatments, and indications for lumbar puncture were analyzed. Febrile seizures were first episodes in 64, simple in 76, and complex in 23 (prolonged, at 30-60 minutes, in 4). The mean age was 20 months. Viral studies in 26 patients were positive in 9 (35%). Bacterial cultures in 100 were positive in 5%, none from CSF. Antibiotics were prescribed in 65%, and antipyretics in 89%. Lumbar puncture was performed in 14 patients; 11 had complex seizures, and 3 simple. Of simple seizure patients, none was aged <12 months, and only 1 was aged <18 months at time of lumbar puncture. Clinical manifestations and complex seizures are the principal indications for lumbar puncture, and not patient age. Viral infection is the most common cause of fever, and bacterial infection is infrequent. Early viral diagnosis should lessen the emphasis on bacterial cultures, and lead to reduced use of empiric antibiotics.

▶ This interesting report extends the discussion on the use of lumbar puncture for first simple febrile seizure as reported in Kimia et al[1] It has been more than 20 years since the first *Haemophilus influenzae* type b conjugate vaccines first appeared on the market to be used in children beginning at 2 months of age. It has been almost a decade now since the pneumococcal conjugate vaccine has been introduced. With both vaccines now being given to more than 90% of infants in the United States, the spectrum of causes of febrile seizures has been altered with fewer and fewer being due to bacterial meningitis. The report of Millichap and Millichap provides information on 100 consecutive childhood patient visits with a diagnosis of febrile seizure treated at the Brody School of Medicine and its East Carolina University affiliated hospital in Greenville, North Carolina. The highest incidence of children presenting with febrile seizures was in the 12- to 18-month age group followed by the 6- to 12-month age group. Only 2% occurred between age 3 and 6 months and just 28% between 2 and 5 years. The most frequent causative infections underlying the febrile seizures were otitis media in 39%, an upper respiratory tract infection in 38% (diagnosed as viral in one-third), pneumonia in 15% (x-ray confirmed in 11%), and influenza in 6%. Infrequent or rare causes included gastroenteritis in 3, urinary tract infection in 2, and varicella in 1. Of those presenting with febrile seizure, just 14% underwent a lumbar puncture. All lumbar punctures were negative for evidence of bacteria or viral meningitis.

The authors of this report suggest that a complex seizure (prolonged, focal, or multiple) is now the main criterion for lumbar puncture in the presence of fever.

Of course, an abnormal neurologic examination would also dictate the need for a lumbar puncture or other signs of infection prompting blood culture or empiric antibiotic treatment. The American Academy of Pediatrics suggests that to avoid the risk of masking bacterial infection, lumbar puncture is strongly considered if the patient has received previous antibiotic treatment. In all cases, guidelines should not subvert clinical judgment.

It is probably worth your time to read the Millichap report in detail. If time is at a premium, just go to the last paragraph of the report. There it is stated that a child age 3 months to 5 years who presents with a first or recurrent febrile seizure should be considered for lumbar puncture if one or more of these indications are present: neurologic signs of meningitis, systemic signs of toxicity, a complex seizure with prolonged postictal obtundation, or pretreatment with an antibiotic. Those are the facts. The disclaimers are that these facts have to be interpreted based on the experience of the treating physician and the certainty of follow-up. Assuming all of these fall on the favorable side of the evaluation, it would seem that lumbar puncture is not indicated for a first simple febrile seizure.

J. A. Stockman III, MD

Reference

1. Kimia AA, Capraro AJ, Hummel D. Utility of lumbar puncture for first simple febrile seizure among children 6-18 months of age. *Pediatrics*. 2009;123:6-12.

Utility of Lumbar Puncture for First Simple Febrile Seizure Among Children 6 to 18 Months of Age

Kimia AA, Capraro AJ, Hummel D, et al (Children's Hosp Boston, MA)
Pediatrics 123:6-12, 2009

Objectives.—American Academy of Pediatrics consensus statement recommendations are to consider strongly for infants 6 to 12 months of age with a first simple febrile seizure and to consider for children 12 to 18 months of age with a first simple febrile seizure lumbar puncture for cerebrospinal fluid analysis. Our aims were to determine compliance with these recommendations and to assess the rate of bacterial meningitis detected among these children.

Methods.—A retrospective cohort review was performed for patients 6 to 18 months of age who were evaluated for first simple febrile seizure in a pediatric emergency department between October 1995 and October 2006.

Results.—First simple febrile seizure accounted for 1% of all emergency department visits for children of this age, with 704 cases among 71 234 eligible visits during the study period. Twenty-seven percent ($n = 188$) of first simple febrile seizure visits were for infants 6 to 12 months of age, and 73% ($n = 516$) were for infants 12 to 18 months of age. Lumbar puncture was performed for 38% of the children ($n = 271$). Samples were available for 70% of children 6 to 12 months of age (131 of 188 children) and 25% of children 12 to 18 months of age (129 of 516 children). Rates of lumbar puncture decreased significantly over time in both age groups. The cerebrospinal fluid white blood cell count was elevated in 10 cases (3.8%). No pathogen was identified in cerebrospinal fluid cultures. Ten cultures (3.8%) yielded a contaminant. No patient was diagnosed as having bacterial meningitis.

Conclusions.—The risk of bacterial meningitis presenting as first simple febrile seizure at ages 6 to 18 months is very low. Current American Academy of Pediatrics recommendations should be reconsidered.

▶ First simple febrile seizure (FSFS) is still fairly common. We see in this report that it accounts for about 1% of all emergency department visits for children ages 6 to 18 months. It was back in 1996 that the American Academy of Pediatrics (AAP) made several very specific recommendations about the definition and management of FSFS. It was defined as a first episode of seizure accompanied by fever, manifested as a primary generalized seizure lasting no longer than 15 minutes and not recurring within 24 hours. It was clearly stated that this definition should not apply to children with known central nervous system infections or underlying seizure disorders. The practice guideline that accompanied the academy report recommended that lumbar puncture (LP) be strongly considered for patients less than 12 months of age and be considered for patients 12 to 18 months of age in order to exclude a diagnosis of bacterial meningitis to be certain that FSFS was not the sole clinical manifestation of this serious disease.[1] Needless to say the AAP recommendations were erring on the side of caution recognizing that seizure is a common presenting sign of bacterial meningitis and that clinical skill and experience may vary significantly among those providers seeing a child with FSFS. At the same time, it was recognized that although seizure is a common symptom among patients presenting with bacterial meningitis, it is quite uncommon for a simple, brief, nonfocal seizure to be the sole manifestation. Also, with the introduction of the 7-valent pneumococcal conjugate vaccine in 2000, the incidence of bacterial meningitis from this organism has appeared to decrease significantly.

The purpose of the report of Kimia et al was to examine the rate of bacterial meningitis among otherwise healthy infants 6 to 18 months of age who presented to a pediatric emergency department with FSFS in the postpneumococcal vaccine era. The study presented is the first that attempts to quantify the risk for bacterial meningitis in the age groups represented in the AAP recommendations in the modern era. The series represents the largest sample of children with FSFS in the 6- to 18-month age group for which concern regarding meningitis should be at its highest. The study identified no cases of bacterial meningitis in the group of children reported. During this same period within the same sample of 70 530 children 6 to 18 months of age without FSFS who were seen in the emergency department, there were 8 cases of bacterial meningitis. In this series, 27% of FSFS presenting to the Boston Children's Hospital emergency room occurred in infants 6 to 12 months of age with 73% occurring in infants 12 to 18 months of age. Lumbar puncture was performed in 38% of the children overall. Please note that the AAP recommendations either strongly recommend or simply recommend lumbar puncture in this age group. They do not dictate that it must be done.

So what should we do with these data? Do they tell us that FSFS is now such a rare presentation of bacterial meningitis that we no longer need to do a lumbar puncture? The authors are quite cautious about going that far. They state that the ability to generalize results from an academic pediatric emergency department to other emergency departments should be questioned. However, the data do indicate that lumbar puncture performance rates for FSFS in general emergency departments are already significantly lower than those seen in the academic emergency department. This fact combined with the finding that is very rare for bacterial meningitis to present as FSFS make the AAP practice parameters recommending that clinicians strongly consider or consider LP for every child with FSFS to have limited use. The authors' final conclusion is that they believe the evidence to recommend LP for FSFS does not exist and that the recommendation should be changed to state simply that meningitis should be considered in the differential diagnosis for any febrile child, and an LP should be performed if there are clinical signs or symptoms of concern. FSFS alone is not such a clinical sign or symptom by itself.

J. A. Stockman III, MD

Reference

1. American Academy of Pediatrics, Provisional Committee on Quality Improvement, Subcommittee on Febrile Seizures. Practice Parameter: the neurodiagnostic evaluation of the child with a first febrile seizure. *Pediatrics*. 1996;97:769-772.

Predictors of cerebrospinal fluid pleocytosis in febrile infants aged 0 to 90 days

Meehan WP 3rd, Bachur RG (Children's Hosp, Boston, MA)
Pediatr Emerg Care 24:287-293, 2008

Background.—Young infants with fever routinely undergo laboratory evaluation, and many are treated with empirical antibiotics even when the infant seems well. The requirement of a lumbar puncture (LP) as part of a routine evaluation is debated; however, administration of antibiotics without an LP can cause concerns for partially treated bacterial meningitis and make subsequent evaluation of the cerebrospinal fluid (CSF) confusing. The ability to predict which febrile infants have a CSF pleocytosis would assist in the decision to perform LP in febrile infants.

Objective.—To develop a model to predict which febrile infants have a CSF pleocytosis.

Methods.—We conducted a retrospective review of febrile children aged 90 days or younger seen in the emergency department. Electronic data sources provided the age of the infant, the triage temperature, and all laboratory values. After univariate analysis, recursive partitioning analysis was performed to develop a decision tree to predict febrile infants at increased risk for CSF pleocytosis, defined as a CSF white blood cell (WBC) count of 25/microL or greater in infants 28 days old or younger and 10/microL or greater in those 29 to 90 days old.

Results.—Two thousand three febrile infants were studied; 176 (8.8%; 95% confidence interval [CI], 7.6%-10.1%) had a CSF pleocytosis. Presentation during the summer season increased the risk of pleocytosis from 5.0% during nonsummer months to 17.4% (95% CI, 14.6%-20.6%). During the nonsummer season, 7.3% (95% CI, 5.6%-9.5%) of febrile infants with a temperature of greater than 38.4 degrees C and a WBC count of greater than 6100/microL had a CSF pleocytosis, as opposed to 2.9% (95% CI, 1.9%-4.4%) of those with lower temperature or lower WBC count. The decision tree has an overall sensitivity of 89% (95% CI, 83%-92%) and a negative predictive value of 97% (95% CI, 96%-98%).

Conclusions.—A significant number of well-appearing febrile infants will have a CSF pleocytosis. A simple decision tree based on objective clinical information can help identify those at greatest risk for CSF pleocytosis.

▶ This report reminds us of something all of us already know and that is that the management of young, well-appearing, febrile infants remains somewhat debatable. We do know that infants younger than 90 days of age who present with fever are at relatively high risk for having an infection, and these are the same infants that are more difficult to assess clinically in comparison with older infants and children. Numerous studies have shown how we might be able to use routine laboratory data to assist us in distinguishing those patients at greatest risk for serious bacterial illness. Numerous studies also tell us, however, that despite efforts to promote standardization of care of febrile young infants, management often deviates from recommended guidelines. One of the greatest inconsistencies in management is the frequency with which lumbar punctures (LPs) are performed.

Most pediatricians use 1 of 2 protocols to manage febrile infants. In the Philadelphia protocol infants 29 to 60 days old with fever (temperature ≥38.0 °C) are considered low risk if they appear well, have no evidence of bacterial infection on examination, and have normal laboratory values, including a white blood cell count of less than 15 000/µL, a band to neutrophil ratio of less than 0.2, a CSF WBC count of less than 8 WBCs per µL, a urinalysis with fewer than 10 WBCs per high power field, a negative chest X-ray when obtained, and in infants with diarrhea, a stool smear with few or no WBCs.[1] The Philadelphia protocol has a negative predictive value of 100%, allowing outpatient management without antibiotics for low-risk infants and inpatient care with parenteral antibiotics for high-risk infants. The Rochester criteria is intended for infants of age 60 days or younger with a rectal temperature of 38.0 °C or greater. Infants studied using the Rochester criteria were defined as low-risk if they were previously healthy, appeared well without focus of infection after history and physical examination, and had normal laboratory values, including a WBC count of greater than 5000/μL and less than 15 000/μL, an absolute band count of 1500/μL or less, urinalysis with 10 WBCs per high power field or less, and for infants with diarrhea, a stool smear with 5 WBCs per high power field or less. Using the Rochester criteria you can expect a negative predictive value of 98.9%.[2] Many care providers point to this protocol as evidence that an LP is not indicated in infants of age 60 days or younger as a routine. The Rochester criteria do state that if parenteral antibiotics are administered, an LP should be performed before the antibiotic administration.

Administration of antibiotics without evaluation of the CSF may lead to complications related to the delayed diagnosis of bacterial meningitis or difficulty interpreting CSF pleocytosis in patients pretreated with antibiotics. A number of studies have shown the inadequacy of history and physical examination to detect serious bacterial illness in this young age group. Despite this, febrile infants are all too often given antibiotics without an LP. When these patients have persistent or worsening clinical findings and an LP is finally performed, the CSF analysis is difficult to interpret and cultures are unreliable. In such cases, the presence of CSF pleocytosis then makes many a care provider think the patient may have bacterial meningitis when in fact the most common cause of CSF pleocytosis is aseptic meningitis or the presence of a concurrent urinary tract infection. When a CSF pleocytosis is discovered after antibiotics have been administered, infants are often subjected to prolonged hospitalization and antibiotic administration.

What Meehan et al have done is to predict what the likelihood is of CSF pleocytosis in an infant who presents with a fever. They used a commonly employed definition of pleocytosis, which is an upper limit of normal of CSF WBC count of 25 cells/μL or greater in patients aged 0 to 28 days and 10 cells/μL or greater in patients aged 29 to 90 days. Aseptic meningitis was defined as CSF pleocytosis and a negative CSF culture for a bacterial pathogen. Bacterial meningitis was defined by a positive CSF culture for a pathogen. Viral studies were not done because these were rarely obtained as part of routine management. In more than 2000 CSF samples that were obtained in febrile infants under 90 days of age, 8.8% had CSF pleocytosis. Only 2.2% of those with pleocytosis were described as ill appearing. Of those seen during summer months, 17.4% had a CSF pleocytosis. This dropped to 5.0% during nonsummer months. From these data, a decision analysis tree was created. On the basis of the decision tree, summer season alone increased the probability of CSF pleocytosis from 8.8% to 17.4% among patients who presented outside the summer season. The 2 greatest risk factors were a temperature greater than 38.4 °C and a white blood cell count greater than 6100/μL, with 7.3% having CSF pleocytosis.

So what does all this mean? What it means is that well-appearing febrile infants aged 90 days or younger frequently have a CSF pleocytosis in the absence of bacterial meningitis. Height of fever, white blood cell count, absolute neutrophil count, and age of the patient are poor individual predictors of CSF pleocytosis. However, when used as part of the decision tree, white blood cell count and height of fever are useful in identifying a group of patients at increased risk of having CSF pleocytosis. As a single predictor, presentation during the summer months increases the frequency of pleocytosis to 17.4%. The authors of this report suggest that the best application of this decision rule that they have developed is for those clinicians currently following guidelines that do not recommend LP. The decision rule would help clinicians who are currently administering antibiotics without first obtaining CSF to selectively perform LP on well-appearing infants who will receive antibiotics and that are high risk for CSF pleocytosis. It is pretty obvious that although bacterial meningitis is rare, 1 in 11 febrile infants age 90 days or younger will have a CSF pleocytosis, including 1 in 6 infants during the summer months. The authors tell us that in circumstances where empirical antibiotics are being considered without LP, the clinician should consider the risk of CSF pleocytosis before initiating antibiotic therapy. Use of the decision tree and its rules can identify those at greatest risk for CSF pleocytosis.

One final comment having to do with the ability to spot seriously ill children, this emanating from Great Britain. A study based on all 957 deaths in children 28 days to 17 years that occurred in England in 2006 found many examples of high quality care including cases where, even though the care was outstanding, a child died. However, the investigation identified avoidable factors in 26% of deaths and potentially avoidable factors in a further 43%. All too often health care practitioners in primary care and in hospitals had difficulty recognizing serious illness in the way children presented. These cases often involved children with febrile illnesses who were assessed by health care providers with little or no experience in the medical care of children. In most instances, there was little pediatric supervision of these providers.

To read more about this, see the results of "Why children die: a pilot study 2006," available at: http://www.cemach.org.uk. In the absence of the ability to have pediatric supervision of all patients, it is suggested that hospital emergency rooms use scoring systems to spot seriously ill children.

J. A. Stockman III, MD

References

1. Backer MD, Bell LM, Avner JR. The efficacy of routine outpatient management without antibiotics in selected infants. *Pediatrics.* 1999;103:627-631.
2. Jaskiewicz JA, McCarthy CA, Richardson AC, et al. Febrile infants at low risk for serious bacterial infection – an appraisal of the Rochester criteria and implications for management. Febrile Infant Collaborative Study Group. *Pediatrics.* 1994;94: 390-396.

Test Characteristics and Interpretation of Cerebrospinal Fluid Gram Stain in Children

Neuman MI, Tolford S, Harper MB, et al (Children's Hosp, Harvard Med School, Boston, MA)
Pediatr Infect Dis J 27:309-313, 2008

Background.—Few data exist regarding the test characteristics of cerebrospinal fluid (CSF) Gram stain among children at risk for bacterial meningitis, especially the rate of false positive Gram stain.

Methods.—We conducted a retrospective cohort study of children seen in the emergency department of Children's Hospital Boston who had CSF obtained between December 1992 and September 2005. Patients who had ventricular shunts, as well as those who received antibiotics before CSF was obtained were excluded. Test characteristics of CSF Gram stain were assessed using CSF culture as the criterion standard. Patients were considered to have bacterial meningitis if there was either: (1) growth of a pathogen, or (2) growth of a possible pathogen noted on the final CSF culture report and the patient was treated with a course of parenteral antibiotics for 7 days or more without other indication.

Results.—A total of 17,569 eligible CSF specimens were collected among 16,036 patients during the 13-year study period. The median age of study subjects was 74 days. Seventy CSF specimens (0.4%) had organisms detected on Gram stain. The overall sensitivity of Gram stain to detect bacterial meningitis was 67% [42 of 63; 95% confidence interval (CI): 54–78] with a positive predictive value of 60% (42 of 70; 95% CI: 48–71). Most patients without bacterial meningitis have negative Gram stain [specificity 99.9% (17,478 of 17,506; 95% CI: 99.8–99.9)] with a negative predictive value of 99.9 (17,478 of 17,499; 95% CI: 99.8–99.9).

Conclusions.—CSF Gram stain is appropriately used by physicians in risk stratification for the diagnosis and empiric treatment of bacterial meningitis in children. Although a positive Gram stain result greatly increases the likelihood of bacterial meningitis; the result may be because of contamination or misinterpretation in 40% of cases and should not, by itself, result in a full treatment course for bacterial meningitis.

▶ No one waits the time it takes to have a culture of cerebrospinal fluid (CSF) return before making a diagnostic decision to treat or not treat for possible bacterial meningitis. Decisions are made not only on the clinical presentation but also, of course, on laboratory tests such as CSF Gram stain, cell count, glucose, and protein, and the presence or absence of CSF pleocytosis. Not surprisingly, patients with a positive CSF Gram stain are routinely assigned to having a high probability of bacterial meningitis. The rub is that from time to time we are faced with a positive Gram stain result in the absence of other strong clinical factors that would lead to a high degree of suspicion for meningitis, which leads all too frequently to wondering whether the Gram stain might be a false positive. At the same time, if a culture comes back negative and the

CSF Gram stain is positive, one wonders if the culture is a false negative. Unfortunately, there are few data regarding the test characteristics of the CSF Gram stain alone in the prediction of bacterial meningitis among children, a reason why this study, performed in the emergency medicine department of Children's Hospital of Boston, was undertaken.

In this study, a retrospective analysis was performed on patients presenting to Children's Hospital of Boston who had CSF obtained between December 1992 and September 2005. Over 18 000 CSF specimens were collected and bacterial growth was detected on culture in 542 CSF specimens (3.1%). Most CSF cultures demonstrating growth were determined to be the result of contamination (88% of the positive culture samples). Just 63 patients met the study definition of bacterial meningitis with the most common pathogen identified as *Streptococcus pneumoniae*. Of all the samples obtained, 0.4% had organisms detected on Gram stain versus the 3.1% of CSF samples that became culture positive. The overall sensitivity of the CSF Gram stain for detecting any growth in culture media was 9.2%. On the other hand, CSF Gram stain demonstrated a specificity of 99.9% with a positive predictive value of 71.4% and a negative predictive value of 97.2% for the detection of any growth in culture. This study therefore affirms that the CSF Gram stain does provide clinical useful information to treating clinicians. Nonetheless, it is also clear that the overall performance of this test in isolation is not ideal.

Decisions regarding treatment and hospitalization of a child suspected of having bacterial meningitis will continue to routinely be made by clinicians based on clinical information. The ill-appearing child or infant should be hospitalized and receive empiric antibiotics. The decision to treat the patient for a full empiric course if the Gram stain is positive, in the face of cultures of blood in CSF that are negative, depends on other factors that impact the probability of bacterial meningitis. These might include the patient's clinical presentation, demographic, and laboratory risk assignment data, including age, clinical presentation and other CSF findings such as the white blood cell count protein, percent neutrophils, and glucose measurements.

The take-home message here is that if the CSF Gram stain is positive, the likelihood is greater than not that the child does in fact have bacterial meningitis. A negative Gram stain should mean little when it comes to the decision to treat or not to treat.

J. A. Stockman III, MD

Exposure to Nontraditional Pets at Home and to Animals in Public Settings: Risks to Children
Pickering LK, and the Committee on Infectious Diseases
Pediatrics 122:876-886, 2008

Exposure to animals can provide many benefits during the growth and development of children. However, there are potential risks associated with animal exposures, including exposure to nontraditional pets in the home and animals in public settings. Educational materials, regulations, and guidelines have been developed to minimize these risks. Pediatricians, veterinarians, and other health care professionals can provide advice on selection of appropriate pets as well as prevention of disease transmission from nontraditional pets and when children contact animals in public settings.

▶ Until this report appeared, this editor was not aware of some of the statistics associated with pet ownership in the United States. While the report focuses on nontraditional pets and exotic animals as pets, the report also highlights the magnitude of "traditional" pet ownership in the United States. For example, were you aware that the percentage of United States households that have 1 or more pets has increased from 56% in 1998 to 63% by the end of 2007? Yes, over 70 million homes have 1 or more pets. Dogs lead in this regard. Dogs are owned by 44.8 million households, cats by 38.4 million, freshwater fish by 14.2 million, birds by 6.4 million, small animals by 6 million, horses by 4.3 million, and saltwater fish by 0.8 million. Total United States pet industry expenditure in 2007 was estimated at more than $40 billion, a figure greater than the initial proposed bailout of the auto industry in the United States.

What Pickering et al have done is to identify original research publications and review articles dealing with infections, injury, and allergies in children resulting from nontraditional pets in the home, including exotic animals, and from animals in public settings using the National Library of Medicine's Med-Line database and the Cochrane Library. Table 1 outlines the animals that were considered as nontraditional pets and/or animals that might be encountered in public settings while Table 2 describes the potential exposures of children to animals in public settings. Importantly, Table 3 provides the guidelines

TABLE 1.—Animals That are Considered Nontraditional Pets and/or Animals That May Be Encountered in Public Settings

Categories	Examples
Amphibians	Frogs, toads, newts, salamanders
Fish	Many types
Mammals: wildlife	Raccoons, skunks, foxes, coyotes, civet cats, tigers, lions, bears, nonhuman primates
Domesticated livestock	Cattle, pigs, goats, sheep
Equines	Horses, mules, donkeys, zebras
Weasels	Ferrets, minks, sables, skunks
Lagomorphs	Rabbits, hares, pikas
Rodents	Mice, rats, hamsters, gerbils, guinea pigs, chinchillas, gophers, lemmings, squirrels, chipmunks, prairie dogs, hedgehogs
Feral animals	Cats, dogs, horses, swine
Reptiles	Turtles, lizards, iguanas, snakes, alligators

(Reprinted from Pickering LK, and the Committee on Infectious Diseases. Exposure to nontraditional pets at home and to animals in public settings: risks to children. *Pediatrics*. 2008;122:876-886.)

TABLE 2.—Potential Exposures of Children to Animals in Public Settings

Area	Animal Involved	Organism
Metropolitan zoo	Elephants, giraffes, rhinoceroses, buffaloes	*M tuberculosis*[56,57]
	Komodo dragons	*Salmonella* serotype *enteritidis*[15]
County or state agricultural fairs	Cattle, calves	E coli O157:H7[38,45,51,64]
	Cattle	*Campylobacter* species[50]
	Reptiles	*Salmonella* species[14]
	Goats	Rabies[62,64]
Farm tours or visits	Cattle, calves	E coli O157[38–40,43,44,46,47,52,62]
	Raw milk	*Campylobacter* species, *Salmonella* species[64]
	Calves	*Cryptosporidium* species, *E coli* O157:H7, *Salmonella* species, *Campylobacter* species[48]
	Sheep, goats, calves	*Cryptosporidium* species[38,53–55,64]
	Sheep	Orf[25]
Livestock exhibits	Cattle	E coli O157[48]
Pet stores	Hamsters, mice, rats	*Salmonella* species[20]
	Kittens	Rabies[61]
	Hamsters	Tularemia,[10] lymphocytic choriomeningitis[21]
	Prairie dogs	Monkeypox[11]
Petting zoos	Cattle, sheep, goats	E coli O157[38,42,49,64]
	Rabbits	*Giardia* species[64]
	Bear cubs	Rabies[63]
Rodeo events	Ponies	Rabies[60]
Fish tanks	Fish	*Mycobacterium* species,[32] *Salmonella* species[33]
Agricultural feed store	Baby poultry (chicks, ducklings, goslings, turkeys)	*Salmonella* species[34]

Editor's Note: Please refer to original journal article for full references.
(Reprinted from Pickering LK, and the Committee on Infectious Diseases. Exposure to nontraditional pets at home and to animals in public settings: risks to children. *Pediatrics*. 2008;122:876-886.)

for prevention of human diseases from nontraditional pets in both the home and public settings.

The bottom line of this report is straightforward. Most nontraditional pets do pose a risk to the health of young children, and their acquisition and ownership should be discouraged in households with young children. By young is meant children under the age of 5. Of course, immunocompromised children of any age and compromised adults should be made aware of the risk of infection related to nontraditional pet ownership. We, as pediatricians, should play a central role in informing families of these risks. In addition, simple and effective advice to avoid illness includes frequent hand washing and the avoidance of direct contact with animals and their environments. Young children should always be supervised closely when in contact with animals in public settings. As importantly, pediatricians should insert themselves when possible into the decision families make about obtaining nontraditional pets. Parents should also be made aware of web sites that provide guidelines for safe pet selection

TABLE 3.—Guidelines for Prevention of Human Diseases From Nontraditional Pets at Home and Exposure to Animals in Public Settings

General
    Wash hands immediately after contact with animals, animal products, or their environment
    Supervise hand-washing for children younger than 5 y
    Wash hands after handling animal-derived pet treats
    Never bring wild animals home, and never adopt wild animals as pets
    Teach children never to handle unfamiliar, wild, or domestic animals even if the animals appear friendly
    Avoid rough play with animals to prevent scratches or bites
    Children should not be allowed to kiss pets or put their hands or other objects into their mouths after handling animals
    Do not permit nontraditional pets to roam or fly freely in the house or allow nontraditional or domestic pets to have contact with wild animals
    Do not permit animals in areas where food or drink are prepared or consumed
    Administer rabies vaccine to mammals as appropriate
    Keep animals clean and free of intestinal parasites, fleas, ticks, mites, and lice
    People at increased risk of infection or serious complications of salmonellosis (eg, children younger than 5 y, older adults, and immunocompromised hosts) should avoid contact with animal-derived pet treats

Animals visiting schools and child-care facilities
    Designate specific areas for animal contact
    Display animals in enclosed cages or under appropriate restraint
    Do not allow food in animal-contact areas
    Always supervise children, especially those younger than 5 y, during interaction with animals
    Obtain a certificate of veterinary inspection for visiting animals and/or proof of rabies immunization according to local or state requirements
    Properly clean and disinfect all areas where animals have been present
    Consult with parents or guardians to determine special considerations needed for children who are immunocompromised or who have allergies or asthma
    Animals not recommended in schools, child-care settings, and hospitals include nonhuman primates, inherently dangerous animals (lions, tigers, cougars, bears, wolfdog hybrids), mammals at high risk of transmitting rabies (bats, raccoons, skunks, foxes, and coyotes), aggressive animals or animals with unpredictable behavior, stray animals with unknown health history, reptiles, and amphibians
    Ensure that people who provide animals for educational purposes are knowledgeable regarding animal handling and zoonotic disease issues

Public settings
    Venue operators must know about risks of disease and injury
        Venue operators and staff must maintain a safe environment
    Venue operators and staff must educate visitors about the risk of disease and injury and provide appropriate preventive measures

Animal specific
    Children younger than 5 y and immunocompromised people should avoid contact in public settings with reptiles, amphibians, rodents, ferrets, baby poultry (chicks, ducklings), and any items that have been in contact with these animals or their environments
    Reptiles, amphibians, rodents, ferrets, and baby poultry (chicks, ducklings) should be kept out of households that contain children younger than 5 y, immunocompromised people, or people with sickle cell disease and should not be allowed in child-care centers
    Reptiles, amphibians, rodents, and baby poultry should not be permitted to roam freely throughout a home or living area and should not be permitted in kitchens or other food-preparation areas
    Disposable gloves should be used when cleaning fish aquariums, and aquarium water should not be disposed in sinks used for food preparation or for obtaining drinking water
    Mammals at high risk of transmitting rabies (bats, raccoons, skunks, foxes, and coyotes) should not be touched by children

(Reprinted from Pickering LK, and the Committee on Infectious Diseases. Exposure to nontraditional pets at home and to animals in public settings: risks to children. *Pediatrics*. 2008;122:876-886.)

and the appropriate handling of pets. As part of a child's routine visit, a history of contact with pets in the home or animals in public settings should take place, and we should always think about such contact as a cause of an unusual illness in a youngster.

J. A. Stockman III, MD

Gene Therapy for Immunodeficiency Due to Adenosine Deaminase Deficiency

Aiuti A, Cattaneo F, Galimberti S, et al (San Raffaele Telethon Inst for Gene Therapy, Milan; University of Milan-Bicocca; et al)
N Engl J Med 360:447-458, 2009

Background.—We investigated the long-term outcome of gene therapy for severe combined immunodeficiency (SCID) due to the lack of adenosine deaminase (ADA), a fatal disorder of purine metabolism and immunodeficiency.

Methods.—We infused autologous CD34+ bone marrow cells transduced with a retroviral vector containing the *ADA* gene into 10 children with SCID due to ADA deficiency who lacked an HLA-identical sibling donor, after nonmyeloablative conditioning with busulfan. Enzyme-replacement therapy was not given after infusion of the cells.

Results.—All patients are alive after a median follow-up of 4.0 years (range, 1.8 to 8.0). Transduced hematopoietic stem cells have stably engrafted and differentiated into myeloid cells containing ADA (mean range at 1 year in bone marrow lineages, 3.5 to 8.9%) and lymphoid cells (mean range in peripheral blood, 52.4 to 88.0%). Eight patients do not require enzyme-replacement therapy, their blood cells continue to express ADA, and they have no signs of defective detoxification of purine metabolites. Nine patients had immune reconstitution with increases in T-cell counts (median count at 3 years, 1.07×10^9 per liter) and normalization of T-cell function. In the five patients in whom intravenous immune globulin replacement was discontinued, antigen-specific antibody responses were elicited after exposure to vaccines or viral antigens. Effective protection against infections and improvement in physical development made a normal lifestyle possible. Serious adverse events included prolonged neutropenia (in two patients), hypertension (in one), central-venous-catheter–related infections (in two), Epstein–Barr virus reactivation (in one), and autoimmune hepatitis (in one).

Conclusions.—Gene therapy, combined with reduced-intensity conditioning, is a safe and effective treatment for SCID in patients with ADA deficiency. (ClinicalTrials.gov numbers, NCT00598481 and NCT00599781.)

▶ The story surrounding gene therapy for immunodeficiency due to adenosine deaminase (ADA) deficiency goes back a couple of decades or so. In the mid-1980s, it became apparent that patients with severe combined immunodeficiency disease (SCID) due to deficiency of ADA when transplanted with human leukocyte antigen (HLA)-matched sibling bone marrow could be cured of their SCID with only a small amount of engrafted marrow, which appears to be able to completely restore the immune system. It became clear then that if the ADA gene could be inserted into even just a modest number of hematopoietic stem cells obtained from a patient with SCID due to ADA deficiency, it might be possible to cure the underlying disease. It took some years before the promise of gene therapy was at hand. Cavazzana-Calvo et al reported immune reconstitution in 5 infants with X-linked SCID who underwent gene therapy in Paris, and Aiuti et al described initial signs of immune reconstitution in 2 infants with SCID due to ADA deficiency in Milan.[1,2] The gene transfer methods used in these 2 studies were similar and involved giving a chemotherapeutic agent, busulfan, intended to make space for the patient's gene-corrected hematopoietic stem cells, permitting enhanced engraftment after reinfusion. With the gene therapy procedure, the patient's stem cells are harvested, genes are inserted, and the stem cells are reinfused to seed into a bone marrow that has been partially depleted of the patient's stem cells with the use of the busulfan, allowing more room for the reinfused stem cells to grow. Since these 2 studies were published, the encouraging results obtained in patients with X-linked SCID have been reproduced in at least 1 other trial carried out in the United Kingdom.[3]

The current report of Aiuti et al, as abstracted, adds to these earlier accomplishments by reporting findings from the extended follow-up of 2 previously studied patients with SCID due to ADA deficiency and an additional 8 patients treated according to the same protocol. Of these 10 patients, 8 have had excellent and persistent immune reconstitution in the absence of enzyme-replacement therapy as documented with the use of multiple laboratory tests and, most importantly, through their continued clinical well-being without the need for protective environment to prevent infection. Among the patients who had excellent recovery was 1 child who was almost 6 years of age at the time of gene therapy. Although this is quite young by most standards, it is still an age at which thymic function, essential to provide the niche for T-cell development, has already declined considerably as compared with infancy. In these patients, essentially all the circulating T-cells and most of the B-cells and natural killer cells have been shown to contain the corrective ADA gene, whereas the levels of ADA-converting granulocytes, monocytes, and bone marrow stem cells or progenitor cells (which are not adversely affected by ADA deficiency) are one-tenth to one-hundredth the levels in the lymphocytes. These findings clearly demonstrate the occurrence of selective amplification of gene-corrected lymphocytes from a quite small number of gene-corrected hematopoietic stem cells.

There are other interesting things to learn from the report of Aiuti et al. None of the patients with SCID due to ADA deficiency have developed long-term problems in contrast to X-linked SCID. Survivors of gene therapy with X-linked SCID seem to run a 20% to 25% risk of developing a T-cell lymphoproliferative syndrome, which presents within 2 to 5 years after the procedure. Investigations have implicated insertional oncogenesis in the pathogenesis of the leukemia-like illness, in which the insertion of the corrective retroviral vector may activate expression of cellular proto-oncogenes. The sharp dichotomy between the absence of this complication in patients with SCID due to ADA deficiency and its occurrence in 25% of patients with X-linked SCID is important to understand if we are to retain the therapeutic efficacy of gene therapy while minimizing its risk. There appear to be significant biological differences between X-linked SCID and SCID due to ADA deficiency.

The outcomes of gene therapy for SCID reported in recent trials are at least as good as, and probably arguably better than, the results reported for bone marrow transplantation. Transplantation of parent or unrelated allogeneic hematopoietic stem cells in infants with SCID who lack HLA matched sibling donors has a success rate of just 50% to 85%. Thus everyone is looking to gene therapy to be the better way to go.

A lot has happened with gene therapy in a relatively short period of time. One can probably bet that a lot more will happen in an even shorter period of time in the coming years. This commentary dealing with the topic of infectious diseases closes with a *Clinical Fact/Curio*, a who-dun-it. You practice in the state of Connecticut and are seeing an 8-year-old who has developed a painless, 1-cm ulcer over the scapula. This child has been treated with amoxicillin-clavulanate and failed to respond. When taking a more careful history, you note that several weeks previously, the patient's father had developed a painless 2-cm papular lesion with surrounding edema. The father was treated with cephalexin and then clindamycin for a presumptive infected spider bite. After several weeks, however, the father's lesion had failed to resolve. It had progressed to an eschar with lymphangitic spread. The clue to the diagnosis is that the father, as a hobby, makes djembe drums. Your diagnosis?

The 2 cases described are indeed real, presenting to the Connecticut Department of Public Health in the summer of 2007. The father underwent a skin biopsy for his skin lesion. Using a polymerase chain reaction, *Bacillus anthracis* was diagnosed. Three days later, his 8-year-old son was similarly diagnosed, although much more promptly. Needless to say, the Federal Bureau of Investigation (FBI) and the Environmental Protection Agency (EPA) quickly became involved because anthrax is a targeted bioterrorism agent.

So what did the FBI, EPA, and the Connecticut Department of Public Health find? They found that the index patient made traditional West African drums (known as djembe drums) by soaking animal hides in water, stretching them over the drum body, then scraping and sanding the drum surface. In June 2007, a contact in New York City told the index patient that he had some new goat hides from Guinea. The index patient purchased 10 of the goat hides, making the transaction on a street corner in New York City. Whether these goat hides were imported legally is not known. The index patient used 3 of the hides to make drums. This was shortly before he developed cutaneous anthrax. Specimens obtained by the FBI and the EPA included samples obtained by swabbing all of the hides and drum heads. This resulted in positive cultures for *B anthracis*. Anthrax pores were also found in the drum maker's car trunk and were also found throughout the house, including in vacuum samples from the house's upstairs hallway. Federal, state, and local officials completed a comprehensive remediation process that included fumigation of the house with chlorine dioxide. The house and work shed behind the house where this fellow made his drums were completely decontaminated.

In case you think this is a totally isolated event, since 2006, a total of 3 unrelated cases of anthrax have been reported from direct occupational association with the djembe drums made from untreated animal hides from West Africa. The first 2 cases were of inhalation anthrax. One occurred in New York City in a drum maker exposed while making a djembe drum from contaminated hides, and the other occurred in a man in Scotland who died of anthrax septicemia after playing or handling djembe drums newly made from contaminated hides. The third case was the father, who purchased his hides from New York City, described in this report.

Few cases of anthrax have been reported in children in the United States because most exposures are acquired occupationally. However, household members can be exposed through cross-contamination of living areas. In 1978, dust samples from vacuum cleaners in the houses of textile mill workers tested positive for *B anthracis*, suggesting that workers carried spores into their homes. A series of cutaneous anthrax cases in a Pennsylvania mill town indicated that 4% of all cases during a 22-year period occurred in household members of mill workers and their families, including children in the families.

Please note that imported animal hides from West Africa, particularly goat hides, remain in demand because they are prized by drum makers for their acoustical quality. Because anthrax outbreaks in livestock frequently occur in West Africa, hides brought into the United States may contain *B anthracis* spores. The Animal and Plant Health Inspection Service of the US Department of Agriculture has the authority to regulate importation of all animal hides, mainly to protect against the introduction of foreign animal diseases into the United States. However, this agency does not mandate screening of imported hides for *B anthracis*; thus, potentially contaminated hides might continue to be imported. Until a process exists for certifying that imported hides from West Africa are free of anthrax, drum makers should follow current published disinfection guidelines to reduce the risk of disease.[4] To read about the cases of anthrax caused by djembe drum making, see the report in *MMWR*.[5]

J. A. Stockman III, MD

References

1. Cavazzana-Calvo M, Hacein-Bey S, de Saint E, et al. Gene therapy of human severe combined immunodeficiency (SCID)-X-1 disease. *Science*. 2000;288: 669-672.
2. Aiuti A, Slavin S, Aker M, et al. Correction of ADA-SCID by stem cell gene therapy combined with nonmyeloablative conditioning. *Science*. 2002;296: 2410-2413.
3. Gaspar HB, Parsley KL, Howe S, et al. Gene therapy of X-linked severe combined immunodeficiency by use of a pseudo-type gammaretroviral vector. *Lancet*. 2004; 364:2181-2187.

4. Russell AD, Yarnych VS, Koulikovski IA. *Guidelines on Disinfection in Animal Husbandry for Prevention and Control of Zoonotic Diseases.* Geneva, Switzerland: World Health Organizations; 1984, http://whqlibdoc.who.int/hq/pre-wholis/who_vph_84.4.pdf; 1984. Accessed July 23, 2009.
5. Cutaneous anthrax associated with drum making using drum hides from West Africa – Connecticut, 2007 [editorial comment]. *MMWR.* 2008;57:628-631.

11 Miscellaneous

Inequalities in healthy life years in the 25 countries of the European Union in 2005: a cross-national meta-regression analysis
Jagger C, Gillies C, Moscone F, et al (Univ of Leicester, UK; et al)
Lancet 372:2124-2131, 2008

Background.—Although life expectancy in the European Union (EU) is increasing, whether most of these extra years are spent in good health is unclear. This information would be crucial to both contain health-care costs and increase labour-force participation for older people. We investigated inequalities in life expectancies and healthy life years (HLYs) at 50 years of age for the 25 countries in the EU in 2005 and the potential for increasing the proportion of older people in the labour force.

Methods.—We calculated life expectancies and HLYs at 50 years of age by sex and country by the Sullivan method, which was applied to Eurostat life tables and age-specific prevalence of activity limitation from the 2005 statistics of living and income conditions survey. We investigated differences between countries through meta-regression techniques, with structural and sustainable indicators for every country.

Findings.—In 2005, an average 50-year-old man in the 25 EU countries could expect to live until 67·3 years free of activity limitation, and a woman to 68·1 years. HLYs at 50 years for both men and women varied more between countries than did life expectancy (HLY range for men: from 9·1 years in Estonia to 23·6 years in Denmark; for women: from 10·4 years in Estonia to 24·1 years in Denmark). Gross domestic product and expenditure on elderly care were both positively associated with HLYs at 50 years in men and women (p<0·039 for both indicators and sexes); however, in men alone, long-term unemployment was negatively associated (p=0·023) and life-long learning positively associated (p=0·021) with HLYs at 50 years of age.

Interpretation.—Substantial inequalities in HLYs at 50 years exist within EU countries. Our findings suggest that, without major improvements in population health, the target of increasing participation of older people into the labour force will be difficult to meet in all 25 EU countries.

Funding.—EU Public Health Programme.

▶ You see very little in the United States written about healthy life years (HLYs). In Europe, beginning in 2004, the European Commission added a measure of health expectancy to the traditional set of structural indicators under the name of HLYs. HLYs actually is a marker of a number of different factors that tell us how many years of life one can expect to be alive and disability-free from the usual impairments associated with aging. This is an important concept since increasing life expectancy does not in itself mean a healthier population. While the report of Jagger et al emanates from Europe and largely deals with adults, children serve as the initial ingredient, as it were, in overall studies of life expectancy. As one can see from Fig 1, if you are a person living to be 50 years of age, your life expectancy at that point is an additional 30.37 years if you are a man living in Italy and 35.37 years if you are a woman living in France (the best odds of long survivorship). On the other hand, if you are a man living in the European Union (EU) and are age 50, your best chance of having the longest healthy life years is if you live in Denmark (an additional 23.64 years). If you are a woman, it is also Denmark at 24.12 years. The shortest life expectancy for men and women who are age 50 occurs for those living in Latvia (21.31 and 20.32 years, respectively). In those same countries, the number of healthy years left to a 50-year old can be counted

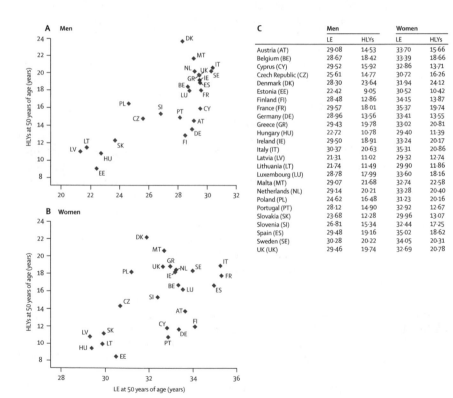

FIGURE 1.—Life expectancy (LE) and healthy life years (HLYs) at 50 years of age for all EU countries HLYs=healthy life years. LE=life expectancy. (A) and (B) show scatter graphs for men and women, respectively. (C) Data for scatter graphs. (Reprinted from Jagger C, Gillies C, Moscone F, et al. Inequalities in healthy life years in the 25 countries of the European Union in 2005: a cross-national meta-regression analysis. *Lancet.* 2008;372:2124-2131, with permission from Elsevier.)

on the fingers of a pair of hands. It is fairly clear that the citizens of the estab-lished European community (15 EU countries) have both longer and healthier lives than do most of the 10 new EU members.

The ultimate trick in life is to die healthy, a statement that is not meant to be an oxymoron. All is well that ends well. This commentary closes with a *Clinical Fact/Curio* presented in the form of a question. Where does the United States now rank in terms of life expectancy in comparison to other countries, and where does it stand among the "most livable" countries in the world? Recently published were rankings of this type. It appears that the United States ranks 42nd in the world for life expectancy, despite spending more on health care per person than any other country, according to a report funded by Oxfam America, the Rockefeller Foundation, and the Conrad Hilton Foundation. Over-all, the United Nation's Human Development index scores showed the United States as the 12th "most livable" country in the world.[1]

J. A. Stockman III, MD

Reference

1. Measure of America [editorial comment]. *Science*. 2008;372:807.

Socioeconomic Inequalities in Health in 22 European Countries

Mackenbach JP, Stirbu I, Roskam A-JR, et al (Univ Med Ctr, Rotterdam, the Netherlands)
N Engl J Med 358:2468-2481, 2008

Background.—Comparisons among countries can help to identify opportunities for the reduction of inequalities in health. We compared the magnitude of inequalities in mortality and self-assessed health among 22 countries in all parts of Europe.

Methods.—We obtained data on mortality according to education level and occupational class from census-based mortality studies. Deaths were classified according to cause, including common causes, such as cardiovas-cular disease and cancer; causes related to smoking; causes related to alcohol use; and causes amenable to medical intervention, such as tubercu-losis and hypertension. Data on self-assessed health, smoking, and obesity according to education and income were obtained from health or multi-purpose surveys. For each country, the association between socioeconomic status and health outcomes was measured with the use of regression-based inequality indexes.

Results.—In almost all countries, the rates of death and poorer self-assessments of health were substantially higher in groups of lower socio-economic status, but the magnitude of the inequalities between groups of higher and lower socioeconomic status was much larger in some coun-tries than in others. Inequalities in mortality were small in some southern European countries and very large in most countries in the eastern and Baltic regions. These variations among countries appeared to be attributable in part to causes of death related to smoking or alcohol use or amenable to medical intervention. The magnitude of inequalities in self-assessed health also varied substantially among countries, but in a different pattern.

Conclusions.—We observed variation across Europe in the magnitude of inequalities in health associated with socioeconomic status. These inequalities might be reduced by improving educational opportunities, income distribution, health-related behavior, or access to health care.

▶ While this report is from Europe, it is of some use to us here in the United States. Specifically, sometimes the easiest way to view ourselves is to look at how others view themselves. The article by Mackenbach et al documents the extraordinary pervasiveness of socioeconomic inequalities in health as well as the varying magnitude of risks among countries of Western and Eastern Europe. The gathering of data from these countries on mortality, morbidity, smoking, and obesity in relation to socioeconomic status allows the authors and us to see the broadest international portrait to date of the association between socioeconomic status and health. Needless to say, the data to some extent surely mirror what we see here in the United States. While the data applied to the effects of these varying factors on adult health, the findings are important to pediatrics because this is the world into which our children will grow unless we do something about it.

So what are the data? First, the results show that in the 16 countries of Eastern and Western Europe that were examined, socioeconomically disadvantaged men and women had higher overall mortality rates than did persons with a higher socioeconomic status. The universal link between social class and mortality is quite remarkable, given the differing disease prevalence and risk factors in these countries. Second, the study shows that the magnitude of risk varies substantially across countries. The ratio of overall mortality rates between those at the opposite end of the socioeconomic spectrum ranges from just over 1.0 (women in Basque country) to nearly 5.0 (men in the Czech Republic). Many of the variations seen are difficult to explain. For example, the risk of death according to class in Nordic countries is greater than that in southern Europe, despite welfare policies in the north that are much better than in Southern Europe, particularly for the most disadvantaged persons. These welfare policies in the northern European countries are aimed at reducing socioeconomic differences. Here in the United States, socioeconomic conditions are usually most strongly related to the risk of cardiovascular disease, yet in countries such as France and Italy, socioeconomic conditions are more strongly related to the risk of cancer than to the risk of cardiovascular disease. Interestingly, Italy and Spain have welfare policies that are significantly less generous and less universal than those of Northern Europe, but they appear to have substantially smaller inequalities in mortality, perhaps partly because of cultural factors, such as the Mediterranean diet and the reluctance of women to take up smoking. Cultural factors seem to have prevented differences in access to material and other resources in these populations from translating into inequalities in lifestyle-related risk factors for mortality.

In an editorial that accompanied this report, Berkman and Epstein note that as we continue to look for ways to reduce socioeconomic differences in health, we must face the reality that there will be no magic bullet.[1] The year 2008 saw a lot of politicking going on during the presidential election run-ups. The presidential candidates focused largely on health insurance and health care as the way to improve health, especially for the most disadvantaged citizens. If there is a lesson to be learned from Europe, this is hardly the magic bullet. Almost all the countries of Eastern and Western Europe have some kind of national health insurance or health care policy, yet wide socioeconomic disparities resulting in health disparities persist in each and every country. Although national health coverage is important for many reasons, none of us should count on it to reduce more than a small part of the socioeconomic, racial, and ethnic disparities we see here in the United States and that underlie much of the health disparity in our population.

This commentary closes with a miscellaneous *Clinical Fact/Curio*. It is estimated that in 2050, there will be 9.1 billion inhabitants of Mother Earth. The question is, how many populated our planet in 1 AD? The answer to this query may be found in a fascinating graph of the likely population of this planet that appeared in the *British Medical Journal* recently.[2] There appears to have been little increase in world population between 160 000 BC and 1000 BC. By 1 AD, the earth's population is estimated to have been 250 million. By 1776, the increase was to 1 billion. By 1945, it was 2.3 billion. In 2006, the world's population was estimated at 6.5 billion. The population growth throughout history shows that world population has roughly quadrupled in the last century. The annual increase in population of about 79 million means that every week an extra 1.5 million people need food and somewhere to live. Every person born adds to greenhouse gas emissions, and escaping poverty is impossible without these emissions increasing.

J. A. Stockman III, MD

References

1. Berkman L, Epstein AM. Beyond healthcare – socioeconomic status and health. *N Engl J Med*. 2008;358:2509-2510.
2. Godlee F. Population control and uncertainty–a doctor's role. *BMJ*. 2008;337: a1076.

Comfort of General Internists and General Pediatricians in Providing Care for Young Adults with Chronic Illnesses of Childhood

Okumura MJ, Heisler M, Davis MM, et al (Univ of California, San Francisco; Univ of Michigan Health System, Ann Arbor; et al)
J Gen Intern Med 23:1621-1627, 2008

Background.—As an increasing number of patients with chronic conditions of childhood survive to adulthood, experts recommend that young adults with chronic conditions transfer from child-focused to adult-focused primary care. Little, however, is known about how comfortable physicians are caring for this population.

Objectives.—To assess the comfort of general internists and general pediatricians in treating young adult patients with chronic illnesses originating in childhood as well as the factors associated with comfort.

Participants.—In a random sample, 1288 of 2434 eligible US general internists and pediatricians completed a mailed survey (response rate = 53%).

Methods.—We measured respondents' comfort level in providing primary care for a patient with sickle cell disease (SCD) or cystic fibrosis (CF). We also measured levels of disease familiarity, training and subspecialty support, as well as individual physician characteristics.

Results.—Fifteen percent of general internists reported being comfortable as the primary care provider for adults with CF and 32% reported being comfortable providing primary care for adults with SCD, compared with 38% of pediatricians for CF (p < .001) and 35% for SCD (p > 0.05). Less than half of general internists felt that their specialty should take primary care responsibility for adult patients with CF and SCD.

Conclusions.—A majority of general internists and pediatricians are not comfortable providing primary care for young adults with chronic illnesses of childhood origin, such as CF and SCD. Efforts to increase treatment comfort among providers may help with the transition to adult-focused care for the growing numbers of young adults with complex chronic conditions.

▶ As more and more pediatric age patients survive into adulthood with complex medical problems including subspecialty ones, the issue of transition of care has become more critical. Obviously, pediatricians are familiar with the management of many of these diseases, but uncomfortable with caring for the child who has become an adult, particularly given the fact that many of these medical conditions begin to be associated with other adult comorbid problems. At the same time, most internists have become inundated with the care of the elderly and when a relatively few young patients in their practices appear with complex problems, they tend to shy away from the latter.

To effectively meet the needs of the growing adult population with chronic conditions of childhood origin, several professional societies have advocated formal "transitioning," defined as the purposeful planned movement of adolescents and young adults with chronic physical and medical conditions from child-centered to adult-oriented health care systems. In 2002, the American Academy of Pediatrics, American College of Physicians-American Society of Internal Medicine, and the American Academy of Family Physicians released a consensus statement that all adults with special care needs deserve an adult-focused primary care physician.[1] It was also suggested in this recommendation that such transitioning could occur as early as 14 years of age, obviously depending on the condition. The report of Okumura et al show just how little has occurred in the last half dozen or more years since the publication of this recommendation in terms of "comfortableness" of internists and pediatricians with dealing with the transitional age patient.

Clearly, the problem of transition of care from pediatric care providers to adult providers is a mounting problem. One example of this is survivors with congenital heart disease. There are now more adult patients with congenital heart disease than there are pediatric patients, a sign of some significant success on our part. Nonetheless, many of these survivors find little reciprocal expertise on the adult side in terms of numbers of specialists who are familiar with the problems they have. This is a remediable issue and it is time to get going on it.

This commentary closes with a *Clinical Fact/Curio* about life expectancy. It is posed in the form of a question. What country in the United Kingdom has the highest rate of spending on health, but the poorest life expectancy? Figures from the Office for National Statistics show that Scotland has the highest health spending in the United Kingdom and the poorest life expectancy. Health and social care spending per head in Scotland ran £2313 ($4543) in 2006-2007, compared with £1915 in England (the lowest). The life expectancy at birth in Scotland was 74.6 years for men and 79.6 years for women, compared with 77.2 years for men and 81.5 years for women in England.[2]

J. A. Stockman III, MD

References

1. American Academy of Pediatrics, American Academy of Family Physicians, American College of Physicians - American Society of Internal Medicine. A consensus statement on healthcare transitions for young adults with special care needs. *Pediatrics*. 2002;110:1304-1306.
2. Scotland's life expectancy lowest in UK [editorial comment]. *BMJ*. 2008;336: 1328.

Awareness and Use of California's Paid Family Leave Insurance Among Parents of Chronically III Children

Schuster MA, Chung PJ, Elliott MN, et al (RAND, Santa Monica, California; et al)
JAMA 300:1047-1055, 2008

Context.—In 2004, California's Paid Family Leave Insurance Program (PFLI) became the first state program to provide paid leave to care for an ill family member.

Objective.—To assess awareness and use of the program by employed parents of children with special health care needs, a population likely to need leave.

Design, Setting, and Participants.—Telephone interviews with successive cohorts of employed parents before (November 21, 2003-January 31, 2004; n = 754) and after (November 18, 2005-January 31, 2006; n = 766) PFLI began, randomly sampled from 2 children's hospitals, one in California (with PFLI) and the other in Illinois (without PFLI).

Response rates were 82% before and 81% after (California), and 80% before and 74% after (Illinois).

Main Outcome Measures.—Taking leave, length of leave, unmet need for leave, and awareness and use of PFLI.

Results.—Similar percentages of parents at the California site reported taking at least 1 day of leave to care for their ill child before (295 [81%]) and after (327 [79%]) PFLI, taking at least 4 weeks before (64 [21%]) and after (74 [19%]) PFLI, and at least once in the past year not missing work despite believing their child's illness necessitated it before (152 [41%]) and after (156 [41%]) PFLI. Relative to Illinois, parents at the California site reported no change from before to after PFLI in taking at least 1 day of leave (difference of differences, −3%; 95% confidence interval [CI], −13% to 7%); taking at least 4 weeks of leave (1%; 95% CI, −9% to 10%); or not missing work, despite believing their child's illness necessitated it (−1%; 95% CI, −13% to 10%). Only 77 parents (18%) had heard of PFLI approximately 18 months after the program began, and only 20 (5%) had used it. Even among parents without other access to paid leave, awareness and use of PFLI were minimal.

Conclusions.—Parents of children with special health care needs receiving care at a California hospital were generally unaware of PFLI and rarely used it. Among parents of children with special health care

TABLE 6.—Reasons for Not Using PFLI Among Employed Parents at California Site (After PFLI Began) Who Had Heard of PFLI But Did Not Use It[a]

Reasons for Not Using PFLI	No. (%) of Parents (n = 57)
You used sick leave, vacation, or other paid time off instead	34 (59)
You did not know about or understand the program	21 (41)
You missed less than the mandatory 1-week waiting period	8 (11)
Your supervisors told you not to take time off even though you were eligible	3 (10)
You were afraid of being demoted or fired	5 (7)
The application process was too difficult or inconvenient	5 (7)
You were afraid of losing good job assignments or opportunities for career advancement	4 (6)
You were afraid that supervisors or coworkers might resent your taking time off	3 (4)
Your employer told you that you were not eligible	1 (2)
Your supervisors or coworkers asked you not to take time off	0

Abbreviation: PFLI, Paid Family Leave Insurance Program.
[a]California site indicates Mattel Children's Hospital, University of California, Los Angeles.

needs, taking leave in California did not increase after PFLI implementation compared with Illinois (Table 6).

▶ It has been 15 years since the federal Family and Medical Leave Act (FMLA) went into effect. FMLA provides job-protected leave for up to 12 weeks after the birth of a child and to care for an immediate family member (spouse, child, or parent) with a serious health condition. Unfortunately, this act has had limited success in part because there has been no provision for paid leave. As part of an effort to correct some of the deficiencies in the federal legislation, several states have adopted their own paid family leave legislation. California is an example. This state was the first to offer a paid leave insurance program. In 2004, nonjob protected family leave for workers caring for a child, spouse, domestic partner, or parent with a serious health condition became available. After missing 1 week of work, employees can receive up to 6 weeks of coverage at 55% of pay (maximum $917 per week) in 2008. Until the report of Schuster et al appeared, we had no information about how the California experience helped parents of chronically ill children. What we learn is the program has not been associated with increased rates of parents taking leave after the legislation was enacted. Eighty-one percent of parents in California and 78% of parents in Illinois with children with special health care needs took 1 or more days of leave to care for an ill child before the legislation, and 79% of parents in California and 79% of parents in Illinois did so afterward. Illinois has no additional provisions for family leave beyond the federal legislation, and thus this state served as the control state. Unfortunately, 18% of California families were unaware of the paid family leave insurance program following its enactment. The study from California shows that despite the documented need to support families with chronically ill children, the state legislation has not been effective in improving that support. Reasons for the lack of effectiveness may include the lack of awareness of the legislation and a perceived lack of protection against job loss or losing career opportunities.

It is important to learn from the California experience. Additional states have either passed or are considering paid family leave legislation. New Jersey's legislation passed in 2008 and is generally similar to California's legislation; Washington State has passed a law similar to California's that will be in place in 2009. Oregon and New York are expected to consider family leave legislation in 2009 as well. If the California legislation serves as a model for other states, its strengths and weaknesses must be carefully analyzed. The strengths include the fact that California's paid leave program includes parents of chronically ill children, has identified a funding source, and covers up to 6 weeks of work leave. Weaknesses are that only 55% of the employee's income is covered, there is not wage protection beyond 6 weeks, and continuing employment is not ensured. Thus, parents will still continue to incur a fair amount of economic stress. At a minimum, future legislation should ensure that use of available state funds will not affect future employment or job opportunities. It is also important to assure employers that paid family leave will not be used frivolously. This requires a specific definition of "a child with serious illness." The latter is discussed in some detail in an editorial that accompanied the report of Schuster et al.[1]

As this commentary closes, another *Clinical Fact/Curio*, this having to do with population statistics. Can you explain why there is a very real possibility that death rates will spike in 2010, but fall in 2011? The answer to this question raises the theoretical issue of the impact of the estate taxes on death rates. The estate tax in the United States falls temporarily to zero in 2010, thanks to legislation passed in the early years of the Bush administration. One observer anticipates ethical problems as the tax bounces back up again to a top rate of 55% in 2011, creating a large financial incentive for people and care providers to orchestrate deaths preferentially during the tax holiday. Almost 2.5 million people nearing the end of their lives could theoretically be affected. Those expecting to die at the end of 2009 might be motivated to accept aggressive life-prolonging treatment to help them survive until 2010. Those in their final illness at the end of 2010 might consider (or be coerced into) an earlier death in return for large financial rewards for their heirs. As the law stood at the beginning of 2010, dying in the wrong year could cost millions of dollars to those with moderate and large estates.

Only time will tell whether there is any impact on estate taxes and death rates. We will all stay tuned.[2]

J. A. Stockman III, MD

References

1. Neff JM. Paid family leave for parents of chronically ill children. *JAMA*. 2008; 300:1080-1081.
2. Tax break could distort care of the dying in the United States [editorial comment]. *Ann Intern Med*. 2008;149:822-824.

Staff-Only Pediatric Hospitalist Care of Patients With Medically Complex Subspecialty Conditions in a Major Teaching Hospital
Bekmezian A, Chung PJ, Yazdani SA (David Geffen School of Medicine at UCLA, Los Angeles)
Arch Pediatr Adolesc Med 162:975-980, 2008

Objective.—To assess cost and length of stay for subspecialty patients on a staff-only general pediatric hospitalist service vs traditional faculty/housestaff subspecialty services in a major teaching hospital.

Design.—Retrospective study of 2 cohort groups: a staff-only general pediatric hospitalist group and subspecialty faculty/housestaff gastroenterology and hematology/oncology groups.

Setting.—Major referral center providing full-spectrum, complex surgical, and subspecialty care including transplantation.

Participants.—Nine hundred twenty-five pediatric patients with gastroenterologic and hematologic/oncologic diseases admitted and discharged between July 1, 2005, and June 30, 2006.

Main Exposure.—Patients with gastroenterologic and hematologic/oncologic diseases were assigned to the hospitalist team when faculty/housestaff teams reached their maximum census of patients per intern.

Main Outcome Measures.—Cost, length of stay, mortality, and readmission to the hospital within 72 hours of discharge.

Results.—Cost averaged $11 000 and $16 500, respectively, for patients on the hospitalist service compared with those on nonhospitalist services. On average, length of stay was 7.2 days and 9.8 days, respectively. In negative binomial regression analyses controlling for subspecialty, demographic data, disease severity, and average daily census, patients on the hospitalist service had 29% lower costs ($P < .05$) and 38% fewer hospital days ($P < .01$) per admission compared with patients on subspecialty faculty/housestaff services, with no clear differences in mortality and readmission rates.

Conclusion.—Compared with the subspecialist faculty/housestaff system, the staff-only pediatric hospitalist system was associated with a marked reduction in cost and length of stay for patients with medically complex subspecialty diseases. In this era of resident duty-hour restrictions and medical complexity of conditions in inpatients, staff-only hospitalist programs may have a vital role in pediatric teaching hospitals.

▶ This is an interesting report that extends our knowledge of the value of pediatric hospitalists. While a number of reports have appeared previously in the literature that document the fact that hospitalists improve costs, and reduce length of stay, this study from Los Angeles is the first to show how well hospitalists perform in a staff only model in which the hospitalist provided care for complex subspecialty conditions. In this model, the hospitalist team, operating at UCLA Hospital and Medical Center that included the Mattel Children's Hospital, provided care for patients Monday through Friday from 8:00 AM to 5:00 PM without daytime coverage from other faculty or house staff. The hospitalist team cared almost exclusively for overflow patients from the gastroenterology and hematology-oncology services, consulting the subspecialist primarily about subspecialty-specific procedures. The roles of the subspecialty attending physician and fellow in the care of hospitalist patients included ordering chemotherapy, ordering immunosuppression for patients with transplants, and performing endoscopy, liver biopsy, bone marrow biopsy, and intrathecal chemotherapy. Otherwise, the hospitalist was responsible for all other day-to-day management of the patients. House staff did cover these patients on nights and weekends, however.

So what do we learn from this report of hospitalists providing care for complex subspecialty patients? We do see a longer length of stay and higher cost in comparison with most other hospitalist studies, but this is likely due to the patient population having a much higher severity of illness given their complex subspecialty diagnoses. However, cost averaged $11 000 and $16 500 respectively for patients on the hospitalist service compared with those on the nonhospitalist services. The length of stay was also shorter (7.2 days vs 9.8 days).

You will have to be the judge of how valid the data are from this report. Obviously, this investigation was carried out at a single medical center with a relatively new hospitalist service. Also, the average daily census per hospitalist service was lower than on the faculty/house staff services, but then again, the hospitalist was acting in isolation in comparison with the teaching services. Nonetheless, the findings from this report suggest that adoption of staff-only hospitalist programs in United States pediatric teaching hospitals may in fact be of some merit. Once fully up to speed on the management of complex subspecialty problems, these hospitalists become extraordinarily invaluable to everyone in the hospital setting.

This commentary closes with another *Clinical Fact/Curio*, this having to do with the miscellaneous topic of systems-based practice. If you are into the design of high efficiency health care systems, recognize that there will be fewer patients showing up for their appointed scheduled office visits on certain days. For example, a recent report from Great Britain has found that attendance at clinics at 2 London hospitals fell by 14% throughout the 2006 World Cup Tournament. Kept appointments fell by 55% on key match days as a result of people not turning up for their routine appointments.[1]

Many in the United States have noticed the same thing. Never try scheduling an appointment for patients whose demographics show that they are addicted to early afternoon soap operas.

J. A. Stockman III, MD

Reference

1. Major football tournament cuts hospital attendance [editorial comment]. *BMJ*. 2007;335:956.

Trends in Pediatric and Adult Bicycling Deaths Before and After Passage of a Bicycle Helmet Law
Wesson DE, Stephens D, Lam K, et al (Texas Children's Hosp, Houston; Hosp for Sick Children Research Inst, Toronto, ON, Canada; Inst for Clinical Evaluative Sciences, Toronto, ON, Canada; et al)
Pediatrics 122:605-610, 2008

Objectives.—The goals were to examine bicycle-related mortality rates in Ontario, Canada, from 1991 to 2002 among bicyclists 1 to 15 years of age and 16 years of age through adulthood and to determine the effect of legislation (introduced in October 1995 for bicyclists <18 years of age) on mortality rates.

Methods.—The average numbers of deaths per year and mortality rates per 100 000 person-years for the prelegislation and postlegislation periods, and the percentage changes, were calculated for each of the 2 age groups (1–15 years and ≥16 years). Differences before and after legislation in the 2 age groups were modeled in a time series analysis.

Results.—There were 362 bicycle-related deaths in the 12-year period (1–15 years: 107 deaths; ≥16 years: 255 deaths). For bicyclists 1 to 15 years of age, the average number of deaths per year decreased 52%, the mortality rate per 100 000 person-years decreased 55%, and the time series analysis demonstrated a significant reduction in deaths after legislation. The estimated change in the number of deaths per month was −0.59 deaths per month. For bicyclists ≥16 years of age, there were only slight changes in the average number of deaths per year and the mortality rate per 100 000 person-years, and the time series analysis demonstrated no significant change in deaths after legislation.

Conclusions.—The bicycle-related mortality rate in children 1 to 15 years of age has decreased significantly, which may be attributable in part to helmet legislation. A similar reduction for bicyclists 16 years of age through adulthood was not identified. These findings support promotion of helmet use, enforcement of the existing law, and extension of the law to adult bicyclists.

▶ This report is from Toronto Canada, but the findings most likely equally apply to the situation south of the Canadian border. Bill 124, an act to amend the highway traffic act requiring all persons under the age of 18 riding a bicycle on a public highway in Toronto to wear a helmet, was passed by the legislature in 1993 with enforcement beginning in the last quarter of 1995. For violators under the age of 16, parents are fined. Sixteen- and 17-year-olds are fined directly. The law does not apply to bicyclists 18 and over.

So did implementation of this helmet law do any good? Indeed it did. The bicycle-related mortality rate for children 1 to 15 years of age decreased from 0.81 deaths per 100 000 person years in 1985-1989 to just 0.27 deaths 100 000 person years in 1995 to 2002. No improvement was seen in the death rate for those 16 and older. Given the fact that little else had been done to improve bicycle riding safety, the reduction in mortality rate in the younger age group seemed to be directly attributable, at least in part, to the introduction of helmet legislation.

The situation in the United States is probably similar to the experience in Canada. Grant and Rutner modeled the effect of helmet legislation on bicycling fatalities in the United States during the period 1975 to 2000, using data from the Fatality Analysis Reporting System.[1] Among children, bicycle fatality rates decreased to one-third over the study period. Among adults, bicycling fatality rates increased modestly. Using regression model analysis, the authors concluded that statewide helmet laws reduce fatality rates by roughly 15%. These findings and others strongly argue for enforcement of the existing law as it applies to bicyclists, at least those in the pediatric age group.

One other comment having to do with safety on the roads, this related to seatbelt use among high school students. A recent report suggests that while the majority (59%) of high school students always use seat belts while driving, a distinct minority (42%) always buckled up as passengers.[2] A fair percentage of passenger deaths in motor vehicle accidents involving teens occur with lack of seat belt use by passengers in the rear seat of motor vehicles. Currently, only a minority of states uniformly require teen motor vehicle occupants in the rear seat to be secured in seat belts. This is a great opportunity to entice our legislatures to be more proactive in tightening up seat belt laws.[3]

J. A. Stockman III, MD

References

1. Grant D, Rutner SM. The effect of bicycle helmet legislation on bicycling fatalities. *J Policy Ann Manag.* 2004;23:595-611.
2. Briggs NC, Lambert EW, Goldzweig IA, Levine RS, Warren RC. Driver and passenger seatbelt use among US high school students. *Am J Prev Med.* 2008; 35:224-228.
3. National Highway Traffic Safety Administration. *Seat Belt Use in 2005–Demographic Results. DT HS 809 969.* Washington, DC: US Department of Transportation; 2005.

Recurrent Rearrangements of Chromosome 1q21.1 and Variable Pediatric Phenotypes
Mefford HC, Sharp AJ, Baker C, et al (Univ of Washington School of Medicine; Univ of Geneva Med School; et al)
N Engl J Med 359:1685-1699, 2008

Background.—Duplications and deletions in the human genome can cause disease or predispose persons to disease. Advances in technologies to detect these changes allow for the routine identification of submicroscopic imbalances in large numbers of patients.

Methods.—We tested for the presence of microdeletions and microduplications at a specific region of chromosome 1q21.1 in two groups of patients with unexplained mental retardation, autism, or congenital anomalies and in unaffected persons.

Results.—We identified 25 persons with a recurrent 1.35-Mb deletion within 1q21.1 from screening 5218 patients. The microdeletions had arisen de novo in eight patients, were inherited from a mildly affected parent in three patients, were inherited from an apparently unaffected parent in six patients, and were of unknown inheritance in eight patients. The deletion was absent in a series of 4737 control persons $(P = 1.1 \times 10^{-7})$. We found considerable variability in the level of phenotypic expression of the microdeletion; phenotypes included mild-to-moderate mental retardation, microcephaly, cardiac abnormalities, and cataracts. The reciprocal duplication was enriched in nine children with mental retardation or autism spectrum disorder and other variable features $(P = 0.02)$. We identified three deletions and three duplications of the 1q21.1 region in an independent sample of 788 patients with mental retardation and congenital anomalies.

Conclusions.—We have identified recurrent molecular lesions that elude syndromic classification and whose disease manifestations must be considered in a broader context of development as opposed to being assigned to a specific disease. Clinical diagnosis in patients with these lesions may be most readily achieved on the basis of genotype rather than phenotype.

▶ This report is a bit of a "hard" read, but an important read for all of us because it teaches us much about recent technology advances in the field of genetics. These recent advances have included the ability now to routinely detect submicroscopic deletions and duplications using comparative genomic hybridization techniques. In the last 10 years or so, we have begun to recognize that the phenotypes associated with imbalances of some regions of the genome can be variable, and modifiers must therefore play an important role in the expression of the genetic abnormality some individuals have. Thus it becomes important to ascertain and describe the specific chromosomal rearrangements that affect the spectrum of phenotypes associated with them. The report of Mefford et al does just that, summarizing the presence of microdeletions and microduplications at a specific region of chromosome 1q21.1 in 2 groups of patients with unexplained mental retardation, autism, or congenital anomalies and in unaffected persons. The investigators have previously described an individual with a deletion of 1q21.1 and another with an overlapping duplication in a series of 390 persons screened by array-based comparative genomic hybridization (CGH) assays. These individuals had global delay, growth retardation, and seizures as well as some degree of facial dysmorphism. The new data reported show that 1q21.1 deletions are associated with a broad array of pediatric developmental abnormalities. The findings show a considerable phenotypic diversity. Among the findings in these patients are heart defects, cataract, müllerian aplasia, autism, and schizophrenia.

So what is the importance of the findings presented in this report? The results do seem to emphasize the significance of rare structural variants in human disease. They further demonstrate the challenges this new information presents. First, large samples of patients and controls are required to show that a specific genetic variant is pathogenic. Although there have been several reports of patients with 1q21.1 deletions in studies of specific diseases, the study reported shows that recurrent 1q21.1 microdeletions are significantly associated with pediatric disease, as shown through systematic comparison of the frequency of rearrangements in affected and unaffected persons. Detailed clinical evaluations of these affected individuals now discloses a much broader spectrum of phenotypes than was anticipated, dispelling any notion of a simple syndromic disease. Needless to say, the phenotypic diversity, incomplete penetrance, and lack of distinct syndromic features associated with 1q21.1 rearrangements will complicate genetic diagnosis and counseling. For those caring for patients with developmental abnormalities, the identification of a 1q21.1 rearrangement by means of a diagnostic array-based CGH should be considered a clinically significant finding and probably an influential genetic factor contributing to the phenotype the patient is presenting with. If one evaluates other family members, one very well may find unaffected persons carrying the same rearrangement. Given the wide spectrum of possible outcomes associated with 1q21.1 rearrangements, such persons should be monitored in the long-term for learning disabilities, autism, or schizophrenia or other neuropsychiatric disorders. A really great challenge is what to do about counseling in the prenatal setting. Although the likelihood of an abnormal outcome is high in an individual with a 1q21.1 rearrangement, our current state of knowledge does not allow us to predict which abnormalities will occur in any given person.

Needless to say, the more we learn about rearrangements of chromosome 1q21.1, the more we learn that we need to learn a lot more. Nonetheless, it is clear that the genetics laboratory capable of performing CGH assays is needed to fully evaluate youngsters with unexplained, but apparently genetic abnormalities.

J. A. Stockman III, MD

Infection and sudden unexpected death in infancy: a systematic retrospective case review
Weber MA, Klein NJ, Hartley JC, et al (Univ College London, UK)
Lancet 371:1848-1853, 2008

Background.—The cause and mechanism of most cases of sudden unexpected death in infancy (SUDI) remain unknown, despite specialist autopsy examination. We reviewed autopsy results to determine whether infection was a cause of SUDI.

Methods.—We did a systematic retrospective case review of autopsies, done at one specialist centre between 1996 and 2005, of 546 infants (aged 7–365 days) who died suddenly and unexpectedly. Cases of SUDI were categorised as unexplained, explained with histological evidence of bacterial infection, or explained by non-infective causes. Microbial isolates gathered at autopsy were classified as non-pathogens, group 1 pathogens (organisms usually associated with an identifiable focus of infection), or group 2 pathogens (organisms known to cause septicaemia without an obvious focus of infection).

Findings.—Of 546 SUDI cases, 39 autopsies were excluded because of viral or pneumocystis infection or secondary bacterial infection after initial collapse and resuscitation. Bacteriological sampling was done in 470 (93%) of the remaining 507 autopsies. 2079 bacteriological samples were taken, of which 571 (27%) were sterile. Positive cultures yielded 2871 separate isolates, 484 (32%) of which showed pure growth and 1024 (68%) mixed growth. Significantly more isolates from infants whose deaths were explained by bacterial infection (78/322, 24%) and from those whose death was unexplained (440/2306, 19%) contained group 2 pathogens than did those from infants whose death was explained by a non-infective cause (27/243, 11%; difference 13·1%, 95% CI 6·9–19·2, p<0·0001 *vs* bacterial infection; and 8·0%, 3·2–11·8, p=0·001 *vs* unexplained). Significantly more cultures from infants whose deaths were unexplained contained *Staphylococcus aureus* (262/1628, 16%) or *Escherichia coli* (93/1628; 6%) than did those from infants whose deaths were of non-infective cause (*S aureus*: 19/211, 9%; difference 7·1%, 95%

CI 2·2–10·8, p=0·005; *E coli*: 3/211, 1%, difference 4·3%, 1·5–5·9, p=0·003).

Interpretation.—Although many post-mortem bacteriological cultures in SUDI yield organisms, most seem to be unrelated to the cause of death. The high rate of detection of group 2 pathogens, particularly *S aureus* and *E coli*, in otherwise unexplained cases of SUDI suggests that these bacteria could be associated with this condition.

▶ As the authors of this report remind us, sudden infant death (SIDS) remains one of the most common presentations of infant death in the postnatal period. While there have been many theories raised as to its etiology, the disorder has remained an enigma. Most SIDS occurs in the age group 7 to 365 days. Investigators have long suspected a role for infection in unexplained SIDS. The most consistent and characteristic feature of unexplained SIDS is the relation of the incidence with age. The number of cases rises rapidly from birth to peak at 8 to 10 weeks, then the number falls such that SIDS deaths are uncommon after 6 months of age and are truly rare by a year postpartum. One could speculate that this age profile is reciprocal to an infant's serum concentration of immunoglobulin that protects against infections by bacteria and bacterial toxins. A long time ago, suspicion focused on *Staphylococcus aureus* and *Escherichia coli* infections as an etiology. These bacteria are commonly present, beginning their colonization of infants early in life. Toxins from *S aureus* and *E coli* interact synergistically with each other and with nicotine to cause death in animal models. Smoking is a known risk factor for SIDS.

Gilbert et al[1] obtained throat swabs from 95 cases of SIDS and 190 healthy age-matched community controls. Curiously, *S aureus*, coliforms, *Streptococcus pneumoniae*, and group B streptococci were more common in samples from infants dying of SIDS. The rub here is that the interpretation of postmortem bacteriology is clearly fraught with problems. For example, while a bacterial isolate from blood or spleen could indicate genuine infection, it could just as well be due to spread from mucosal surfaces at the time of death or during active resuscitation. Translocation of bacteria from mucosal surfaces is also possible after death if the body is not appropriately stored. Worse yet, contamination of samples is quite common at autopsy. What Weber et al now show are data regarding bacteriological results from 507 cases of SIDS. Collected over 10 years, this series includes 379 cases of unexplained SIDS, 72 cases of which appear to be specific causes of SIDS not due to infection, and 56 cases of SIDS diagnosed due to infection on the basis of postmortem histology. Deaths caused by infection were in slightly older children than those in the other 2 groups, but the age distributions of the unexplained SIDS group and the explained noninfection group were the same. This is important because bacterial mucosal carriage is strongly age dependent. The bacterial isolates were classified into 3 groups: (1) nonpathogens; (2) group 1 pathogens, which are organisms usually associated with a recognizable focus of infection; and (3) group 2 pathogens, which are organisms known to cause septicemia without an obvious cause. The data show that group 2 pathogens were more common in the explained infection group and the unexplained

SIDS group than in the explained SIDS noninfection group. In particular, *S aureus* and *E coli* were more commonly found in the unexplained SIDS group than in cases of noninfective explained.

Even the authors of this report stress that association does not mean causation, but if one takes this work together with previous studies, there is some support for the idea that *S aureus* and *E coli* could have causal roles at least in some cases of unexplained SIDS.

Most evidence now indicates that death in unexplained SIDS is often rapid, with a transition from well-being to death in less than 1 hour in many cases. If bacteria have a role in the causation of SIDS, this points to a direct action of bacterial toxins on cardiorespiratory activity or neural control. Soon we will know more about this. The new science of proteomics offers fascinating techniques to recognize bacterial protein products in human bodily fluids. Using proteomics, investigators will soon be investigating this potential aspect of causation of SIDS.

J. A. Stockman III, MD

Reference

1. Gilbert R, Rudd P, Bery PJ, et al. Combined effect of infection and heavy wrapping of the risk of sudden infant death in infancy. *Arch Dis Child*. 1992;67:171-177.

Sudden Infant Death Syndrome: Changing Epidemiologic Patterns in California 1989-2004

Chang R-KR, Keens TG, Rodriguez S, et al (Harbor-UCLA Med Ctr, Torrance, CA; Univ of Southern California, Los Angeles)
J Pediatr 153:498-502, 2008

Objective.—To evaluate the changes of sudden infant death syndrome (SIDS) epidemiology in California.

Study Design.—We used 1989 to 2004 California statewide death registry data. SIDS cases were selected by "age of decedent" <1 year and "cause of death" listed as SIDS.

Results.—We identified 6303 cases (61% males) of SIDS. SIDS incidence rate decreased by 77%, from 1.38 per 1000 births in 1989 to 0.31 per 1000 births in 2004. No further decrease in SIDS incidence was noted from 2002 to 2004. The incidence rate was highest among blacks (2.02 per 1000 births) and lowest in Asian/Pacific Islanders (0.46 per 1000 births). The overall median age at death was 82 days, with no significant change over time. However, the peak age at death shifted from 2 months of age in 1989 to 2001 to 3 months of age in 2002 to 2004. Seasonal variation in the incidence of SIDS was attenuated. The difference in incidence rates between weekdays and weekends increased over the study period.

Conclusions.—The incidence rate of SIDS declined in California from 1989 to 2001, with no further decline after 2002. Several epidemiologic changes were noted: The peak age of SIDS death shifted from 2 months

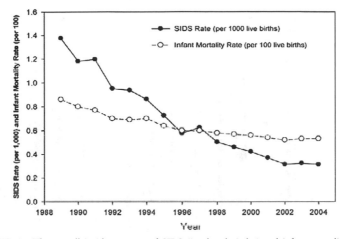

FIGURE 1.—The overall incidence rates of SIDS (in closed circles) and infant mortality (in open circles) in California, 1989-2004. The SIDS incidence rate is calculated as per 1000 live births on the y-axis, infant mortality rate is calculated as per 100 live births on the y-axis. (Reprinted from Chang R-KR, Keens TG, Rodriguez S, et al. Sudden infant death syndrome: changing epidemiologic patterns in California 1989-2004. *J Pediatr.* 2008;153:498-502, with permission from Elsevier.)

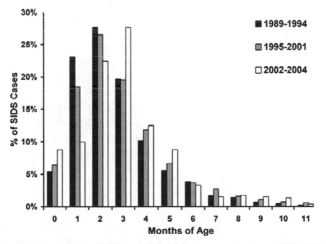

FIGURE 4.—Peak age at death of SIDS cases in California, comparing 3 eras: 1989–1994, 1995–2001, and 2002–2004. (Reprinted from Chang R-KR, Keens TG, Rodriguez S, et al. Sudden infant death syndrome: changing epidemiologic patterns in California 1989-2004. *J Pediatr.* 2008;153:498-502, with permission from Elsevier.)

to 3 months of age; seasonal variation diminished; and weekday to weekend difference became more pronounced.

▶ The goal of this study reported from California was to examine the sudden infant death syndrome (SIDS) incidence rates among California infants over the period 1989 to 2004 in order to evaluate the changes in SIDS epidemiology

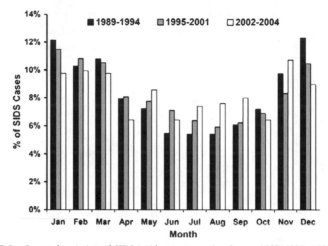

FIGURE 5.—Seasonal variation of SIDS incidence, comparing 3 eras: 1989–1994, 1995–2001, and 2002–2004. (Reprinted from Chang R-KR, Keens TG, Rodriguez S, et al. Sudden infant death syndrome: changing epidemiologic patterns in California 1989-2004. *J Pediatr*. 2008;153:498-502, with permission from Elsevier.)

before and a decade after the launch of the national Back-to-Sleep campaign. The hypothesis was that one would find changes in epidemiologic trends of SIDS once the sleep positioning component risk was diminished. As suspected as a result of the Back-to-Sleep program, there was a progressive and steady decrease in SIDS rates, which actually began shortly before the Back-to-Sleep campaign was initiated, presumably due to an increased awareness of the risk of prone sleeping among the more highly educated portions of the populations of California. Notably, although the SIDS incidence decreased significantly during the 1990s, a plateau was reached around the year 2002 with no further significant decline observed. One might think that the Back-to-Sleep campaign therefore had reached its maximal effectiveness, but it is also possible that given the success of the Back-to-Sleep campaign, less attention and funding for research and intervention has occurred in the interval recent years. One other possibility is that the Back-to-Sleep campaign worked for certain types of causes of SIDS, but other causes persist, an important component of the information provided by this report. This is consistent with the observation that the age of peak SIDS incidence by month of age shifted from 2 months (third month of life) to 3 months of age (fourth month of life) in the period before and after the Back-to-Sleep program, allowing the speculation that this change of peak incidence age may reflect the heterogeneity of the underlying etiologies of SIDS and the alterations of contributions by various etiologies with the implementation of the Back-to-Sleep campaign. One could hypothesize that the Back-to-Sleep campaign (Figs 1, 4, and 5) affected the respiratory causes of SIDS but not other potential causes such as those that might be cardiac or metabolic based.

The bottom line from this report is that in the post Back-to-Sleep period, we have hit a brick wall and that it is incumbent upon us to define other causes of

SIDS if we are going to achieve greater gains in preventing this problem. We know what some of these are already including deprived socioeconomic status, maternal smoking during pregnancy, co-sleeping, or bed-sharing. Surely there are other risk factors as well.

A report of Fu et al provides us with some new insights about risk factors for SIDS.[1] These investigators looked at demographic information and infant care practices among 708 mothers of infants age 0 to 8 months and found that a total of 48.6% of mothers room-shared without bed sharing, 32.5% bed-shared, and 18.9% slept in separate rooms. They also found that compared with infants who slept in separate rooms, infants who room-shared without bed-sharing were more likely to be Hispanic (odds ratio 2.58) and younger (3.66). Compared with infants who bed-shared, infants who room-shared without bed-sharing were more likely to be 0 to 1 month old and less likely to be African-American. In the aggregate, approximately one-third of mothers and infants bed-share despite the fact that this is known to increase the risk of SIDS.

In the United States, SIDS remains the third most common cause of death in infants and the most common cause of death in infants 1 month to 1 year of age. The greatest risk of SIDS remains in low-income populations where the mother is still a teen. We need to learn more about why parents bed-share in order to effectively identify appropriate interventions to change typical and customary practices of infants sleep location in certain populations.

J. A. Stockman III, MD

Reference

1. Fu LY, Colson ER, Corwin MJ, et al. Infants–sleep location: associated maternal and infant characteristics with sudden infant death syndrome prevention recommendations. *J Pediatr.* 153:503-508.

Use of a Fan During Sleep and the Risk of Sudden Infant Death Syndrome
Coleman-Phox K, Odouli R, Li D-K (Kaiser Permanente Northern California, Oakland)
Arch Pediatr Adolesc Med 162:963-968, 2008

Objective.—To examine the relation between room ventilation during sleep and risk of sudden infant death syndrome (SIDS).

Design.—Population-based case-control study.

Setting.—Eleven California counties.

Participants.—Mothers of 185 infants with a confirmed SIDS diagnosis and 312 randomly selected infants matched on county of residence, maternal race/ethnicity, and age.

Intervention.—Fan use and open window during sleep.

Main Outcome Measure.—Risk of SIDS.

Results.—Fan use during sleep was associated with a 72% reduction in SIDS risk (adjusted odds ratio [AOR], 0.28; 95% confidence interval [CI], 0.10-0.77). The reduction in SIDS risk seemed more pronounced in adverse sleep environments. For example, fan use in warmer room temperatures was associated with a greater reduction in SIDS risk (AOR, 0.06; 95% CI, 0.01-0.52) compared with cooler room temperatures (0.77; 0.22-2.73). Similarly, the reduction associated with fan use was greater in infants placed in the prone or side sleep position (AOR, 0.14; 95% CI, 0.03-0.55) vs supine (0.84; 0.21-3.39). Fan use was associated with a greater reduction in SIDS risk in infants who shared a bed with an individual other than their parents (AOR, 0.15; 95% CI, 0.01-1.85) vs with a parent (0.40; 0.03-4.68). Finally, fan use was associated with reduced SIDS risk in infants not using pacifiers (AOR, 0.22; 95% CI, 0.07-0.69) but not in pacifier users (1.99; 0.16-24.4). Some differences in the effect of fan use on SIDS risk did not reach statistical significance.

Conclusion.—Fan use may be an effective intervention for further decreasing SIDS risk in infants in adverse sleep environments.

▶ This report looks at an interesting new piece of information that if implemented might actually further decrease the incidence of sudden infant death syndrome (SIDS). It has been hypothesized for some time that rebreathing exhaled carbon dioxide trapped near an infant's airway by bedding could be one of the possible mechanisms for SIDS, particularly in settings of soft bedding, covering of the head during sleep, and the use of the prone sleep position. It does not take a rocket scientist to understand that inadequate ventilation would facilitate such pooling of carbon dioxide around an infant's mouth and nose. In this regard, increased movement of air in the sleeping room of an infant could theoretically decrease the accumulation of carbon dioxide around the infant's nose and mouth and therefore reduce the risk of rebreathing. In a related way, data shows that the use of a pacifier significantly reduces the risk of SIDS with one possible explanation for this being that sucking movements help to maintain air passages in sleep environments with decreased airflow, such as sleeping with the head covered or on soft bedding. On the basis of all these suppositions, the authors of this report examine whether improved ventilation by use of a fan or an open window might affect the risk of SIDS. The investigators analyzed data from a population-based case-control study of risk factors for SIDS that included detailed information on sleep environment.

The data from this report show that fan use during the last sleep was associated with a significantly reduced incidence of SIDS risk. Although it is impossible to know the exact underlying mechanism of the observed association, the findings are consistent with the hypothesis that reducing rebreathing might reduce the risk of SIDS. Presumably, the increased air turbulence resulting from fan use prevents the accumulation of carbon dioxide around an infant's nose and mouth. Because previous studies have not looked at the association of fan use and SIDS incidence, the findings from this report emanating from California provide the first epidemiologic evidence of the benefit of fan use in reducing SIDS risk.

It would be interesting to see if there is any regional variation that might relate to fan use and the incidence of SIDS. This editor lives in the southern United States where ceiling fans are fairly pervasive, even in homes that are air conditioned. It would be interesting to repeat the study from California to see if such regional differences in SIDS rates might be based on the prevalence of fan use. This is a study waiting to happen. In the meantime, it will also be interesting to see if this report stimulates parents of newborns to stop at their local hardware store and pick up a fan or 2 for their baby's room. Who would have thought that an old-fashioned fan might be all it takes to help reduce an infant's risk of SIDS?

J. A. Stockman III, MD

Quality of Care of Children in the Emergency Department: Association with Hospital Setting and Physician Training

Dharmar M, Marcin JP, Romano PS, et al (Univ of California Davis, Sacramento; et al)
J Pediatr 153:783-789, 2008

Objective.—To investigate differences in the quality of emergency care for children related to differences in hospital setting, physician training, and demographic factors.

Study Design.—This was a retrospective cohort study of a consecutive sample of children presenting with high-acuity illnesses or injuries at 4 rural non-children's hospitals (RNCHs) and 1 academic urban children's hospital (UCH). Two of 4 study physicians independently rated quality of care using a validated implicit review instrument. Hierarchical modeling was used to estimate quality of care (scored from 5 to 35) across hospital settings and by physician training.

Results.—A total of 304 patients presenting to the RNCHs and the UCH were studied. Quality was lower (difference = -3.23; 95% confidence interval [CI] = -4.48 to -1.98) at the RNCHs compared with the UCH. Pediatric emergency medicine (PEM) physicians provided better care than family medicine (FM) physicians and those in the "other" category (difference = -3.34, 95% CI = -5.40 to -1.27 and -3.12, 95% CI = -5.25 to -0.99, respectively). Quality of care did not differ significantly between PEM and general emergency medicine (GEM) physicians in general, or between GEM and PEM physicians at the UCH; however, GEM physicians at the RNCHs provided care of lesser quality than PEM physicians at the UCH (difference = -2.75; 95% CI = -5.40 to -0.05). Older children received better care.

Conclusions.—The quality of care provided to children is associated with age, hospital setting, and physician training.

▶ It is difficult to decide what to do with the information from this report. The study that forms the basis of this report looked at outcomes of the most seriously ill children presenting to 4 regional rural emergency rooms and compared that care with respect to outcomes to a pediatric tertiary referral center in the emergency room. As one would suspect, the more sophisticated the environment and the more highly trained the physician personnel were in pediatric emergency care, the better the outcomes. Of course, it is hard to expect equivalent care under these circumstances. Were the local care adequate, what is the need for a tertiary center?

This report was accompanied by an interesting editorial that provided detailed information on the data emanating from this study.[1] This editorial noted that while there were differences in the numerical scoring of quality care indicators between rural hospitals and the urban center, in both instances, the absolute score was clearly within the "acceptable" range of quality of care. While the data statistically and numerically prove that care in the rural setting provided by nonpediatric emergency physicians is inferior, the real question is whether it is substantially different enough to be clinically relevant given the fact that the care itself was "adequate."

It is unlikely that there will ever be sufficient numbers of pediatric emergency medicine specialists to staff all of the emergency rooms in the United States that provide care for children. It is even less likely that there would be sufficient numbers of individuals who have undergone combined adult emergency medicine and pediatric emergency medicine training. A training pathway for the latter does exist, but the numbers of folks taking this training are extremely small. What this means is that we will continue to need to rely on the skills of adult emergency physicians who are required to provide care for children. It is incumbent upon those who do have pediatric emergency training to be involved with educational programs that maximize the skills of our adult emergency medicine counterparts. It is possible to close the quality gap.

This commentary closes with a miscellaneous *Clinical Fact/Curio*. What do gecko feet and a new surgical tape have in common? The answer is that both are incredibly sticky and adhere well. Sticky gecko feet have provided the inspiration for a totally new surgical adhesive. The tape has been put to the test in an animal model of hernia surgery and is better than any previous prototypes, which generally work well only in dry conditions. This "gecko" variety of tape uses a synthetic polymer called PGSA that works when wet and can be "doped" with whatever is the wound healing medication du jour to accelerate healing. The sheet of PGSA is engineered into nanoscale conical pillars, similar to the fibrillar arrays that cover the bottom of geckos' feet, which allow attachment to vertical surfaces. Those engineering this tape have one more step, and that is to figure out how to get the stuff off after wounds have healed.[2]

J. A. Stockman III, MD

References

1. McCabe JB. Quality pediatric emergency care: everywhere, all the time. *J Pediatr.* 2008;153:738-740.
2. Mahdavi A, Ferreira L, Sundback C, et al. A biodegradable and biocompatible gecko-inspired tissue adhesive. *Proc Natl Acad Sci.* 2008;105:2307-2312.

Performance during Internal Medicine Residency Training and Subsequent Disciplinary Action by State Licensing Boards

Papadakis MA, Arnold GK, Blank LL, et al (Univ of California at San Francisco; American Board of Internal Medicine, Philadelphia, PA; Culliton Group, Washington, DC)
Ann Intern Med 148:869-876, 2008

Background.—Physicians who are disciplined by state licensing boards are more likely to have demonstrated unprofessional behavior in medical school. Information is limited on whether similar performance measures taken during residency can predict performance as practicing physicians.

Objective.—To determine whether performance measures during residency predict the likelihood of future disciplinary actions against practicing internists.

Design.—Retrospective cohort study.

Setting.—State licensing board disciplinary actions against physicians from 1990 to 2006.

Participants.—66171 physicians who entered internal medicine residency training in the United States from 1990 to 2000 and became diplomates.

Measurements.—Predictor variables included components of the Residents' Annual Evaluation Summary ratings and American Board of Internal Medicine (ABIM) certification examination scores.

Results.—2 performance measures independently predicted disciplinary action. A low professionalism rating on the Residents' Annual Evaluation Summary predicted increased risk for disciplinary action (hazard ratio, 1.7 [95% CI, 1.3 to 2.2]), and high performance on the ABIM certification examination predicted decreased risk for disciplinary action (hazard ratio, 0.7 [CI, 0.60 to 0.70] for American or Canadian medical school graduates and 0.9 [CI, 0.80 to 1.0] for international medical school graduates). Progressively better professionalism ratings and ABIM certification examination scores were associated with less risk for subsequent disciplinary actions; the risk ranged from 4.0% for the lowest professionalism rating to 0.5% for the highest and from 2.5% for the lowest examination scores to 0.0% for the highest.

Limitations.—The study was retrospective. Some diplomates may have practiced outside of the United States. Nondiplomates were excluded.

Conclusion.—Poor performance on behavioral and cognitive measures during residency are associated with greater risk for state licensing board actions against practicing physicians at every point on a performance continuum. These findings support the Accreditation Council for Graduate Medical Education standards for professionalism and cognitive performance and the development of best practices to remediate these deficiencies.

▶ One of the serious problems that we ultimately must face in medicine is why too many "bad apples" creep through our educational system into practice and then stay in practice. To say this differently, medical schools graduate virtually all who enroll. Residency training programs pass on to the certification process virtually all who enter residency training. The certification process weeds out perhaps only about 6% or 7%. State licensing boards then are faced with the task of monitoring the profession. Would it not be nice to understand who is at greatest likelihood for unsuitability to become a physician at the start of this process?

The Accreditation Council for Graduate Medical Education (ACGME) has historically accredited residency training programs. This accreditation is based on the ability of a program to adequately educate residents. In 1999, the ACGME endorsed as a measure of a program's accomplishment residents' success in achieving educational outcomes. The ACGME designated 6 competencies as measures of a residency program's effectiveness, one of which was professionalism. Much thought has now gone into how best to teach and measure professionalism across the specialties during graduate medical education. Of course, once a resident leaves an accredited program and is in clinical practice, the maintenance of certification program for those who are able to become certified serves as an instrument for continuing measurement of professionalism, along with state licensure. Previous studies have shown that physicians who are disciplined by state licensing boards are more likely to have demonstrated unprofessional behavior in medical school.[1] What has been missing is an understanding of whether similar predictions of future problems could be found during residency training. The report of Papadakis et al attempts to address this.

Papadakis et al studied a cohort of all physicians who entered internal medicine residency training in the United States between 1990 and 2000 and who subsequently became Diplomates of the American Board of Internal Medicine (ABIM). These investigators took advantage of the fact that the same criteria are used to assess residents' performance throughout the United States. In addition, internal medicine residents receive a grade for professionalism, unlike medical students, whose professionalism component may be embedded in the overall grade of their clerkship. Almost 67 000 internal medicine training program graduates who became Diplomates of the ABIM were able to be tracked down. Data on these individuals were compared with information provided by the Federation of State Medical Boards (FSMB) that reports licensing actions. Compared with nondisciplined ABIM diplomates, diplomates who were disciplined had lower ratings on their ABIM Resident's Evaluation Summary, had more unsuccessful attempts and lower scores on the internal medicine certification examination, and were less likely to be certified in an internal medicine subspecialty.

So what are the limitations of this study? Most residents who had poor performance measures during residency training turn out not to be disciplined by a licensing board. Thus unprofessional behavior during residency training, while a risk factor for licensing actions, is a weak signal for the relatively rare event of a subsequent disciplinary action. These residency performance measures are predictors but are not adequate screening tests in and of themselves for subsequent disciplinary action.

So what are the implications of these findings? The authors of this report remind us that it is reassuring that most physicians will not get into trouble with their state licensing boards, and it is probable that many residents who receive lower professionalism ratings subsequently resolve the basis for these low ratings. Recognize, however, that licensing actions taken by state medical boards are designed only to detect egregious behavior. Thus, a state licensing board disciplinary action is probably a very insensitive measure of overall competency as things now stand. Please note that the National Alliance for Physician Competence has promulgated a "white paper" that is a guide to describing the characteristics of a truly competent physician. The FSMB initially organized the process of gathering disparate groups from within medicine to create these guidelines. Public input was also obtained. The FSMB has also defined, in another white paper on maintenance of licensure, a process of evaluating as part of periodic license renewal the same 6 general competencies that are assessed during residency training and as part of maintenance of certification. The intent is clear. That intent is that state licensing boards over time will do more than simply require money for renewal of a medical license. Competencies will be assessed as part of relicensure.

Unfortunately, there is no perfect system now and there probably never will be one that can weed out all the "bad apples." Unfortunately, a small but real number of individuals within our profession should not be practicing medicine. The good news, however, is that the vast majority of physicians embrace all the elements embodied within the definition of professionalism.

J. A. Stockman III, MD

Reference

1. Papadakis MA, Teherani A, Banach MA, et al. Disciplinary action by medical boards and prior behavior in medical school. N Engl J Med. 2005;353:2673-2682.

Clinical Inactivity Among Pediatricians: Prevalence and Perspectives

Freed GL, Dunham KM, Switalski KE (Univ of Michigan, Ann Arbor)
Pediatrics 123:605-610, 2009

Introduction.—During their careers, physicians may have periods of clinical inactivity for a variety of reasons. Concerns have been raised about the impact of clinical inactivity on the growing physician workforce shortage. It is unknown how these periods of clinical inactivity impact physician competence and patient safety. With this study we sought to determine the rates of clinical inactivity, the duration of periods of inactivity, professional activities during those periods, and the perspective of pediatricians regarding future requirements of competency for return to clinical practice.

Patients and Methods.—A random sample of 6757 American Board of Pediatrics diplomates aged ≤65 years received a structured questionnaire by mail. The survey explored the prevalence of and reasons for clinical

TABLE 3.—Primary Reason for Longest Period of Clinical Inactivity ($N = 552$)

Variable	Provide Care to My Children, % (n)	Career Change to Nonclinical, % (n)	Sabbatical, % (n)	Personal Health Issues, % (n)	P
Overall	41 (225)	31 (173)	10 (53)	9 (49)	NA
Gender					
Male	3 (5)	62 (95)	11 (17)	8 (13)	<.0001[a]
($N = 154$)					
Female	55 (220)	20 (78)	9 (36)	9 (36)	
($N = 398$)					
Female physicians					
Generalist	59 (201)	16 (55)	9 (29)	9 (30)	.0014[a]
($N = 339$)					
Subspecialist	32 (19)	39 (23)	12 (7)	10 (6)	
($N = 59$)					
Faculty status					
Full-time faculty	20 (15)	50 (38)	13 (10)	10 (8)	.0018[a]
($N = 76$)					
Part-time, adjunct, and nonfaculty ($N = 470$)	44 (208)	29 (135)	9 (43)	8 (39)	

NA indicates not applicable. Comparisons between male generalists and subspecialists showed no statistically significant differences.

[a] $P < .05$ for male versus female pediatricians, female generalists versus female subspecialists, and full-time faculty versus part-time, adjunct, and nonfaculty.

(Reprinted from Freed GL, Dunham KM, Switalski KE, et al. Clinical inactivity among pediatricians: prevalence and perspectives. *Pediatrics.* 2009;123:605-610.)

inactivity and perspectives on the return to clinical practice. Clinical inactivity was defined as a period of absence of ≥ 12 months from any direct or consultative clinical care.

Results.—The response rate was 74%. Of respondents, 88% ($n = 4176$) were currently engaged in pediatric clinical care. Twelve percent ($n = 554$) indicated that they had experienced a period of clinical inactivity lasting ≥ 12 months. Women were more likely than men (16% vs 7%) to have had periods of clinical inactivity. Controlling for gender, generalists were no more likely than subspecialists to report a past period of clinical inactivity. More than one third of the respondents ($n = 1672$ [36%]) agreed that pediatricians who return from clinical inactivity after >1 year should undergo a competency evaluation.

Conclusions.—Almost 1 in 8 pediatricians has suspended clinical care for ≥ 1 year, and a similar proportion of respondents were inactive at the time of our survey. Currently, all of these physicians may maintain both their licensure and board certification during these periods. The impact of clinical inactivity on patient care and patient safety is unknown (Table 3).

▶ Previous studies have been reported from the American Academy of Pediatrics telling us about the frequency with which pediatricians take time off from practice. One recent survey from the academy that looked at 1158 pediatricians over the age of 50 found that 22% of women and 6.5% of men had taken an extended leave of absence of 6 months or more from clinical practice at some point earlier in their careers. The amount of clinical activity within a subspecialty is an important issue when it comes to workforce planning. Clinical inactivity is also of some importance related to patient safety concerns. The issue is that when one takes time off for extended periods from clinical practice, one might be unable to maintain one's level of clinical competence to the same degree as one who is continuously in practice. This is something that the state medical licensing boards are beginning to pay some attention to.

The report of Freed et al gives us an update on the clinical activity/inactivity profile of certified pediatricians by examining a random sample of 6757 Diplomates of the American Board of Pediatrics who are age 65 years or younger. This survey had an amazing 74% response rate. In the survey, 88% of the responders were currently engaged in clinical practice as defined by any degree of direct and/or consultative care. One in 8 pediatricians, however, had suspended the provision of clinical care for more than a year during the course of their careers. Women were twice as likely as men to have done this. Even though these individuals were clinically inactive, more than half reported that they maintained an active medical license to practice and/or board certification during these periods of clinical inactivity. The table shows the primary reason for the longest period of clinical activity observed in this study. Time off to provide care to children was the most common reason given followed by a career change to a nonclinical position, followed then by a sabbatical or a personal health concern.

It is interesting to note that the data from this report are not substantially different than data from the American Board of Internal Medicine's survey of board-certified internists. If one looks at a cross section of all internists, one finds that 1 in 5 internists at any point in time are not clinically active, again defined as any degree of direct and/or consultative patient care.

According to data from the American Medical Association, the number of inactive physicians in the United States is in fact increasing. Between 1980 and 2004, the proportion of physicians categorized as inactive almost doubled from 5.5% to 10.4%.[1] The issue of clinical inactivity has become of growing importance to state licensing authorities. The state licensing authorities are under the umbrella of the Federation of State Medical Boards (FSMB). The medical boards are in the process of attempting to determine whether inactive clinicians should have the same licensure status and privileges as those who are active. This is a difficult determination because there is no consensus as to whether there should be a specific and defined educational or testing process for inactive physicians who wish to return to an active status. The state licensing boards, however, do feel increasing responsibility for reporting to the public whether a licensed physician is actually caring for patients and if not, for how long.

J. A. Stockman III, MD

Reference

1. American Medical Association. *Physician characteristics and distribution in the United States: 2006 Edition.* Chicago, IL: American Medical Association; 2006.

Protecting the Public: State Medical Board Licensure Policies for Active and Inactive Physicians

Freed GL, Dunham KM, Abraham L, et al (Univ of Michigan, Ann Arbor)
Pediatrics 123:643-652, 2009

Objective.—The purpose of this research was to explore state physician licensing board policies and regulation of active, inactive, and retired licenses.

Methods.—We conducted structured telephone interviews from January to March 2007 with representatives of all 64 state allopathic and osteopathic medical licensing boards in the United States. All of the licensing boards participated.

Results.—Only 34% of state licensing boards query physicians regarding clinical activity at both initial licensure and renewal. The majority of boards allow physicians to hold or renew an unrestricted active license to practice medicine, although they may not have cared for a patient in years. Only 1 board requires a minimum number of patient visits to maintain an active license. Five boards allow physicians with inactive licenses to practice some form of medicine, whereas 7 boards allow physicians with retired licenses to practice. Few states have any mechanism to assess the competency of clinically inactive physicians who return to active practice.

Conclusions.—The number of inactive physicians in the United States is growing. Currently, state medical board policies do not address the issue of continuing competence in license renewal. Greater medical safety concerns on the part of the public will likely lead to calls for greater accountability by state licensing authorities.

▶ The report of Freed et al tells us about a study of all 64 state allopathic and osteopathic medical licensing boards and the policies they have in place regarding clinically inactive physicians. What we see is that only 34% of state licensing boards currently actually ask physicians about their level of clinical activity at the time of initial licensure. The significant majority of boards in the United States allow physicians to hold and renew an unrestricted active license to practice medicine, although they may not have cared for a patient in many years. Just 42% of state boards request information from physicians about their clinical activity at relicensure, but only one state at the time of relicensure requires a minimum number of patient visits per year to maintain an active license.

So how important is this issue of clinical inactivity when it comes to quality of care? Although there are no studies that have examined the clinical outcome of patients whose physicians returned to practice after periods of inactivity, there are a number of studies that have examined whether the frequency of care provided for a specific diagnoses or the performance of certain procedures is associated with better outcomes. We know, for example, that those who take care of adult patients with myocardial infarction have better outcomes if they have higher patient volumes. Research has shown that the volume and frequency of care provided for specific conditions in hospitals and emergency departments also have an important impact on accuracy of diagnosis, frequency of surgical complications, and patient survival. Research has also raised concerns about the clinical acumen of physicians who practice part-time, much less those who experience periods of total clinical inactivity. For example, Freeman found a substantial variation in outcomes of endoscopy based on the ongoing case volume of an individual endoscopist.[1] In the aggregate, what studies there are suggest that even once-competent physicians may be at risk of losing both diagnostic and procedural skills during a period of inactivity. Unfortunately, there is little data regarding clinical activity and outcomes in pediatric care providers who are working within what otherwise is known as a "cognitive" discipline.

In order to partially address the issue of competency related to clinical inactivity, the Federation of State Medical Boards (FSMB) formed a committee several years ago known as the Maintenance of Licensure Committee. This group came to the conclusion that the current practices regarding both license renewal and the identification and licensing of inactive physicians is no longer acceptable to the public. In 2008, the Maintenance of Licensure Committee developed a model policy for state regulations that would require physicians to demonstrate their continuing competence on a periodic basis. The FSMB has recommended to the states that the licensing boards collect information regarding physician practice status (scope, type, status, and clinical activity) at the point of initial licensure and at license renewal. The report suggests that if a physician has had no evidence of clinical activity for a period of 2 years or longer, that physician wishing to practice again must engage in a practice reentry program in order to assure the public that their skills are up to date. The FSMB also indicated that physician participation in specialty board maintenance of certification programs is an acceptable standard for meeting the maintenance of licensure requirements. This assessment is currently used only by the New Mexico medical board and only for licensure by endorsement. Other than this instance, no state requires either specialty board certification or recertification for initial license, license renewal, or reactivation. This shows how minimal the state requirements are at the present time.

Should the recommendations of the FSMB be embraced by the various state and territorial medical licensing boards, there will be a sea of change in the requirements for relicensure. Physicians will have to demonstrate competencies in all areas of their practice. When it comes to assessment of knowledge, a secure examination will need to be administered once every 10 years. Again, the FSMB has stated that participation in maintenance of certification programs would otherwise meet the state requirements. It will take quite some time before the recommendations of the FSMB are implemented because each state has its own legislative process authorizing such requirements. Chances are, however, with the greater emphasis seen these days on patient safety and quality, we will see this change occurring across the country.

As this commentary closes, another *Clinical Fact/Curio*, this having to do with medicine in general. Do you know why Benjamin Franklin (1706-1719) was called Dr Franklin? Benjamin Franklin assumed the moniker "Dr" in 1759, not because he had finished medical training, but because the University of Saint Andrews in Scotland awarded him an honorary doctorate that recognized his contributions to understanding electricity. Although Franklin did not receive formal instruction in medicine and never claimed to be a clinician, he might also have appropriately had the title of Doctor in the medical sense because licensing did not exist in the colonies and in so many diverse ways, he actually behaved like a physician, including the founding of the first hospital in the United States, Pennsylvania Hospital in 1752.

Among Franklin's other medical accomplishments was the use of electric therapy for various conditions. In 1740, scientists had already discovered how to store static electricity in foil-coated glass bottles. In 1850, using these latent Leyden jars to electrocute a turkey, which he would later roast for Christmas, Franklin accidentally, shocked himself, causing his body to shake violently. This and other electrical accidents suggested to him possible therapeutic values for electricity. Franklin began treating paralyzed patients with 3 times daily shocks to their affected extremities to see if he could strengthen a patient's muscles. Indeed, limbs seemed to strengthen somewhat, but the sessions were too painful and the benefits too short lived to be acceptable. Interestingly, some patients with other conditions did seem to improve, and Franklin's experiments are considered by some to be an early example of electroconvulsive therapy for psychiatric problems. Franklin did recommend electrical therapy for insane people.

In addition to the above, Franklin designed a urethral catheter, this to help his brother who had a bladder stone. Franklin also described the "dangles," a wrist drop from radial neuropathy, in printers who dried lead types in front of a fire, thus describing one clinical manifestation of lead poisoning. He also observed that no moss grew on eaves stained with the drippings from roofs painted with white lead, and he also noted that a family developed dry belly ache after drinking rainwater collected from a leaded roof.

Additionally, Benjamin Franklin was a strong supporter of variolation to prevent small pox. Also, when he became tired of using 2 spectacles for his hyperopia and presbyopia, he had a single pair of glasses cut, each lens being divided in half, thus inventing the bifocal lens. In 1760, he observed that if you place a dark cloth on snow, the snow would melt faster, thus describing the effect of color on heat absorption. Franklin then proposed an important practical application, that is, on hot days people should wear white, rather than dark, clothing, especially when participating in strenuous exercise! He later described the beneficial effects of evaporative cooling with water and alcohol. In the area of dermatology, he described many of the clinical features of psoriasis, a condition that he had for more than 14 years and that eventually resulted in psoriatic patches covering almost his entire body, except for his hands and face. Interestingly, after a severe attack of polyarticular gout, the lesions permanently disappeared.

One could go on and on about the medical achievements of "Dr" Franklin. His contributions to medicine, although a small part of his numerous and diverse accomplishments, may have been among his most satisfying.[2]

J. A. Stockman III, MD

References

1. Freeman ML. Training and competent in gastrointestinal endoscopy. *Rev Gastroenterol Disord.* 2001;1:73-76.
2. Hirschmann JV. Benjamin Franklin in medicine. *Ann Intern Med.* 2005;143:832-834.

Alcohol consumption and alcohol counselling behaviour among US medical students: cohort study

Frank E, Elon L, Naimi T, et al (Univ of British Columbia, Vancouver; Emory Univ Rollins School of Public Health, Atlanta, GA; Natl Ctr for Chronic Disease Prevention and Health Promotion, Atlanta, GA)
BMJ 337:a2155, 2008

Objective.—To determine which factors affect alcohol counselling practices among medical students.

Design.—Cohort study.

Setting.—Nationally representative medical schools (n = 16) in the United States.

Participants.—Medical students who graduated in 2003.

Interventions.—Questionnaires were completed (response rate 83%) at the start of students' first year (n = 1846/2080), entrance to wards (typically during the third year of training) (n = 1630/1982), and their final (fourth) year (n = 1469/1901).

Main Outcome Measures.—Previously validated questions on alcohol consumption and counselling.

Results.—78% (3777/4847) of medical students reported drinking in the past month, and a third (1668/ 4847) drank excessively; these proportions changed little over time. The proportion of those who believed alcohol counselling was highly relevant to care of patients was higher at entrance to wards (61%; 919/1516) than in final year students (46%; 606/1329). Although students intending to enter primary care were more likely to believe alcohol counselling was highly relevant, only 28% of final year students (391/1393) reported usually or always talking to their general medical patients about their alcohol consumption. Excessive drinkers were somewhat less likely than others to counsel patients or to think it relevant to do so. In multivariate models, extensive training in alcohol counselling doubled the frequency of reporting that alcohol counselling would be clinically relevant (odds ratio 2.3, 95% confidence interval 1.6 to 3.3) and of reporting doing counselling (2.2, 1.5 to 3.3).

Conclusions.—Excessive drinking and binge drinking among US medical students is common, though somewhat less prevalent than among comparably aged adults in the US general population. Few students usually discussed alcohol use with patients, but greater training and confidence about alcohol counselling predicted both practising and believing in the relevance of alcohol counselling. Medical schools should consider routinely training students to screen and counsel patients for alcohol misuse and consider discouraging excessive drinking.

▶ The data from this report are important because they tell us a great deal about the youngest within our medical profession, the average United States medical student and his or her drinking habits. It has been estimated that somewhere between 10% and 12% of physicians in the United States will develop a substance abuse disorder, the most common of which is alcoholism. Data from the McLellan et al report, which evaluates the effectiveness of United States state physician health programs in treating physicians with substance abuse disorders, verify that alcoholism comprises 50% of drug problems related to substance abuse in physicians.[1] Clearly, this problem can be traced back to much earlier in life. The report of Frank et al is based on surveys done at 16 United States medical schools on first-year medical students, third-year medical students, and students completing their fourth year.

The findings from this report show that most medical students reported drinking alcohol in the preceding month (78%) with some 34% noting that they had drunk excessively (24% of women and 43% of men). These proportions changed little over time in medical school. Those moving into nonprimary care disciplines were more likely to have drunk excessively even when adjusted for sex disparity in specialty choice. A large percentage drank at the "binge" level (that is 5 or more drinks for men or 4 or more drinks for women). Nearly half of fourth-year students considered alcohol counseling highly relevant to their intended specialty area. Thus, one's own history of alcohol consumption becomes a variable in the likely manner in which this counseling might actually take place. Medical students' personal and clinical attitudes about alcohol can have important implications for their current care of patients.

This editor has never been in an environment where a medical school has done much to educate a medical student about his or her own drinking habit and the implications of the latter toward subsequent clinical practice. If medical students were better educated about drinking and screening and counseling for alcohol misuse, they might be more likely to adhere to clinical prevention guidelines and be better equipped to identify and reduce excessive drinking among their patients. In this regard, a trip to the doctor should begin at home when it comes to a physician. While the prevalence of binge drinking among United States medical students is somewhat lower than in their peers of comparable age in the general population, the prevalence of this problem is still quite high.[1]

This commentary closes with another *Clinical Fact/Curio* regarding medical education. In the United States, all medical school applicants are now screened to see if they have a police record. The question is, did such screening prevent the acceptance of a student to a first-year medical school class in Stockholm recently? The answer is no. The Karolinska Institute, in Stockholm, recently expelled a first-year medical student who had been admitted the previous year without knowing he had served time in prison for murder with a firearm. The story ignited a parliamentary discussion in Sweden about the need to better screen medical students. The Institute first learned of the student's violent past through anonymous tips. Tipsters, who also notified news organizations, alleged that the 31-year-old medical student had been a Nazi sympathizer convicted of a murder in 1999 under his former name. The convicted felon had been released from prison in early 2007, after serving 6.5 years of an 11-year murder sentence. As it turned out, despite the widespread, although not universal, sentiment in the medical community that a murderer should not be admitted to medical school, the university could not legally revoke the individual's admission on the grounds that he was a convicted murderer. In reviewing the individual's application, however, the Institute learned that his high school transcript had been falsified to show his current surname in place of his former name, giving the university legal grounds for his ultimate expulsion. Thus it is, in Stockholm, that if you legally change your name, but fraudulently fail to disclose that, you can be kicked out of medical school, but not so if you are a murderer.[2] Obviously, this individual would not have been admitted had officials known he was a murderer. It should be noted that in Sweden, after pedophiles were found to be working in daycare centers a few years ago, Sweden adopted a new law mandating that schools and daycare centers check criminal records of all applicants.

J. A. Stockman III, MD

References

1. McLellan AT, Skipper GS, Campbell M, DuPont RL. Five-year outcomes in a cohort study of physicians for substance abuse disorders in the United States. *BMJ*. 2008;337:1154-1158.
2. Stafford N. Karolinska expels student after finding murder conviction. *BMJ*. 2008; 336:240.

Five year outcomes in a cohort study of physicians treated for substance use disorders in the United States

McLellan AT, Skipper GS, Campbell M, et al (Treatment Res Inst, Philadelphia, PA; Alabama Physician Assistance Program, Montgomery; Inst for Behavior and Health, Rockville, MD)
BMJ 337:a2038, 2008

Objective.—To evaluate the effectiveness of US state physician health programmes in treating physicians with substance use disorders.

Design.—Five year, longitudinal, cohort study.

Setting.—Purposive sample of 16 state physician health programmes in the United States.

Participants.—904 physicians consecutively admitted to one of the 16 programmes from September 1995 to September 2001.

Main Outcome Measures.—Completion of the programme, continued alcohol and drug misuse (regular urine tests), and occupational status at five years.

Results.—155 of 802 physicians (19.3%) with known outcomes failed the programme, usually early during treatment. Of the 647 (80.7%) who completed treatment and resumed practice under supervision and monitoring, alcohol or drug misuse was detected by urine testing in 126 (19%) over five years; 33 (26%) of these had a repeat positive test result. At five year follow-up, 631 (78.7%) physicians were licensed and working, 87 (10.8%) had their licences revoked, 28 (3.5%) had retired, 30 (3.7%) had died, and 26 (3.2%) had unknown status.

Conclusion.—About three quarters of US physicians with substance use disorders managed in this subset of physician health programmes had favourable outcomes at five years. Such programmes seem to provide an appropriate combination of treatment, support, and sanctions to manage addiction among physicians effectively.

▶ Reported in Frank et al[1] is the high prevalence of binge drinking among United States medical students, including among women students. Because excessive alcohol consumption represents about 50% of drug problems requiring treatment in addiction programs for physicians, alcoholism is a particularly important problem among our peers. In this report of McLellan et al, the primary drug problems included alcohol (50%), opiates (36%), stimulants (8%), and other miscellaneous substances (6%). Some 50% of physicians entering a treatment program report misusing more than 1 substance and almost 15% report a history of intravenous drug abuse. The average duration of substance abuse before entering any treatment program was 5 years.

What McLellan et al have done is to report on a retrospective longitudinal cohort study from 1995 through 2001 of all 904 physicians consecutively admitted to 16 physician health programs designed to treat doctors with substance abuse. Of the 802 physicians with known outcomes, some 20% failed to complete their contracted period of treatment and supervision. More than half of these voluntarily stopped practicing medicine and relinquished their license to practice. An additional one-quarter had their licenses revoked owing to relapse. The remainder either died (some from suicide) or otherwise were lost to follow-up. Five years out from treatment, almost 80% of the remaining physicians completing their treatment were licensed and either practicing medicine or working in a nonclinical capacity. Thus, of the total at a five-year follow-up, 78% were still employed in good standing, but 15% had stopped practicing medicine (11% involuntarily) and 4% had died.

The report of McLellan et al obviously has a good news, bad news aspect to it. The good news is that the combination of identification, intervention, treatment, support, and monitoring by physician health programs is almost 80% effective in rehabilitating most addicted physicians, at least over a 5-year period. The bad news is that a fair percentage of physicians never satisfactorily complete the program or fall off the wagon within a year or two. Given that many physicians have had a problem for several years before the problem is overtly identified, the more we can do to recognize these physicians early, the more we can do to help them.

J. A. Stockman III, MD

Reference

1. Frank E, Elon L, Naimi T, et al. Alcohol consumption and alcohol counseling behaviour among US medical students: cohort study. *BMJ*. 2008;337:a2155.

Educational Debt and Reported Career Plans among Internal Medicine Residents

McDonald FS, West CP, Popkave C, et al (Mayo Clinic, Rochester, MN; American College of Physicians, Philadelphia, PA)
Ann Intern Med 149:416-420, 2008

Background.—Physicians often enter the workplace with substantial debt. The relationship between debt and reported career plans among internal medicine residents is unknown.

Objective.—To determine distributions of educational debt among internal medicine residents and associations of debt with reported career plans.

Design.—Cross-sectional survey using data from the annual Internal Medicine In-Training Examination Residents Questionnaire completed by U.S. categorical internal medicine residents.

Setting.—Categorical internal medicine residencies in the United States.

Participants.—22 563 residents in their third (final) year of residency, representing 74.1% of all eligible U.S. categorical internal medicine residents from 2003 through 2007.

Measurements.—Distributions of educational debt were tabulated. Proportions of residents choosing career plans were calculated for various levels of debt.

Results.—International medical graduates represented 48.7% of the cross section and had considerably less debt than U.S. medical graduates: 53.8% of U.S. medical graduates had debt of $100 000 or greater and 60.2% of international medical graduates had none. U.S. medical graduates with debt of $100 000 to $150 000 dollars were less likely than those with no debt to choose a subspecialty career (57.5% vs. 63.5%). U.S. medical graduates with debt of $50 000 to $99 999 were more likely than those with no debt to choose a hospitalist career (8.5% vs. 6.2%), and this preference increased with increasing debt level (10.0% for those with >$150 000 debt). These associations are more pronounced for U.S. medical graduates than for international medical graduates.

Limitation.—The study addressed total educational debt, but not when it was incurred, and did not allow inferences related to causality.

Conclusion.—Educational debt is associated with differences in reported career plans among internal medicine residents.

▶ There has been a lot of data to suggest that there is a relationship between how a medical student chooses a particular specialty career and their level of educational indebtedness. The Association of the American Medical Colleges has reported that in 2003, more than 81% of United States medical graduates had educational debt, with a median debt of $100 000 for graduates of public medical schools and $135 000 for graduates of private medical schools. In 2007, more than one-third of United States medical graduates had a debt greater than $150 000. The report of McDonald et al examines whether the level of indebtedness in any way affected the choice of a final career among internal medicine residents. This study is important because it has some potential correlation between what we are seeing occurring in pediatrics.

Upon the completion of residency training, internists may choose to enter the workforce immediately as general internists or hospitalists or they may continue with fellowship training in a subspecialty. While compensation during fellowship training is substantially less than that received by a general internist in practice or a hospitalist, after fellowship training, many subspecialists can more than double their compensation relative to those in general internal medicine positions where additional training is not required. On the other hand, the sooner you enter the workforce, the quicker you can start to manage your debt. Debt has been hypothesized to influence this decision. In order to study this, investigators took data from the annual internal medicine in-training examination residents' questionnaire completed by United States categorical internal residents in their third (final) year of residency. Data from this survey showed that international medical school graduates (representing not quite 50% of those finishing training) had considerably less debt than United States medical graduates. Some 54% of United States medical graduates had debt of $100 000 or greater, while 60% of international medical school graduates had no debt. United States medical school graduates with a debt of $100 000 to $150 000 were less likely than those with no debt to choose a subspecialty career. United States medical graduates with a debt of $50 000 to $100 000 were more likely than those with no debt to choose a hospitalist career, and this preference increased with increasing debt level. The lower magnitude of educational debt seen in international medical school graduates presumably is the result of the lesser educational cost, prior to residency training incurred outside the United States.

This editor lives in Durham, North Carolina, commonly known as the "City of Medicine." This is because of the presence of a large medical center that is very productive of physicians in training. Many of these physicians stay in the local community, but you are more likely to encounter snow in July here than running into a general internist. I used to think that people went into high-paying disciplines just to make a lot of money (a phenomenon once referred to as "scoping for dollars"). Lately in pediatrics, there has been a marked increase in subspecialty training. One wonders if this could be partially explained in the same way as appears to be true in internal medicine.

A great deal has been written about medical education in the past few years. This commentary closes with a *Clinical Fact/Curio* having to do with just how satisfied medical students are with their sex lives. A recent survey from the University of California at San Francisco provides the information.[1] It appears that many medical students in fact are quite dissatisfied with their sex lives. The results of the survey showed that 28% of male students are dissatisfied with their sex lives, 30% have erectile dysfunction, and 6% have low sex desire.

Almost two-thirds of female medical students (63%) appear to be at high risk of sexual dysfunction.

It is tough to know what to make of the findings of this report from the University of California at San Francisco. If there is a silver lining to the findings, it is that perhaps there is more time for these students to study.

J. A. Stockman III, MD

Reference

1. Shindel AW, Ferguson GG, Nelson CJ, Brandes SB. The sexual lives of medical students: a single institution survey. *J Sex Med*. 2008;5:796-803.

Handedness Effects on Procedural Training in Pediatrics

Damore D, Rutledge J, Pan S, et al (New York Presbyterian Hosp/Weill Cornell Med Ctr; New York Presbyterian Hosp/Children's Hosp of New York; et al)
Clin Pediatr 48:156-160, 2009

Objective.—To determine handedness effects on procedural training.

Patients and Methods.—Pediatric trainees and attendings from 3 institutions participated in a Web-based survey examining whether handedness affected learning procedures, the hand used to perform procedures, and if handedness training was received.

Results and Conclusions.—Of 778 physicians, 39% completed surveys, and 11% wrote with their left hand. Learning procedures were affected in left-handed physicians (60% vs 7.7%; odds ratio [OR] = 17.9; 95% confidence interval [CI] = 7.9-40.1), and they used their non-dominant or both hands to perform procedures (48.6% vs 21%; OR = 3.6; 95% CI = 1.7-7.4). Few physicians received handedness training (20% vs 10.7%; P = .16). Left-handed physicians were affected learning lumbar puncture (29% vs 4%; OR = 10.0; 95% CI = 3.8-26.4), intubation (36% vs 5%; OR = 11.0; 95% CI = 4.4-27.4), and suturing (32% vs 4%; OR = 11.7; 95% CI = 4.5-30.5).

▶ A lot has been written about handedness in the surgical literature, but little is to be found in the pediatric medical literature. About 1 in 10 people in developed countries will write with their left hand. In some instances, being left-handed may be an advantage. Advantages for left-handed individuals have been seen in some sports, but not in others.[1,2] Interestingly, left-handed men who attended college have been found to earn more than similarly trained right-handed males, whereas left-handed women with college education have not been shown to have increased earnings.[3]

The report of Damore et al looked at the influence of handedness on physician procedural training. It is well known that left-handed surgical residents tend to be more reactive to stress, more cautious, and have somewhat different technical skills (rated lower). Before the report of Damore et al, the effects of right- and left-handedness had not been studied in pediatric training. What we see from this report is that of 778 pediatric trainees who were surveyed, 11% wrote with their left hand. An excess number of left-handed pediatricians in training felt that their handedness did affect learning. Few indicated that they received any handedness training during their residency. Being left-handed did affect performance during lumbar puncture, intubation, and suturing, however.

It is difficult to tell whether or not anything should be done differently during training as a result of the information provided by the Damore et al report. Most left-handed individuals, physicians included, seem to do perfectly well in society. Curiously, starting in one's mid-50s, many left-handed people start writing with their right hand such that by age 65, only 5% of the population is using their left hand to write. Gosh knows what this means.

This commentary closes with a miscellaneous *Clinical Fact/Curio*, one posed in the form of a question. What is the historical origin of the word "surgery?" The answer is that "surgery" is from the Greek word, *kheirourgia*, made up of *kheir* (hand) and *erg* (work). The term appeared in English in the 14th century from the Latin, *chirurgia*, by way of old French, *serurgien*. The word *surgeon* came into more common usage in the 16th century when healing metaphors central to Christianity began to appear. For example, *Coverdale's Bible* of 1835 talks of the "the lord of thy surgione" (Exodus 15:26). In the 18th century, run-of-the-mill surgeons turned themselves into surgeon-apothecaries and then general practitioners. By the 19th century, the room where these men saw their patients began to be called a "surgery." In the United Kingdom, after World War II, the term was borrowed by members of parliament who had weekly surgeries for their constituents.

J. A. Stockman III, MD

References

1. Holtzen DW. Handedness in professional tennis. *Int J Neurosci.* 2000;105:101-119.
2. Wood CJ, Aggleton JP. Handedness in "fastball" sports: do left-handers have an innate advantage? *Br J Psychol.* 1989;80:227-240.
3. Ruebeck CS, Harrington JE, Moffitt R. Handedness and earnings. NBER working paper series. www.NBER.org/papers/w12387; July 2006. Accessed July 25, 2008.

Effect of 80-Hour Workweek on Continuity of Care
McBurney PG, Gustafson KK, Darden PM (Med Univ of South Carolina, Charleston)
Clin Pediatr 47:803-808, 2008

Work limitations were mandated (2003) to increase safety and improve resident lifestyle. Is clinic continuity affected? Medical University of South Carolina pediatric residents' records for 6 months of 2002 (before regulation) and 2003 (after regulation) were reviewed. Continuity for physician formula, *t* tests, and multivariate linear regression were used. Continuity was calculated for 44 residents (2002) and 45 residents (2003). Mean continuity was 54% (2002) and 53% (2003; $P = .5$); continuity for well-child care visits was 78% (2002) and 73% (2003; $P = .047$). Continuity decreased most for interns (52% [2002], 47% [2003] for all visits; 76%, 67% for well-child care visits). In the multivariate model, year did not predict continuity. When only well-child care visits were considered, year showed a trend toward significance ($P = .07$): 2003 had less continuity. Compared with third-year residents, interns had 8% points less continuity for all visits (6% points less for well-child care visits). Continuity can be maintained despite regulations. Interns are most vulnerable.

▶ It is now almost 6 years since the reduction in resident work hours was mandated by the Accreditation Council for Graduate Medical Education (ACGME). In the interim period, there has been relatively little in the way of information about the impact of the current 80-hour workweek requirement. This report suggests that there has been some reduction in patient continuity on the part of residents in training. A report by Landrigan et al looked at the outcomes of the reduced work hour requirement in 3 large pediatric training programs populated by over 200 residents.[1] It was observed that although scheduling changes were made in each program to accommodate the ACGME standards, 24- to 30-hour shifts remained fairly common and the frequency of residents' on-call remained largely unchanged. At the same time there was no change in residents' measured work hours or sleep hours and no change in the overall rate of medication errors. Rates of motor vehicle crashes, occupational exposures, depression, and self-reported medical errors and overall ratings of work and educational experience did not change. The conclusion of this report was that without more widespread action by policy makers, professional organizations, hospital leaders, and program directors to implement such evidence-based work hour limits, the ACGME's laudable goal of reducing the negative effects of sleep loss on resident education and on the safety and well-being of patients and residents is likely to remain elusive.

Much of the impetus for reducing resident work hours comes from the British Isles. The European Working Time Directive was produced by the Council of the European Union back in 1993 and was incorporated into British law in 1998. This law requires a reduction in the maximum number of resident working hours to 56 hours by 2007 and a planned further reduction to 48 hours in 2009 as well as the need for a minimum of allowed 11 hours rest in any 24-hour period. This law, by the way, applies to all workers in Great Britain, not just residents in training. The Royal College of Surgeons' survey of junior doctors in 2005 suggested that since the implementation of the directive, three-quarters of residents think that continuity of care has deteriorated and 90% think that direct contact with patients has decreased. The organization of junior doctors also indicated that a 48-hour workweek was incompatible with surgical training.

A recent editorial on the European Working Time Directive strongly suggests that the directive is not achieving any of its presumed goals for residents in training and that quality of life has not improved, training in fact has deteriorated, and for most patients, medical care is no safer.[2] This editorial calls on the British government in collaboration with other European countries facing similar problems to abandon the tightening of maximum working hours from 56 to 48 hours.

As this commentary closes, another *Clinical Fact/Curio*, this having to do with sleep deprivation and residency training. In the European Union, careful data are compiled related to the 48-hour European Working Time Directive that has been legislated to improve sleep and possibly patient safety among "resident" trainees. Data from the European Union published in January 2009 showed that during a total of 4782 patient days involving 481 admissions, 32.7% fewer medical errors occurred during the intervention period of shorter work hours than during a traditional rotation (27.6 errors vs 41.0 errors per 1000 patient days, $P = .006$). Unfortunately for "proving" that the reduction in work hours had a direct cause and effect relationship on a reduction in medical errors, many other processes were being put in place at the time to increase patient safety, making it difficult to identify the specific impact of any one factor, including the reduction in resident working hours.[3]

J. A. Stockman III, MD

References

1. Landrigan CP, Fahrenkopf AM, Lewin D, et al. Effects of the accreditation council for graduate medical education duty hour limits on sleep, work hours, and safety. *Pediatrics.* 2008;122:250-258.
2. Cairns H, Hendry B, Leather A, et al. Outcomes of the European working time directive. from 56 to 48 hours is a step too far. *BMJ.* 2008;337:421-422.
3. Shorter working week reduces safety incidents [editorial comment]. *BMJ.* 2009; 338:374.

Pediatric surgery workforce: population and economic issues
Nakayama DK, Newman KD (Mercer Univ School of Medicine, Macon, GA; Children's Hosp Natl Med Ctr, Washington, DC)
J Pediatr Surg 43:1426-1431, 2008

Background.—Whether a shortage of pediatric surgeons exists in the United States, such as those observed in the total physician and general surgical workforces, is an important issue that will affect decisions regarding training, credentialing, and reimbursement. Our goal was to update information regarding the demand and supply of pediatric surgeons.

Methods.—Online American Pediatric Surgical Association (APSA) membership directory gave numbers of pediatric surgeons and their residence by metropolitan statistical areas (MSA), defined by the US census. Population and economic data were obtained from appropriate US government agencies.

Results.—There were 835 APSA members and 375 MSA. Eliminated were 86 MSA (with 12 APSA members) with incomplete data, 14 MSA (0 members) with populations less than 100,000, and 25 members with listed locations outside an MSA. The remaining 798 members and 275 MSA comprised the study. The number of APSA members in an MSA correlated closely with MSA population ($R^2 = 0.836$) and 2006 births ($R^2 = 0.767$). Metropolitan statistical areas without an APSA member had a smaller population and birth rate than those with one or more members ($P = .0001$). An MSA with 1 APSA member had a higher population ($P = .0003$) and births per APSA member ratios ($P = .0014$) than MSA with 2 and 3 or more members. The presence of a medical school or a pediatric training program had no effect on population or births-to-APSA member ratios. There was no correlation between numbers of APSA members and state GDP or state GDP per capita. We used a low, medium, and high threshold to predict the need for pediatric surgeons based upon population per APSA member ± 1 SD (272,466 ± 163,386) to predict a need of 82 to 1344 pediatric surgeons, an increase in the APSA membership by 10% to 168%.

Conclusion.—Based on population estimates and APSA membership, a current shortage of pediatric surgeons exists. Measures should be taken to address this workforce issue.

▶ It does not take a workforce study to know that we are short of pediatric surgeons. Our current production line yields just 20 to 30 such surgeons a year, given the limited number of training positions and interest in this specialty. We see in this report that the ratio of population to pediatric surgeons is roughly 200 000 to 1. The average number of job postings for open pediatric surgeon positions has not decreased over the last 10 years. There are 3 openings for every pediatric surgeon who exits pediatric surgery fellowship. You can argue whether it is appropriate for smaller hospitals and small- to moderate-sized towns to have a pediatric surgeon on staff, but most of the open positions are not in such hospitals. The consequence of these shortages is that surgeons with primarily adult practices continue to extend their practice to include infants and children. This is not necessarily the best situation for children, but it is better than no one offering their services. It is one thing for an adult surgeon to fix a pyloric stenosis or remove an appendix in a child. It is another thing to deal with Hirschsprung's disease, esophageal and tracheal abnormalities, and multiple congenital anomalies. The problem of the shortage of pediatric surgeons must be solved.

While on the topic of things surgical, were you aware that Dr Michael DeBakey's life was saved by something he invented? Indeed it was. DeBakey had the unique experience of being saved by a procedure he had devised. In late 2005, at the age of 98, DeBakey suffered a dissecting aortic aneurysm, and after initially refusing surgery, was eventually operated on, becoming the oldest survivor of his own operation. A Dacron graft, like the one he had pioneered, was implanted. DeBakey himself did not think the surgery was survivable, thus his reluctance to have it performed, but his pain became so intolerable he undertook the risk. Interestingly, when DeBakey decided to experiment with materials for arterial grafts in the 1950s, he went to a department store in Houston, Texas to get some nylon for this purpose. The clerk informed him that they were out of nylon, but had a new fabric called Dacron. DeBakey bought a yard. Using techniques he had learned at his mother's knee, he made the material into arterial patches at his wife's sewing machine. A colleague had been able to buy nylon about the same time, but unfortunately in the latter experimentation, it deteriorated in the body when the surgeon tried to use it. To say this differently, luck is a good partner. After Dacron proved long lasting in vascular grafts, DeBakey won the 1963 Lasker Award for his work and the same material was used to save his life. Dr DeBakey passed away in 2008.

This commentary closes with a miscellaneous *Clinical Fact/Curio*. What undergraduate school is the most likely alma mater for those earning a PhD in the United States? The answer is that a recent study found the most likely undergraduate alma mater for Americans earning a PhD in 2006 is Tsinghua University in China. Peking University, its neighbor in the Chinese capitol, ranks second. Between 2004 and 2006, those 2 schools overtook the University of California at Berkeley as the source of the most fertile training ground for United States PhDs. South Korea's Seoul National University occupies fourth place behind Berkeley, followed then by Cornell University and the University of Michigan at Ann Arbor.

These statistics were compiled by the Commission on Professionals in Science and Technology from a survey conducted by the United States National Science Foundation. The data reflect the fact that 37% of doctoral recipients from United States universities are not citizens of this country. UC Berkeley retains its top ranking for the number of undergraduates who went on to earn PhDs over the past 10 years. Its total (4298) is not that far ahead of Seoul's 3020.[1]

J. A. Stockman III, MD

Reference

1. Mervis J. Top PhD feeder schools are now Chinese. *Science*. 2008;321:185.

Electromagnetic Interference From Radio Frequency Identification Inducing Potentially Hazardous Incidents in Critical Care Medical Equipment
van der Togt R, van Lieshout EJ, Hensbroek R, et al (VU Univ, Amsterdam, the Netherlands; Univ of Amsterdam, the Netherlands; TNO Netherlands Organization for Applied Scientific Research, Leiden; et al)
JAMA 299:2884-2890, 2008

Context.—Health care applications of autoidentification technologies, such as radio frequency identification (RFID), have been proposed to improve patient safety and also the tracking and tracing of medical equipment. However, electromagnetic interference (EMI) by RFID on medical devices has never been reported.

Objective.—To assess and classify incidents of EMI by RFID on critical care equipment.

Design and Setting.—Without a patient being connected, EMI by 2 RFID systems (active 125 kHz and passive 868 MHz) was assessed under controlled conditions during May 2006, in the proximity of 41 medical devices (in 17 categories, 22 different manufacturers) at the Academic Medical Centre, University of Amsterdam, Amsterdam, the Netherlands. Assessment took place according to an international test protocol. Incidents of EMI were classified according to a critical care adverse events scale as hazardous, significant, or light.

Results.—In 123 EMI tests (3 per medical device), RFID induced 34 EMI incidents: 22 were classified as hazardous, 2 as significant, and 10 as light. The passive 868-MHz RFID signal induced a higher number of incidents (26 incidents in 41 EMI tests; 63%) compared with the active 125-kHz RFID signal (8 incidents in 41 EMI tests; 20%); difference 44% (95% confidence interval, 27%-53%; $P < .001$). The passive 868-MHz RFID signal induced EMI in 26 medical devices, including 8 that were also affected by the active 125-kHz RFID signal (26 in 41 devices; 63%). The median distance between the RFID reader and the medical device in all EMI incidents was 30 cm (range, 0.1-600 cm).

Conclusions.—In a controlled nonclinical setting, RFID induced potentially hazardous incidents in medical devices. Implementation of RFID in the critical care environment should require on-site EMI tests and updates of international standards.

▶ We are hearing more and more about radiofrequency identification devices (RFID) these days. These are used in anti theft clips in retail merchandising, in security access cards, and even for electronic toll collection. The devices are quickly making their way into our health care systems. For example, RFIDs can be embedded into surgical sponges for tracking during an operation. They can be placed in endoscopic capsules to help assess where those capsules are along the GI tract. They can be built into the end of endotracheal tubes allowing external monitoring of where that tube is located. We have also seen the development of a syringe-implantable glucose-sensing RFID microchip. Of course, these chips are also being used as identification devices for our pets.

There are two types of RFIDs: passive and active. RFID technology is based on 2 components: tags and readers. Tags are manufactured as either passive or active, and use radio waves to communicate their identity and possible other information to nearby readers (Fig 1). Passive RFID tags do not have internal power, but rather are activated by the electromagnetic field generated by the external reader, transmitting information back to the reader. The electromagnetic field can cover a distance ranging from 1 cm to 50 cm to 10 m to 30 m. Active RFID tags are operated by batteries and can broadcast information, such as identity or product temperature, without being activated by the reader. The active tag can broadcast over a distance of 50 m to 100 m. The reader is often also called a scanner.

The report from the Netherlands is an important one. It was designed to determine whether RFID technology might interfere with other medical devices

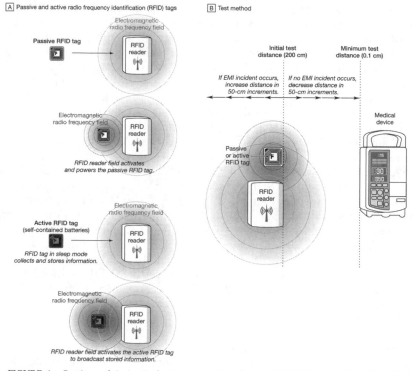

FIGURE 1.—Passive and Active Radio Frequency Identification (RFID) Tags and Test Methods. A, Active RFID tags contain batteries and are able to collect, store, and broadcast information without activation by an RFID reader. To save power, some active RFID tags are in sleep mode and can be awakened by a reader to start broadcasting. B, EMI indicates electromagnetic interference. The same test method was used for both passive and active tags. (Reprinted from van der Togt R, van Lieshout EJ, Hensbroek R, et al. Electromagnetic interference from radio frequency identification inducing potentially hazardous incidents in critical care medical equipment. *JAMA.* 2008;299:2884-2890. Copyright 2008 American Medical Association. All rights reserved.)

commonly found, for example, in critical care units. Indeed, interference turned out to be quite common. In 123 tests of electromagnetic interference, RFIDs induced 34 malfunctions of equipment, the majority of which would be considered hazardous malfunctions. The median distance at which all RFID incidents occurred was just 30 cm with a considerable range up to 600 cm. RFID devices were capable of shutting down infusion pumps, inactivating internal pacemakers, turning off ventilators, causing intra-aortic balloon pumps to malfunction and other assorted, potentially lethal, effects.

Only time will tell how far RFID technology will progress and what the unintended consequences will be in medical settings. If you thought cell phones in ICUs were bad, RFIDs may be very bad. If you want to learn more about taming the technology beast, see the editorial with the same name that accompanied the RFID report.[1] It is well worth reading.

As this commentary closes, another *Clinical Fact/Curio*, this having to do with medical schools. There is an increasing trend in the United States to attribute names to medical schools in addition to that of the host university. As of the beginning of 2009, 19 of 126 United States medical schools (approximately 15%) have such names. Some include the names of famous scientists such as the Albert Einstein College of Medicine of Yeshiva University, politicians (F. Edward Hebert School of Medicine of the Uniformed Services University of the Health Sciences), and religious figures such as San Juan Bautista School of Medicine. Some 15 medical schools have changed their names based on a gift and 10 of these 15 schools have been renamed in the last decade. Of the 15 medical schools named after donors, the median initial gift for naming rights was $95 million (range $8 million to $100 million). Eight of the schools are private and 7 are public. In one recent name change, which occurred in January 2007, Brown University announced that the Warren Alpert Foundation donated $100 million to the school that was then renamed the Warren Alpert Medical School of Brown University. Some schools actually drop the name of an individual to morph into a different named medical school. For example, Bowman Gray School of Medicine of Wake Forest University, after 57 years, has become the Wake Forest University School of Medicine. The latter name change reflects both the strong ties of the medical school to the university as well as its desire to distance the school and its name from the tobacco industry (Mr Gray was the former president of R.J. Reynolds Tobacco Company). The James H. Quillen College of Medicine of East Tennessee State University was originally the Quillen-Dishner College of Medicine from 1978 to 1989. Rumors concerning alleged objectionable activity by the benefactor, Dr Paul Dishner, led the university to remove his name from the school. Other universities and their names have survived controversy. Brown University was named after Nicholas Brown, Jr, in 1804, the Brown family having been instrumental in moving the former College of Rhode Island from Newport to its current location in Providence. The Brown family accumulated enormous wealth in trade with China, in farming, and from investments in the slave trade during the 1760s through 1780s. Brown University completed a detailed study in 2001 that addressed naming the school in honor of a family in which some members were involved in the slave trade. No change in name was forthcoming.

There are several examples of "push-backs" from groups that approve the naming rights to schools, hospitals, and other health facilities. The University of Iowa recently rejected a $15 million gift from Wellmark Corporation to rename the School of Public Health because the faculty felt there were ethical and moral issues related to working in a school named after a for-profit health insurance company. The Children's Hospital in Columbus, Ohio was renamed after Columbus-based Nationwide Insurance in exchange for a donation of $50 million over 10 years. One wonders what would happen if in time Nationwide Insurance, whose slogan is the company is "on your side" was ever determined not to be the latter.

You can see from the provided list some schools that have been named after benefactors. In 2007 dollar equivalents, the cost to have a medical school in your own name varies from a low of slightly over $10 million to about one-quarter of a billion dollars. While none of these amounts is exactly chump change, one wonders whether some of these "named" medical schools will regret the decisions they have made.[2]

J. A. Stockman III, MD

References

1. Berwick DM. Taming the technology beast. *JAMA.* 2008;299:2898-2899.
2. Loeffler JS, Halperin EC. Selling a medical school's name. Ethical and practical dilemmas. *JAMA.* 2008;300:1937-1938.

School	Year	Amount, $ in Millions	2007 Amount, $ in Millions[b]
Schools Named After Benefactors[a]			
Warren Alpert Medical School, Brown University	2007	100	100
Boonshoft School of Medicine, Wright State University	2005	28.5	31.1
Sanford School of Medicine, University of South Dakota	2005	20	21.8
Miller School of Medicine, University of Miami	2004	100	112.5
Roy J. and Lucille A. Carver College of Medicine, University of Iowa	2002	90	105.7
Feinberg School of Medicine, Northwestern University	2002	75	88.1
David Geffen School of Medicine, University of California, Los Angeles	2000	200	246.7
Joan C. Edwards School of Medicine, Marshall University	2000	65	80.2
Brody School of Medicine, East Carolina University	1999	8	10.1
Keck School of Medicine, University of Southern California	1999	110	139.4
Weill Cornell Medical College, Cornell University	1998	200	257.7
Robert Wood Johnson Medical School, University of Medicine and Dentistry of New Jersey	1986	16	30.4
Quillen-Dishner College of Medicine, East Tennessee State University[c]	1978	14	47.4
Pritzker School of Medicine, University of Chicago	1968	12	73.8
Bowman Gray School of Medicine, Wake Forest University[d]	1941	0.75	11

[a]All data were taken from Web sites of the various institutions.
[b]2007 dollar conversion was performed by the Federal Reserve Bank of Minneapolis Consumer Price Index Calculator.
[c]School renamed in 1989 to James H. Quillen College of Medicine.
[d]School renamed in 1998 to Wake Forest University School of Medicine.

12 Musculoskeletal

Age-related patterns of injury in children involved in all-terrain vehicle accidents
Kellum E, Creek A, Dawkins R, et al (Univ of Tennessee-Campbell Clinic, Memphis)
J Pediatr Orthop 28:854-858, 2008

Background.—All-terrain vehicle (ATV) accidents are considerable sources of morbidity and mortality for children and adolescents. This study was done to investigate the types and severity of injuries and the role of age and body mass index on the types of fractures sustained in children younger than 16 years.

Methods.—A retrospective chart review was done on 96 consecutive children who sustained injuries in ATV-related accidents during a 30-month period. Sixty-four patients were boys and 32 were girls. The mean age of the children was 11.0 years. To determine differences in fracture type, Glasgow Coma Scale, Pediatric Trauma Score, and length of hospitalization, the 96 patients were divided into 2 groups: group A, 54 children (56%) 12 years or younger, and group B, 42 children (44%) 13 years or older.

Results.—Sixty-one children (64%) required hospital admission. No statistically significant difference between the 2 groups was noted. Fifty-four (56%) children required surgical treatment. One fatality occurred. No statistically significant differences between the 2 groups were noted regarding the Glasgow Coma Scale and the Pediatric Trauma Score. Orthopaedic injuries were the most common, occurring in 58 (60%) children, followed by head injury in 34 (35%) and intraabdominal/intrathoracic injuries in 23 (24%). Nineteen (20%) children had more than 1 system involved, and 1 had 3 systems involved. Sixty-eight fractures occurred in 58 children (38 in group A and 30 in group B) including 9 open fractures. As expected, older children had a significantly increased body mass index compared with younger children (P < 0.02). Age-related patterns of fracture were observed. Younger children (≤12 years) were more likely to sustain an isolated fracture (odds ratio 2.9, P < 0.02) and were more likely to sustain a lower extremity fracture (odds ratio 3.2, P < 0.03), specifically a femoral fracture (odds ratio 6.5, P < 0.01), than older children (≥13 years). Older children were more likely to sustain a pelvic fracture (odds ratio 1.108, P < 0.04).

Conclusions.—To our knowledge, this is the first study to evaluate age-related patterns of fractures in ATV-related accidents. It is our hope that increased awareness of the severity and types of injuries and fracture patterns will lead to more rapid diagnosis and help to bring about improved safety measures, increased public awareness, and even legislation concerning the use of ATVs by children.

Level of Evidence.—Level IV.

▶ All-terrain vehicle (ATV) injuries continue on the rise. This report of Kellum et al is important because it describes and confirms that ATV accidents are a significant source of morbidity and mortality in children and adolescents and also demonstrates that musculoskeletal injuries are common and that children frequently have associated injuries of the head, chest, and abdomen. Clearly, children younger than 12 years represent a greater proportion of those injured, and when injured are more likely to have fractures. Lower extremity fractures, and in particular femoral fractures, are more common in younger children, whereas pelvic fractures are more common in older children. The figures in the original article show the likeliest areas of the body to be injured in an ATV accident.

While on the topic of orthopedic injuries and orthopedics in general, please recognize that we are now in a situation where we are desperately short of pediatric orthopedic surgeons. Back in the 1990s, studies suggested that there were excess numbers of orthopedic surgeons in general in the United States and predicted that by the year 2010 there would be a serious oversupply. This has not occurred. In fact, we do not have enough orthopedic surgeons to meet current demands for care. When it comes to pediatric orthopedics, of the 45 pediatric orthopedic fellowship positions in the United States and Canada, an average of just 27 positions fill each year. Many of the physicians who train in North America are foreign medical graduates who may not be able to continue to practice on our shores upon completion of their fellowship. Add to that the fact that more than 50% of medical students are now women, who seldom select orthopedic surgery, and you see the nature of the problem. One way to address the current work shortage is described by Ward et al.[1] This article suggests the use of mid-level providers in the pediatric orthopedic office setting. There are many common musculoskeletal problems that can be seen by nurse practitioners and physician assistants trained in the practice of pediatric orthopedics. These problems include in-toeing, out-toeing, bowlegs, knock-knees, anterior knee pain, and so on. Given the fact that half of all billings done by pediatric orthopedic surgeons originate in the office setting, you can see how the use of mid-level practitioners will help address the shortage of people who need to be in the operating room.

This commentary closes with a *Clinical Fact/Curio* about the musculoskeletal system. The word amputation is derived from the Latin *putare*, literally meaning to prune. Thus the word, despite its gory medical implications, has its origins in horticulture. It should be noted that amputation was rarely practiced by surgeons in antiquity. It was only in the 17th century that the word amputation entered the English language. Previous to this, someone who operated to remove a body part would have talked of "dismembering." From around 1600, both gardeners and surgeons used the term equally. In John Woodall's *Surgion's Mate* (1617), he described amputation as "the most lamentable part of Chirurgery." Soon the word amputation entered the medical literature and was applied not just to amputations of the limb, but also any body part. For example, a mastectomy was previously known as "the amputation of the breast." Allegedly, the great surgeon, Robert Liston, set a record by amputating a leg in less than 30 seconds. Incidentally, the amputation also included the accidental severing of 2 fingers of his assistant's hand.[2]

J. A. Stockman III, MD

References

1. Ward WT, Eberson CP, Otis SA, et al. Pediatric orthopedic practice management: the role of mid-level providers. *J Pediatr Orthop.* 2008;28:795-798.
2. Lawrence C. Historical word: amputation. *Lancet.* 2008;371:1065.

Mechanical supports for acute, severe ankle sprain: a pragmatic, multicentre, randomised controlled trial

Lamb SE, Marsh JL, Hutton JL, et al (Univ of Warwick, Coventry, UK)
Lancet 373:575-581, 2009

Background.—Severe ankle sprains are a common presentation in emergency departments in the UK. We aimed to assess the effectiveness of three different mechanical supports (Aircast brace, Bledsoe boot, or 10-day below-knee cast) compared with that of a double-layer tubular compression bandage in promoting recovery after severe ankle sprains.

Methods.—We did a pragmatic, multicentre randomised trial with blinded assessment of outcome. 584 participants with severe ankle sprain were recruited between April, 2003, and July, 2005, from eight emergency departments across the UK. Participants were provided with a mechanical support within the first 3 days of attendance by a trained health-care professional, and given advice on reducing swelling and pain. Functional outcomes were measured over 9 months. The primary outcome was quality of ankle function at 3 months, measured using the Foot and Ankle Score; analysis was by intention to treat. This study is registered as an International Standard Randomised Controlled Trial, number ISRCTN37807450.

Results.—Patients who received the below-knee cast had a more rapid recovery than those given the tubular compression bandage. We noted clinically important benefits at 3 months in quality of ankle function with the cast compared with tubular compression bandage (mean difference 9%; 95% CI $2 \cdot 4$–$15 \cdot 0$), as well as in pain, symptoms, and activity. The mean difference in quality of ankle function between Aircast brace and tubular compression bandage was 8%; 95% CI $1 \cdot 8$–$14 \cdot 2$, but there were little differences for pain, symptoms, and activity. Bledsoe boots offered no benefit over tubular compression bandage, which was the least effective treatment throughout the recovery period. There were no significant differences between tubular compression bandage and the other treatments at 9 months. Side-effects were rare with no discernible differences between treatments. Reported events (all treatments combined) were cellulitis (two cases), pulmonary embolus (two cases), and deep-vein thrombosis (three cases).

Interpretation.—A short period of immobilisation in a below-knee cast or Aircast results in faster recovery than if the patient is only given tubular compression bandage. We recommend below-knee casts because they show the widest range of benefit.

Funding.—National Co-ordinating Centre for Health Technology Assessment.

▶ Virtually no youngster gets out of childhood/the teen years without having experienced a strain, sprain, or a fracture. When it comes to ankle sprains in particular, little has been written about the very best way these should be managed. The report of Lamb et al presents a randomized trial in which the investigators aimed to evaluate the effects of 4 different types of immobilization devices (TubiGrip compression bandage, Bledsoe boot, Aircast brace, and below-knee cast) on the outcome of patients recovering from severe ankle sprains. The bottom line was that a below-knee cast for 10 days resulted in more rapid resolution of symptoms, including pain and the greatest recovery of self-reported ankle function at 3-month follow-up compared with the other 3 treatments. This finding is likely to be viewed as controversial because consensus recommendations in recent decades have been toward functional treatment of ankle sprains. These recommendations emphasize little, if any, immobilization, early return to weight bearing, and progressive range of motion, balance, and coordination exercises.

Most of us have been taught to believe that ankle sprains are innocuous injuries with little or no lasting consequences, when in fact lingering symptoms, self-reported disability, lower levels of physical activity, and recurrent ankle sprains are often reported for months and sometimes years after initial ankle sprain injury. Adult data suggest that 30% of patients with an initial ankle sprain will develop chronic ankle instability or repetitive giving way of the ankle during functional activities.[1] Some also believe that severe and repetitive ankle sprains can lead to an increased risk of ankle osteoarthritis. These long-term problems point to the need for a more solid consensus on the best way to manage common sprains.

Lamb et al have presented provocative results that show the benefits of 10 days of below-knee casting in patients with ankle sprains. Pediatric age patients were included in this report, although most of these patients were well into their teen years. It should be noted that while short-term benefits were identified in 3 months, by 9 months no differences were seen among the management techniques.

In a commentary that accompanied this report, Hertel suggested 1 reason that the below-knee cast was associated with diminished symptoms and pain and increased function at 3 months postsprain was that better ligamentous healing occurred with the period of immobilization.[2] Clearly, the findings reported by Lamb et al are unexpected and deserving of further consideration.

J. A. Stockman III, MD

References

1. Kerkhoff SGM, Struijs PA, Martl RK, et al. Functional treatments for acute ruptures of the lateral ankle ligament: a systematic review. *Acta Orthop Scand.* 2003;74:69-77.
2. Hertel J. Immobilization for acute severe ankle sprain. *Lanet.* 2008;373:524-525.

Patterns of skeletal fractures in child abuse: systematic review
Kemp AM, Dunstan F, Harrison S, et al (Cardiff Univ, UK)
BMJ 337:a1518, 2008

Objectives.—To systematically review published studies to identify the characteristics that distinguish fractures in children resulting from abuse and those not resulting from abuse, and to calculate a probability of abuse for individual fracture types.

Design. Systematic review.

Data Sources.—All language literature search of Medline, Medline in Process, Embase, Assia, Caredata, Child Data, CINAHL, ISI Proceedings, Sciences Citation, Social Science Citation Index, SIGLE, Scopus, TRIP, and Social Care Online for original study articles, references, textbooks, and conference abstracts until May 2007.

Study Selection.—Comparative studies of fracture at different bony sites, sustained in physical abuse and from other causes in children <18 years old were included. Review articles, expert opinion, postmortem studies, and studies in adults were excluded.

Data Extraction and Synthesis.—Each study had two independent reviews (three if disputed) by specialist reviewers including paediatricians, paediatric radiologists, orthopaedic surgeons, and named nurses in child protection. Each study was critically appraised by using data extraction sheets, critical appraisal forms, and evidence sheets based on NHS Centre for Reviews and Dissemination guidance. Meta-analysis was done where possible. A random effects model was fitted to account for the heterogeneity between studies.

Results.—In total, 32 studies were included. Fractures resulting from abuse were recorded throughout the skeletal system, most commonly in infants (<1 year) and toddlers (between 1 and 3 years old). Multiple fractures were more common in cases of abuse. Once major trauma was excluded, rib fractures had the highest probability for abuse (0.71, 95% confidence interval 0.42 to 0.91). The probability of abuse given a humeral fracture lay between 0.48 (0.06 to 0.94) and 0.54 (0.20 to 0.88), depending on the definition of abuse used. Analysis of fracture type showed that supracondylar humeral fractures were less likely to be inflicted. For femoral fractures, the probability was between 0.28 (0.15 to 0.44) and 0.43 (0.32 to 0.54), depending on the definition of abuse used, and the developmental stage of the child was an important discriminator. The probability for skull fractures was 0.30 (0.19 to 0.46); the most common fractures in abuse and non-abuse were linear fractures. Insufficient comparative studies were available to allow calculation of a probability of abuse for other fracture types.

Conclusion.—When infants and toddlers present with a fracture in the absence of a confirmed cause, physical abuse should be considered as a potential cause. No fracture, on its own, can distinguish an abusive from a non-abusive cause. During the assessment of individual fractures, the site, fracture type, and developmental stage of the child can help to determine the likelihood of abuse. The number of high quality comparative research studies in this field is limited, and further prospective epidemiology is indicated.

▶ This systematic review of fractures in child abuse by Kemp et al is a truly rigorous attempt to derive meaningful conclusions from a diverse and highly heterogeneous literature. If there is a bottom line to the message from this report, it is that the site or type of fracture can never in and of itself distinguish between an abusive episode and an accident. A number of other factors need to be taken into account, including age. The child's age is very important—a fracture of the humerus should obviously be viewed differently in a 2-month-old child than in a 15-year-old football player, and abuse may be seriously considered in a young child with a serious injury if no history that correlates with the injury is given or if a care provider's history differs from one telling to another. Perhaps the most important finding from this report is that rib fractures, regardless of the type, tend to be highly specific for abuse in the absence of an overt traumatic or organic cause.

It may be worthwhile reading this report in some detail because it does synthesize a wide body of literature from international publications dealing with child abuse. The report also identifies many deficiencies in the scientific research published to date and also identifies the methodological limitations in the field of child abuse.

J. A. Stockman III, MD

Pediatric Heelys injuries
Aarons C, Iobst C, Lopez M (Univ of Miami, FL)
J Pediatr Orthop 28:502-505, 2008

Background.—To determine the incidence and severity of injuries caused by Heelys.

Methods.—A retrospective review of all fractures presenting to an orthopaedic emergency room at a metropolitan children's hospital during a 90-day period. The type of fracture, mechanism of injury, and management were recorded for each patient. For those injuries related to the use of Heelys, further data were collected including total number of visits, cast changes, and cost. Each Heelys patient/family was contacted and answered a questionnaire detailing their use of Heelys and the events surrounding the injury.

Results.—A total of 953 patients with fractures were evaluated for 90 days. Sixteen patients with 17 fractures (1.68%) were identified as being related to the use of Heelys. This compares to the incidence of fractures in our sample from basketball (6.19%), bicycle (4.41%), football (4.09%), monkeybars (3.78%), skateboarding (3.25%), soccer (2.62%), baseball (2.52%), and trampoline (2.31%). The average age of each Heelys patient was 8.9 years, and 13 patients were girls. There were 16 upper extremity and 1 lower extremity fracture. No patient needed operative treatment or admission. Average number of follow-up visits was 1.6, with an average of 1.4 casts per patient. Average cost per patient was $1368. Ninety-two percent of the Heelys injuries occurred outdoors. Fifty-four percent of children were being supervised when they fell, but only 31% were wearing any safety equipment. Sixty-two percent of parents were not aware that safety equipment was recommended. All 13 parents indicated that they would not purchase another pair of Heelys, and only 23% of the children wanted to keep using Heelys after the injury.

Conclusions.—The incidence of Heelys injuries (1.68%) was relatively low compared with other common childhood play activities. The fractures were mostly in the upper extremity, and no fracture required surgical intervention or admission to the hospital. Sixty-two percent of the parents were not aware that safety equipment was recommended, and only 31% of the children were wearing safety equipment.

▶ The title of this report caught me off guard. This editor obviously is not "hip." I thought the word "Heelys" might be an eponym, or perhaps a misspelling of "Healy," implying that a pediatric Healys injury might be the result of being struck by a British automobile. Obviously I missed the introduction for the 2000 Christmas shopping season of Heelys, the shoe that is designed to appear as regular sneakers, but which have the option to install a single or double wheel in the heel. The construction of the shoe is such that the wearer can transition from walking to heeling simply by shifting his or her weight. Heeling position is to place one foot in front of the other and shift the weight to the wheel portion of the sole. If case balance is lost, shifting the weight to the front of the sole will stop all motion. Although use of Heelys seems simple, the question asked by these authors is just how safe they are.

The authors of this report studied all patients with fractures seen in the orthopaedic emergency room at Miami Children's Hospital over a 3-month period. A total of 953 fractures were observed during that timeframe. Of these, 17 fractures related to using Heelys. This equates to Heelys causing 1.68% of all fractures seen in a pediatric emergency room at least in Miami. The average cost of a Heelys fracture was $2467, a fairly expensive price to pay for a pair of wheeled sneakers. The majority of the fractures were of the upper extremity.

The findings from this report indicate that the public is not getting the message that safety equipment is required while wearing Heelys. Heelys do carry a warning label in this regard. Also, there is a warning on the sole of the shoe that states removal of the sticker acts as a release of liability of the company. It should also be noted that there have been anecdotal reports of significant spine and head injuries related to the use of Heelys.

Heelys are now being sold all over the country and in fact, all over the world. By 1988, more than 4.5 million pairs had been sold and Heelys have quickly become part of pop culture. According to their web site, Heelys are even worn by National Basketball Association superstar Shaquille O'Neal (size 22).[1]

If there is a bottom line here, it is indeed that safety equipment should be worn by anyone using Heelys, unless you are so well "heeled" that you are willing not only to be injured, but to pick up a several thousand dollar emergency room tab.

J. A. Stockman III, MD

Reference

1. Heeling Sports Ltd. Web site., http://www.heelys.com/hsl_background_inform ation.pdf. Accessed July 27, 2008.

Ultrasound hip evaluation in achondroplasia

De Pellegrin M, Moharamzadeh D (IRCCS San Raffaele Hosp, Milan, Italy)
J Pediatr Orthop 28:427-431, 2008

Background.—During the period from 1985 to 2006, 22 children (44 hips) affected by achondroplasia were ultrasonographically evaluated.

Methods.—The patients' age at examination ranged from 7 days to 29 months. The hip ultrasound (US) examination was performed, according to Graf's method, using a Siemens Sonoline sonogram with linear 5.0- and 7.5-MHz probes. In all the hips, the alpha angle was impossible to be measured because the medial margin of the ilium was not ultrasonographically detectable. The ultrasonographic findings included the following: configuration of the acetabular bony rim, configuration of the acetabular roof, echogenicity of the head and acetabular cartilage, bony coverage percentage of the femoral head according to Morin et al, beta angle according to Graf, dynamic hip instability, and presence of the proximal femoral ossific nucleus.

Results.—All hips had a sharp acetabular bony rim, a horizontal acetabular roof, thickened acetabular cartilage, and normal echogenicity. The femoral head was well centered and deeply contained in the acetabular fossa. The mean coverage was 86.7% (range: 78%-90%) and showed progressively larger values with increasing age. The mean value of the beta angle was 20 degrees (range: 8 degrees-38 degrees). The value of the beta angle tended to decrease as age increased. No difference was observed between the right and the left hip in both measurements. All hips were stable. The ossific nucleus was present in 5 children.

Conclusions.—The characteristic findings in hip ultrasonography in children with achondroplasia can aid in its early diagnosis because ultrasound can anatomically detect the altered development of the achondroplastic acetabulum.

▶ All of us know that achondroplasia is the most common form of dwarfism. The significant majority of cases occur sporadically. While for most babies born with dwarfism, physical findings are present at birth, for others, the findings are quite equivocal. For those diagnosed based on physical findings, the most frequent characteristics include a large head and a wide face with prominent frontal region, a chest which is normal in length, but which is flat with flared costal margins. The hands are broad with a shorter middle finger. The lower limbs, which are often bowed, have an overabundance of skin. The primary morphologic anomaly in achondroplasia occurs in the growth plate: the cell columns are short and disordered, with the proliferative zone being the most severely affected.

As noted, the clinical features of achondroplasia may not be fully apparent at birth. Interestingly, however, since the introduction of screening using ultrasound of the hip for screening diagnosis of developmental dysplasia, newborn infants with achondroplasia are being picked up with the findings described in the De Pellegrin et al report. The many skeletal findings that would be expected to be seen in an individual affected with achondroplasia may not show up with standard radiographs at birth because there is a large amount of cartilage present in normal newborns, particularly in the achondroplastic newborn skeleton. Thus plain films may miss the diagnosis, but ultrasound can detect cartilaginous abnormalities, which are almost universally seen in infants with achondroplasia. Thus, it is that purely by coincidence when ultrasound is used to screen for neonatal signs of developmental dysplasia of the hip, a diagnosis of achondroplasia might in fact be made.

While on the topic of neonatal developmental dysplasia of the hip, please recognize that maternal hyperthyroidism has now been described to predispose to an increased risk of developmental dysplasia of the hip.[1] The incidence of developmental dysplasia in infants born to mothers with Graves disease appears to be increased some 10 to 30 times normal. Thyroid hormone's role in bone maturation and muscle development is well described and apparently having too much thyroid hormone during embryogenesis can do a job on an infant's hips in utero. The study, which reported the relationship between neonatal developmental dysplasia of the hip and maternal hyperthyroidism, also showed that the risk of developmental dysplasia of the hip is significantly elevated in babies born of mothers who had hyperemesis during pregnancy. The reasons for the latter relationship remain unclear.

J. A. Stockman III, MD

Reference

1. Ishikawa N. The relationship between neonatal developmental dysplasia of the hip and maternal hyperthyroidism. *J Pediatr Orthop.* 2008;28:432-434.

Age-appropriate body mass index in children with achondroplasia: interpretation in relation to indexes of height

Hoover-Fong JE, Schulze KJ, McGready J, et al (Johns Hopkins Univ, Baltimore, MD; et al)
Am J Clin Nutr 88:364-371, 2008

Background.—Achondroplasia is the most common short stature skeletal dysplasia, with an estimated worldwide prevalence of 250 000. Body mass index (BMI)–for-age references are required for weight management guidance for children with achondroplasia, whose body proportions are unlike those of the average stature population.

Objective.—This study used weight and height data in a clinical setting to derive smoothed BMI-for-age percentile curves for children with achondroplasia and explored the relation of BMI with its components, weight and height.

Design.—This was a longitudinal observational study of anthropometric measures of children with achondroplasia from birth through 16 y of age.

Results.—The analysis included 1807 BMI data points from 280 children (155 boys, 125 girls) with achondroplasia. As compared with the BMI of peers of average stature, the BMI in children with achondroplasia is higher at birth, lacks a steep increase in infancy and a later nadir between 1 and 2 y of age, and remains substantially higher through 16 y of age in both sexes. Patterns of change in height and weight in children with achondroplasia are unique in that there is no overlap in the height distribution after 6 mo of age and no spike in height velocity during infancy or puberty—the 2 periods of greatest linear growth in individuals of average stature.

Conclusions.—Sex- and age-specific BMI curves are available for children with achondroplasia (birth to 16 y of age) for health surveillance and future research to determine associations with health outcomes (eg, cardiovascular disease, diabetes, and indication for and outcome of surgery).

▶ This author is old enough to recall a time when we did not have normative growth curves for children with many genetic disorders, including Down syndrome and achondroplasia. Of course we now have these available, but we are still learning about other related aspects of growth. This report from Baltimore provides the first BMI-for-age growth curves for children with achondroplasia using data obtained longitudinally over decades of clinical practice. Needless to say, such reference curves are important to clinical practice in order to provide the type of medical care we should for this population of youngsters. Excess weight takes its toll on everyone, but children with certain disorders can be at exceptional risk for being overweight. For example, overweight children with achondroplasia are more susceptible to obstructive sleep apnea, genu varus, spinal stenosis, and lordosis. In addition, morbidity and mortality studies of those affected with achondroplasia show a higher than expected age- and sex-matched risk of cardiovascular events.

What we learn from this report is that BMI is substantially higher in children with achondroplasia than in peers and that patterns of change in BMI with age differ between individuals with achondroplasia and their peers of average stature. Clearly references for BMI derived from children of average stature are not applicable to the achondroplastic population because of the dramatic differences in body proportions, such that nearly all children with achondroplasia would be considerably overweight if evaluated against the norm of those with an average stature. BMI tends to overestimate body fatness in populations with disproportionately long trunk and short limb length even in other normal populations such as in Asian and Inuit populations. At the same time, body fatness is underestimated by BMI in populations with long limbs such as Australian Aborigines. Achondroplasia represents an extreme of the former body type, thus justifying condition-specific BMI curves such as those reported in the study from Baltimore.

Chances are reasonably good that any large general pediatric practice will have one or more children with achondroplasia in that practice. Although skeletal dysplasias are relatively uncommon, it is estimated that more than a quarter of a million worldwide have achondroplasia since this is the most prevalent form of dwarfism. If you do have a patient in your clinical practice with achondroplasia, you would do well to note the BMI-for-age growth charts from the manuscript abstracted and put these in your patient's chart. They will serve you and your patient well.

J. A. Stockman III, MD

Asymmetric loads and pain associated with backpack carrying by children
Macias BR, Murthy G, Chambers H, et al (Univ of California-San Diego)
J Pediatr Orthop 28:512-517, 2008

Background.—Shoulder and back pain in school children is associated with wearing heavy backpacks. Such pain may be attributed to the magnitude of the backpack load and the manner by which children distribute the load over their shoulders and back. The purpose of this study is to quantify the pressures under backpack straps of children while they carried a typical range of loads during varying conditions.

Methods.—Ten healthy children (aged, 12-14 years) wore a backpack loaded at 10%, 20%, and 30% body weight (BW). Backpacks were carried under 2 conditions, low on back or high on back. Pressure sensors (0.1 mm thick) measured pressures beneath the shoulder straps.

Results.—When walking with the backpack straps over both shoulders, contact pressures were significantly greater in the low-back condition than in the high-back condition (P = 0.004). In addition, when children carried the backpack in the low-back condition, mean pressures (± SE) over the right shoulder were as follows: 98 ± 31, 153 ± 48, and 170 ± 54 mm Hg at 10%, 20%, and 30% BW, respectively, which were significantly higher (P < 0.001) than those over the left shoulder (46 ± 14, 92 ± 29, and 90 ± 29 mm Hg, respectively). Perceived pain with the backpack over 1 shoulder was significantly greater (P = 0.002) than that for donning with both shoulders in the low-back condition.

Conclusions.—Pressures at 10%, 20%, and 30% BW loads on the right or left shoulder, during low-back or high-back conditions, are higher than the pressure thresholds (approximately 30 mm Hg) to occlude skin blood flow. Furthermore, asymmetric and high pressures exerted for extended periods of time may help explain the shoulder and back pain attributed to backpacks.

▶ This report contains a lot of information that this editor was not aware of with respect to backpack carrying by children. For example, did you know that the average child who uses a backpack loads it up to somewhere between 10% and 22% of their body weight? Did you know that when a youngster donning a backpack with a 20% body weight load, he or she is producing a skin contact pressure over the shoulder that ranges from 70 to 110 mm Hg, a pressure that directly correlates with back pain? Were you aware that almost three-quarters of children wearing a backpack use only 1 shoulder strap rather than the both that are provided with the backpack and that use of 1 shoulder strap significantly alters posture when wearing the backpack? All these statistics and points are made in this report that comes from the Department of Orthopedic Surgery at the Children's Hospital Health Center in San Diego, California.

This study from California looks at the impact of carrying a backpack in various positions. It was observed that carrying a backpack in the low back position generates higher contact pressures than carrying the backpack load in a high back position. Interestingly, regardless of the carrying position, contact pressures on the right shoulder are always higher than those on the left shoulder (Fig in the original article). The higher contact pressures over the right shoulder are probably due to posture. It is likely that subjects alter their posture by elevating their right shoulder, thereby increasing the contact pressure and loading on the right shoulder to support the backpack load. This study and others report that shoulder and spinal angles significantly increase when wearing a backpack with 1 strap compared with wearing a backpack with 2 straps. Interestingly, handedness bears no relationship to this higher right shoulder pressure load. One additional finding from this report is that low back pain was significantly more common if a youngster wears a backpack with 1 shoulder strap as opposed to 2.

Needless to say, avoiding the use of heavy backpacks can prevent some shoulder-related injuries in children and low back pain. Also needless to say, children should properly place a backpack with both straps over both shoulders to minimize local high pressures. Furthermore, children should wear backpacks above their hips and maximize the contact area between the backpack and the upper body.

This editor went to grade school in the decade following World War II. The only backpacks anyone wore at that time were surplus army ones, which were just large enough for a couple of school books and some notebooks, nothing of the size that is currently used by grade- and high-school students. Most of these kids look like they're going camping for a month or have packed a couple of parachutes.

J. A. Stockman III, MD

Changing trends in acute osteomyelitis in children: impact of methicillin-resistant Staphylococcus aureus infections

Saavedra-Lozano J, Mejías A, Ahmad N, et al (Univ of Texas Southwestern Med Ctr, Dallas)
J Pediatr Orthop 28:569-575, 2008

Background.—Staphylococcus aureus remains the most common etiologic agent of acute osteomyelitis in children. Recently, methicillin-resistant S. aureus (MRSA) has emerged as a major pathogen.

Methods.—Records of all children admitted with acute osteomyelitis from January 1999 to December 2003 were reviewed. For the comparative analysis, the study population was evenly distributed in 2 periods: period A, January 1999 to June 2001; n = 113; and period B, July 2001 to December 2003; n = 177. In addition, clinical findings of MRSA osteomyelitis were compared with non-MRSA osteomyelitis, including methicillin-sensitive S. aureus infections.

Results.—Two hundred ninety children (60% male subjects) with acute osteomyelitis were identified. Median (25th-75th percentile) age at diagnosis was 6 years (range, 2-11 years). Significant clinical findings included the following: localized pain (84%), fever (67%), and swelling (62%). Affected bones included the following: foot (23%), femur (20%), tibia (16%), and pelvis (7%). Thirty-seven percent of blood cultures were positive, and a bacterial isolate was obtained in 55% of cases. Bacteria most frequently isolated included the following: methicillin-sensitive S. aureus (45%) (57% in period A vs 40% in period B), MRSA (23%) (6% in A vs 31% in B; P < 0.001), Streptococcus pyogenes (6%), and Pseudomonas aeruginosa (5%). Children with MRSA compared with those with non-MRSA osteomyelitis had significantly greater erythrocyte sedimentation rate and C-reactive protein values on admission and increased length of hospital stay, antibiotic therapy, and overall rate of complications. We observed significant changes in antibiotic therapy related to increased use of agents with activity against MRSA.

Conclusions.—Methicillin-resistant S. aureus was isolated more frequently in the second study period and was associated with worse clinical outcomes.

▶ Until recently, the management of acute osteomyelitis acquired in the community (which is true of the vast majority of cases) was less problematic because almost all *Staphylococcus aureus* were found to be susceptible to traditional β-lactam antibiotics. Only in the last few years, however, has community-acquired methicillin-resistant *S aureus* (MRSA) become not only a major pediatric problem in the United States and elsewhere, but also a problem when it comes to specific infections such as osteomyelitis. There has been little, though, in the way of information about whether youngsters with MRSA-related osteomyelitis have a different set of characteristics in terms of outcomes in comparison with children with infection due to nonresistant *S aureus*. The authors of this report from the University of Texas in Dallas designed a study to examine the characteristics of acute myelitis in children in the period before the spike up in MRSA infections and in a more recent period as well. The goal was to determine whether MRSA osteomyelitis might have a more severe presentation and worse outcome. The investigators were able to classify 4 populations of patients with osteomyelitis: those with MRSA, those with methicillin-sensitive *S aureus*, those with non-*S aureus* infection, but with positive culture for other organisms, and those with osteomyelitis in whom the cultures were negative.

So what did these investigators find? They observed that according to most parameters, children with MRSA osteomyelitis had a worse outcome, including more days of fever, complications, duration of antibiotic therapy, presence of arthritis, need for surgery, days to normalization of CRP and ESR, and days of hospitalization. For those patients who had positive blood cultures, those with MRSA had positive blood cultures significantly longer than those cases with methicillin-sensitive *S aureus*. Children with negative culture osteomyelitis far and away had the most benign outcomes. In terms of prognostic features, anemia at presentation was more frequently associated with a poor prognosis. Interestingly, a delay of 2 days or more in the initiation of appropriate antibiotic therapy had no impact on outcomes. This implies that MRSA infection can be so severe when it causes osteomyelitis that even early antibiotic treatment does not confer a significantly better set of outcomes.

The findings from this report also showed a couple of other interesting observations. MRSA osteomyelitis was significantly more prevalent in black children (44.4% vs 13.9%) in comparison with methicillin-sensitive *S aureus*-related osteomyelitis. This has been described in other reports. Also, Hispanic children were less likely to have MRSA osteomyelitis, a new finding in the literature. Last, one bacterial organism seemed to have a far better outcome than expected. This was osteomyelitis caused by *Kingella kingae*. This is an interesting organism that seems to be increasingly reported these days. It is an organism that is difficult to isolate and frequently takes longer to identify, but fortunately, has a better prognosis associated with it in most cases.

J. A. Stockman III, MD

Abatacept in children with juvenile idiopathic arthritis: a randomised, double-blind, placebo-controlled withdrawal trial

Ruperto N, for the Paediatric Rheumatology INternational Trials Organization (PRINTO) and the Pediatric Rheumatology Collaborative Study Group (PRCSG) (IRCCS G Gaslini, PRINTO, Genoa, Italy; et al)
Lancet 372:383-391, 2008

Background.—Some children with juvenile idiopathic arthritis either do not respond, or are intolerant to, treatment with disease-modifying anti-rheumatic drugs, including anti-tumour necrosis factor (TNF) drugs. We aimed to assess the safety and efficacy of abatacept, a selective T-cell cos-timulation modulator, in children with juvenile idiopathic arthritis who had failed previous treatments.

Methods.—We did a double-blind, randomised controlled withdrawal trial between February, 2004, and June, 2006. We enrolled 190 patients aged 6–17 years, from 45 centres, who had a history of active juvenile idio-pathic arthritis; at least five active joints; and an inadequate response to, or intolerance to, at least one disease-modifying antirheumatic drug. All 190 patients were given 10 mg/kg of abatacept intravenously in the open-label period of 4 months. Of the 170 patients who completed this lead-in course, 47 did not respond to the treatment according to predefined Amer-ican College of Rheumatology (ACR) paediatric criteria and were excluded. Of the patients who did respond to abatacept, 60 were randomly assigned to receive 10 mg/kg of abatacept at 28-day intervals for 6 months, or until a flare of the arthritis, and 62 were randomly assigned to receive placebo at the same dose and timing. The primary endpoint was time to flare of arthritis. Flare was defined as worsening of 30% or more in at least three of six core variables, with at least 30% improvement in no more than one variable. We analysed all patients who were treated as per protocol. This trial is registered, number NCT00095173.

Findings.—Flares of arthritis occurred in 33 of 62 (53%) patients who were given placebo and 12 of 60 (20%) abatacept patients during the double-blind treatment (p—0·0003). Median time to flare of arthritis was 6 months for patients given placebo (insufficient events to calculate IQR); insufficient events had occurred in the abatacept group for median time to flare to be assessed (p=0·0002). The risk of flare in patients who continued abatacept was less than a third of that for controls during that double-blind period (hazard ratio 0·31, 95% CI 0·16–0·95). During the double-blind period, the frequency of adverse events did not differ in the two treatment groups. Adverse events were recorded in 37 abatacept recip-ients (62%) and 34 (55%) placebo recipients (p=0·47); only two serious adverse events were reported, both in controls (p=0·50).

Interpretation.—Selective modulation of T-cell costimulation with abatacept is a rational alternative treatment for children with juvenile idio-pathic arthritis.

Funding.—Bristol-Myers Squibb.

▶ Systemic-onset juvenile idiopathic arthritis is a subtype of chronic childhood arthritis of unknown cause, manifested by spiking fever, erythematous skin rash, pericarditis, and hepatosplenomegaly. While half of patients given nonsteroidal anti-inflammatory agents or steroids will have a significant response, the other half continue to show progressive involvement of increasing number of joints and severe functional disability, often with striking growth impairment. Even if steroids do work, their long-term use frequently leads to various disorders including iatrogenic Cushing's disease, growth suppression, bone fracture, and cataract.

One major development in rheumatology was the introduction of biological-response modifiers. Tumor necrosis factor alpha (TNFα) concentrations are increased in serum and synovial fluid of children with juvenile idiopathic arthritis, and these levels correlate with disease activity. With this recognition, children who have not responded to traditional therapies, including metho-trexate, have been given antitumor necrosis factor (anti-TNF). However, as is true of adults with rheumatoid arthritis, some patients with juvenile idiopathic arthritis do not respond or become intolerant to this therapy. An alternative to anti-TNF therapy is the agent abatacept. This is human fusion protein that consists of the extracellular domain of cytotoxic T-lymphocyte-associated antigen (CTLA)-4, also known as cytotoxic T-lymphocyte-associated antigen, which interferes with CD28 binding to CD80 or CD86 and leads to

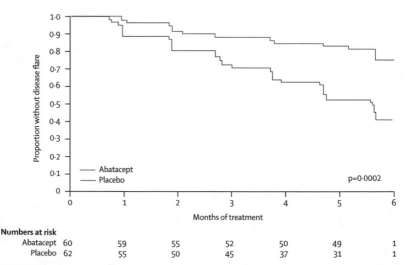

FIGURE 4.—Proportion of patients without disease flare during the 6-month double-blind period Kaplan–Meier analysis of the time to disease flare during the double-blind withdrawal period. p value represents the comparison of the time to disease flare between the abatacept and placebo groups. (Reprinted from Ruperto N, for the Paediatric Rheumatology INternational Trials Organization (PRINTO) and the Pediatric Rheumatology Collaborative Study Group (PRCSG). Abatacept in children with juvenile idiopathic arthritis: a randomised, double-blind, placebo-controlled withdrawal trial. *Lancet.* 2008;372:383-391, with permission from Elsevier.)

a down-modulation of activated T-cells. Trials in adult rheumatoid arthritis have shown that abatacept will induce improvement in disease and health-related quality of life, inhibiting progression of structural damage in patients who did not respond to other more commonly used therapies.

This report from Cincinnati and countries south of our borders looked at the efficacy and safety of abatacept compared with placebo in children and adolescents with juvenile idiopathic arthritis, children who either did not respond or became intolerant to other disease-modifying antirheumatic drugs, including some patients who had failed anti-TNF treatment. The report shows that more than half of youngsters on the placebo had a flare of their arthritis during the study period, while only 20% of those managed with abatacept did so (Fig 4). Furthermore, the time to first flare was markedly extended in those on abatacept. The drug seemed to be as well tolerated as any other form of antirheumatic therapy.

We seem to be reading a lot these days about disease-modifying agents for the treatment of refractory juvenile idiopathic arthritis. Recently, a report appeared showing the clinical benefits of tocilizumab, an anti-interleukin-6-receptor monoclonal antibody given to children aged 2 to 19 years with disease refractory to conventional treatment. As many as 90% of these youngsters responded favorably.[1] Needless to say, therapy of juvenile idiopathic arthritis with agents such as abatacept and tocilizumab represent quite sophisticated management.

An article recently appearing in *Archives of Pediatrics and Adolescent Medicine* showed that most patients with suspected new-onset juvenile rheumatoid arthritis do not obtain prompt care from an arthritis specialist.[2] There may be lots of reasons for this slow rate of rheumatology consultation. Of special concern is the possibility of the current severe shortage of rheumatologists being the cause. Possible solutions to the difficulties posed include improved medical education and the implementation of good screening techniques to help primary care physicians identify probable juvenile rheumatoid arthritis. More accurate triage by pediatric rheumatologists would also help so that they are not inundated with youngsters who really do not need the sophisticated expertise that they are capable of providing.

This commentary closes with a *Clinical Fact/Curio* related to the musculoskeletal system, specifically juvenile idiopathic arthritis. The mother of a child with juvenile idiopathic arthritis wants to know if her child would be benefitted by eating a lot of celery. In fact, celery, green peppers, and chamomile contain generous amounts of luteolin. Luteolin has anti-inflammatory properties as was recently demonstrated. Luteolin given to mice in drinking water definitively reduces levels of inflammatory markers in the blood. Authors of a study suggest that luteolin has a potential as a powerful treatment for inflammatory conditions, particularly of the brain.[3]

J. A. Stockman III, MD

References

1. Yokota S, Imagawa T, Mori M, et al. Efficacy and safety of tocilizumab in patients with systemic-onset juvenile idiopathic arthritis: a randomized, double-blind, placebo-controlled, withdrawal phase III trial. *Lancet.* 2008;371:998-1006.
2. Feldman DE, Abernatsky S, Abrahamowicz M, et al. Consultation with an arthritis specialist for children with suspected juvenile rheumatoid arthritis. A population-based study. *Arch Pediatr Adolesc Med.* 2008;162:538-543.
3. Jang S, Kelley KW, Johnson RW. Luteolin reduces IL-6 production in microglia by inhibiting JNK phosphorylation and activation of AP-1. *Proc Natl Acad Sci.* 2008; 105:7534-7539.

Autologous bone marrow transplantation in autoimmune arthritis restores immune homeostasis through CD4$^+$CD25$^+$Foxp3$^+$ regulatory T cells

Roord STA, de Jager W, Boon L, et al (Univ Med Ctr, Utrecht, Wilhelmina Children's Hosp, Utrecht)

Blood 111:5233-5241, 2008

Despite the earlier use of potent immunosuppressive or cytostatic drugs and the recent emergence of biologicals as treatment for human autoimmune diseases (AIDs), some patients still remain unresponsive to treatment. To those severely ill patients, autologous bone marrow transplantation (aBMT) is applied as a last resource, leading to disease remission in a majority of patients. The underlying mechanism of action of aBMT is still largely unknown. Here, we showed that regulatory T cells (Tregs) play a role in the natural disease course of proteoglycan-induced arthritis (PGIA) and in disease remission by aBMT. aBMT led to an initial phase of rapid disease improvement corresponding with a relative increase in CD4$^+$CD25$^+$ T cells. At this time, the CD4$^+$CD25$^+$ cells did not yet show an increase in Foxp3 expression and showed less potent suppression. After this initial improvement, disease relapsed but stabilized at a level below the severity before aBMT. This second phase was actively regulated by potently suppressive CD4$^+$CD25$^+$Foxp3$^+$ Tregs. This work provided further insight into the role of Tregs in restoration of the immune balance by aBMT and can open the way to explore therapeutic interventions to further improve treatment of AID and disease relapses.

▶ In the last decade, several thousand patients worldwide have undergone autologous hematopoietic stem cell transplantation (HSCT) as a therapy for refractory autoimmune diseases, including systemic sclerosis, multiple sclerosis, systemic lupus, Crohn disease, and rheumatoid arthritis. Human autoimmune diseases are often difficult to treat and a cause of major disability. In recent years, treatment has become increasingly more aggressive, with the earlier use of potent immunosuppressive or cytostatic drugs. These drugs and alternative therapies are based on a generalized and nonspecific inhibition of immune response and inflammation and usually have considerable side effects. More often they are not curative. In autoimmune arthritis, such as rheumatoid arthritis

(RA) and juvenile idiopathic arthritis (JIA), considerable progress has been made by the introduction of immunotherapy with biologic agents, which aims to interfere with the molecular processes that are involved in the immune-mediated pathogenesis of these autoimmune disorders.

Despite the progress that has been made to date in treatment methods of autoimmune diseases in both adults and children, some patients are still unresponsive. For those severely ill children, autologous bone marrow transplantation using HSCT methods has been the last resource. The results of HSCT in JIA are remarkably good. It induces drug-free disease remission in the majority of JIA patients during follow-up of 12 to 60 months after transplantation. It is questionable whether the achieved disease remission will be long lasting, as the assumed genetic predisposition does not change with autologous transplantation. Anecdotally, severe relapse of disease has been seen after many years of full remission following HSCT.

One critical question that investigators must address is exactly how HSCT does its job so that HSCT can be modified to induce sustained disease-free survival and, ideally, cure most patients with autoimmune diseases. The report of Roord et al sheds light on this topic. In this respect, the contributory role of Treg reconstitution as identified by Roord et al points to a promising future for the field. These investigators have shown in a mouse model that depleting CD25+ cells will yield a 100% incidence of arthritic symptoms, strongly supporting the protective role of naturally occurring Tregs. In the mouse model, when there was adequate Treg repopulation, the arthritis resolved. The opposite occurred when there was not reconstitution. It will be of interest to determine whether methods can be found to further improve Treg reconstitution. There are laboratory methods to do this.

While we are awaiting further information on how to improve HSCT as part of the management of JIA, recognize that even absent new information, HSCT can be helpful for those children with severely debilitating disease who are refractory to standard approaches to managing the disorder.

J. A. Stockman III, MD

Differentation of Post-Streptococcal Reactive Arthritis from Acute Rheumatic Fever

Barash J, Mashiach E, Navon-Elkan P, et al (The Hebrew Univ, Jerusalem, Israel; et al)
J Pediatr 153:696-699, 2008

Objective.—To perform a retrospective study comparing clinical and laboratory aspects of patients with acute rheumatic fever (ARF) and patients with post-streptococcal reactive arthritis (PSRA), to discern whether these are 2 separate entities or varying clinical manifestations of the same disease.

Study Design.—We located the records of 68 patients with ARF and 159 patients with PSRA, whose diseases were diagnosed with standardized criteria and treated by 8 pediatric rheumatologists in 7 medical centers, using the Israeli internet-based pediatric rheumatology registry. The medical records of these patients were reviewed for demographic, clinical, and laboratory variables, and the data were compared and analyzed with univariate, multivariate, and discriminatory analysis.

Results.—Four variables were found to differ significantly between ARF and PSRA and serve also as predictors: sedimentation rate, C-reactive protein, duration of joint symptoms after starting anti-inflammatory treatment, and relapse of joint symptoms after cessation of treatment. A discriminative equation was derived that enabled us to correctly classify >80% of the patients.

Conclusion.—On the basis of simple clinical and laboratory variables, we were able to differentiate ARF from PSRA and correctly classify >80% of the patients. It appears that ARF and PSRA are distinct entities.

▶ There is not one among us who has not faced the difficulty of trying to figure out whether a particular patient with arthritis and a recent group A streptococcal infection might or might not have acute rheumatic fever as opposed to the more common poststreptococcal reactive arthritis (PSRA). While the definition of the latter is fairly straightforward, arthritis in one or more joints, associated with a recent group A streptococcal infection in a subject who does not fulfill the Jones criteria for the diagnosis of acute rheumatic fever, the rub is trying to be absolutely sure about the fulfillment, or lack of fulfillment, of the Jones criteria. If one reads the literature carefully, one will see that some believe that PSRA is actually just a part of the spectrum of acute rheumatic fever, but obviously most practitioners seem to consider it a different entity. A few of those who seem to have PSRA may go on to develop a carditis, which would make the clinical scenario suggestive of acute rheumatic fever.

More than 15 years ago, Deighton tried to sort all of this out by proposing very specific features of PSRA: onset within 10 days of group A streptococcal infection (as opposed to 2-3 three weeks in acute rheumatic fever); prolonged or recurrent arthritis (in contrast to acute rheumatic fever in which the arthritis lasts for usually only a few days to a few weeks); and slow and partial response to aspirin (whereas in acute rheumatic fever the response to aspirin is usually, albeit not always, not quite dramatic).[1] Arthritis (acute onset, usually nonmigratory, affecting any joint, persistent or recurrent), poor responsivity to aspirin or nonsteroidal anti-inflammatory drugs, evidence of preceding group A streptococcal infection, and failure to fulfill the Jones criteria for diagnosis of acute rheumatic fever have been recently restated as characteristics of PSRA.[2]

The report of Barash et al relooks at a slightly different way of sorting out PSRA from acute rheumatic fever. A total of 159 patients with PSRA and 68 patients with acute rheumatic fever for whom there was sufficient analyzable data were identified. Acute rheumatic fever was diagnosed according to the revised Jones criteria, and PSRA was diagnosed in cases of arthritis involving one or more joints associated with proven group A streptococcal infection in a patient not fulfilling the Jones criteria. Clinical and laboratory data were examined retrospectively, and the characteristics of these data were compared between the acute rheumatic fever group and the PSRA group. There was little or no difference in these 2 groups when it came to age and other geographic and demographic data. The groups did not differ in the proportion of positive throat cultures at the onset of joint disease, and there was no significant difference in the levels of antistreptolysin O antibody titers.

So what were the differences between those previously diagnosed with acute rheumatic fever and PSRA? One difference was the remarkably higher erythrocyte sedimentation rates and the levels of C-reactive protein in the acute rheumatic fever group. Also, patients with acute rheumatic fever had significantly more active joints with almost 80% having migratory arthritis in contrast to just one-third of patients with PSRA. There was no difference in the joints involved except that large joints in the upper extremities were more frequently involved in acute rheumatic fever. Arthritis was symmetrical in 40% of patients with acute rheumatic fever and in just 22% of patients with PSRA. As one might suspect, no patient with PSRA had clinical evidence of carditis, whereas 60% of those with acute rheumatic fever did. Two patients in the PSRA group, however, did have prolonged P-R intervals. The interval from onset of pharyngitis to the onset of arthritis was 15.1 days for those with acute rheumatic fever versus 14.6 days for those with PSRA. As expected, the time for resolution of joint symptoms in response to anti-inflammatory treatment was significantly shorter in acute rheumatic fever patients versus those with PSRA (2.18 days vs 6.73 days, respectively) (Table 2).

If you are really into math, the authors of this report from Italy provide a fascinating formula, which can be used to discriminate between acute rheumatic fever and PSRA in those in whom there might be some difficulty, clinically, in making this distinction. By using multivariate, backward, stepwise logistic regression, 4 variables were found to be significant diagnostic discriminators between acute rheumatic fever and PSRA: erythrocytes sedimentation rate, C-reactive protein, duration of joint symptoms in response to treatment with anti-inflammatory medications, and a relapse of joint symptoms after cessation of anti-inflammatory treatment (Table 2). By using discriminate analysis, the authors calculated this prediction equation: $-1.568 + 0.015 \times$ sedimentation rate $+ 0.02 \times CRP - 0.162 \times$ days to resolution of joint symptoms $-2.04 \times$ return of joint symptoms (yes $= 1$, no $= 0$). If the value turns out to be >0, the patient is classified as having acute rheumatic fever; otherwise,

TABLE 2.—Significant Predictors of Acute Rheumatic Fever by Using Stepwise Logistic Regression

Variable	Odds Ratio	95% CI	Significance
ESR	1.015	1.000-1.031	0.043
CRP	1.016	1.004-1.028	0.007
Days to disappearance of joint symptoms	0.565	0.389-0.820	0.003
Relapse after cessation of treatment (yes/no)	0.026	0.002-0.390	0.008

(Reprinted from Barash J, Mashiach E, Navon-Elkan P, et al. Differentation of post-streptococcal reactive arthritis from acute rheumatic fever. *J Pediatr.* 2008;153:696-699.)

the patient is classified as having PSRA. This formula gives a 79% sensitivity rate (correct classification as acute rheumatic fever) and 87.5% specificity rate (correct classification as PSRA).

On the basis of this study, it can be accepted that acute rheumatic fever and PSRA appear to be 2 distinct entities with the former having a more acute presentation, with fever, acute phase responses in the laboratory, and a greater number of joints involved as well as a higher frequency of cardiac involvement. Also acute rheumatic fever has a much quicker response to treatment with respect to joint symptoms. The course of arthritis is shorter than in PSRA. Were PSRA simply to be part of the spectrum of acute rheumatic fever, one would have expected the joints to have at least have responded similarly. They do not.

The next time you see a patient who has a streptococcal infection who subsequently develops joint symptoms, think of this report of Barash, look up the formula, and run the numbers. A positive value equals acute rheumatic fever. A negative value equals PSRA.

J. A. Stockman III, MD

References

1. Deighton C. Beta-hemolytic streptococci and reactive arthritis in adults. *Ann Rheum Dis.* 1993;52:475-482.
2. Ayoub EM, Ahmed S. Update on the complications of group A streptococcal infections. *Curr Probl Pediatr.* 1997;27:90-101.

Bone Metabolism in Adolescent Athletes With Amenorrhea, Athletes With Eumenorrhea, and Control Subjects

Christo K, Prabhakaran R, Lamparello B, et al (Massachusetts General Hosp and Harvard Med School, Boston; et al)
Pediatrics 121:1127-1136, 2008

Objective.—We hypothesized that, despite increased activity, bone density would be low in athletes with amenorrhea, compared with athletes with eumenorrhea and control subjects, because of associated hypogonadism and would be associated with a decrease in bone formation and increases in bone-resorption markers.

Methods.—In a cross-sectional study, we examined bone-density measures (spine, hip, and whole body) and body composition by using dual-energy radiograph absorptiometry and assessed fasting levels of insulin-like growth factor I and bone-turnover markers (N-terminal pro-peptied of type 1 procollagen and N-telopeptide) in 21 athletes with amenorrhea, 18 athletes with eumenorrhea, and 18 control subjects. Subjects were 12 to 18 years of age and of comparable chronologic and bone age.

Results.—Athletes with amenorrhea had lower bone-density z scores at the spine and whole body, compared with athletes with eumenorrhea and control subjects, and lower hip z scores, compared with athletes with eumenorrhea. Lean mass did not differ between groups. However, athletes

with amenorrhea had lower BMI z scores than did athletes with eumenorrhea and lower insulin-like growth factor I levels than did control subjects.
Levels of both markers of bone turnover were lower in athletes with amenorrhea than in control subjects. BMI z scores, lean mass, insulin-like
growth factor I levels, and diagnostic category were important independent predictors of bone mineral density z scores.

Conclusions.—Although they showed no significant differences in lean
mass, compared with athletes with eumenorrhea and control subjects,
athletes with amenorrhea had lower bone density at the spine and whole
body. Insulin-like growth factor I levels, body-composition parameters,
and menstrual status were important predictors of bone density. Follow-
up studies are necessary to determine whether amenorrhea in athletes
adversely affects the rate of bone mass accrual and therefore peak bone
mass.

▶ Menstrual difficulties are quite common in high school athletes. Data
suggest that as many as almost 25% of young women in high school who
participate in significant athletic activities will experience amenorrhea
compared with their peers. This prevalence, of course, varies depending on
the type, intensity, and duration of exercise. The highest risk of amenorrhea is
found in athletes who are the most trim. Activities such as diving, ballet, track
running, gymnastics, swimming, and cheerleading tend to have the leanest
young women as participants, and these disciplines have the highest probability
of being associated with amenorrhea. Several of these disciplines are ones also
associated with the greatest risk of stress fractures. Thus, any potential association between amenorrhea and low bone mineral density would place such
athletes at greatest risk. It should also be recognized that maximal bone mass
accrual occurs between 11 and 14 years of age in girls, with 90% of peak
bone mass being achieved by the end of the second decade. It is this very
age that one wishes that one could optimize and maximize bone mineral density
as a protective factor throughout the rest of one's life.

The study of Christo et al examines bone mineral density, levels of bone
formation and bone-resorption markers, and predictors of bone mineral density
and bone-turnover markers in adolescent athletes with amenorrhea, athletes
with eumenorrhea, and control subjects of comparable maturity. Lower bone-
density measures were found in adolescent athletes with amenorrhea compared
with athletes who had normal menstrual cycles. These findings raise serious
concerns regarding the deleterious effects of a hypogonadal state on bone
metabolism, despite the known beneficial effects of exercise, particularly
high-impact load and weight bearing exercises on bone mass.

Needless to say that because as many as one-quarter of high school athletes
may have menstrual irregularities and because the adolescent years are a critical
time for bone mass accrual, the data from this report are highly significant.
Athletes with amenorrhea have lower bone mineral density not only in comparison with athletes with normal menstrual cycles, but also in comparison with
nonathletic control subjects with normal menstruation. Therefore, in addition
to the beneficial effects of exercise on bone density being lost in girls who

develop amenorrhea, amenorrhea may actually be truly deleterious to bone health. In this report, although lean mass in athletes with normal menstrual cycles was somewhat greater than in athletes with amenorrhea and control subjects, these differences were not statistically significant. Thus, it may be that amenorrhea, separate from nutritional status, related to low estrogen levels, is the culprit.

This report obviously is highly worrisome. Unfortunately, the report sheds no light on what can or should be done to deal with the problem of poor bone mineral metabolism in young athletic women. Both girls and boys have only one shot at fully mineralizing their bones, and this shot occurs at the sweet spot in life where one would like to see teens engaged in sporting activities. It should also be noted that men can also get osteoporosis, particularly later in life. This is particularly common in thin men who have been physically inactive throughout much of their life.[1] The report of osteoporosis in thin men showed that a self-assessment screening tool based on questions related to age and weight had a greater sensitivity in picking up osteoporosis in comparison with other commonly used assessment tools such as calcaneal ultrasound.

This commentary closes with a *Clinical Fact/Curio* that illustrates how gullible men are when it comes to sports-enhancing drugs. Men who receive a shot that might or might not contain growth hormone are more likely than women to believe it is the real thing, a new study finds. In fact, men who received placebo shots actually scored higher on a jumping test, findings reported this past summer at a meeting of the Endocrine Society of Australia. Similar findings were not observed in women receiving such a placebo.[2]

J. A. Stockman III, MD

References

1. Editorial comment. Older, thinner men are at risk of osteoporosis. *Ann Intern Med.* 2008;148:685-701.
2. Seppa N. Wishful thinking. *Sci News.* July 19, 2008;8.

Chronic fatigue syndrome in children aged 11 years old and younger

Davies S, Crawley E (Southmead Hosp, Bristol, UK; Centre for Child and Adolescent Health, Cotham Hill, UK)
Arch Dis Child 93:419-422, 2008

Children in primary school can be very disabled by chronic fatigue syndrome or ME (CFS/ME). The clinical presentation in this age group (under 12 years old) is almost identical to that in older children.

Aim.—To describe children who presented to the Bath paediatric CFS/ME service under the age of 12 years.

Method.—Inventories measuring fatigue, pain, functional disability, anxiety, family history and symptoms were collected prospectively for all children presenting to the Bath CFS/ME service between September 2004 and April 2007. Data from children who presented to the service under the age of 12 are described and compared to those who presented at age 12 or older.

Results.—178 children (under the age of 18) were diagnosed as having CFS/ME using the RCPCH criteria out of 216 children assessed. The mean age at assessment for children with CFS/ME was 14.5 years old (SD 2.9). Thirty-two (16%) children were under 12 years at the time of assessment, four children were under 5 years and the youngest child was 2 years old. Children under 12 were very disabled with mean school attendance of just over 40% (average 2 days a week), Chalder fatigue score of 8.29 (CI 7.14 to 9.43 maximum possible score = 11) and pain visual analogue score of 39.7 (possible range 0–100). Comparison with children aged 12 or older showed that both groups were remarkably similar at assessment. Twenty-four out of the 26 children with complete symptom lists would have been diagnosed as having CFS/ME using the stricter adult Centers of Disease Control and prevention (CDC) criteria.

Conclusion.—Disability in the under-12 age group was high, with low levels of school attendance, high levels of fatigue, anxiety, functional disability and pain. The clinical pattern seen is almost identical to that seen in older children, and the majority of children would also be diagnosed as having CFS/ME using the stricter adult definition.

► As much as is written about the chronic fatigue syndrome in older teens and young and older adults, there is very little in the literature about the condition in young teens and those in the preteen and earlier years of life. The latter is the focus of this report, which provides important information in this regard. The report represents the first detailed study describing primary school aged children with the chronic fatigue syndrome. Some 32 children fulfilling the criteria

TABLE 2.—Symptom List

Symptoms	Under 12 Years No With Symptom (%)	Over 12 Years No With Symptom (%)	p Value
Post-exertional malaise	26/26 (100)	135/140 (96.4)	1
Unrefreshing sleep	24/26 (92)	134/140 (95.7)	0.6
Subjective memory problems	21/28 (75)	116/139 (83.6)	0.29
Headaches	21/26 (80.8)	106/141 (75.2)	0.6
Muscle pain	19/27 (70.4)	103/141 (73.1)	0.82
Abdominal pain	16/26 (61.5)	68/138 (49.3)	0.29
Tender lymph nodes	13/26 (50)	62/140 (44.3)	0.67
Joint pain	16/27 (59.2)	94/140 (67.1)	0.51
Sore throat	16/26 (61.5)	80/140 (57.1)	0.83
Dizziness	13/26 (50)	79/137 (57.7)	0.52
Nausea	14/27 (51.9)	81/139 (58.3)	0.67
Noise sensitivity	10/26 (38.5)	48/136 (35.3)	0.82
Light sensitivity	7/27 (25.9)	33/136 (24.3)	0.81
Hypersensitivity to touch	1/26 (3.85)	20/137 (14.6)	0.2

(Courtesy of Davies S, Crawley E. Chronic fatigue syndrome in children aged 11 years old and younger. *Arch Dis Child.* 2008;93:419-421. BMJ Publishing Group Ltd.)

for the disorder were reported. The chronic fatigue syndrome in this series was defined as "generalized fatigue persisting after routine tests and investigations have failed to identify an obvious underlying cause." The functional definition used is consistent with the Centers for Disease Control definition, which requires an individual to have 6 months of fatigue and 4 additional symptoms.

What we learn from this study is that youngsters even as young as 2 years of age may fulfill the definitional requirement for having the chronic fatigue syndrome. Obviously, the diagnosis in youngsters who are preschool age is very difficult as subjective description of symptoms is less reliable. In the British report, the diagnosis was made on what appears to be disabling fatigue. In those preteens meeting the definition of chronic fatigue syndrome, associated problems other than fatigue included unrefreshing sleep, memory problems, headaches, muscle, and abdominal pains. For the full list of symptoms, see the table (Table 2).

You will have to be the one to decide whether there is such a thing as chronic fatigue syndrome at young ages. There are common medical conditions that can present with what appears to be the chronic fatigue syndrome and you should be looking for these conditions (thyroid disorders, viral infection, including EBV, etc).

As this comment closes, another *Clinical Fact/Curio*, having to do with how the human musculoskeletal system can be used to generate energy. Soon, Tokyo's harried train commuters may not only have to buy their tickets, but also generate the energy needed to punch them. East Japan Railway is testing a floor system that harvests energy from the footsteps of people walking through ticket gates. The flooring is fitted with piezoelectric elements that convert the mechanical stress from a pedestrian's weight into little blips of electricity. Twenty-five square meters of piezoelectric flooring are expected to generate 1400 kilowatt-seconds of power per day, enough to light a 40-watt LED bulb for 17 hours. It is not much, but it is expected that similar equipment is fully capable of powering automated ticket gates and information boards. As of early 2009, a 2-month pilot system was being tested at Tokyo Station, where 70 000 train riders surge through the ticket gates daily.[1]

J. A. Stockman III, MD

Reference

1. Power walking [editorial comment]. *Science*. 2009;323:315.

13 Neurology and Psychiatry

Low Iron Storage in Children and Adolescents with Neurally Mediated Syncope

Jarjour IT, Jarjour LK (Baylor College of Medicine, Houston, TX)

J Pediatr 153:40-44, 2008

Objective.—To investigate whether neurally mediated syncope (NMS) is associated with low iron storage or serum ferritin (SF).

Study design.—206 children evaluated between 2000 and 2004 for probable syncope at a tertiary care Pediatric Neurology Clinic were included in a retrospective study. Serum ferritin (SF), iron, total iron binding capacity, and hemoglobin were measured prospectively after initial history taking and physical examination, along with other diagnostic testing. We defined iron deficiency (ID) as SF <12 μg/L, and low iron storage as SF ≤25 μg/L.

Results.—Among 106 included patients with syncope, 71 had NMS and 35 had other causes of syncope. Patients with NMS, when compared with those with other causes of syncope, had a higher prevalence of low-iron storage (57% vs 17%, $P < .001$) and lower mean values of SF (27 vs 46 μg/L, $P < .001$), transferrin saturation (23 vs 31 %, $P < .01$), and hemoglobin (13.3 vs 14 g/dL, $P < .05$). Only patients with NMS had ID (15%), anemia (11%), or ID with anemia (7%).

Conclusions.—Low iron storage or serum ferritin is associated with NMS and is a potentially pathophysiologic factor in NMS.

▶ There are lots of reasons why youngsters faint. In fact syncope is quite common throughout childhood, and is particularly true in adolescence. The most common type of syncope in children and adolescents is neurally mediated syncope. Most of the literature refers to the latter as the "simple faint," which accounts for about 3-quarters or more of children with syncope. This is not to say that other causes of syncope should not be thought of, however. Other causes of syncope include cardiogenic syncope, acute hypovolemia, hyperventilation, and rarely, vertebral basilar transient ischemic attacks, in which syncope is associated with focal neurologic deficits.

Clinicians have been hampered by the lack of available treatments for children who have simple faint. It is known, however, that breath-holding spells, which some consider as a form of simple faint in early childhood are amenable to a trial of iron therapy. Based on the theory that iron deficiency might be a cause of simple faint, Jarjour and Jarjour undertook a study to assess iron status in over 100 patients with syncope. Of those with simple faint, almost 60% showed evidence of low serum ferritin values.

There are a number of nonhematologic consequences of iron deficiency that I have commented on previously. It is not clear why these manifestations of iron deficiency occur and do so often in the absence of anemia. Iron is essential for the proper functioning of many iron-dependent enzymes, particularly those involved with the synthesis and degradation of catecholamines. Interestingly, high plasma norepinephrine levels have been found in patients with postural tachycardia syndrome, many of whom have neurally mediated syncope.[1]

The next time you see a child or adolescent with unexplained syncope for which there does not seem to be a defined etiology, at least think about the possibility of iron deficiency. We learned that lesson awhile back when it came to the management of breath-holding spells. You may surprise yourself with how quickly and how well your patients get better with a tincture of iron. There is not much iron needed to replenish enzyme systems, which recover very quickly with just a dab of treatment. In fact, just a little dab will do you, in terms of the nonhematologic manifestations of iron deficiency, although more iron will be needed to replete iron stores.

This commentary closes with a *Clinical Fact/Curio* regarding neurology. It is posed in the form of a question. Would you believe that scientists have actually asked the question "do good sperm predict a good brain?" What is the story behind this? The issue raised is whether high-quality brains and high-quality sperm travel together. Some scientists wonder if there is a "latent fitness factor" that would cause evolutionarily desirable traits, both physical and mental, to be correlated with one another. Researchers from the University College London, the University of New Mexico, and the University of Delaware decided to test the question by looking for a correlation between IQ and sperm quality, the latter a direct measure of reproductive fitness. They obtained data on sperm quantity, motility, and density from a health study of 425 veterans aged 31 to 44 years and compared the data with results of the vets' intelligence tests. After correcting for factors such as drug use, they found a positive correlation. Even more interesting is that these scientists considered this an area worthy of further pursuit.[2]

J. A. Stockman III, MD

References

1. Grubb BP, Kanjawal Y, Kosinski DJ. The postural tachycardia syndrome: concise guide to diagnosis and management. *J Cardiovasc Electrophysiol.* 2006;17: 108-112.
2. Do good sperm predict a good brain? [editorial comment]. *Science.* 2008;321:487.

The influence of different food and drink on tics in Tourette syndrome

Müller-Vahl KR, Buddensiek N, Geomelas M, et al (Hannover Med School, Germany)
Acta Paediatr 97:442-446, 2008

Aim.—Tourette syndrome (TS) is characterized by waxing and waning motor and vocal tics. Because standard medication often remains unsatisfactory, many patients seek alternative medicine. The aim of this study was to increase experience about the influence of food and drinks in TS.

Methods.—A standardized questionnaire was sent to 887 people recruited from our Tourette outpatient clinic and the German TS self aid group. Respondents should assess whether 32 different foods influenced their tics.

Results.—Two hundred twenty-four questionnaires could be used for analyses. A significant positive correlation (tic deterioration) was found for caffeine and theine containing drinks such as coke ($p < 0.001$), coffee ($p < 0.001$) and black tea ($p < 0.001$) as well as for preserving agents ($p < 0.001$), refined sugar ($p < 0.001$) and sweeteners ($p < 0.001$). A significant negative correlation (tic improvement) was not found.

Conclusions.—Results from this first survey investigating the influence of special foods and drinks on tics demonstrated that 34% and 47% of responders, respectively, assessed that coffee and coke deteriorate tics. It, therefore, can be speculated that caffeine may further stimulate an already overactive dopaminergic system in TS and thus increases tics. However, from these preliminary data, no further general recommendations regarding special diets and food restrictions can be made.

▶ There have been a lot of mysteries surrounding what influences the severity of tics in Tourette syndrome. Anecdotal reports have appeared about the success of special diets in Tourette syndrome and some on the fringe have said that nicotine, alcohol, cannabis, and tetrahydrocannabinol might actually improve tics. Only 1 previous study has actually attempted to properly investigate the influence of nutritional supplements in patients with Tourette syndrome.[1] In the latter report, almost 90% of 115 responders had used 1 or more nutritional supplements. Most using these reported some improvement in their symptoms. Obviously, this was not a controlled study. Most of us are aware of the poor quality of the literature possibly linking foods and additives in causing behavioral disorders such as attention deficit hyperactivity disorder (ADHD). The purpose of the study reported by Müller-Vahl et al was to look at the influence of foods and drinks on tics in patients suffering from Tourette syndrome. The most common treatment for tics in this disorder are dopamine receptor blocking drugs that can be associated with side effects and often are ineffective. The study was conducted by mailing a detailed standardized survey to a large group of individuals with Tourette syndrome asking them to write the influence of 32 different foods, drinks, and diets on their tics.

It is tough to know whether or not to believe the data from this report because they represent self-reported observations. The findings demonstrated that a group of those who did respond noted that cola, coffee, black tea, preserving agents, white sugars, and sweeteners seemed to exacerbate the frequency of tics. In some respects, as questionable as the findings are with respect to caffeine, they seem to make sense. An earlier report suggested that caffeine did increase tic frequency.[2] Caffeine will potentiate the effects of dopamine agonists. Thus, there may be some sense to the belief that caffeine can make problems worse for individuals with tics.

What makes less sense is whether ingesting preserving agents and refined sugars would make tics worse. Unfortunately, preserving agents and refined sugars have a bad rap when it comes to health in general. This might cause one to think that these agents might deteriorate tics.

In summary, the data from this survey investigating the influence of special foods on tics in Tourette syndrome noted that 34% and 47% of responders, respectively, assessed that coffee and cola will deteriorate tics. Obviously, this is not a controlled study. One needs to be done to verify these findings. It seems of little harm, however, to see if a reduction in the consumption of beverages and foods that contain caffeine might be of help in selected patients. Given the limitations of the design of this study, it is difficult to say more than this.

As this commentary closes, another *Clinical Fact/Curio*, this having to do with neurology. Most syndromes have a nonsyndrome name that is as commonly, if not more commonly, used to identify the associated disorder. For example, Kawasaki disease is also known as mucocutaneous lymph node syndrome. There are a few syndromes, however, for which there really is no commonly available "nonsyndrome" name. One of these is Tourette's syndrome, but there once was. Tourette's syndrome is named after the French neurologist Georges Gilles de la Tourette, who in 1885 identified a combination of multiple motor tics and involuntary vocalizations. He called this distinct disorder convulsive tic disease with coprolalia, the latter disorder name not having stuck very well throughout the last century or so. According to Gilles de la Tourette, the illness began with childhood motor and vocal tics that over time increased in number and variety with the eventual appearance of coprolalia (convulsive cursing). This disease, he proposed, had a "degenerative" cause in which the afflicted inherited a nervous system weakened by the cumulative effects of the preceding generation's immoral behaviors.

To read more about the background on Tourette's syndrome and the current thinking of the differences between a syndrome and a disease, see the excellent commentary by Kushner.[3]

J. A. Stockman III, MD

References

1. Mantel BJ, Meyers A, Tran QY, Rogers S, Jacobson JS. Nutritional supplements and complementary alternative medicine in Tourette syndrome. *J Child Adolesc Psychopharmacol.* 2004;14:582-589.
2. Davis RE, Osorio I. Childhood caffeine tic syndrome. *Pediatrics.* 1998;101:e4.
3. Kushner HI. The art of medicine. History as a medical tool. *Lancet.* 2008;371: 552-553.

A case-control evaluation of the ketogenic diet versus ACTH for new-onset infantile spasms

Kossoff EH, Hedderick EF, Turner Z, et al (Johns Hopkins Med Insts, Baltimore, MD)
Epilepsia 49:1504-1509, 2008

Purpose.—ACTH is currently the standard first-line therapy for new-onset infantile spasms, but it has significant side effects. We hypothesized the ketogenic diet (KD), previously reported as beneficial for intractable infantile spasms, would have similar efficacy, but better tolerability than ACTH when used first-line.

Methods.—We conducted a retrospective chart review of all infants started on the KD (n − 13) and high-dose ACTH (n = 20) for new-onset infantile spasms at our institution since 1996.

Results.—Infants were spasm-free in 8 of 13 (62%) infants treated with the KD within 1 month, compared to 18 of 20 (90%) treated initially with ACTH, $p − 0.06$. When effective, median time to spasm freedom was similar between ACTH and the KD (4.0 vs. 6.5 days, p = 0.18). Those treated with ACTH were more likely to have a normal EEG at 1 month (53% vs. 9%, p = 0.02), however, use of the KD led to EEG normalization within 2–5 months in all eight who became spasm-free. In the five children in whom the KD was unsuccessful, four became spasm-free subsequently with ACTH or topiramate immediately. Side effects (31% vs. 80%, p = 0.006) and relapse rate after initial success (12.5% vs. 33%, p = 0.23) were lower with the KD.

Discussion.—In this retrospective study, the KD stopped spasms in nearly two-thirds of cases, and had fewer side effects and relapses than ACTH. ACTH normalized the EEG more rapidly, however. Further prospective study of the KD as, with a 2-week time limit if unsuccesful, first-line therapy for infantile spasms is warranted.

▶ The search has been on for some time for new and better agents to help manage infantile spasms. Back in 2004, the American Academy of Neurology and Child Neurology Society practice parameter concluded that adrenocorticotropic hormone (ACTH) was "probably" effective for new-onset infantile spasms. It also indicated that vigabatrin was "possibly" effective in this regard.[1] The same report indicated that all other treatments had insufficient evidence for their use. Unfortunately, since 2004, vigabatrin is no longer licensed. ACTH is remarkably expensive and at one point was costing up to $80 000 for a one-month supply.[2] For these reasons, old-time approaches to the management of infantile spasms are being relooked at, including the ketogenic diet.

The ketogenic diet, as we all know, is a high fat, low carbohydrate diet used for intractable childhood epilepsy. Although not without any side effects, the side effects of a ketogenic diet are generally minor and transient and can be dealt with without having to completely discontinue the diet. For some it is not very palatable, but because infantile spasms by definition begin in infancy and because infants generally eat whatever they are given, it is not too hard for a baby to be kept on a ketogenic diet.

The authors of this report from Johns Hopkins tested whether a ketogenic diet or ACTH would work best for new onset infantile spasms. After one month of treatment, 62% of infants treated with a ketogenic diet were spasm free, compared with 90% of those treated with ACTH. The median time to spasm freedom was slightly more rapid with ACTH (4.0 days) compared with the ketogenic diet (6.5 days). In infants treated with the ketogenic diet, correction of the EEG was unlikely in comparison with ACTH, which commonly improved the EEG. With respect to developmental outcomes, there was no difference in those treated with a ketogenic diet compared with those managed with ACTH. Poor developmental outcomes (moderate to severe delays) were noted in 38% of those initially managed with a ketogenic diet compared with 35% of those in the ACTH group. In terms of side effects, irritability was reported in 60% of those receiving ACTH, a group that also experienced excessive weight gain in 30% and insomnia in 10%. Side effects among those treated with the ketogenic diet included gastroesophageal reflux, constipation, poor formula tolerability, and weight loss, each occurring in 1 infant.

So what is the bottom line? In general, one can say that the ketogenic diet is safe and well tolerated and reasonably effective as a first-line therapy for infantile spasms. All in all, about two-thirds of infants treated with a ketogenic diet became spasm-free, doing so within 18 days of beginning the diet. ACTH, on the other hand, had a higher likelihood of a spasm-free response after 1 month of therapy, although the 90% spasm-free outcome at this point was somewhat higher than expected based on the literature. Use of the ketogenic diet did require longer treatment duration to normalize the EEG even in those infants who were clinically spasm free. This suggests that a clinical response is much more likely before the EEG proves. In terms of acceptability by parents, most families were more likely to accept a change in formula rather than the demands of giving their infants intramuscular injections.

It is hard to say whether the tried and true approach of using ACTH for infantile spasms will likely change by virtue of this report. The investigators from Hopkins believe that future studies are needed to nail down the true potential of a ketogenic diet, but in the meantime, there is great hope that an alternative other than ACTH may be in the wings.

This commentary closes with a *Clinical Fact/Curio* about neurology, specifically the nonpharmacologic management of seizures. There is a folk tradition of using smelly shoes as a first measure in epilepsy, particularly in some poor countries. A recent study shows that such an approach may not be entirely without merit.[3] Investigators in India have documented that strong olfactory stimuli can decrease the epileptic threshold and interfere with seizure activity in the limbic system.

While it may look a little bit odd, the next time you see someone have a seizure and do not know what to do about it at the moment, hopefully your own smelly shoes might just do the trick. If not, you might try borrowing our family pug, Oliver. His breath would stop a locomotive, much less a simple fit.

J. A. Stockman III, MD

References

1. Mackay MT, Weiss SK, Adams-Webber T, et al. Practice parameter: medical treatment of infantile spasms: report of the American Academy of Neurology and the Child Neurology Society. *Neurol.* 2004;62:1668-1681.
2. Questcor press release. Union City, CA: Questcor Pharmaceuticals; August, 2007.
3. Jaseja H. Scientific basis behind traditional practice of application of "shoe-smell" in controlling epileptic seizures in the eastern countries. *Clin Neurol Neurosurg.* 2008;110:535-538.

Hypothermia Therapy after Traumatic Brain Injury in Children

Hutchison JS, for the Hypothermia Pediatric Head Injury Trial Investigators and the Canadian Critical Care Trials Group (Hosp for Sick Children, Toronto, ON; et al)
N Engl J Med 358:2447-2456, 2008

Background.—Hypothermia therapy improves survival and the neurologic outcome in animal models of traumatic brain injury. However, the effect of hypothermia therapy on the neurologic outcome and mortality among children who have severe traumatic brain injury is unknown.

Methods.—In a multicenter, international trial, we randomly assigned children with severe traumatic brain injury to either hypothermia therapy (32.5°C for 24 hours) initiated within 8 hours after injury or to normothermia (37.0°C). The primary outcome was the proportion of children who had an unfavorable outcome (i.e., severe disability, persistent vegetative state, or death), as assessed on the basis of the Pediatric Cerebral Performance Category score at 6 months.

Results.—A total of 225 children were randomly assigned to the hypothermia group or the normothermia group; the mean temperatures achieved in the two groups were $33.1 \pm 1.2°C$ and $36.9 \pm 0.5°C$, respectively. At 6 months, 31% of the patients in the hypothermia group, as compared with 22% of the patients in the normothermia group, had an unfavorable outcome (relative risk, 1.41; 95% confidence interval [CI], 0.89 to 2.22; $P = 0.14$). There were 23 deaths (21%) in the hypothermia group and 14 deaths (12%) in the normothermia group (relative risk, 1.40; 95% CI, 0.90 to 2.27; $P = 0.06$). There was more hypotension ($P = 0.047$) and more vasoactive agents were administered ($P<0.001$) in the hypothermia group during the rewarming period than in the normothermia group. Lengths of stay in the intensive care unit and in the hospital and other adverse events were similar in the two groups.

Conclusions.—In children with severe traumatic brain injury, hypothermia therapy that is initiated within 8 hours after injury and continued for 24 hours does not improve the neurologic outcome and may increase mortality.

▶ For some time now, it has been suspected that inducing hypothermia either in an adult or a child who has sustained traumatic brain injury might improve short- and long-term outcomes. Indeed there are animal studies, albeit in rodents, which document this. Before the report of Hutchison et al appeared, there were 2 previous clinical trials involving a total of 96 children with severe traumatic brain injury reporting the effects of hypothermia therapy.[1,2] Unfortunately, these 2 trials did not have sufficient numbers of patients to tell us whether there might have been significant improvements in survival or neurologic recovery. The report of Hutchison et al attempted to overcome this problem by enrolling more than 200 youngsters (average age 10 years) who had a traumatic brain injury. Half of the patients served as controls while the other half had hypothermia induced at an average of 6 hours following the brain insult. Core body temperature was lowered to about 33°C for 24 hours.

The bottom line from this study carried out at 17 centers in 3 countries is that moderate hypothermia therapy (32°C-33°C) initiated within 8 hours after injury and maintained for 24 hours, did not improve the functional outcome at 6 months. Purely coincidentally, while this study was being undertaken in children, the results of a large study of hypothermia therapy in 392 adults with severe traumatic brain injury were published.[3] This investigation also did not show meaningful benefits in the rate of survival or functional outcomes, and in fact documented more complications, such as critical hypotension in adults who were treated with hypothermia for 48 hours, than in those who were managed with normothermia (Fig 2). These data are consistent with several systematic reviews of hypothermia treatment.

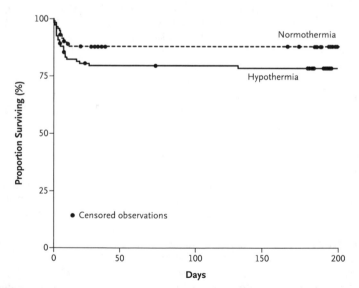

FIGURE 2.—Kaplan–Meier Estimates of Survival. The causes of death in the hypothermia group were brain death (4 patients), brain trauma (12), brain ischemia (1), hypoxia resulting from severe lung injury (3), and septic shock (1), with unknown causes in 2 patients. The causes of death in the normothermia group were brain death (2 patients), brain trauma (9), and brain ischemia (2), with an unknown cause in 1 patient. (Reprinted from Hutchison JS, for the Hypothermia Pediatric Head Injury Trial Investigators and the Canadian Critical Care Trials Group. Hypothermia therapy after traumatic brain injury in children. *N Engl J Med.* 2008;358:2447-2456. Copyright 2008 Massachusetts Medical Society. All rights reserved.)

Please recognize that hypothermia therapy may be of benefit in some adults and newborns with hypoxic-ischemic brain injury.[4,5]

It is hard to say whether the collaborative study authored by Hutchison et al will wind up being the definitive one in terms of documentation that hypothermia is of little or no value in the management of acute traumatic brain injury in children. There was a significant limitation to the study—the mean time to initiation of hypothermia was 6.3 hours. It is plausible that hypothermia therapy might be more effective if it were initiated earlier. Animal studies showing its effectiveness were based on hypothermia being instituted within 15 minutes of the onset of the trauma. Obviously, it would be technically difficult to attempt to induce hypothermia in a very short period of time following brain injury in a youngster.

Until and unless something dramatic occurs with hypothermia therapy, it is clear now, at least according to the parameters of the Hutchison et al study, that it is not worth the trouble.

Recently, a new specialty certifying board was formed in the field of sleep medicine.

This commentary closes with a *Clinical Fact/Curio* on this topic. There are mountains of evidence to show that sleep does enhance memory. Investigators in Germany have now struck a positive blow for power napping by showing that falling asleep for just 6 minutes is enough to significantly enhance memory. This is the shortest period of sleep found to affect mental functioning to date.[6] In the German study subjects reported to a sleep laboratory at 1 PM. They were given 2 minutes to memorize a list of 30 words and then were tested on their recall an hour later. In the interim, they either stayed awake or took a 6-minute or longer nap. Those who napped actually slept an average of 35 minutes. With no sleep, subjects recalled an average of under 7 words. A short 6-minute nap clearly raised this average quite significantly and an even longer nap in deep sleep raised the average still further. It is suspected that the experiment reveals a process of memory consolidation that begins even before sleep that could continue after waking from a very brief sleep.

A sleeping brain is not merely on standby; it runs through a suite of complex and orderly activities. One of these is a flow of neural activity from the hippocampus, where short-term memories are formed, then to the cortex, where the memories are stored in more durable forms—a possible reason people can remember things better on awakening. Other studies have shown that slumber is especially important for doing clever stuff with recently acquired information such as extracting the gist of what has been learned, combining facts in interesting ways, and dealing with one's recent emotions. This type of "executive thinking" is particularly impaired by sleep loss. This is something for residents in training to be aware of, given the recent debates on numbers of hours that such trainees should work, or not work.

Please be aware that until recently, sleep researchers generally overlooked the value of naps, perhaps because certain societies such as the United States frown on afternoon snoozes. If you want to earn your boss's displeasure, try such a memory enhancing activity. However, short sleeps are in fact the norm in most other mammalian species. Getting all your sleep in a monolithic block is quite unusual except among infants and the elderly.

J. A. Stockman III, MD

References

1. Biswas SK, Bruce DA, Sklar FH, Bokovoy JL, Sommerauer JF. Treatment of acute traumatic brain injury in children with moderate hypothermia improves intracranial hypertension. *Crit Care Med.* 2002;30:2742-2751.
2. Adelson PD, Ragheb J, Kaneb P, et al. Phase II clinical trial of moderate hypothermia after severe traumatic brain injury in children. *Neurosurg.* 2005;56: 740-754.
3. Clifton GL, Miller ER, Choi SC, et al. Lack of effect of induction of hypothermia after acute brain injury. *N Engl J Med.* 2001;344:556-563.
4. Gluckman PD, Wyatt JS, Azzopardi D, Ballard R, Edwards AD, Ferriero DM. Selective head cooling with mild systemic hypothermia after neonatal encephalopathy; multicentre randomized trial. *Lancet.* 2005;365:663-670.
5. Bernard SA, Gray TW, Buist MD, et al. Treatment of comatose survivors of out of hospital cardiac arrest with induced hypothermia. *N Engl J Med.* 2002;346: 557-563.
6. Whitfield J. Naps for better recall. *Scientific Am.* May, 2008;320.

Nonsurgical treatment of deformational plagiocephaly: a systematic review
Xia JJ, Kennedy KA, Teichgraeber JF, et al (The Methodist Hosp Res Inst, Houston, TX)
Arch Pediatr Adolesc Med 162:719-727, 2008

Objective.—To evaluate and summarize the evidence comparing nonsurgical therapies in the treatment of infants with deformational plagiocephaly.

Data Sources.—Scientific articles and abstracts published in English between January 1978 and August 2007 were searched from 5 online literature databases, along with a manual search of conference proceedings.

Study Selection.—Studies were selected and appraised for methodological quality by 2 reviewers independently using a Critical Appraisal Skills Programme form (cohort criteria).

Interventions.—Molding helmet therapy vs head repositioning therapy.

Main Outcome Measure.—Success rate of the treatment.

Results.—A total of 3793 references were retrieved. There were no randomized controlled trials. Only 7 cohort studies met the inclusion criteria. Five of the 7 studies presented evidence that molding therapy is more effective than repositioning, even with the biases favoring the repositioning groups. In the molding groups, the asymmetry was more severe and the infants were older. The infants who failed to respond to repositioning therapy were also switched to molding therapy. The treatment outcomes from the other 2 studies were difficult to assess because of flaws in their study design. Finally, the relative improvement of using molding therapy was calculated from one study. It was about 1.3 times greater than with repositioning therapy.

Conclusion.—The studies showed considerable evidence that molding therapy may reduce skull asymmetry more effectively than repositioning therapy. However, definitive conclusions on the relative effectiveness of these treatments were tempered by potential biases in these studies. Further research is warranted.

▶ Deformational plagiocephaly (DP) is the misshaping of the head and possibly the face as a result of prenatal and/or postnatal external molding pressure to the malleable and growing skull. The prevalence of DP varies between 6.1% to 13% at birth, 16% to 22.1% at 6 to 7 weeks, and some 20% by 4 months of age. By 12 months of age, approximately 7% of babies will manifest some degree of DP.[1] The specific causes of DP are fairly varied and include a restrictive intrauterine environment, premature birth, assisted vaginal delivery, prolonged labor, unusual birth position, multiple birth, and primiparity. DP, of course, does not have to be present at birth and can develop in the first few months of life. Nonvarying nursing habits, nonvarying head position when awake or asleep, supine sleeping position, positional preference, developmental delay, and lower activity level are all risk factors for the development of plagiocephaly. While the true physical consequences of deformational plagiocephaly are minor, this head-molding deformation does have the potential to induce negative physical and psychosocial effects. Parents fear that unattractive facial characteristics will lead to adverse effects such as teasing and poor self-perception. Conservative strategies to prevent or treat positional preference and DP are parent counseling, counterpositioning, physical therapy, and orthotic devices.

Xia et al reviewed the world's literature to see whether or not surgical treatments for DP were effective, and if so, which ones were most effective. This report is especially timely. Because the American Academy of Pediatrics recommendations were made back in 1992 that infants be placed on their back to sleep to reduce the risk of sudden infant death, there has been a literal "explosion" in the incidence of DP. What Xia et al found, unfortunately, was that there were no randomized controlled studies in the treatment of DP, but we do have some clues from data in the literature. The age at which treatment is begun and the severity of plagiocephaly are key considerations in whether the infant should be treated by repositioning or by more active molding therapy. The general consensus from the literature is that repositioning is preferred over molding therapy in patients 4 months or younger and in whom the severity is moderate or less. In patients 6 months or older, or in patients with more than moderate asymmetry regardless of age, molding therapy is preferred. In patients between 4 and 6 months of age, the treatment of choice remains controversial.

The bottom line to the Xia et al report is that we need to learn more about the treatment of DP. The authors of this report make 4 specific recommendations: there is a need to undertake a rigorously designed clinical trial on the evaluation of molding versus repositioning therapy; uniform evaluation criteria for treatment outcome must be defined; the cost-effectiveness of molding therapy must be included in any future evaluation; finally, we need to learn more about treatment options for infants older than 12 months who have not been adequately managed by that age.

At the time this meta-analysis appeared, a randomized controlled trial was reported on the effect of pediatric physical therapy on DP in children with positional preference.[2] A 4-month program of pediatric physical therapy to treat the problem did in fact reduce the prevalence of severe DP that had positional preference as its cause.

J. A. Stockman III, MD

References

1. Hutchison BL, Hutchison LA, Thompson JM, Mitchell EA. Plagiocephaly and brachycephaly in the first two years of life: a prospective cohort study. *Pediatrics.* 2004;114:970-980.
2. van Vlimmeren LA, van der Graaf Y, Boere-Boonekamp MM, L'Hoir MP, Helders PJ, Engelbert RH. Effect of pediatric physical therapy on deformational plagiocephaly in children with positional preference. a randomized controlled trial. *Arch Pediatr Adolesc Med.* 2008;162:712-718.

Effect of Simvastatin on Cognitive Functioning in Children With Neurofibromatosis Type 1: A Randomized Controlled Trial

Krab LC, de Goede-Bolder A, Aarsen FK, et al (Erasmus MC Univ Med Ctr, Rotterdam, the Netherlands; et al)
JAMA 300:287-294, 2008

Context.—Neurofibromatosis type 1 (NF1) is among the most common genetic disorders that cause learning disabilities. Recently, it was shown that statin-mediated inhibition of 3-hydroxy-3-methylglutaryl coenzyme A reductase restores the cognitive deficits in an NF1 mouse model.

Objective.—To determine the effect of simvastatin on neuropsychological, neurophysiological, and neuroradiological outcome measures in children with NF1.

Design, Setting, and Participants.—Sixty-two of 114 eligible children (54%) with NF1 participated in a randomized, double-blind, placebo-controlled trial conducted between January 20, 2006, and February 8, 2007, at an NF1 referral center at a Dutch university hospital.

Intervention.—Simvastatin or placebo treatment once daily for 12 weeks.

Main Outcome Measures.—Primary outcomes were scores on a Rey complex figure test (delayed recall), cancellation test (speed), prism adaptation, and the mean brain apparent diffusion coefficient based on magnetic resonance imaging. Secondary outcome measures were scores on the cancellation test (standard deviation), Stroop color word test, block design, object assembly, Rey complex figure test (copy), Beery developmental test of visual-motor integration, and judgment of line orientation. Scores were corrected for baseline performance, age, and sex.

Results.—No significant differences were observed between the simvastatin and placebo groups on any primary outcome measure: Rey complex figure test ($\beta = 0.10$; 95% confidence interval [CI], −0.36 to 0.56);

cancellation test ($\beta = -0.19$; 95% CI, -0.67 to 0.29); prism adaptation (odds ratio $= 2.0$; 95% CI, 0.55 to 7.37); and mean brain apparent diffusion coefficient ($\beta = 0.06$; 95% CI, -0.07 to 0.20). In the secondary outcome measures, we found a significant improvement in the simvastatin group in object assembly scores ($\beta = 0.54$; 95% CI, 0.08 to 1.01), which was specifically observed in children with poor baseline performance ($\beta = 0.80$; 95% CI, 0.29 to 1.30). Other secondary outcome measures revealed no significant effect of simvastatin treatment.

Conclusion.—In this 12-week trial, simvastatin did not improve cognitive function in children with NF1.

Trial Registration.—isrctn.org Identifier: ISRCTN14965707.

▶ Most pediatricians are not sufficiently familiar with the molecular basis of neurofibromatosis type 1 (NF1) to expect that a statin would in any way help with the management of the disorder. In fact, there is a very plausible reason to think that statins could, at least theoretically, improve the neurocognitive functioning of these kids.

NF1, as we all know, is a fairly common autosomal-dominant genetic disorder caused by a mutation in the gene encoding neurofibromin, a protein that activates the hydrolysis of a substance known as RAS-bound guanosine triphosphate. In addition to the neurocutaneous manifestations of NF1, as well as problems in fine and gross motor functioning, frequently one also sees the occurrence of cognitive disabilities. For example, children with NF1 have a lower mean IQ (usually in the range of 86-94) with particular deficits in visual-spatial skills, nonverbal long-term memory, executive functioning, and attention. These problems can seriously impact school performance of children with NF1. Laboratory studies have suggested that the abnormal brain functioning is a result of difficulties with RAS transforming activity in the brain. This activity requires isoprenylation, an activity which can be blocked by statins via a mechanism that is very similar to its effect on the rate-limiting enzyme pathway in which cholesterol is synthesized. Importantly, treatment of mice that are bred with a model of NF1 with a statin for just a few days has been shown to reverse the cognitive deficits these mice manifest.

It is on the basis of these laboratory and animal findings that Krab et al decided to treat more than 60 children, ranging in age from 11 to 15 years, with a statin to see whether their cognitive functioning would improve over a period of several months. Unfortunately, there was no improvement in either neurologic or cognitive functioning.

Despite the negative findings from this report, further clinical trials using statins in NF1 do seem warranted. One would love to do such a clinical trial at a much younger age, at a time when the brain is significantly more plastic. As most of us know, however, statins are not approved for use for its intended condition (hypercholesterolemia) in children younger than 8 years of age. The use of statins in very young children has not been studied. Given the rare, but often very complicated, side effects of statins, a clinical trial of statins in very young children would have to be undertaken with great caution.

If you want to learn more about statins in the management of cardiovascular health in children, including its use beginning at 8 years of age, see this summary of lipid screening and cardiovascular health in children from the American Academy of Pediatrics.[1]

J. A. Stockman III, MD

Reference

1. Daniels SR, Greer FR. Committee on Nutrition. Lipid screening and cardiovascular health in childhood. *Pediatrics.* 2008;122:198-208.

Differential diagnosis of congenital muscular dystrophies
Klein A, Clement E, Mercuri E, et al (Univ Children's Hosp Zurich, Switzerland; Imperial College, London, UK; et al)
Eur J Paediatr Neurol 12:371-377, 2008

Congenital muscular dystrophies (CMDs) are defined by signs of muscle weakness in the first 6 months of life with myopathic changes in muscle biopsy. The progress in the last decade has helped to make molecular and genetic diagnoses in the majority of patients fulfilling these criteria. In a number of patients a definite diagnosis cannot be reached and these individuals are often grouped together as "merosin positive" congenital muscular dystrophy. In the last 5 years, 25 patients referred for assessment as possible congenital muscular dystrophy have been found to have alternative diagnoses. This paper aims to highlight these conditions as the common differentials or more difficult to diagnoses to consider in patients presenting as CMD.

▶ It has only been in the last 15 years that the diagnosis of congenital muscular dystrophies has become more specific. In 1995, the discovery that approximately half of patients with congenital muscular dystrophy were lacking in an extracellular protein called merosin allowed the first attempt at classifying these dystrophies. Classification has been based on immunohistochemical findings, which have more recently been complemented by genetic studies. It is now possible to pursue a molecular genetic diagnosis in 13 different forms of congenital muscular dystrophy. When immunohistochemical findings and molecular studies are normal in a child with a myopathic or dystrophic muscle biopsy and there are no additional features such as cores, inclusions or rods, suggesting a congenital myopathy, a definite diagnosis is often difficult to reach. This report from Switzerland, the United Kingdom, and Italy illustrates the possible differential diagnosis in a group of patients with an initial diagnosis of congenital muscular dystrophy in whom a different diagnosis was subsequently reached. The most common diagnosis was that of early and severe presentation of laminopathies.

You will have to read this article in some detail if you are interested in the muscular dystrophies. It is a bit of a tough read. It highlights the problems neurologists have in reaching a final diagnosis in suspected cases of congenital muscular dystrophy. You should also be aware that studies are under way looking at genetic engineering as a possible treatment of certain forms of muscular dystrophy. These trials are based on some impressive studies in genetically modified rodents where manipulation of individual genes has increased muscle mass, muscle strength, or running endurance depending on the gene that was being manipulated. Reviews of these animal studies have also suggested that such genetic manipulations could theoretically improve human athletic performance. Recently, there has been speculation that at some point in time athletes could use genetic modification to enhance their athletic prowess. If you are interested in reading more about this, see the interesting commentary by Wells.[1]

J. A. Stockman III, MD

Reference

1. Wells D. Genetic engineering in athletes. Safeguards are needed before the hypothetical threat becomes a reality. *BMJ.* 2008;337:63-64.

Prevalence of enuresis and its association with attention-deficit/ hyperactivity disorder among U.S. children: results from a nationally representative study

Shreeram S, He JP, Kalaydjian A, et al (Natl Insts of Health, Bethesda, MD)
J Am Acad Child Adolesc Psychiatry 48:35-41, 2009

Objective.—There are no published nationally representative prevalence estimates of enuresis among children in the United States using standardized diagnostic criteria. This study sets out to describe the prevalence, demographic correlates, comorbidities, and service patterns for enuresis in a representative sample of U.S. children.

Method.—The diagnosis of enuresis was derived from parent-reported data for "enuresis, nocturnal" collected using the computerized version of the Diagnostic Interview Schedule for Children (C-DISC 4.0) from a nationally representative sample of 8- to 11-year-old children (n = 1,136) who participated in the 2001-2004 National Health and Nutrition Examination Surveys.

Results.—The overall 12-month prevalence of enuresis was 4.45%. The prevalence in boys (6.21%) was significantly greater than that in girls (2.51%). Enuresis was more common at younger ages and among black youth. Attention-deficit/hyperactivity disorder (ADHD) was strongly associated with enuresis (odds ratio 2.88; 95% confidence interval 1.26-6.57). Only 36% of the enuretic children had received health services for enuresis.

Conclusions.—Enuresis is a common condition among children in the United States. Few families seek treatment for enuresis despite the potential for adverse effects on emotional health. Child health care professionals should routinely screen for enuresis and its effects on the emotional health of the child and the family. Assessment of ADHD should routinely include evaluation for enuresis and vice versa. Research on the explanations for the association between enuresis and ADHD is indicated.

▶ There is actually a code in the *International Classification of Diseases and Related Health Problems*, 10th edition (ICD-10) that defines enuresis. The definition is bedwetting that occurs at a frequency of twice per month in the past 3 months for children 5 and 6 years of age and once per month in the past 3 months for children ages 7 years or older. *DSM-IV*, however, requires a bedwetting frequency of twice per week for 3 consecutive months or the presence of clinically significant distress or impairment, irrespective of age of the child. Even with these definitions, there is a striking lack of data on the prevalence of enuresis in children in the United States. The only study of a nationally representative sample found that 10.1% of children wet the bed at least once during the previous 12 months.[1] Another study, which followed a birth cohort of more than 800 children in Baltimore for 12 years, reported a 19% prevalence of nighttime wetting at 8 years and 8% at 12 years.[2] More recently, a 3- to 7-year prospective study of a community sample in North Carolina yielded a prevalence of 5.11% using the *DSM-III* defined enuresis and a 3.8% for the *DSM-IV* defined enuresis.[3] We all know that enuresis is approximately twice as common in boys as in girls and that ultimately the diagnosis is one that one outgrows with just 2% of adults having enuresis.

The report of Shreeram et al is an important one because it represents the first nationally representative estimate of the prevalence of enuresis in the United States based on totally standardized diagnostic criteria. Using these strict criteria, it was observed that 4.45% of United States children 8 to 11 years of age have enuresis. That represents a fairly high percentage of the childhood population. Enuresis appears to peak at 8 years of age using current diagnostic criteria. Also seen in this study was a 2.7-fold greater probability of having enuresis if you were a boy. The most important aspect of this report, however, relates to the high association between enuresis and the comorbid presence of attention-deficit/hyperactivity disorder (ADHD). If one has enuresis in childhood, the probability of also having ADHD raises almost some 3-fold.

The authors of this report obviously were unable to produce any firm reasons why there might be an association between enuresis and ADHD. They speculate that the relationship might be due to a common etiologic pathway underlying the 2 conditions or possibly due to "causal" relations in which the nonresolution or treatment of one disorder increases the risk for the other. Developmental and epidemiological studies are needed to better understand the comorbidity between enuresis and other psychiatric disorders and the possible role of enuresis in the development or nonresolution of these other disorders. Recent studies have noted that atomoxetine, a medication that is approved for the treatment of ADHD, has been found to decrease the frequency of bedwetting among children with enuresis who have ADHD.[4] Thus, if you have a child with ADHD who is also enuretic, you might try treating the ADHD fairly aggressively first to see what might happen.

This commentary closes with a *Clinical Fact/Curio* related to a neurologic disorder presenting as an occupational hazard. It appears that slaughterhouse workers who inhale pig-brain particles are at risk for contracting a nerve-damaging illness. More than 20 individuals have been diagnosed with the mysterious disease, which causes nondescript pain, weakness, fatigue, and paralysis. The first case appeared in 2004 at a Minnesota slaughterhouse. Since then, at least 18 workers from that same plant, Quality Pork Processors, have been diagnosed with similar signs and symptoms. Pork plants in Indiana and Nebraska have had the same problems. Neurologists at the Mayo Clinic in Rochester, Minnesota have reported new ways to diagnose this illness clinically by systematically cataloging the signs and symptoms of what is still an unnamed disorder.

If it were not for the fact that pig brain-associated neurologic disease is so serious, this editor would opt for simply calling it "Oink-Oink disease."[5]

J. A. Stockman III, MD

References

1. Byrd RS, Weitzman M, Lanphear NE, Auinger P. Bedwetting in US children: epidemiology and related behavior problems. *Pediatrics.* 1996;98:414-419.
2. Oppel WC, Harper PA, Rider RV. Social, psychological and neurological factors associated with nocturnal enuresis. *Pediatrics.* 1968;42:627-641.
3. Costello EJ, Mustillo S, Erkanli A, Keeler G, Angold A. Prevalence and development of psychiatric disorders in childhood and adolescence. *Arch Gen Psychiatr.* 2003;60:837-844.
4. Shatkin JP. Atomoxetine for the treatment of pediatric nocturnal enuresis. *J Child Adolesc Psychopharmacol.* 2004;14:443-447.
5. Danger from pig brains [editorial comment]. *Sci News.* May 10, 2008;11.

Childhood Attention-Deficit/Hyperactivity Disorder and the Emergence of Personality Disorders in Adolescence: A Prospective Follow-Up Study

Miller CJ, Flory JD, Miller SR, et al (Univ of Windsor, Ontario, Canada; Queens College; et al)

J Clin Psychiatry 69:1477-1484, 2008

Objectives.—Adults with attention-deficit/hyperactivity disorder (ADHD) experience considerable functional impairment. However, the extent to which comorbid Axis II personality disorders contribute to their difficulties and whether such comorbidities are associated with the childhood condition or the persistence of ADHD into adulthood remain unclear.

Method.—This study examined the presence of personality disorders in a longitudinal sample of 96 adolescents diagnosed with ADHD when they were 7 through 11 years old, as compared to a matched, never ADHD–diagnosed, control group (N = 85). Participants were between 16 and 26 years old at follow-up. On the basis of a psychiatric interview, the ADHD group was subdivided into those with and without persistent ADHD. Axis II symptoms were assessed by using the Structured Clinical Interview for DSM-IV Axis II Personality Disorders. Data were analyzed using logistic regression, and odds ratios (ORs) were generated. The study was conducted from 1994 through 1997.

Results.—Individuals diagnosed with childhood ADHD are at increased risk for personality disorders in late adolescence, specifically borderline (OR = 13.16), antisocial (OR = 3.03), avoidant (OR = 9.77), and narcissistic (OR = 8.69) personality disorders. Those with persistent ADHD were at higher risk for antisocial (OR = 5.26) and paranoid (OR = 8.47) personality disorders but not the other personality disorders when compared to those in whom ADHD remitted.

Conclusion.—Results suggest that ADHD portends risk for adult personality disorders, but the risk is not uniform across disorders, nor is it uniformly related to child or adult diagnostic status.

▶ A recent epidemiologic study has found that nearly 40% of children with attention-deficit/hyperactivity disorder (ADHD) will have persisting symptoms significant enough for a diagnosis of ADHD in adulthood, making ADHD one of the most common chronic disorders in our population.[1] Studies of adults with ADHD have shown elevated levels of moodiness, anxiety, and substance abuse disorders. In addition, adults with ADHD are frequently characterized by affective volatility, occupational instability, poor social relationships, and impulsive and self-destructive behaviors that may or may not be related to the actual presence of ADHD. Additionally, numerous studies have shown an association between childhood ADHD and adult antisocial personality disorder, but only a limited number of studies have examined associations between childhood ADHD and other adult personality disorders.

The primary goal of the investigation of Miller et al was to assess personality disorders in a longitudinal sample of adolescents who were diagnosed with ADHD during childhood. The study also attempted to determine the degree to which personality disorder diagnoses were linked to the persistence of ADHD symptoms into young adulthood as opposed to the childhood condition per se. The underlying hypothesis was that as compared with matched controls, individuals diagnosed with ADHD in childhood would be more likely to be diagnosed with a personality disorder in late adolescence. Indeed that is exactly what was found. Specifically, diagnoses of avoidant, narcissistic, borderline, and/or antisocial personality disorders were found to be more common. In addition, those individuals in whom ADHD persisted were at substantially elevated risk for antisocial and paranoid personality disorders when compared with those in whom ADHD resolved, findings consistent with previous studies suggesting increased risk for antisocial personality disorder and other types of personality disorders in children and adolescents with ADHD. The authors of this report are careful to note that the presence of adolescent antisocial personality disorder is not directly linked to the presence of childhood ADHD, nor is it strongly related to childhood comorbidity psychopathology. Instead, the persistence of ADHD appears to be a marker and strongly predictive of later antisocial personality disorders. The authors suggest that it may be that children with ADHD interact with their families and other significant individuals in such a way that these relationships increase the likelihood of developing a personality disorder. They also suggest that it may be that abnormal interpersonal interactions that are potentiated by childhood ADHD become risk factors within the personality of the individual, and that these distorted relationships may be the beginning of future personality disorders.

Obviously, not every youngster with ADHD is going to grow up to be an adult with a personality disorder, but if you believe the data from this report, and you probably should, those with ADHD are at somewhat greater risk for a diagnosis of a personality disorder by late adolescence. For these reasons we should be mindful of possible co-occurring ADHD and personality disorders. The relationship is also one additional very good reason for making sure that children with ADHD are properly treated. It is a lot easier to nip an emerging personality disorder in the bud early on than later in life.

J. A. Stockman III, MD

Reference

1. Kessler RC, Adler LA, Barkley J, et al. Patterns and predictors of attention-deficit/-hyperactivity disorder persistence into adulthood: Results from the National Comorbidity Survey Replication. *Biol Psychiatr.* 2005;57:1442-1451.

Stimulant Therapy and Risk for Subsequent Substance Use Disorders in Male Adults With ADHD: A Naturalistic Controlled 10-Year Follow-Up Study

Biederman J, Monuteaux MC, Spencer T, et al (Massachusetts General Hosp, Boston)
Am J Psychiatry 165:597-603, 2008

Objective.—The extant literature does not provide definite answers pertaining to whether stimulant treatment increases, decreases, or does not affect the risk for subsequent substance use disorders in youths with attention deficit hyperactivity disorder (ADHD). The authors examined the association between stimulant treatment in childhood and adolescence and subsequent substance use disorders (alcohol, drug, and nicotine) into the young adult years.

Method.—The authors conducted a 10-year prospective follow-up study. One hundred forty male Caucasian children with ADHD, ages 6 to 17, were examined at baseline. Of these, 112 (80%) were reassessed at the 10-year follow-up (mean age at follow-up = 22 years). Assessments were made using Cox proportional hazards survival models. All models were adjusted for conduct disorder, since conduct disorder is a potent predictor of subsequent substance use disorders.

Results.—Of the 112 ADHD subjects who were reassessed at the 10-year follow-up, 82 (73%) had been treated previously with stimulants and 25 (22%) were undergoing stimulant treatment at the time of the follow-up assessment. There were no statistically significant associations between stimulant treatment and alcohol, drug, or nicotine use disorders.

Conclusions.—The findings revealed no evidence that stimulant treatment increases or decreases the risk for subsequent substance use disorders in children and adolescents with ADHD when they reach young adulthood.

▶ This is not the first study to look at an association between childhood attention deficit hyperactivity disorder (ADHD) and adult substance abuse. Numerous studies have suggested that ADHD is significantly associated with adolescent and adult substance abuse disorders. Animal studies have raised concern regarding stimulant treatment because of findings of sensitization to the effects of drugs in general. The sensitization hypothesis, a neuroadaptational model, maintains that exposure to stimulants results in dopamine system alterations, which in turn increase sensitivity to the reinforcing effects of the previously experienced substance. Behavioral sensitization has been demonstrated in numerous mammalian species, including nonhuman primates, and has been found to be long lasting. Consistent with this model, some studies have suggested there may be a causal link between stimulant treatment and childhood and later substance use disorder. The potential role of stimulants in the pathogenesis of substance abuse later in life could be a major public health concern. Stimulant use is now widespread, and these medications are increasingly prescribed to younger and younger children. More than a dozen studies have examined the association between stimulant treatment of ADHD and substance abuse disorder and, with one exception,[1] have not found a significant positive relationship. No study has examined the association between age at first exposure to stimulants and later substance abuse disorder.

A report of Mannuzza et al did look at whether age and initiation of stimulant treatment in children with ADHD is related to subsequent development of substance abuse disorders.[2] The authors conducted a prospective longitudinal study of 176 methylphenidate-treated boys (ages 6-12) with ADHD, but without conduct disorder. The participants in the study were followed up in late adolescence (mean age of 18.4 years) and adulthood (mean age 25.3 years). The risk of developing substance abuse was significantly associated with age at methylphenidate treatment; specifically, the later the treatment, the greater the chances of developing substance abuse disorder. The principal value of this finding is that it challenges the position that early exposure to stimulants represents particular risk to children with ADHD.

The report of Biederman et al examines the association between stimulant treatment in childhood and adolescents and subsequent substance abuse disorder into young adulthood by the conduct of a 10-year prospective follow-up study. They found no statistically significant associations between stimulant treatment and alcohol, drug, or nicotine use disorders. There was also no association between the duration of stimulant treatment and subsequent substance abuse disorders. These findings support the hypothesis that stimulant treatment does not in itself increase the risk for subsequent substance abuse disorders. To date, this study represents the most methodologically rigorous assessment concerning the question of whether stimulant treatment increases the risk for subsequent substance abuse disorders with follow-up into adult years, while adjusting for conduct disorder, testing of a diverse set of substance outcomes, using DSM criteria to define case status, and employing proportional hazards survival models. The present results fail to replicate earlier published findings of these same authors, which detected a positive effect of stimulant treatment. The most likely factor to account for this discrepancy is the additional information gained through continued follow-up.

The bottom line here is that as far as most studies show, concerns among clinicians and parents about future substance abuse disorder problems arising when prescribing stimulants to children with ADHD do not have much merit. Unfortunately, naysayers in this regard will point to numerous potential conflicts of interest of individuals who carry out studies on stimulant use because, as can be seen in the conflict of interest acknowledgments following most articles, most investigators do receive research support from the pharmaceutical industry. The latter does not mean that such research is not appropriately conducted, just that it will always be in the shadow of suspicion by some.

J. A. Stockman III, MD

References

1. Lambert NM, Hartsough CS. Prospective study of tobacco smoking and substance dependence among samples of ADHD and non-ADHD participants. *J Learn Disabil.* 1998;31:533-544.
2. Mannuzza S, Klein RG, Truong NL, et al. The age of methylphenidate treatment initiation in children with ADHD and later substance abuse: prospective follow up into adulthood. *Am J Psychiatr.* 2008;165:604-609.

Hypericum perforatum (St John's Wort) for Attention-Deficit/Hyperactivity Disorder in Children and Adolescents: A Randomized Controlled Trial

Weber W, Vander Stoep A, McCarty RL, et al (Bastyr Univ, Kenmore, WA; Children's Hosp and Regional Med Ctr; et al)
JAMA 299:2633-2641, 2008

Context.—Stimulant medication can effectively treat 60% to 70% of youth with attention-deficit/hyperactivity disorder (ADHD). Yet many parents seek alternative therapies, and *Hypericum perforatum* (St John's wort) is 1 of the top 3 botanicals used.

Objective.—To determine the efficacy and safety of *H perforatum* for the treatment of ADHD in children.

Design, Setting, and Participants.—Randomized, double-blind, placebo-controlled trial conducted between March 2005 and August 2006 at Bastyr University, Kenmore, Washington, among a volunteer sample of 54 children aged 6 to 17 years who met *Diagnostic and Statistical Manual of Mental Disorders* (Fourth Edition) criteria for ADHD by structured interview.

Intervention.—After a placebo run-in phase of 1 week, participants were randomly assigned to receive 300 mg of *H perforatum* standardized to 0.3% hypericin (n = 27) or a matched placebo (n = 27) 3 times daily for 8 weeks. Other medications for ADHD were not allowed during the trial.

Main Outcome Measures.—Performance on the ADHD Rating Scale–IV (range, 0-54) and Clinical Global Impression Improvement Scale (range, 0-7), and adverse events.

Results.—One patient in the placebo group withdrew because of an adverse event. No significant difference was found in the change in ADHD Rating Scale–IV scores from baseline to week 8 between the treatment and placebo groups: inattentiveness improved 2.6 points (95% confidence interval [CI], −4.6 to −0.6 points) with *H perforatum* vs 3.2 points (95% CI, −5.7 to −0.8 points) with placebo ($P = .68$) and hyperactivity improved 1.8 points (95% CI, −3.7 to 0.1 points) with *H perforatum* vs 2.0 points (95% CI, −4.1 to 0.1 points) with placebo ($P = .89$). There was also no significant difference between the 2 groups in the percentage of participants who met criteria for improvement (score ≤2) on the Clinical Global Impression Improvement Scale (*H perforatum*, 44.4%; 95% CI, 25.5%-64.7% vs placebo, 51.9%; 95% CI, 31.9%-71.3%; $P = .59$). No difference between groups was found in the number of participants who experienced adverse effects during the study period (*H perforatum*, 40.7%; 95% CI, 22.4%-61.2% vs placebo, 44.4%; 95% CI, 25.5%-64.7%; $P = .78$).

Conclusion.—In this study, use of *H perforatum* for treatment of ADHD over the course of 8 weeks did not improve symptoms.

Trial Registration.—clinicaltrials.gov Identifier: NCT00100295.

▶ This report is important for 2 reasons. It is the first study of *Hypericum perforatum* (St. John's wort) for attention-deficit/hyperactivity disorder (ADHD) in children and adolescents. Also, it is an extraordinarily noteworthy example of a high-quality randomized controlled trial evaluating a specific complementary and alternative medicine (CAM) therapy in children. Weber et al report the results of an 8-week randomized, placebo-controlled, double-blind trial of St. John's wort in 54 children aged 6 through 17 years who met the criteria for a diagnosis of ADHD and who were not receiving any other ADHD-related treatments, including drugs during the study period. Changes in ADHD symptoms as measured by the ADHD Rating Scale IV, changes in global functioning as rated on the clinical global impression improvement scale, and safety as rated by the Monitoring of Side Effects Scale were the primary outcomes. The research showed no significant differences on any of the efficacy measures or the frequency of adverse effects in those assigned to receive 3 mg of *H perforatum* 3 times daily for 8 weeks versus a control group receiving placebo.

ADHD is a diagnosis especially prone to the use of CAM by parents. Here in the United States, the most common herbal treatments used by children with ADHD are St. John's wort, *Echinacea*, and *Ginkgo*. St. John's wort is also commonly used to treat depression. Pharmacologically it inhibits reuptake of serotonin, norepinephrine, and dopamine. The only medication with highly similar actions is bupropion hydrochloride, which is sometimes used by those caring for children and adolescents to treat ADHD. Please note that bupropion is not believed to strongly inhibit serotonin reuptake and is not approved by the United States Food and Drug Administration (FDA) for this indication. In the last 10 years, a new nonstimulant selective norepinephrine reuptake inhibitor, atomoxetine, was approved by the FDA for the treatment of ADHD in children and adolescents. It was on the basis that St. John's wort is believed to act as a norepinephrine reuptake inhibitor that the study, which appeared in *JAMA*, was undertaken, albeit for naught because no benefit was found.

The report of Weber et al is the first placebo-controlled trial of St. John's wort in children and adolescents. Unfortunately, too many CAM studies fail to meet the threshold of adequate clinical design. In a extraordinarily well-written editorial on the topic of the quality of efficacy research in complementary and alternative medicine, Chan notes that ultimately increased attention to and emphasis on deepening a rigorous evidence-base for all healthcare practices will benefit patients and family and that the time for bad science, whether in conventional or unconventional medicine is past. There is a lot of wisdom in these words.[1]

One final comment about ADHD and "alternative" treatments. Eliminating food colorings and preservatives is regarded by some as an "alternative" treatment rather than a "standard" treatment (stimulant drugs) for ADHD. A recent randomized, placebo-controlled trial in 297 children aged 3 to 9 years provides evidence of increased hyperactive behavior after the children ate a mixture of food colorings and a preservative (sodium benzoate).[2] A recent review of all studies looking at food colorings and preservatives and their effects on ADHD has concluded that there is a small but real relationship between the two.[3] The meta-analysis does show that dietary elimination of colorings and preservatives provides a statistically significant benefit and in view of the fact that such elimination diets are relatively harmless, perhaps they are worth trying to see if there is any benefit in a particular patient. However, it should rightfully be pointed out that ADHD has multifactorial causes and exclusively focusing on food additives may detract from the provision of adequate treatment for children with the disorder.

J. A. Stockman III, MD

References

1. Chan E. Quality of efficacy research in complementary and alternative medicine. *JAMA.* 2008;299:2685-2686.
2. McCann D, Barrett A, Cooper A, et al. Food additives and hyperactive behaviour in 3-year-old and 8/9-year-old children in the community: a randomized, double-blinded, placebo-controlled trial. *Lancet.* 2007;370:1560-1567.
3. Kemp A. Food additives and hyperactivity: Evidence supports a trial period of eliminating colourings and preservatives from the diet. *BMJ.* 2008;336:1144.

Absence of Preferential Looking to the Eyes of Approaching Adults Predicts Level of Social Disability in 2-Year-Old Toddlers With Autism Spectrum Disorder

Jones W, Carr K, Klin A (Yale Univ School of Medicine; Yale Child Study Ctr, New Haven, CT)
Arch Gen Psychiatry 65:946-954, 2008

Context.—Within the first week of life, typical human newborns give preferential attention to the eyes of others. Similar findings in other species suggest that attention to the eyes is a highly conserved phylogenetic mechanism of social development. For children with autism, however, diminished and aberrant eye contact is a lifelong hallmark of disability.

Objective.—To quantify preferential attention to the eyes of others at what is presently the earliest point of diagnosis in autism.

Design.—We presented the children with 10 videos. Each video showed an actress looking directly into the camera, playing the role of caregiver, and engaging the viewer (playing pat-a-cake, peek-a-boo, etc). Children's visual fixation patterns were measured by eye tracking.

Participants.—Fifteen 2-year-old children with autism were compared with 36 typically developing children and with 15 developmentally delayed but nonautistic children.

Main Outcome Measure.—Preferential attention was measured as percentage of visual fixation time to 4 regions of interest: eyes, mouth, body, and object. Level of social disability was assessed by the Autism Diagnostic Observation Schedule.

Results.—Looking at the eyes of others was significantly decreased in 2-year-old children with autism ($P < .001$), while looking at mouths was increased ($P < .01$) in comparison with both control groups. The 2 control groups were not distinguishable on the basis of fixation patterns. In addition, fixation on eyes by the children with autism correlated with their level of social disability; less fixation on eyes predicted greater social disability ($r = -0.669$, $P < .01$).

Conclusions.—Looking at the eyes of others is important in early social development and in social adaptation throughout one's life span. Our results indicate that in 2-year-old children with autism, this behavior is already derailed, suggesting critical consequences for development but also offering a potential biomarker for quantifying syndrome manifestation at this early age.

▶ The average person might think that the reasons why someone cannot look someone else in the eye is either because that individual is terribly shy, or that they are lying. Now we see there is a third reason and that is that if you are a toddler and fail to look at an observer in the eye, you just may well have some component of an autism spectrum disorder. One of the developmental milestones that we all use is that by 3 months of age, an infant will look more at a person's eyes that at any other part of the face and at a person's face more than anywhere else on the body. This is

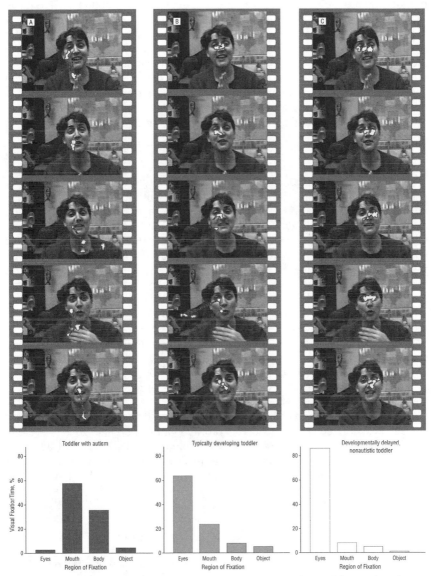

FIGURE 2.—Example visual scanpaths and fixation time summaries for 3 toddlers watching the same video of an actress playing the role of a caregiver. Each frame shows 2 seconds of eye-tracking data overlaid on a single still image (the still image on which data are plotted is the midpoint of the 2-second window of plotted data). Saccades are plotted as thin white lines with white dots, while fixation data are plotted as larger white dots. A, Data from a toddler with autism. B, Data from a typically developing toddler. C, Data from a developmentally delayed but nonautistic toddler. Bar graphs show percentages of fixation time to each region of interest (eyes, mouth, body, and object). Bar graphs are for individual children for a single movie (and thus include no error bars). Eye-tracking data were recorded at 60 Hz. (Reprinted from Jones W, Carr K, Klin A. Absence of preferential looking to the eyes of approaching adults predicts level of social disability in 2-year-old toddlers with autism spectrum disorder. *Arch Gen Psychiatry.* 2008;65:946-954. Copyright 2008, American Medical Association. All rights reserved.)

part of a normal developmental process in which infants engage preferentially with what is social in the environment about them. The situation is different in infants and toddlers with autism. By definition, autism in part is a disorder defined by altered engagement with the social world. Features of autism include deficits in social interaction and communication as well as the presence of repetitive behaviors and restricted interest lacking in social exchange value. As part of the evaluation for autism, the clinician should take note of whether a child focuses on other people, whether there is reduced interaction with others, failure to respond to one's name, and inability to engage in imitative games.

The authors of this report hypothesized that altered looking patterns—less looking at the eyes and increase looking at mouth, body, and object areas might indicate reliable quantifiers of social disability and altered engagement with the social world in autism. Specifically, the authors designed a study to answer the following questions: Is looking at the eyes of approaching adults altered in children with autism by the age of 2 years, and do such alterations relate to the child's level of social disability? To carry out this study, 15 toddlers with autism spectrum disorders, 36 typically developing children, and 15 toddlers with developmental delays, but without autism, were evaluated. The children were shown 10 video clips, each presenting an actress looking directly into the camera and playing the role of a caregiver, entreating the viewing toddler by engaging in childhood games such as pat-a-cake. Visual fixation patterns were measured with eye-tracking equipment that permitted a recording of exactly where a child was looking. The group of toddlers with autism fixated significantly less on the eye region relative to the typically developing group and the developmentally delayed, nonautistic group. The autism group tended to fix significantly more often on the mouth region rather than on the eyes of the actresses (Fig 2).

In the case of a toddler with autism spectrum disorder, this early-altered course of experience is likely to have a profound impact on later social development. Failure to look at the eyes of others during critical windows of development and looking at other parts of the world instead suggest an altered path for learning about the world. The authors of this report suggest that because the eye region of the face is critical for extraction of expression information, if a child has less experience observing and reacting to the eyes of others, that child is very likely to develop less expertise about social cues conveyed by the eyes resulting in a set of cascading effects on further socialization. The authors are probably right in this assessment.

Yes, the inability to look someone squarely in the eyes can have many causes. Autism spectrum disorder is just one, but a very important one, if you are a 2-year-old. Remember this as part of your screening for this important problem.

J. A. Stockman III, MD

Correlates of Accommodation of Pediatric Obsessive-Compulsive Disorder: Parent, Child, and Family Characteristics

Peris TS, Bergman RL, Langley A, et al (UCLA Semel Inst for Neuroscience and Human Behavior, Los Angeles, CA)
J Am Acad Child Adolesc Psychiatry 47:1173-1181, 2008

Objective.—Pediatric obsessive-compulsive disorder (OCD) is a chronic, impairing condition associated with high levels of family accommodation (i.e., participation in symptoms). Understanding of factors that may engender accommodation of pediatric OCD is limited. This study conducted exploratory analyses of parent-, child-, and family-level correlates of family accommodation, considering both behavioral and affective components of the response.

Method.—The sample included 65 youths (mean age 12.3 years, 62% male) with OCD and their parents who completed a standardized assessment battery composed of both clinical and self-report measures (e.g., Children's Yale-Brown Obsessive Compulsive Scale, Brief Symptom Inventory).

Results.—Family accommodation was common, with the provision of reassurance and participation in rituals the most frequent practices (occurring on a daily basis among 56% and 46% of parents, respectively). Total scores on the Family Accommodation Scale were not associated with child OCD symptom severity; however, parental involvement in rituals was associated with higher levels of child OCD severity and parental psychopathology and with lower levels of family organization. Comorbid externalizing symptomatology and family conflict were associated with parent report of worse consequences when not accommodating.

Conclusions.—Although these findings must be interpreted in light of potential type I error, they suggest that accommodation is the norm in pediatric OCD. Family-focused interventions must consider the parent, child, and family-level variables associated with this familial response when teaching disengagement strategies.

▶ This report reminds us that pediatric obsessive-compulsive disorder (OCD) is among the most common psychiatric disorders of childhood affecting somewhere between 0.5% and 2% of youngsters. The report also shows us how poorly parents deal with their offspring who have this disorder, frequently providing accommodation rather than effective parenting. Accommodation is the process by which a family member assists or actually participates in the patient's rituals, a phenomenon particularly well documented in the OCD literature. The report of Peris et al shows that family accommodation is quite common in the form of reassurance or actual participation in patient rituals, occurring on a daily basis among almost 50% of parents. Parents in this study acknowledged verbal reassurance, facilitation of avoidance, and actual participation in rituals as the most common manifestations of accommodation for their child's OCD. These responses are troubling both because they are likely to shape and maintain OCD symptoms and because they are directly at odds with exposure-based treatments currently indicated for pediatric OCD. Parent accommodation fundamentally adds to the burden of disease and fosters further family stress. For some parents, it is all too easy to give in.

It is unfortunate that parents of youngsters with OCD all too often make the situation worse for their affected child. It is likely that these parents have simply given up, and in fact give in to the way in which their child goes about their daily routine. On a related topic, if you want to see the latest update on neuro-psychiatric disorders associated with streptococcal infection that can present with OCD, see a recent case-control study.[1] Using health insurance claims data, investigators compared the occurrence of streptococcal infection in children ages 4 to 13 years with OCD, Tourette syndrome, or newly diagnosed tic disorder. Supporting earlier claims of a relationship, subjects with newly diag-nosed OCD, Tourette syndrome, or tic disorder were more likely than controls to have had a diagnosis of streptococcal infection in the previous year (odds ratio 1.54). There has been a lot of controversy about the relationship of strepto-coccal infection and neuropsychiatric disorders, but this most recent report seems to underscore the real possibility of a linkage.

J. A. Stockman III, MD

Reference

1. Leslie DL, Kozma L, Martin A. Neuropsychiatric disorders associated with strep-tococcal infection: a case-control study among privately insured children. *J Am Acad Child Adolesc Psychiatry.* 2008;47:1166-1172.

Cognitive Behavioral Therapy, Sertraline, or a Combination in Childhood Anxiety

Walkup JT, Albano AM, Piacentini J, et al (Johns Hopkins Med Insts, Baltimore; New York State Psychiatric Inst–Columbia Univ Med Ctr; Univ of California, Los Angeles; et al)

N Engl J Med 359:2753-2766, 2008

Background.—Anxiety disorders are common psychiatric conditions affecting children and adolescents. Although cognitive behavioral therapy and selective serotonin-reuptake inhibitors have shown efficacy in treating these disorders, little is known about their relative or combined efficacy.

Methods.—In this randomized, controlled trial, we assigned 488 children between the ages of 7 and 17 years who had a primary diagnosis of separation anxiety disorder, generalized anxiety disorder, or social phobia to receive 14 sessions of cognitive behavioral therapy, sertraline (at a dose of up to 200 mg per day), a combination of sertraline and cogni-tive behavioral therapy, or a placebo drug for 12 weeks in a 2:2:2:1 ratio. We administered categorical and dimensional ratings of anxiety severity and impairment at baseline and at weeks 4, 8, and 12.

Results.—The percentages of children who were rated as very much or much improved on the Clinical Global Impression–Improvement scale were 80.7% for combination therapy (P<0.001), 59.7% for cognitive behavioral therapy (P<0.001), and 54.9% for sertraline (P<0.001); all therapies were superior to placebo (23.7%). Combination therapy was superior to both monotherapies (P<0.001). Results on the Pediatric Anxiety Rating Scale documented a similar magnitude and pattern of response; combination therapy had a greater response than cognitive behavioral therapy, which was equivalent to sertraline, and all therapies were superior to placebo. Adverse events, including suicidal and homicidal ideation, were no more frequent in the sertraline group than in the placebo group. No child attempted suicide. There was less insomnia, fatigue, sedation, and restlessness associated with cognitive behavioral therapy than with sertraline.

Conclusions.—Both cognitive behavioral therapy and sertraline reduced the severity of anxiety in children with anxiety disorders; a combination of the two therapies had a superior response rate. (ClinicalTrials.gov number, NCT00052078.)

▶ Anyone practicing pediatrics knows how common anxiety disorders are in children. Many children with anxiety disorders will show global signs of anxiety, but may also show separation anxiety and social phobia as well. Data from the literature suggest that these disorders taken together affect somewhere between 5% and 20% of children and adolescents. More commonly than not, the disorders are not recognized for what they are by families and care providers. This is not a good situation because failure to identify these problems early in life can lead to increased rates of anxiety disorders, depression, and even substance abuse later in life as well as to educational underachievement.

The report of Walkup et al on the Child-Adolescent Anxiety Multimodal Study (CAMS) addresses the need for early diagnosis and treatment for these disorders. CAMS represents a large multicenter trial that was designed to address current gaps in the treatment literature by evaluating the relative efficacy of cognitive behavioral therapy, sertraline, a combination of the 2 therapies, and a placebo drug. The study was designed as a 2-phase, multicenter, randomized, controlled trial for children and adolescents between the ages of 7 and 17 years who had separation or generalized anxiety disorder or social phobia. Phase I of the study included a 12-week trial of short-term treatment comparing cognitive behavioral therapy, sertraline, and their combination with a placebo drug. Phase II was a 6-month open extension for patients who had a response in phase I. Cognitive behavioral therapy involved 14 sessions each for 60 minutes, which included review and ratings of the severity of a youngster's anxiety, response to treatment, and adverse events. Pharmacotherapy involved 8 sessions of 30 to 60 minutes each that included review and ratings of the severity of subjects' anxiety, the response to treatment, and adverse events. Sertraline (Zoloft) and matching placebo were administered on a fixed-flexible schedule beginning with 25 mg per day and adjustments of up to 2 mg per day by week 8 of the report.

Although early randomized, control trials have demonstrated the effectiveness of the individual treatments (antidepression medications and cognitive behavioral therapy) used in this study, CAMS was a useful study in that it compared the 2 monotherapies, examined their combination, and revealed several interesting findings. First, the 2 monotherapies were equally effective. Medication therapy did kick in earlier in terms of positive results when compared with cognitive behavioral therapy. Combination therapy, however, appeared to be superior to either of the 2 monotherapies alone, and the absolute difference between the combination therapy and placebo was a striking difference.

Currently, it is highly unlikely that most children with persistent anxiety therapies are getting adequately treated. A commentary on this report by Emslie suggests that from a public health perspective, it is crucial that effective treatments be available for children who need them with anxiety disorders.[1] The commentary also reminds us that partial treatment frequently is as good as no treatment at all in that residual symptoms actually increase the likelihood of relapse and that partial treatment often masks the fact that children are not truly improved. When it comes down to what is the best treatment for any one child, it is clear that all 3 of the treatment options described in this report can be recommended, but a combination treatment is the most likely to produce the best long-term outcome, but one must take into consideration a family's treatment preferences, treatment availability, cost, and the time burden associated with cognitive behavioral therapy.

J. A. Stockman III, MD

Reference

1. Emslie GJ. Pediatric anxiety-under-recognized and undertreated. *N Engl J Med.* 2008;359:2835-2836.

Cost-Effectiveness of Treatments for Adolescent Depression: Results From TADS

Domino ME, Burns BJ, Silva SG, et al (Univ of North Carolina at Chapel Hill; Duke Univ, Durham, NC; Duke Univ Med Ctr, Durham, NC; et al)
Am J Psychiatry 165:588-596, 2008

Objective.—While the evidence base for treatments for adolescent depression is building, little is known about the relative efficiency of such treatments. Treatment costs are a relevant concern given the competing demands on family and health care budgets. The authors evaluated the cost-effectiveness of three active treatments among adolescents with major depressive disorder.

Method.—Volunteers (N = 439) ages 12 to 18 with a primary diagnosis of major depressive disorder participated in a randomized, controlled trial conducted at 13 U.S. academic and community clinics from 2000 to 2004. Subjects included those participants who did not drop out and had evaluable outcome and cost data at 12 weeks (N = 369). Subjects were randomly assigned to 12 weeks of either fluoxetine alone (10–40 mg/

day), CBT alone, CBT combined with fluoxetine (10–40 mg/day), or placebo (equivalent to 10–40 mg/day). Both placebo and fluoxetine were administered double-blind; CBT alone and CBT in combination with fluoxetine were administered unblinded. Societal cost per unit of improvement on the Children's Depression Rating Scale—Revised and cost per quality-adjusted life year (QALY) were compared.

Results.—Results ranged from an incremental cost over placebo of $24,000 per QALY for treatment with fluoxetine to $123,000 per QALY for combination therapy treatment. The cost-effectiveness ratio for CBT treatment was not evaluable due to negative clinical effects. The models were robust on a variety of assumptions.

Conclusions.—Both fluoxetine and combination therapy are at least as cost-effective in the short-term as other treatments commonly used in primary care (using a threshold of $125,000/QALY). Fluoxetine is more cost-effective than combination therapy after 12 weeks of treatment.

▶ Many are not aware that a study has been going on for some time known as the Treatment for Adolescents with Depression Study (TADS). TADS is a multicenter, randomized, masked clinical trial designed to evaluate the effectiveness of cognitive-behavioral therapy (CBT), the drug fluoxetine, and their combination for the treatment of major depressive disorder in adolescents.[1] Stage I of TADS compared 4 groups randomly assigned to 12 weeks of treatment with fluoxetine alone, CBT alone, combination therapy, or medical management with pill placebo. The report of Domino et al extracts data from TADS to tell us the cost-effectiveness of these various forms of treatment for adolescent depression.

What we learn from this report is that in the short term, treatment with fluoxetine costs only slightly more than a placebo (median difference of $101 in total cost over 12 weeks). Fluoxetine was better than placebo in terms of improved outcomes. Interestingly, CBT was neither an effective nor cost-effective option at 12 weeks into the study. Combination therapy had the highest total cost, but the greatest improvement in Children's Depression Rating Scale. The cost, however, was $123 000 per quality-adjusted life year (QALY). The implication of these results is that fluoxetine is more cost-effective based on short-term outcomes. Combination therapy would be only recommended over fluoxetine if the additional clinical improvement were worth the markedly higher cost.

Please note that the results reported involve only short-term (12 weeks) cost outcomes. If that is the aim, the greatest bang for the buck comes from taking a pill. This commentary closes with a *Clinical Fact/Curio* about antidepressants. In the fish world, baby is just another word for lunch because it behooves aquatic larvae to be able to move about quickly and to be ever-vigilant. Data now suggest that such fish embryos or hatchlings who are in water polluted with pharmaceuticals in trace concentration are much more likely to become food. It is apparent that tons of medications end up in the environment each year. Much of these have been excreted by patients in their urine, while sometimes leftover pills are flushed down the toilet. Because water treatment plants are not designed to remove pharmaceuticals, the water these plants release generally carries a wide array of drug residues, albeit in trace amounts. In 2006, a pair of chemists reported that antidepressants downstream of a water treatment plant were showing up in trace amounts in the brains of fish. It was also shown that exposure to specific antidepressants affect larval flathead minnows. Fish exposed as hatchling embryos to trace concentrations of antidepressants do not react as quickly to normal stimuli signaling a possible predator. This laid-back reaction could prove to be a death sentence. Studies have shown that antidepressants can impair a fish's ability to eat, to avoid being eaten, and perhaps to attract a mate. Unfortunately, the effects of antidepressants on fish vary by type of fish. For example, hybrid striped bass exposed to the same pharmaceutical brew are not much affected and freely scarf down flathead minnows who mope along as a consequence of exposure to the same antidepressants.

If all of this sounds like a fish story, read the report by Raloff.[2]

J. A. Stockman III, MD

References

1. Treatment for adolescents with depression study team. Treatment for adolescents with depression study (TADS): rationale, design, and methods. *J Am Acad Child Adolesc Psychiatr.* 2003;42:531-542.
2. Raloff J. Antidepressants make for sad fish: drugs may effect feeding, swimming and mate-attracting. *Sci News.* December 20, 2008;15.

Burnout and Suicidal Ideation among U.S. Medical Students

Dyrbye LN, Thomas MR, Massie FS, et al (Mayo Clinic, Rochester, MN; Univ of Alabama School of Medicine, Birmingham; et al)
Ann Intern Med 149:334-341, 2008

Background.—Little is known about the prevalence of suicidal ideation among U.S. medical students or how it relates to burnout.

Objective.—To assess the frequency of suicidal ideation among medical students and explore its relationship with burnout.

Design.—Cross-sectional 2007 and longitudinal 2006 to 2007 cohort study.

Setting.—7 medical schools in the United States.

Participants.—4287 medical students at 7 medical schools, with students at 5 institutions studied longitudinally.

Measurements.—Prevalence of suicidal ideation in the past year and its relationship to burnout, demographic characteristics, and quality of life.

Results.—Burnout was reported by 49.6% (95% CI, 47.5% to 51.8%) of students, and 11.2% (CI, 9.9% to 12.6%) reported suicidal ideation within the past year. In a sensitivity analysis that assumed all nonresponders did not have suicidal ideation, the prevalence of suicidal ideation in the past 12 months would be 5.8%. In the longitudinal cohort, burnout ($P < 0.001$ for all domains), quality of life ($P < 0.002$ for each domain), and depressive symptoms ($P < 0.001$) at baseline predicted suicidal ideation over the following year. In multivariable analysis, burnout and low mental quality of life at baseline were independent predictors of suicidal ideation over the following year. Of the 370 students who met criteria for burnout in 2006, 99 (26.8%) recovered. Recovery from burnout was associated with markedly less suicidal ideation, which suggests that recovery from burnout decreased suicide risk.

Limitation.—Although response rates (52% for the cross-sectional study and 65% for the longitudinal cohort study) are typical of physician surveys, nonresponse by some students reduces the precision of the estimated frequency of suicidal ideation and burnout.

Conclusion.—Approximately 50% of students experience burnout and 10% experience suicidal ideation during medical school. Burnout seems to be associated with increased likelihood of subsequent suicidal ideation, whereas recovery from burnout is associated with less suicidal ideation.

▶ With all that has been written about work hours and the positive and negative impacts on resident training here in the United States, little has been written about whether a reduction in work hours might improve the stress that some residents find themselves under. Stress is clearly a part of training and not all of this is related to work hours. What we see in this report is that even before residency training, there are psychological problems that individuals have during medical school. The study demonstrates a high prevalence of recent suicidal ideation in medical students with as many as 1 in 9 having thought of suicide in the past year. In fact, the rate of suicidal ideation runs almost twice what one would expect in an age-matched population in the United States. A strong linkage was observed between burnout and a desire to commit suicide. At the same time, recovery from burnout was shown to be associated with a dramatic decrease in the likelihood of suicidal ideation. Please note that this is not the first study to suggest that medical students have a problem with contemplating suicide. Givens et al surveying all medical students at a private United States medical school found that 6.2% reported contemplating suicide during their medical school training period.[1]

It is clear that all medical schools should have in place student support services and wellness programs as well as systems to optimize the learning environment. All of these tend to help diminish medical student burnout. Medical schools should also be aware that common negative life events can trigger stress that medical students are already under. Serious personal illness or death of a close family member, for example, can be enough to tip a student over.

The data from this report should not be ignored. The study has significant validity compared with previous reports in that all medical students at the Mayo Medical School, University of Washington School of Medicine, University of Chicago Pritzker School of Medicine, University of Minnesota, University of Alabama School of Medicine and the University of San Diego School of Medicine as well as the Uniformed Services University of Health Sciences were included in the surveys that were part of this report. It is critical that practical ways to identify students at risk need to be developed. Suicide is not rare among our progeny.

J. A. Stockman III, MD

Reference

1. Givens JL, Tjia J. Depressed medical students use of mental health services and barriers to use. *Acad Med.* 2002;77:918-921.

Common genetic determinants of schizophrenia and bipolar disorder in Swedish families: a population-based study
Lichtenstein P, Yip BH, Björk C, et al (Karolinska Institutet, Stockholm, Sweden; et al)
Lancet 373:234-239, 2009

Background.—Whether schizophrenia and bipolar disorder are the clinical outcomes of discrete or shared causative processes is much debated in psychiatry. We aimed to assess genetic and environmental contributions to liability for schizophrenia, bipolar disorder, and their comorbidity.

Methods.—We linked the multi-generation register, which contains information about all children and their parents in Sweden, and the hospital discharge register, which includes all public psychiatric inpatient admissions in Sweden. We identified 9 009 202 unique individuals in more than 2 million nuclear families between 1973 and 2004. Risks for schizophrenia, bipolar disorder, and their comorbidity were assessed for biological and adoptive parents, offspring, full-siblings and half-siblings of probands with one of the diseases. We used a multivariate generalised linear mixed model for analysis of genetic and environmental contributions to liability for schizophrenia, bipolar disorder, and the comorbidity.

Findings.—First-degree relatives of probands with either schizophrenia (n = 35 985) or bipolar disorder (n = 40 487) were at increased risk of these disorders. Half-siblings had a significantly increased risk (schizophrenia: relative risk [RR] $3\cdot6$, 95% CI $2\cdot3$–$5\cdot5$ for maternal half-siblings, and $2\cdot7$, $1\cdot9$–$3\cdot8$ for paternal half-siblings; bipolar disorder: $4\cdot5$, $2\cdot7$–$7\cdot4$ for maternal half-siblings, and $2\cdot4$, $1\cdot4$–$4\cdot1$ for paternal half-siblings), but substantially lower than that of the full-siblings (schizophrenia: $9\cdot0$, $8\cdot5$–$11\cdot6$; bipolar disorder: $7\cdot9$, $7\cdot1$–$8\cdot8$). When relatives of probands with bipolar disorder were analysed, increased risks for schizophrenia existed for all relationships, including adopted children to biological parents with bipolar disorder. Heritability for schizophrenia and bipolar disorder was 64% and 59%, respectively. Shared environmental effects were small but substantial (schizophrenia: $4\cdot5$%, $4\cdot4$%–$7\cdot4$%; bipolar disorder: $3\cdot4$%, $2\cdot3$%–$6\cdot2$%) for both disorders. The comorbidity between disorders was mainly (63%) due to additive genetic effects common to both disorders.

Interpretation.—Similar to molecular genetic studies, we showed evidence that schizophrenia and bipolar disorder partly share a common genetic cause. These results challenge the current nosological dichotomy between schizophrenia and bipolar disorder, and are consistent with a reappraisal of these disorders as distinct diagnostic entities.

▶ Some believe that schizophrenia and bipolar disorder are linked with a common cause while others believe the entities represent entirely different processes. Still others envision a shared causative factor for part of each disorder. A common cause has been suggested by molecular genetic studies by the existence of an intermediate phenotype (schizoaffective disorder), which shares diagnostic features of both disorders, and by evidence that similar endophenotypes (eg, brain white matter density) are associated with both disorders. Thus far, evidence from genetic epidemiological studies has been mixed, partly because of small sample sizes. This is where the report published in the *Lancet* becomes so important.

Lichtenstein et al provide information from the largest family study of schizophrenia and bipolar disorder ever undertaken. They studied more than 2 million nuclear families, which are identified from the Swedish population and hospital discharge registers. The results are clear: first-degree relatives of probands with schizophrenia or bipolar disorder have an increased risk of both disorders. Moreover, evidence from half-siblings and adopted away relatives among the Swedish families suggests that this effect is mainly due to genetic factors. From these data, it is reasonable therefore to conclude that schizophrenia and bipolar disorder partly share a common genetic cause. These findings are critically important to the care of children because if this information holds up, kids born in families with schizophrenia and bipolar disorder are at significant risk of 1 or both of these problems.

It is interesting to see back in history how schizophrenia and bipolar disorder became separate entities. More than 100 years ago, Emil Kraepelin split the nonorganic (so-called functional) psychoses into 2 disorders and thereby created a dichotomous approach to classification that persists today. He distinguished the disorders on the basis of differences in course and outcome with dementia praecox, now known as schizophrenia, characterized by relentlessly deteriorating mental function, whereas manic depressive insanity, now known as bipolar disorder, was seen as an essentially relapsing and remitting disorder of affect with full recovery between episodes. Although Kraepelin himself came to question the validity of this strict dichotomy, it has settled in concrete in the American Psychiatric Association's *Diagnostic and Statistical Manual of Mental Disorders* and the World Health Organization's international classification of diseases. As a result, it is widely but erroneously assumed that the 2 disorders are discrete, natural disease entities with distinct pathogenesis, which can be identified by current operational diagnostic conventions. To this day, this belief has survived despite the fact that, although typical schizophrenia and bipolar disorder are often seen in many patients who have both psychotic and affective symptoms over the course of their illnesses, and it is not uncommon for patients to receive both diagnoses at different times. Unfortunately, most in the mental health field believe that these 2 disorders tend to breed true. That is to say that in families with schizophrenia, there is an increased risk of schizophrenia. In families with bipolar disorder, there is an increased risk of bipolar disorder.

Based on the information from the report of Lichtenstein et al, we now must ask whether clinical practice and research can continue to be best served by persistence in basing our diagnoses on the binary concept of separating schizophrenia from bipolar disorder. While keeping these disorders distinct helps us to think we are doing a better job with the types of drugs we use for each, perhaps we should be a little more open-minded about overlapping pathological processes. It is especially timely to consider this issue now because efforts to reformulate the American Psychiatric Association's *Diagnostic and Statistical Manual of Mental Health Disorders* (V) and the World Health Organization's international classification of diseases (XI) are under way. From the pediatric point of view, the bottom line is that the similar molecular genetic findings seen in schizophrenia and bipolar disorder means that when we see either of these diseases in a family, the risk of both increases in siblings and subsequent generations.

J. A. Stockman III, MD

Enuresis as a premorbid developmental marker of schizophrenia
Hyde TM, Deep-Soboslay A, Iglesias B, et al (Univ of Maryland, Baltimore; et al)
Brain 131:2489-2498, 2008

There is comparatively little information about premorbid maturational brain abnormalities in schizophrenia (SCZ). We investigated whether a history of childhood enuresis, a well-established marker of neurodevelopmental delay, is associated with SCZ and with measures of brain abnormalities also associated with SCZ. A Diagnostic and Statistical Manual of Mental Disorders (DSM-IV) based history of enuresis, volumetric brain MRI scans and neuropsychological testing were obtained in patients with SCZ, their non-psychotic siblings (SIB) and non-psychiatric controls (NC). The subjects were 211 patients (79.6% male), 234 of their SIB (43.2% male) and 355 controls (39.2% male). Frequency of enuresis was compared across groups and correlated with cognitive measures. Total and regional brain volumes were determined using voxel-based morphometry on matched subsets of probands ($n = 82$) with or without enuresis ($n = 16$, $n = 66$, respectively) and controls ($n = 102$) with or without enuresis ($n = 11$, $n = 91$, respectively). Patients with SCZ had higher rates of childhood enuresis (21%) compared with SIB (11%; $\chi^2 = 6.42$, $P = 0.01$) or controls (7%; $\chi^2 = 23.65$, $P < 0.0001$) and relative risk for enuresis was increased in SIB ($\lambda_S = 2.62$). Patients with enuresis performed worse on two frontal lobe cognitive tests [Letter Fluency ($t = 1.97$, $P = 0.05$, df $= 200$) and Category Fluency ($t = 2.15$, $P = 0.03$, df $= 200$)] as compared with non-enuretic patients. Voxel-based morphometry analysis revealed grey matter volume reductions in several frontal regions (right BA 9, right BA 10 and bilateral BA 45) and right superior parietal cortex (BA 7) in patients with a history of enuresis as compared with non-enuretic patients (all $t > 3.57$, all $P < 0.001$). The high frequency of childhood enuresis associated with SCZ and abnormalities in prefrontal function and structure in patients with a childhood history of enuresis suggest that childhood enuresis may be a premorbid marker for neurodevelopmental abnormalities related to SCZ. These findings add to the evidence implicating prefrontal dysmaturation in this disorder, potentially related to genetic risk factors.

▶ This is a chilling report. Few studies have explored the relationship between a history of childhood enuresis and schizophrenia, but if one looks back in the literature, one can see that almost 100 years ago Kraepelin anecdotally referred to obstinate nocturnal enuresis in childhood in cases of dementia praecox, the old term for schizophrenia.[1] The acquisition of bladder control, particularly at night, has been used as an important and well-established developmental neurological milestone, usually occurring around 4 years of age. Rates of enuresis in otherwise healthy children range from 10% among 6-year-olds to 5% among 10-year-olds and, of course, are higher in boys than girls as is true of the relative proportion of schizophrenia in the childhood and adult population. Absent any definitive cause, the inability to have volitional bladder control by the time of entry to school has been felt to represent a neurodevelopmental abnormality.

There have been several studies that have explored the relationship between childhood enuresis and other psychiatric or developmental disorders. For example, studies have found increased rates of enuresis in children with attention deficit hyperactivity disorder, childhood Tourette's syndrome, and adult bipolar disorder. Some have also suggested that enuresis is associated with an increased risk of adolescent suicidal behavior and conduct problems.

The study reported from Maryland represents the first comprehensive analysis of the potential link between a history of childhood enuresis and adult onset schizophrenia. A total of 800 subjects participated in research funded by the National Institutes of Mental Health in this regard. The data from the study suggest that adult patients with schizophrenia do have a much higher rate of previous childhood enuresis (21%) in comparison with their healthy siblings (11%) or with normal controls (7%). This study is also the only one in the literature that has looked at adults with schizophrenia and a history of enuresis examined with both neuropsychological testing and structural brain imaging. The data from this report should not be used to say that childhood enuresis is a determinative and specific risk factor for schizophrenia, as most children with enuresis certainly do not develop this psychiatric disorder. The study did reveal that those with a history of enuresis have a higher probability of showing abnormal brain scans, specifically with decreased gray matter on frontal imaging.

If the data from this report hold up, they suggest a view that childhood enuresis is a general reflection in some instances, of maturational neurodevelopmental abnormalities that impede the acquisition of normal developmental milestones and that in some, this is a marker for a predisposition to psychiatric disorders. Although one can speculate, without any degree of certainty, about the relationship between childhood enuresis and schizophrenia, it does seem clear that childhood enuresis is much more common in schizophrenic adults than in controls. It is entirely possible that there may be an inherited component to childhood enuresis in families of patients with schizophrenia. At a minimum, the study does underscore the potential concept of schizophrenia being associated with early developmental difficulties, particularly those related to structural abnormalities of the frontal lobe.

This comment closes with a *Clinical Fact/Curio* about a neurologic disorder. What do beauticians, pharmacists, morticians, chemists, laboratory technicians, physicians, veterinarians, dentists, fire fighters, photographers, and printers have in common—something that increases their risk for a certain disease? The answer is that exposure to formaldehyde may increase an individual's risk of developing amyotrophic lateral sclerosis (ALS). Investigators have analyzed data from the American Cancer Society's Cancer Prevention Study II, which includes more than one million individuals. Participants in the study reported their exposure to 12 classes of chemicals. They were followed up to 15 years. The researchers identified 617 men and 539 women who died of ALS during that period. Surprisingly, no statistical increased risk of ALS was found among participants who reported regular pesticide exposure compared with those who did not. However, the investigators did find that individuals who reported formaldehyde exposure had a 34% higher risk of the disorder in comparison with those who reported no such exposure. Also found was a strong dose-response relationship between formaldehyde exposure and ALS. For example, those exposed to formaldehyde for up to 4 years had a 50% greater risk of dying of the disorder compared with those who were not exposed. Those with 4 to 10 years of exposure had more than twice the risk of dying from ALS than those who were unexposed. Those with more than 10 years of exposure had 4 times the risk. Those in certain occupations were more likely to report formaldehyde exposure, including beauticians, pharmacists, morticians, chemists, laboratory technicians, physicians, veterinarians, dentists, fire fighters, photographers, printers, and nurses. Individuals with these occupations had a 30% higher rate of ALS than a comparable control population.[2]

J. A. Stockman III, MD

References

1. Kraepelin E. *Dementia Praecox*. New York, NY: Churchill Livingstone, Inc; 1987: 1919-1971.
2. Kuehn BM. Researchers identify neurological risks. *JAMA*. 2008;299:2375-2376.

14 Newborn

Cumulative Live-Birth Rates after In Vitro Fertilization
Malizia BA, Hacker MR, Penzias AS (Boston IVF, Waltham, MA; Beth Israel
Deaconess Med Ctr and Harvard Med School, Boston, MA)
N Engl J Med 360:236-243, 2009

Background.—Outcomes of in vitro fertilization (IVF) treatment are
traditionally reported as pregnancies per IVF cycle. However, a couple's
primary concern is the chance of a live birth over an entire treatment
course.

Methods.—We estimated cumulative live-birth rates among patients
undergoing their first fresh-embryo, nondonor IVF cycle between 2000
and 2005 at one large center. Couples were followed until either discontinuation of treatment or delivery of a live-born infant. Analyses were stratified according to maternal age and performed with the use of both
optimistic and conservative methods. Optimistic methods assumed that
patients who did not return for subsequent IVF cycles would have the
same chance of a pregnancy resulting in a live birth as patients who
continued treatment; conservative methods assumed no live births
among patients who did not return.

Results.—Among 6164 patients undergoing 14,248 cycles, the cumulative live-birth rate after 6 cycles was 72% (95% confidence interval [CI],
70 to 74) with the optimistic analysis and 51% (95% CI, 49 to 52) with
the conservative analysis. Among patients who were younger than 35
years of age, the corresponding rates after six cycles were 86% (95%
CI, 83 to 88) and 65% (95% CI, 64 to 67). Among patients who were
40 years of age or older, the corresponding rates were 42% (95% CI, 37
to 47) and 23% (95% CI, 21 to 25). The cumulative live-birth rate
decreased with increasing age, and the age-stratified curves (<35 vs. ≥40
years) were significantly different from one another (P<0.001).

Conclusions.—Our results indicate that IVF may largely overcome infertility in younger women, but it does not reverse the age-dependent decline
in fertility (Fig 2).

► This study reports accurate evidence-based estimates of the likelihood that
a couple presenting for in vitro fertilization (IVF) will have a pregnancy resulting
in a live birth. One would have thought that this information would have been
available already, but actually there is little in this regard. What does exist is
a commonly used statistic, the outcome per cycle according to maternal age.
The primary reason for the use of this cross-sectional statistic is the simplicity

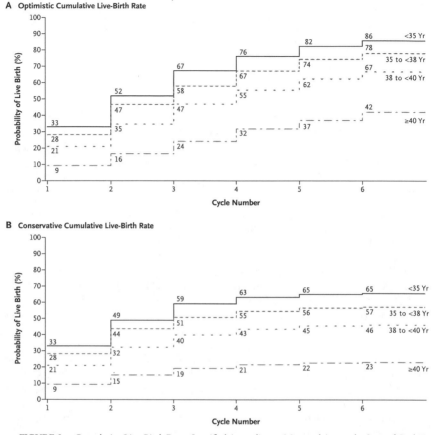

A Optimistic Cumulative Live-Birth Rate

B Conservative Cumulative Live-Birth Rate

FIGURE 2.—Cumulative Live-Birth Rates Stratified According to Maternal Age at the Start of Cycle 1. Panel A shows the optimistic cumulative live-birth rates stratified according to age. These rates are based on the assumption that patients who did not return for treatment had the same chance of a pregnancy resulting in a live birth as those who remained in treatment. Panel B shows the conservative cumulative live-birth rates stratified according to age. These rates are based on the assumption that patients who did not return for subsequent IVF cycles had no chance of a pregnancy resulting in a live birth. In both panels, the age-stratified curves are significantly different from one another (P<0.001). These optimistic and conservative rates reflect the best-case and worst-case estimates, respectively, of the cumulative live-birth rate for each age group in the population. (Reprinted from Malizia BA, Hacker MR, Penzias AS. Cumulative live-birth rates after in vitro fertilization. *N Engl J Med*. 2009;360:236-243. Copyright 2009 Massachusetts Medical Society. All rights reserved.

with which it can be calculated. Data in the literature basically list the IVF outcomes as pregnancies per cycle rather than the likelihood that a woman starting the process is likely to have a successful pregnancy resulting in a live birth. The report of Malizia et al tells us about the cumulative live-birth rates among more than 6000 patients undergoing multiple IVF cycles using both fresh and frozen embryos in a single large center. The cumulative live-birth rate in this population was between 51% and 72%. The higher (optimistic) esti-mate of the cumulative live-birth rate, which assumes that women who did not return for subsequent IVF cycles had the same chance of a pregnancy resulting in a live birth as those who remained in treatment, was probably an overestimate. It is likely that the true IVF success rate more closely approximates the lower range noted in this report.

This report also reminds us that there is a natural decline in fertility with age, both in the general population and in the population with decreased fertility. The age-stratified cumulative live-birth rates decreased with increasing age. Interestingly, the birth rates seen in this report among women 39 years of age or younger who were treated with up to 6 cycles of IVF appeared to be similar to or higher than those reported in the general population, suggesting that IVF overcomes infertility in younger women. However, women 40 years of age or older should be informed that IVF does not completely reverse the age-dependent decrease in fertility. Fig 2 shows the live-birth rate stratified according to maternal age.

Finally, we have a meaningful cumulative live-birth rate to answer a couple's primary question—what is the chance that IVF will result in a baby? Fig 2 provides the answer to this question and as with so many questions, the answer is "it depends."

J. A. Stockman III, MD

Effects of technology or maternal factors on perinatal outcome after assisted fertilisation: a population-based cohort study
Romundstad LB, Romundstad PR, Sunde A, et al (St Olavs Univ Hosp, Trondheim, Norway; Norwegian Univ of Science and Technology, Trondheim; et al)
Lancet 372:737-743, 2008

Background.—Research suggests that singleton births following assisted fertilisation are associated with adverse outcomes; however, these results might be confounded by factors that affect both fertility and pregnancy outcome. We therefore compared pregnancy outcomes in women who had singleton pregnancies conceived both spontaneously and after assisted fertilisation.

Methods.—In a population-based cohort study, we assessed differences in birthweight, gestational age, and odds ratios (OR) of small for gestational age babies, premature births, and perinatal deaths in singletons (gestation ≥22 weeks or birthweigh ≥500 g) born to 2546 Norwegian women (>20 years) who had conceived at least one child spontaneously and another after assisted fertilisation among 1 200 922 births after spontaneous conception and 8229 after assisted fertilisation.

Findings.—In the whole study population, assisted-fertilisation conceptions were associated with lower mean birthweight (difference 25 g, 95% CI 14 to 35), shorter duration of gestation (2·0 days, 1·6 to 2·3) and increased risks of small for gestational age (OR 1·26, 1·10 to 1·44), and perinatal death (1·31, 1·05 to 1·65) than were spontaneous conceptions. In the sibling-relationship comparisons, the spontaneous versus the assisted-fertilisation conceptions showed a difference of only 9 g (−18 to 36) in birthweight and 0·6 days (−0·5 to 1·7) in gestational age. For assisted fertilisation versus spontaneous conception in the sibling-relationship comparisons, the OR for small for gestational age was 0·99 (0·62 to 1·57) and that for perinatal mortality was 0·36 (0·20 to 0·67).

Interpretation.—Birthweight, gestational age, and risks of small for gestational age babies, and preterm delivery did not differ among infants of women who had conceived both spontaneously and after assisted fertilisation. The adverse outcomes of assisted fertilisation that we noted compared with those in the general population could therefore be attributable to the factors leading to infertility, rather than to factors related to the reproductive technology.

▶ Pediatricians need to be aware of what currently is available to couples who have had fertility problems. Pregnancies resulting from assisted fertilization sometimes result in offspring that require neonatal intensive care. Thus, the report of Romundstad et al should be on our reading list. These investigators address an important question: is impaired perinatal outcome in infants born after assisted reproductive technology (ART) an effect of the technology or is the result of maternal or even paternal factors that have resulted in the diminished fertility these couples have experienced?

What these investigators did was to compare the outcome of pregnancies with ART with a conventional control group of pregnancies from the general population, and confirmed the poorer perinatal outcome in infants born as singletons. They avoided the trap of trying to evaluate outcomes of multiple pregnancies that result from ART. The investigators included a second control group by comparing perinatal outcomes in singletons after spontaneous versus in vitro conceptions, in the same women. Using sibship comparisons, the investigators analyzed data from consecutive deliveries of first-born and second-born infants: some women have an ART conception followed by a spontaneous conception or vice versa. With the siblings as controls, the differences between ART and spontaneously conceived infants disappeared. Similar results were found for birth weight, length of gestation, or odds ratios of small for gestational age, and the risk of perinatal mortality was even lower after ART conceptions. The conclusion was that the adverse outcomes in ART pregnancies are likely to be better explained as an effect of maternal factors than as a result of the technology itself.

The Romundstad et al report is a truly elegant study because it helps to pinpoint the cause of the perinatal problems experienced by the offspring of pregnancies initiated by ART. The problem lies largely with the mothers of these babies, not with the ART. Women who conceive after ART are often of advanced age, primiparous, and likely to deliver multiple infants. The outcome data in children born with ART are generally derived from meta-analyses of studies with control groups from the general population and are adjusted for maternal age, parity, multiple births, year of birth, and type of fertility treatment. Singletons have an increased risk of both short- and long-term health problems, including poor perinatal outcome, increased risk of malformations, chromosomal aberrations, and cerebral palsy compared with spontaneously conceived children. This has been shown in other studies. Obviously additional risks are seen with multiple births following ART.

The greatest problem that lies truly at the heart of ART is the increase in multiple delivery rates, which run as high as 23%. Some are addressing the issue of multiple pregnancies related to in vitro fertilization by selective single-embryo transfer.

For a number of reasons, the number of newborns that are being delivered as a result of conception after ART is increasing. While a reduction in the number of multiple births has led to improvements in outcomes, it is important for us to gain an improved biological understanding of the underlying reasons why infertility and ovarian stimulation in and of itself might have adverse effects on the rates of infant morbidity and mortality.

For more on the topic of neonatal outcome following ART, see the excellent editorial on this topic by Andersen et al.[1]

J. A. Stockman III, MD

Reference

1. Andersen AN, Pimborg A, Loft A. Neonatal outcome in singletons conceived after ART. *Lancet.* 2008;372:694-695.

Clomifene citrate or unstimulated intrauterine insemination compared with expectant management for unexplained infertility: pragmatic randomised controlled trial

Bhattacharya S, Harrild K, Mollison J, et al (Univ of Aberdeen; Univ of Oxford; et al)
BMJ 337.a716, 2008

Objective.—To compare the effectiveness of clomifene citrate and unstimulated intrauterine insemination with expectant management for the treatment of unexplained infertility.

Design.—Three arm parallel group, pragmatic randomised controlled trial.

Setting.—Four teaching hospitals and a district general hospital in Scotland.

Participants.—Couples with infertility for over two years, confirmed ovulation, patent fallopian tubes, and motile sperm.

Intervention.—Expectant management, oral clomifene citrate, and unstimulated intrauterine insemination.

Main Outcome Measures.—The primary outcome was live birth. Secondary outcome measures included clinical pregnancy, multiple pregnancy, miscarriage, and acceptability.

Results.—580 women were randomised to expectant management (n=193), oral clomifene citrate (n=194), or unstimulated intrauterine insemination (n=193) for six months. The three randomised groups were comparable in terms of age, body mass index, duration of infertility, sperm concentration, and motility. Live birth rates were 32/193 (17%), 26/192 (14%), and 43/191 (23%), respectively. Compared with expectant management, the odds ratio for a live birth was 0.79 (95% confidence interval 0.45 to 1.38) after clomifene citrate and 1.46 (0.88 to 2.43) after unstimulated intrauterine insemination. More women randomised to clomifene citrate (159/170, 94%) and unstimulated intrauterine insemination (155/162, 96%) found the process of treatment acceptable than those randomised to expectant management (123/153, 80%) (P=0.001 and P<0.001, respectively).

Conclusion.—In couples with unexplained infertility existing treatments such as empirical clomifene and unstimulated intrauterine insemination are unlikely to offer superior live birth rates compared with expectant management.

Trial Registration.—ISRCT No: 71762042.

▶ As mentioned elsewhere, it is important for us to be aware of the impact on newborns of assisted reproductive technology (ART). The report of Bhattacharya et al helps us with several understandings. These investigators' randomized controlled trial compared the use of clomifene citrate or intrauterine insemination for 6 months with expectant management in almost 600 women with unexplained infertility. The authors found no significant difference in the live birth rate between the 2 groups. Although the study did not include intrauterine insemination with ovarian stimulation as an intervention, the beneficial effect of this treatment relative to expectant management has already been questioned. A systematic review of the use of in vitro fertilization as another alternative in unexplained fertility has found that it significantly increases the risk of clinical pregnancy in comparison with expectant management.[1] The importance of this report is that one can compare clomifene citrate and intrauterine insemination against watchful waiting, the results are the same. Watchful waiting, of course, is a lot less expensive and much less likely to result in the delivery of twins or multiple births with all the complications the latter entails.

Given the fact that 1 in 7 couples trying to have a child fails to conceive after 1 year of regular unprotected intercourse, the information from this report is most important. Traditionally, treatment of infertility proceeds in a stepwise manner, starting with low-cost risk intervention such as stimulation of ovulation with clomifene citrate and unstimulated intrauterine insemination, both of which we now know work as well as simply waiting the problem out a bit. When such treatments fail, clinicians usually recommend intrauterine insemination with ovarian stimulation and then move on to in vitro fertilization. As a direct result of the lack of evidence, many couples with unexplained infertility endure (and even request) expensive, potentially hazardous, and often unnecessary treatments. It appears that multiple cycles of intrauterine insemination without ovarian stimulation in couples with unexplained infertility are likely to be a waste of time. Obviously, we need more high-quality clinical trials to guide policy makers and health care providers in order to devise optimum treatment regimens. An editorial that accompanied the report abstracted suggests that in the meantime, appropriate selection of couples for different treatment pathways is critical and that if a woman is under 36 and the duration of infertility is less than 3 years, 6 to 12 months of expectant management would seem to be justified, particularly so if the woman has been previously pregnant. Older age, a longer duration of infertility and lack of pregnancy after expectant management should be regarded as indications for a more proactive treatment.[2] Admittedly, the choice of the first-line treatment will need to be individualized according to the couple's expectations and available resources. On the basis of the best evidence currently available, in vitro fertilization seems to be the most cost-effective intervention after tincture of time has failed to achieve pregnancy.

For a comprehensive review of ART approaches, see the excellent summary of this topic by Right et al that appeared in *Morbidity and Mortality Weekly Report* in mid 2008.[3]

J. A. Stockman III, MD

References

1. Pandian Z, Bhattacharya S, Vale L, et al. In vitro fertilization for unexplained sub fertility. *Cochrane Database Syst Rev.* 2005;2:CD003357.
2. El-Toukhy TA, Khaliaf Y. The treatment of unexplained infertility. Should be tailored to the patient's expectations, centers experience, and available resources. *BMJ.* 2008;337:362-363.
3. Right VC, Chang J, Jeng G, et al. Assisted reproductive technology surveillance – United States, 2005. *MMWR.* 2008;57:1-23.

Intensive Care for Extreme Prematurity — Moving Beyond Gestational Age

Tyson JE, for the National Institute of Child Health and Human Development Neonatal Research Network (Univ of Texas Med School at Houston; et al)

N Engl J Med 358:1672-1681, 2008

Background.—Decisions regarding whether to administer intensive care to extremely premature infants are often based on gestational age alone. However, other factors also affect the prognosis for these patients.

Methods.—We prospectively studied a cohort of 4446 infants born at 22 to 25 weeks' gestation (determined on the basis of the best obstetrical estimate) in the Neonatal Research Network of the National Institute of Child Health and Human Development to relate risk factors assessable at or before birth to the likelihood of survival, survival without profound neurodevelopmental impairment, and survival without neurodevelopmental impairment at a corrected age of 18 to 22 months.

Results.—Among study infants, 3702 (83%) received intensive care in the form of mechanical ventilation. Among the 4192 study infants (94%) for whom outcomes were determined at 18 to 22 months, 49% died, 61% died or had profound impairment, and 73% died or had impairment. In multivariable analyses of infants who received intensive care, exposure to antenatal corticosteroids, female sex, singleton birth, and higher birth weight (per each 100-g increment) were each associated with reductions in the risk of death and the risk of death or profound or any neurodevelopmental impairment; these reductions were similar to those associated with a 1-week increase in gestational age. At the same estimated likelihood of a favorable outcome, girls were less likely than boys to receive intensive care. The outcomes for infants who underwent ventilation were better predicted with the use of the above factors than with use of gestational age alone.

Conclusions.—The likelihood of a favorable outcome with intensive care can be better estimated by consideration of four factors in addition to gestational age: sex, exposure or nonexposure to antenatal corticosteroids, whether single or multiple birth, and birth weight. (ClinicalTrials. gov numbers, NCT00063063 and NCT00009633.)

▶ Prematurity still remains the principal cause of morbidity and mortality among those who inhabit our neonatal intensive care units. A recent review of the management and outcomes of very low birth weight infants reminds us that some 12.5% of births here in the United States are preterm (occurring before 37 weeks gestation).[1] Most define very low birth weight as those infants weighing 1500 g or less at birth and those with extreme prematurity as weighing 1000 g or less, accounting for 1.5% and 0.7% of live births, respectively. In the report of Tyson et al, extreme prematurity was defined as being born before 25 weeks. Whether or not to initiate or forgo intensive care for extremely premature infants has remained a topic of some controversy with some intensive care units providing care to everyone who crosses their threshold while others are selective on the basis of gestational-age thresholds. For example, care is likely to be routinely administered at 25 weeks gestation, but may or may not be provided at 23 to 24 weeks and then only with parental agreement. Most nurseries will provide "comfort care" for infants born at 22 weeks or earlier. What this report does is to look at the evidence, pro and con, providing support for or against these various decisions. What we learn is that the current widespread use of gestational-age thresholds, in and of themselves, may not be appropriate in deciding whether to administer intensive care to extremely premature babies.

So what are the factors that should be taken into account when trying to decide which infant is sufficiently mature to be viable and to have at least a fair shot at normality if they survive? We learn from this report that female sex, exposure to prenatal steroids, being a single birth, and increased birth weight (per 100 g increment) each are associated with benefits similar to those of an increase in gestational age of approximately 1 week. Interestingly, race or ethnic group had no significant association with outcomes. You would think that with the precision we now have with prenatal ultrasonographic assessment of gestational age that information provided by prenatal ultrasounds could be thrown into this equation. Estimates based on ultrasonographic examinations have been reported to have an error (± 2 SD) of approximately 4 days at 12 to 14 weeks and 7 days at 14 to 22 weeks. Please note, estimates of prematurity based on ultrasonographic examinations are in fact subject to both systematic and random error. Their accuracy has generally been assessed in relatively healthy populations evaluated by ultrasonographers who are aware of other indicators of pregnancy length. In fact, error under field conditions at 20 to 30 weeks gestation may be as great as 2 weeks. For many extremely premature infants, the measurement error in assessing pregnancy length is more than the 1- to 2-week difference in gestational age that could change treatment decisions with the use of current gestational-age thresholds. Thus, data from prenatal ultrasounds should be used with great caution in trying to determine gestational age as a criterion for giving or not giving supportive therapy to an extremely premature baby.

You will have to decide whether the information provided by this report can be translated in any meaningful way into nurseries that you may be associated with. The report suggests that barring any major therapeutic advances, the findings from this report indicate that extending intensive care to all of the most immature infants would entail considerable suffering, resource use, and cost to benefit only a small proportion of surviving infants. The cost of neonatal care is estimated to run approximately $3400 per hospital day (2007 US dollars). Exactly when are the burdens of intensive care justified by the likelihood of benefit? Traditional estimates are based on the proportion of births of infants in the highest risk groups with good outcome, but because some infants die without receiving intensive care, this approach underestimates the likelihood of a benefit from intensive care. Deciding when to administer intensive care, Paris suggests that "the best one can do is to make a human judgment based on probabilities."[2] Consideration of multiple factors, not just gestational age, is likely to promote treatment decisions that are less arbitrary, more individualized, and more transparent to care providers and parents. If you want to look at a simple web-based tool that allows clinicians to use the findings from this report in estimating the likelihood that intensive care will benefit individual infants, go to the following web site: www.nichd.nih.gov/neonatalestimates. For a complete review of the topic of the management and outcomes of very low birth weight infants, see the commentary of Eichenwald and Stark.[3]

J. A. Stockman III, MD

References

1. Eichenwald EC, Stark AR. Management and outcomes of very low birth weight. *N Engl J Med.* 2008;358:1700-1711.
2. Paris JJ. Resuscitation decisions for "fetal infants". *Pediatrics.* 2005;115:1415.
3. Eichenwald EC, Stark AR. Management and outcomes of very low birth weight. *N Engl J Med.* 2008;358:1700-1712.

Long-Term Medical and Social Consequences of Preterm Birth
Moster D, Lie RT, Markestad T (Univ of Bergen, Norway; et al)
N Engl J Med 359:262-273, 2008

Background.—Advances in perinatal care have increased the number of premature babies who survive. There are concerns, however, about the ability of these children to cope with the demands of adulthood.

Methods.—We linked compulsory national registries in Norway to identify children of different gestational-age categories who were born between 1967 and 1983 and to follow them through 2003 in order to document medical disabilities and outcomes reflecting social performance.

Results.—The study included 903,402 infants who were born alive and without congenital anomalies (1822 born at 23 to 27 weeks of gestation, 2805 at 28 to 30 weeks, 7424 at 31 to 33 weeks, 32,945 at 34 to 36 weeks, and 858,406 at 37 weeks or later). The proportions of infants who survived and were followed to adult life were 17.8%, 57.3%, 85.7%, 94.6%, and 96.5%, respectively. Among the survivors, the prevalence of having cerebral palsy was 0.1% for those born at term versus 9.1% for those born at 23 to 27 weeks of gestation (relative risk for birth at 23 to 27 weeks of gestation, 78.9; 95% confidence interval [CI], 56.5 to 110.0); the prevalence of having mental retardation, 0.4% versus 4.4% (relative risk, 10.3; 95% CI, 6.2 to 17.2); and the prevalence of receiving a disability pension, 1.7% versus 10.6% (relative risk, 7.5; 95% CI, 5.5 to 10.0). Among those who did not have medical disabilities, the gestational age at birth was associated with the education level attained, income, receipt of Social Security benefits, and the establishment of a family, but not with rates of unemployment or criminal activity.

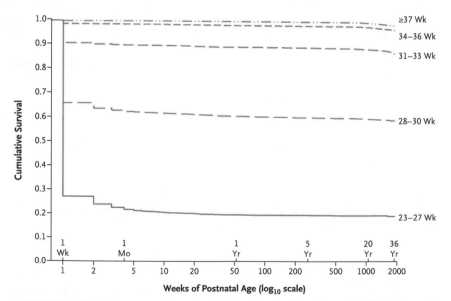

FIGURE 2.—Survival curves according to gestational age. (Reprinted from Moster D, Lie RT, Markestad T. Long-term medical and social consequences of preterm birth. *N Engl J Med*. 2008;359:262-273. Copyright 2008 Massachusetts Medical Society. All rights reserved.)

Conclusions.—In this cohort of people in Norway who were born between 1967 and 1983, the risks of medical and social disabilities in adulthood increased with decreasing gestational age at birth.

▶ A recent report by Field et al from Great Britain examined the survival of extremely premature babies comparing a period of 1994-1999 with 2000-2005. It was found that the survival of infants born at 24 and 25 weeks of gestation significantly increased. There appeared to be no improvement in survival for infants born at 23 weeks. Care for infants born at 22 weeks remained unsuccessful with no viable infants described.[1] The information from this British report was studied by the British House of Commons Select Committee in its review of legislation regarding gestational age limits for abortion. Current United Kingdom legislation limits abortion to before 24 weeks gestation unless there are specific medical issues. The United Kingdom Abortion Act of 1967 was amended in 1990 to lower the age limit from 28 to 24 weeks, a change that was influenced by the Royal College of Obstetricians and Gynecologists report that noted significant improvements in the survival of infants born preterm. Based on the current information that was provided to it, proposals to lower the 24-week deadline for abortion were rejected in the House of Commons. As one might suspect, decisions involving late abortion and the care of extremely preterm infants continue to be based on strongly held beliefs.

So what does all this have to do with the report of Moster et al? In this study involving almost 1 million infants who were born alive between 1967 and 1983 without congenital anomalies, 18% born at 23 to 27 weeks of age made it to adulthood, 57% born at 28 to 30 weeks made it to adulthood, 86% born at 31 to 33 weeks survived, and over 95% born past this gestational age survived (Fig 2). The likelihood of having cerebral palsy was 9% for those born at 23 to 27 weeks of gestation, and the risk of mental retardation was 4.4% at these gestational ages (Table 2). These data relate to babies born in Norway. The findings are consistent with those of previous studies showing that very preterm birth is associated with specific difficulties in the areas of motor, cognitive, behavioral, psychological, and social function among preschool and school-aged children, problems that persist into adulthood at a small but real level.

The survival rates among children with the lowest gestational ages in this report increased over time and did coincide with an increased prevalence of cerebral palsy. Among preterm survivors, however, the prevalence of cerebral palsy may be decreasing, but at the same time, younger and younger babies are surviving.

When it comes to the debate regarding abortion, including the debate within that deals with the lower gestational age limit for legal abortion, you can bet that both sides within this debate will view the data from Norway in different ways. It is clear that more and more increasingly preterm babies are capable of surviving, albeit with a small but real risk of disability. If the age limit for legal abortion is based on viability absent the consequences of surviving a very early birth, then these data are quite significant in terms of the debate.

TABLE 2.—Medical Disabilities According to Gestational Age at Birth*

Disability	Subjects		P Value for Trend
	No./Total no.(%)	Relative Risk (95% CI)	
Cerebral palsy†			<0.001
23 Wk to 27 wk 6 days	33/362 (9.1)	78.9 (56.5−110.0)	
28 Wk to 30 wk 6 days	101/1,686 (6.0)	45.8 (37.1−56.5)	
31 Wk to 33 wk 6 days	125/6,591 (1.9)	14.1 (11.6−17.2)	
34 Wk to 36 wk 6 days	112/32,187 (0.3)	2.7 (2.2−3.3)	
≥37 Wk	1,110/853,309 (0.1)	1.0 (reference)	
Mental retardation†			<0.001
23 Wk to 27 wk 6 days	16/362 (4.4)	10.3 (6.2−17.2)	
28 Wk to 30 wk 6 days	30/1,686 (1.8)	4.2 (2.9−6.0)	
31 Wk to 33 wk 6 days	64/6,591 (1.0)	2.1 (1.7−2.8)	
34 Wk to 36 wk 6 days	223/32,187 (0.7)	1.6 (1.4−1.8)	
≥37 Wk	3,578/853,309 (0.4)	1.0 (reference)	
Schizophrenia†			0.12‡
23 Wk to 27 wk 6 days	2/362 (0.6)	4.5 (0.7−16.5)‡	
28 Wk to 30 wk 6 days	2/1,686 (0.1)	0.9 (0.1−3.2)‡	
31 Wk to 33 wk 6 days	15/6,591 (0.2)	1.4 (0.8−2.5)	
34 Wk to 36 wk 6 days	61/32,187 (0.2)	1.3 (1.0−1.7)	
≥37 Wk	1,152/853,309 (0.1)	1.0 (reference)	
Autism spectrum†			0.002‡
23 Wk to 27 wk 6 days	2/362 (0.6)	9.7 (1.5−36.2)‡	
28 Wk to 30 wk 6 days	6/1,686 (0.4)	7.3 (2.7−17.6)‡	
31 Wk to 33 wk 6 days	3/6,591 (0.05)	1.0 (0.2−3.0)‡	
34 Wk to 36 wk 6 days	11/32,187 (0.03)	0.8 (0.4−1.4)	
≥37 Wk	403/853,309 (0.05)	1.0 (reference)	
Disorders of psychological development, behavior, and emotion†			<0.001
23 Wk to 27 wk 6 days	9/362 (2.5)	10.5 (5.6−19.9)	
28 Wk to 30 wk 6 days	12/1,686 (0.7)	2.9 (1.6−5.2)	
31 Wk to 33 wk 6 days	23/6,591 (0.3)	1.4 (0.9−2.2)	
34 Wk to 36 wk 6 days	108/32,187 (0.3)	1.5 (1.2−1.8)	
≥37 Wk	1,798/853,309 (0.2)	1.0 (reference)	
Other major disabilities†§			<0.001
23 Wk to 27 wk 6 days	15/362 (4.1)	19.6 (11.9−32.2)	
28 Wk to 30 wk 6 days	37/1,686 (2.2)	9.3 (6.6−13)	
31 Wk to 33 wk 6 days	35/6,591 (0.5)	2.3 (1.7−3.3)	
34 Wk to 36 wk 6 days	110/32,187 (0.3)	1.5 (1.2−1.8)	
≥37 Wk	1,916/853,309 (0.2)	1.0 (reference)	
Any medical disability severely affecting working capacity¶			<0.001
23 Wk to 27 wk 6 days	38/359 (10.6)	7.5 (5.5−10.0)	
28 Wk to 30 wk 6 days	138/1,674 (8.2)	4.8 (4.1−5.7)	
31 Wk to 33 wk 6 days	272/6,548 (4.2)	2.2 (2.0−2.5)	
34 Wk to 36 wk 6 days	781/32,062 (2.4)	1.4 (1.3−1.5)	
≥37 Wk	14,286/850,437 (1.7)	1.0 (reference)	

*All analyses are adjusted for sex, year of birth, multiple births, single motherhood, maternal age, mother's level of education, father's level of education, and whether parents were immigrants.

†This category of diagnosis is extracted from the primary medical diagnoses registered in the National Insurance Scheme as the reasons for giving disability benefits (Table 1 of the Supplementary Appendix).

‡Relative risk, confidence interval, and P value were based on exact logistic regression, adjusting for calendar year and sex because of small numbers.

§Other major disabilities include blindness, low vision, hearing loss, and epilepsy.

¶Disability affecting working capacity was assessed by the National Insurance Scheme as the working capacity of a person 18 years of age or older that was permanently reduced by at least 50% owing to any medical condition. Children who died before their 18th birthday were excluded from this analysis.

(Reprinted from Moster D, Lie RT, Markestad T. Long-term medical and social consequences of preterm birth. *N Engl J Med*. 2008;359:262-273.)

As mentioned earlier, however, age of viability is only one component, and in many people's minds, a small component, of the overall debate.

J. A. Stockman III, MD

Reference

1. Field DJ, Dorling JS, Manktelow BN, Draper ES. Survival of extremely premature babies in a geographically defined population: prospective cohort study of 1994-1999 compared with 2000-2005. *BMJ.* 2008;336:1221-1223.

Increased Risk of Adverse Neurological Development for Late Preterm Infants

Petrini JR, Dias T, McCormick MC, et al (Perinatal Data Ctr, White Plains, NY; Harvard School of Public Health, Boston, MA; et al)
J Pediatr 154:169-176, 2009

Objective.—To assess the risks of moderate prematurity for cerebral palsy (CP), developmental delay/mental retardation (DD/MR), and seizure disorders in early childhood.

Study Design.—Retrospective cohort study using hospitalization and outpatient databases from the Northern California Kaiser Permanente Medical Care Program. Data covered 141 321 children $\geq$30 weeks born between Jan 1, 2000, and June 30, 2004, with follow-up through Jun 30, 2005. Presence of CP, DD/MR, and seizures was based on *International Classification of Diseases, Ninth Revision codes* identified in the encounter data. Separate Cox proportional hazard models were used for each of the outcomes, with crude and adjusted hazard ratios calculated for each gestational age group.

Results.—Decreasing gestational age was associated with increased incidence of CP and DD/MR, even for those born at 34 to 36 weeks gestation. Children born late preterm were >3 times as likely (hazard ratio, 3.39; 95% CI, 2.54-4.52) as children born at term to be diagnosed with CP. A modest association with DD/MR was found for children born at 34 to 36 weeks (hazard ratio, 1.25; 95% CI, 1.01-1.54), but not for children in whom seizures were diagnosed.

Conclusions.—Prematurity is associated with long-term neurodevelopmental consequences, with risks increasing as gestation decreases, even in infants born at 34 to 36 weeks.

▶ This is another report reminding us that it is best to be born at term when it comes to an increased risk of adverse neurological development. Making it to near term is not good enough. The recent rise in preterm birth has occurred throughout the industrialized world, but has been particularly marked in the United States. Most of the increase in preterm birth here and elsewhere is attributable to increases in late preterm birth, primarily between 34 and 36 weeks of gestation. Advances in neonatal care, including intensive care, have markedly improved the survival throughout preterm gestational age range, but these advances may have led many obstetricians and neonatologists to consider late preterm births to be risk free. They are not. It is clear that even 34- to 36-week-old infants are at increased risk for mortality in both the neonatal and postnatal periods. Obviously, the relative risks (vs infants born at term) are modest compared with infants born at less than 32 weeks, but the much larger and increasing numbers of birth at late preterm gestational ages now translate into a significant impact on overall infant mortality. In this regard, the current study by Petrini et al fills an important gap in our knowledge.

Petrini et al present data from the Northern California Kaiser Permanente Medical Care Program and show a three-fold increased risk of cerebral palsy and a modestly but significantly increased risk of developmental delay, mental retardation, or both in children who were born 34 to 36 weeks of age. If nothing else is learned from this report, it is that we as care providers must be aware and more vigilant of potential neurocognitive problems in the follow-up of infants born near term. A good bit of births at this age are the result of ovulation stimulation and multiple embryo transfer and the rising rate of routine labor induction. In a commentary that accompanied the Petrini et al report, Kramer poses the question of whether more frequent induction might be doing more harm than good.[1] He noted that the issue of how much labor induction is too much can only be adequately addressed with a randomized trial of labor induction at 34 to 36 weeks for specific maternal or fetal indications. In the meantime, it is suggested that obstetricians, pediatricians, and other care providers should inform pregnant women of the long-term risk associated with late preterm birth and should take those risks into account when making decisions about ovulation stimulation, multiple embryo transfer and labor induction. These are wise cautions.

J. A. Stockman III, MD

Reference

1. Kramer MS. Late preterm birth: appreciable risk, rising incidence. *J Pediatr.* 2009; 154:159-160.

Aggressive vs. Conservative Phototherapy for Infants with Extremely Low Birth Weight

Morris BH, Oh W, Tyson JE, et al (Univ of Texas Med School, Houston; Brown Univ, Providence, RI, et al)
N Engl J Med 359:1885-1896, 2008

Background.—It is unclear whether aggressive phototherapy to prevent neurotoxic effects of bilirubin benefits or harms infants with extremely low birth weight (1000 g or less).

Methods.—We randomly assigned 1974 infants with extremely low birth weight at 12 to 36 hours of age to undergo either aggressive or conservative phototherapy. The primary outcome was a composite of death or neurodevelopmental impairment determined for 91% of the infants by investigators who were unaware of the treatment assignments.

Results.—Aggressive phototherapy, as compared with conservative phototherapy, significantly reduced the mean peak serum bilirubin level (7.0 vs. 9.8 mg per deciliter [120 vs. 168 μmol per liter], P<0.01) but not the rate of the primary outcome (52% vs. 55%; relative risk, 0.94; 95% confidence interval [CI], 0.87 to 1.02; P = 0.15). Aggressive phototherapy did reduce rates of neurodevelopmental impairment (26%, vs. 30% for conservative phototherapy; relative risk, 0.86; 95% CI, 0.74 to 0.99). Rates of death in the aggressive-phototherapy and conservative-phototherapy groups were 24% and 23%, respectively (relative risk, 1.05; 95% CI, 0.90 to 1.22). In preplanned subgroup analyses, the rates of death were 13% with aggressive phototherapy and 14% with conservative phototherapy for infants with a birth weight of 751 to 1000 g and 39% and 34%, respectively (relative risk, 1.13; 95% CI, 0.96 to 1.34), for infants with a birth weight of 501 to 750 g.

Conclusions.—Aggressive phototherapy did not significantly reduce the rate of death or neurodevelopmental impairment. The rate of neurodevelopmental impairment alone was significantly reduced with aggressive phototherapy. This reduction may be offset by an increase in mortality among infants weighing 501 to 750 g at birth. (ClinicalTrials.gov number, NCT00114543.)

▶ The controversy about whether a modest elevation of total serum bilirubin is harmful or not has been raised for some time. Most believe that modest elevations of bilirubin are in fact not harmful and that overly aggressive use of phototherapy in fact may do more harm than good. Addressing such a complex issue of the interrelationship between phototherapy, bilirubin levels, and long-term outcome is not an uncomplex task and requires a massive commitment of many institutions willing to provide data. That in fact is the source of the data for this report, which emanates from members of the Eunice Kennedy Shriver National Institute of Child Health and Human Development Neonatal Research Network whose chair is at the University of Cincinnati. The investigators randomly assigned almost 2000 infants with extremely low birth weight (501-1000 g) at 12 to 36 hours of age to undergo either aggressive or conservative phototherapy. For infants in the aggressive-phototherapy group, phototherapy was initiated at enrollment when the bilirubin level was expected to be approximately 5 mg/deciliter. For infants with a birth weight of 501 to 750 g, the aggressive phototherapy was continued or restarted whenever the bilirubin was found to be 5 mg/ deciliter or higher. For infants with a birth weight of 751 to 1000 g, the aggressive phototherapy was continued or restarted whenever the bilirubin level was found to be 5 mg/deciliter or higher during the first 7 days after birth and 7 mg/deciliter or higher during the next 7 days. Conservative phototherapy was initiated, continued, or restarted whenever the bilirubin level was 8 mg/deciliter or higher for infants weighing 501 to 750 g at birth and 10 mg/deciliter or higher for infants weighing 751 to 1000 g at birth.

So what were the findings of this report? In this multicenter trial, the investigators found no significant difference in the rate of death or neurodevelopmental outcome (the primary outcome) at 18 to 22 months of corrected age between neonates randomly assigned to receive aggressive phototherapy as compared with those assigned to receive conservative phototherapy as previously defined. However, the use of aggressive phototherapy significantly reduced the overall rate of neurodevelopmental impairment in infants with birth weights of 751 to 1000 g. In fact, for infants with a birth weight of 501 to 750 g, the possibility that increased mortality might offset any potential benefits of aggressive therapy probably means that we should be dialing back on our aggressivity when it comes to these very tiny babies. Interestingly, this report reminds us that a little bilirubin is actually possibly good for us because it is a potent antioxidant.

On a peripherally related subject having to do with hyperbilirubinemia, it has been observed that the use of intravenous immunoglobulin (IVIG) is capable of reducing the need for exchange transfusion as a therapeutic modality to prevent kernicterus.[1] While IVIG therapy does not remove circulating antibodies like exchange transfusion, it does interfere with the hemolytic process, thus reducing the need for exchange transfusion to keep bilirubin levels down.

J. A. Stockman III, MD

Reference

1. Huizing KMN, Roislien J, Hansen TWR. Intravenous immune globulin reduces the need for exchange transfusion in Rhesus and ABO incompatibility. *Acta Paediatr.* 2008;97:1362-1365.

Early Insulin Therapy in Very-Low-Birth-Weight Infants
Beardsall K, Vanhaesebrouck S, Ogilvy-Stuart AL, et al (Univ of Cambridge; Cambridge Univ Hosp Natl Health Service Found Trust; Univ of Leuven, Belgium; et al)
N Engl J Med 359:1873-1884, 2008

Background.—Studies involving adults and children being treated in intensive care units indicate that insulin therapy and glucose control may influence survival. Hyperglycemia in very-low-birth-weight infants is also associated with morbidity and mortality. This international randomized, controlled trial aimed to determine whether early insulin replacement reduced hyperglycemia and affected outcomes in such neonates.

Methods.—In this multicenter trial, we assigned 195 infants to continuous infusion of insulin at a dose of 0.05 U per kilogram of body weight per hour with 20% dextrose support and 194 to standard neonatal care on days 1 to 7. The efficacy of glucose control was assessed by continuous glucose monitoring. The primary outcome was mortality at the expected date of delivery. The study was discontinued early because of concerns about futility with regard to the primary outcome and potential harm.

Results.—As compared with infants in the control group, infants in the early-insulin group had lower mean ($\pm$SD) glucose levels (6.2 $\pm$ 1.4 vs. 6.7 $\pm$ 2.2 mmol per liter [112 $\pm$ 25 vs. 121 $\pm$ 40 mg per deciliter], P = 0.007). Fewer infants in the early-insulin group had hyperglycemia for more than 10% of the first week of life (21% vs. 33%, P = 0.008). The early-insulin group had significantly more carbohydrate infused (51 $\pm$ 13 vs. 43 $\pm$ 10 kcal per kilogram per day, P<0.001) and less weight loss in the first week (standard-deviation score for change in weight, -0.55 ± 0.52 vs. -0.70 ± 0.47; P = 0.006). More infants in the early-insulin group had episodes of hypoglycemia (defined as a blood glucose level of <2.6 mmol per liter [47 mg per deciliter] for >1 hour) (29% in the early-insulin group vs. 17% in the control group, P = 0.005), and the increase in hypoglycemia was significant in infants with birth weights of more than 1 kg. There were no differences in the intention-to-treat analyses for the primary outcome (mortality at the expected date of delivery) and the secondary outcome (morbidity). In the intention-to-treat analysis, mortality at 28 days was higher in the early-insulin group than in the control group (P = 0.04).

Conclusions.—Early insulin therapy offers little clinical benefit in very-low-birth-weight infants. It reduces hyperglycemia but may increase hypoglycemia (Current Controlled Trials number, ISRCTN78428828.)

▶ Most of us are aware that in very low birth weight infants (those weighing < 1500 g) the incidence of hyperglycemia tends to be quite high. Reports in the literature show this incidence to range anywhere from 20% to 85%.[1] The issue is whether these infants would benefit from insulin therapy and better management of their blood sugars. This has been looked at in adults who are critically ill who also have problems regulating their blood sugar. Early studies suggested that improved glucose control would reduce morbidity and mortality, but subsequent studies have shown modest effects, if any, from insulin therapy. In newborns, hyperglycemia tends to be a frequent complication of intravenous alimentation, but until the report of Beardsall et al appeared, the use of insulin in this population has remained largely controversial.

Exactly why preterm babies are not able to regulate their blood glucose remains largely unknown. Infants can mount hormonal response to stress that is quite similar to what you see in older critically ill patients and it has been suggested that very low birth weight infants have, as is true of older adults with a reduced ability to produce insulin, a defective beta-cell processing of proinsulin to insulin, resulting in elevated levels of proinsulin, which is significantly less active than insulin itself. Add to this the fact that small infants have an inability to suppress hepatic glucose production in response to glucose infusion and a decreased uptake of glucose secondary to a limited mass of insulin-sensitive tissues such as muscle and fat and you see the potential multifactorial basis of the hyperglycemia that preterm low birth weight infants have.

What Beardsall et al have done is to report on a large, open-label, randomized, controlled trial of early continuous insulin infusion in very-low-birth-weight infants. This was a large prospective multi-center trial designed to investigate whether insulin infusions begun on the first day of life improve glucose control and affect mortality and morbidity. The study unfortunately had to be discontinued by the Oversight Safety Monitoring Board following the study before complete enrollment occurred. The study was stopped because of safety concerns related to an excess dilatation of the cerebral ventricles and parenchymal lesions seen on cranial ultrasound images as well as a trend toward more deaths in the early-insulin group. The results that were obtained were otherwise largely negative. While there was better control of glucose levels in the early-insulin group, there was no difference in the primary outcome, death before expected date of delivery (14.4% in the early insulin group versus 9.4% in the control group). Worrisome was that there was a higher mortality in the early insulin group at 28 days of age (11.9% versus 5.7%) and an increased incidence of hypoglycemia as well as abnormalities detected on cranial ultrasound images.

Most of us are more than aware of the problems associated with routine, intermittent bedside glucose monitoring. The study of Beardsall et al simply confirms this. As compared with intermittent glucose monitoring, a much higher incidence of hypoglycemia was observed with the use of continuous glucose monitoring (30% versus 8.8% in the early-insulin group and 17% versus 1.6% in the control group). Chances are that the actual incidence of hypoglycemia may have been underestimated in this study since episodes of hypoglycemia lasting more than 1 hour would not have been reported.

When hyperglycemia is detected in very low birth weight infants (as defined by a plasma glucose concentration > 150 mg/deciliter), one begins to think about lowering that blood sugar. Most in reality do not initiate some management technique until the blood sugar rises above 180 mg/deciliter. Control of blood sugar can be accomplished either by reducing the glucose infusions that the infant is receiving or by administering insulin. The report of Beardsall et al provides a very strong cautionary note about the use of continuous insulin therapy to control glucose levels. The inference is that one probably would best consider the use of continuous insulin therapy only in infants with severe hyperglycemia (plasma glucose concentrations > 250 mg/deciliter). Until even larger studies provide the much needed evidence of the short-term and long-term benefit and safety of continuous insulin therapy in very low birth weight or extremely low birth weight infants, it would seem wise to use this therapy with great caution, if at all.

J. A. Stockman III, MD

Reference

1. Hay E. Hyperglycaemia in the very preterm baby. *Semin Fetal Neonatal Med.* 2005;10:377-387.

A Randomized, Controlled Trial of Magnesium Sulfate for the Prevention of Cerebral Palsy

Rouse DJ, for the Eunice Kennedy Shriver NICHD Maternal–Fetal Medicine Units Network (Univ of Alabama at Birmingham; et al)
N Engl J Med 359:895-905, 2008

Background.—Research suggests that fetal exposure to magnesium sulfate before preterm birth might reduce the risk of cerebral palsy.

Methods.—In this multicenter, placebo-controlled, double-blind trial, we randomly assigned women at imminent risk for delivery between 24 and 31 weeks of gestation to receive magnesium sulfate, administered intravenously as a 6-g bolus followed by a constant infusion of 2 g per hour, or matching placebo. The primary outcome was the composite of stillbirth or infant death by 1 year of corrected age or moderate or severe cerebral palsy at or beyond 2 years of corrected age.

Results.—A total of 2241 women underwent randomization. The baseline characteristics were similar in the two groups. Follow-up was achieved for 95.6% of the children. The rate of the primary outcome was not significantly different in the magnesium sulfate group and the placebo group (11.3% and 11.7%, respectively; relative risk, 0.97; 95% confidence interval [CI], 0.77 to 1.23). However, in a prespecified secondary analysis, moderate or severe cerebral palsy occurred significantly less frequently in the magnesium sulfate group (1.9% vs. 3.5%; relative risk, 0.55; 95% CI, 0.32 to 0.95). The risk of death did not differ significantly between the groups (9.5% vs. 8.5%; relative risk, 1.12; 95% CI, 0.85 to 1.47). No woman had a life-threatening event.

Conclusions.—Fetal exposure to magnesium sulfate before anticipated early preterm delivery did not reduce the combined risk of moderate or severe cerebral palsy or death, although the rate of cerebral palsy was reduced among survivors. (ClinicalTrials.gov number, NCT00014989.)

▶ Until I read this report, I was not aware that magnesium sulfate might have neuroprotective effects on babies born preterm. Magnesium sulfate, of course, has been used for many years to delay active labor, although studies done in recent times seem to indicate that it is ineffective for this indication. It does seem to work, however, to help treat and prevent eclampsia. Some studies have shown that preterm infants whose mothers received magnesium sulfate have reductions in the prevalence of cerebral palsy as compared with infants of untreated mothers. Not all studies have documented this, however. A Cochrane review of the world's literature did not show any significant effect of magnesium sulfate on either death or cerebral palsy, but did show a significant reduction in the rate of substantial gross motor dysfunction.[1]

The report of Rouse et al is significant in that it tells us the results of a multicenter, placebo-controlled, randomized trial of over 200 women at risk for preterm birth between 24 and 31 weeks of gestation who were randomly assigned to receive either intravenous magnesium sulfate or a placebo. Only women at risk of premature rupture of membranes or advanced preterm labor were included. Women with hypertension or preeclampsia were excluded. As compared with the placebo group, the magnesium sulfate group had significantly reduced rates of cerebral palsy overall (4.2% versus 7.3%) and the distribution of severity of cerebral palsy differed. The issue that is not resolved with this report is whether women threatening labor should be given magnesium sulfate routinely to provide a neuroprotective effect for their offspring. Again, magnesium sulfate has been documented not to be an effective agent in forestalling the onset of labor in those without preeclampsia or eclampsia. An editorial that accompanied this article by Stanley et al advises caution about recommending magnesium sulfate administration as a routine procedure in preterm deliveries.[2] This editorial indicates that we need to learn a lot more about the overall effects of this drug and how it works.

J. A. Stockman III, MD

References

1. Doyle LW, Crowther CA, Middleton P, Marret S, Rouse D. Magnesium sulfate for women at risk of preterm birth for neuroprotection of the fetus. *Cochrane Database Syst Rev.* 2009;1:CD004661.
2. Stanley FJ, Crowther C. Antenatal magnesium sulfate for neuro-protection before preterm birth? *N Engl J Med.* 2008;359:962-963.

Neuroprotective Effects of the Nonpsychoactive Cannabinoid Cannabidiol in Hypoxic-Ischemic Newborn Piglets

Alvarez FJ, Lafuente H, Rey-Santano MC, et al (Univ of Aberdeen, Scotland)
Pediatr Res 64:653-658, 2008

To test the neuroprotective effects of the nonpsychoactive cannabinoid cannabidiol (CBD), piglets received i.v. CBD or vehicle after hypoxia-ischemia (HI: temporary occlusion of both carotid arteries plus hypoxia). Nonhypoxic-ischemic sham-operated piglets remained as controls. Brain damage was studied by near-infrared spectroscopy (NIRS) and amplitude-integrated electroencephalography (aEEG) and by histologic assessment (Nissl and FluoroJadeB staining). In HI+vehicle, HI led to severe cerebral hemodynamic and metabolic impairment, as reflected in NIRS by an increase in total Hb index (THI) and a decrease in the fractional tissue oxygenation extraction (FTOE); in HI+CBD the increase of THI was blunted and FTOE remained similar to SHAM. HI profoundly decreased EEG amplitude, which was not recovered in HI+vehicle, indicating cerebral hypofunction; seizures were observed in all HI+vehicle. In HI+CBD, however, EEG amplitude recovered to 46.4 ± 7.8% baseline and seizures appeared only in 4/8 piglets (both $p < 0.05$). The number of viable neurons decreased and that of degenerating neurons increased in HI+vehicle; CBD reduced both effects by more than 50%. CBD administration was free from side effects; moreover, CBD administration was associated with cardiac, hemodynamic, and ventilatory beneficial effects. In conclusion, administration of CBD after HI reduced short-term brain damage and was associated with extracerebral benefits.

▶ What Alvarez et al have shown is that a certain cannabinoid, cannabidiol, is capable of protecting a newborn piglet brain from global hypoxia ischemia by improving hemodynamic and metabolic function in the brain in the early hours after injury. Cannabidiol-treated piglets showed fewer seizures suggesting that the drug may also act as an anticonvulsant, although this effect may be due to the less severe injury seen in the treated piglet. Importantly, there was a return of the electroencephalogram (EEG) to baseline normal findings much sooner in newborn piglets that were treated with cannabidiol following exposure to hypoxia. In humans, such early EEG recovery has been associated with significantly improved outcomes. Thus it does appear that cannabidiol will protect against early brain injury at least in this animal model. No side effects were seen with the drug. Perhaps, it is too soon to recommend a human clinical trial with cannabidiol until the pharmacology and drug distribution are better understood, but it is not inconceivable that similar findings might be found in the human infant.

Recently, cannabinoids have been implicated in a variety of positive brain developmental processes even though cannabinoids are thought to be associated with some deleterious effects as well. In humans, maternal use of cannabis is associated with cognitive deficits during pregnancy, but not uniformly so. Cannabidiol is an interesting cannabinoid that does not evoke the psychoactive properties of its cousin cannabinoids. It was cannabidiol that seemed to have a beneficial protective effect in the newborn piglet. Thus it is that not all forms of "pot" may necessarily be bad for you, depending on the time in life you are exposed.

While on the topic of things that can be inhaled, are you aware that there are more than 1 billion tobacco users worldwide with a third of these individuals living in China? It has been estimated that the number of years of life lost by a smoker is 15. For more on smoking-attributable mortality, years of potential life lost and productivity losses, see the report in *MMWR*.[1]

J. A. Stockman III, MD

Reference

1. Centers for Disease Control and Prevention (CDC). Smoking-attributable mortality, years of potential life lost, and productivity losses – United States, 2000-2004. *MMWR*. 2008;57:1226-1228.

Childhood outcomes after prescription of antibiotics to pregnant women with spontaneous preterm labour: 7-year follow-up of the ORACLE II trial

Kenyon S, Pike K, Jones DR, et al (Univ of Leicester, UK; et al)
Lancet 372:1319-1327, 2008

Background.—The ORACLE II trial compared the use of erythromycin and/or amoxicillin–clavulanate (co-amoxiclav) with that of placebo for women in spontaneous preterm labour and intact membranes, without overt signs of clinical infection, by use of a factorial randomised design. The aim of the present study—the ORACLE Children Study II—was to determine the long-term effects on children after exposure to antibiotics in this clinical situation.

Methods.—We assessed children at age 7 years born to the 4221 women who had completed the ORACLE II study and who were eligible for follow-up with a structured parental questionnaire to assess the child's health status. Functional impairment was defined as the presence of any level of functional impairment (severe, moderate, or mild) derived from the mark III Multi-Attribute Health Status classification system. Educational outcomes were assessed with national curriculum test results for children resident in England.

Findings.—Outcome was determined for 3196 (71%) eligible children. Overall, a greater proportion of children whose mothers had been prescribed erythromycin, with or without co-amoxiclav, had any functional impairment than did those whose mothers had received no erythromycin (658 [42·3%] of 1554 children *vs* 574 [38·3%] of 1498; odds ratio 1·18, 95% CI 1·02–1·37). Co-amoxiclav (with or without erythromycin) had no effect on the proportion of children with any functional impairment, compared with receipt of no co-amoxiclav (624 [40·7%] of 1523 *vs* 608 [40·0%] of 1520; 1·03, 0·89–1·19). No effects were seen with either antibiotic on the number of deaths, other medical conditions, behavioural patterns, or educational attainment. However, more children whose mothers had received erythromycin or co-amoxiclav developed cerebral palsy than did those born to mothers who received no erythromycin or no co-amoxiclav, respectively (erythromycin: 53 [3·3%] of 1611 *vs* 27 [1·7%] of 1562, 1·93, 1·21–3·09; co-amoxiclav: 50 [3·2%] of 1587 *vs* 30 [1·9%] of 1586, 1·69, 1·07–2·67). The number needed to harm with erythromycin was 64 (95% CI 37–209) and with co-amoxiclav 79 (42–591).

Interpretation.—The prescription of erythromycin for women in spontaneous preterm labour with intact membranes was associated with an increase in functional impairment among their children at 7 years of age. The risk of cerebral palsy was increased by either antibiotic, although the overall risk of this condition was low.

Funding.—UK Medical Research Council.

▶ The ORACLE I trial assessed the use of amoxicillin-clavulanate 375 mg or erythromycin 250 mg, or both, or placebo, 4 times a day for 10 days until birth, whichever was sooner in women presenting with preterm rupture of the fetal membranes (PROM). That particular collaborative study showed that erythromycin would indeed decrease the risk of the composite primary outcome (death or major cerebral abnormality or chronic neonatal lung disease). The use of erythromycin was also associated with prolongation of pregnancy and reductions in neonatal morbidity compared with women who did not receive erythromycin, and now is a recommended practice in most centers. It should be noted that amoxicillin-clavulanate was not associated with any change in the primary outcomes. However, although women who received this antibiotic combination had prolonged pregnancy compared with those who did not receive any antibiotic, its use was associated with a significantly higher incidence of neonatal necrotizing enterocolitis.

The ORACLE II study compared the use of erythromycin and/or amoxicillin-clavulanate with that of placebo in women with PROM in order to determine the long-term effects on children who were exposed in utero to these antibiotics. In ORACLE II, the administration of antibiotics to women with PROM produced no demonstrable benefit, and indeed the difficulty of diagnosing preterm labor accurately was shown by the fact that 63.5% of women in the control group in this study actually delivered after 37 weeks gestation. The positive finding of a small benefit from erythromycin in PROM in singletons may have been due to chance alone. The clinical significance of the short-term benefits (less oxygen dependence at 28 days, fewer major cerebral abnormalities on cerebral ultrasound, and fewer positive blood cultures) was also debatable. Amoxicillin-clavulanate produced no such benefits and was again associated with an increase in necrotizing enterocolitis.

In the study abstracted, the ORACLE II investigators presented outcomes 7 years out from birth. Reassuringly, the short-term gains from giving erythromycin in PROM have not been counterbalanced by any significant long-term disadvantage. However, neither has there been any persistent advantage. Meanwhile, there has been a substantial increase in prescriptions for peripartum erythromycin, unfortunately, with no specific microbiological surveillance of the consequences. In some areas, there has been a significant rise in the number of isolates of erythromycin-resistant group B streptococcus. Worrisome, however, is that this report documents an increased risk of cerebral palsy in offspring who had been exposed to antibiotics in utero. The increase in risk was anywhere from $1.6\times$ to $1.9\times$. The mechanism of this effect is unclear, but when subclinical infection is provoking labor, treatment with low doses of an oral antibiotic might only suppress rather than eradicate infection from the amniotic fluid and uterine cavity. Suppression without eradication might prolong the pregnancy, thus allowing continued fetal exposure to a damaging environment. The doses of antibiotics used in ORACLE II were too small and the route inappropriate for proper treatment of in utero infection.

If there is a lesson to be learned from the ORACLE II report, it is that contrary to popular opinion ("might as well give them, they don't do any harm"), antibiotics are not risk-free. As we have seen, there is an increased risk of necrotizing enterocolitis with the use of low-dose antibiotics as part of the management of PROM. Now we learn that there is possibly an increased risk of neurologic damage. While the chance of this occurrence is small, it is greater than one might have otherwise expected. The trick will be to figure out which mothers with PROM indeed are actively infected, recognizing that low-dose oral antibiotics are insufficient in such circumstances to protect a baby.

To learn more about the ORACLE studies, see the results of the ORACLE I trial.

J. A. Stockman III, MD

Neurodevelopmental Outcomes of Preterm Infants Fed High-Dose Docosahexaenoic Acid: A Randomized Controlled Trial

Makrides M, Gibson RA, McPhee AJ, et al (Children's Hosp and Flinders Med Centre, Adelaide, Australia; Univ of Adelaide, Australia; et al)
JAMA 301:175-182, 2009

Context.—Uncertainty exists about the benefit of dietary docosahexaenoic acid (DHA) on the neurodevelopment of preterm infants.

Objective.—To determine the effect of meeting the estimated DHA requirement of preterm infants on neurodevelopment at 18 months' corrected age.

Design, Setting, and Participants.—Randomized, double-blind controlled trial enrolling infants born at less than 33 weeks' gestation from April 2001 to October 2005 at 5 Australian tertiary hospitals, with follow-up to 18 months.

Intervention.—High-DHA (approximately 1% total fatty acids) enteral feeds compared with standard DHA (approximately 0.3% total fatty acids) from day 2 to 4 of life until term corrected age.

Main Outcome Measures.—Bayley Mental Development Index (MDI) at 18 months' corrected age. A priori subgroup analyses were conducted based on randomization strata (sex and birth weight <1250 g vs ≥1250 g).

Results.—Of the 657 infants enrolled, 93.5% completed the 18-month follow-up. Bayley MDI scores did not differ between the high- and standard-DHA groups (mean difference, 1.9; 95% confidence interval [CI], −1.0 to 4.7). The MDI among girls fed the high-DHA diet was higher than girls fed standard DHA in unadjusted and adjusted analyses (unadjusted mean difference, 4.7; 95% CI, 0.5-8.8; adjusted mean difference, 4.5; 95% CI, 0.5-8.5). The MDI among boys did not differ between groups. For infants born weighing less than 1250 g, the MDI in the high-DHA group was higher than with standard DHA in the unadjusted comparison (mean difference, 4.7; 95% CI, 0.2-9.2) but did not reach statistical significance following adjustment for gestational age, sex, maternal education, and birth order (mean difference, 3.8; 95% CI, −0.5 to 8.0). The MDI among infants born weighing at least 1250 g did not differ between groups.

Conclusion.—A DHA dose of approximately 1% total fatty acids in early life did not increase MDI scores of preterm infants overall born earlier than 33 weeks but did improve the MDI scores of girls.

Trial Registration.—anzctr.org.au Identifier: ACTRN12606000327583.

▶ The story relating docosahexaenoic acid (DHA) to brain development in the infant goes back a long way. DHA is a long chain of polyunsaturated fatty acid and has been of particular interest because it is a major lipid in the brain with specific structural and functional roles. An inadequate nutrient supply of DHA has been hypothesized to contribute to poor developmental outcome. Entry of DHA into the brain and nervous system is greatest during the last trimester of pregnancy. Postmortem studies have shown that average full body accumulation of DHA during this time is in excess of 50 mg/kg/d, which is equivalent to a dietary DHA content of approximately 1% of total fatty acids. Once a preterm baby is born, however, they must rely on the relatively low levels of DHA supplied by human milk or that supplemented in infant formulas. These constitute just 0.2% to 0.35% total fatty acids. Preterm infants have a significantly greater requirement for DHA than do their peer term counterparts.

The few studies that have been undertaken to date looking at whether DHA supplementation might help a preterm baby have produced conflicting results. Makrides et al conducted a randomized controlled trial to study the long-term efficacy of high-dose dietary DHA in the preterm infant. The study was designed to reflect the feeding practices of most neonatal units, where expressed breast milk is the nutrition of choice. In this study, lactating women received tuna oil supplements to increase the DHA concentration of their milk. Preterm infant formula with a matching DHA composition was used if there was insufficient breast milk. The study itself was a randomized, double-blind, controlled trial involving more than 600 preterm infants. High DHA (approximately 1% total fatty acids) diets were compared with standard DHA diets (approximately 0.3% total fatty acids) given from day 2 to 4 of life until term-corrected age. Outcomes were assessed using the Bailey Mental Developmental Index (MDI) performed at 18 months corrected age to determine whether high-dose DHA supplementation would improve developmental quotient.

So did DHA help? The answer was no. The trial reported was designed to resolve uncertainties about the putative role of dietary DHA in improving the developmental outcomes of children born preterm recognizing that previous trials were limited by insufficient dose or lack of power. With all these problems tended to, the developmental outcomes of these preterm infants were no better than expected with a standard amount of DHA in the diet. If there is any ray of hope with DHA based on the findings of this report, it is that there was some improvement in MDI scores of girls, which would suggest that high-dose interventions might be appropriate in future studies. Given the fact that there is no alternative therapy for cognitive delay that we know of these days, it is clear that further studies are warranted. As of now, DHA does not seem to be the magic bullet.

J. A. Stockman III, MD

Maternal caffeine intake during pregnancy and risk of fetal growth restriction: a large prospective observational study
CARE Study Group (Univ of Leicester, UK)
BMJ 337:a2332, 2008

Objective.—To examine the association of maternal caffeine intake with fetal growth restriction.

Design.—Prospective longitudinal observational study.

Setting.—Two large UK hospital maternity units.

Participants.—2635 low risk pregnant women recruited between 8-12 weeks of pregnancy.

Investigations.—Quantification of total caffeine intake from 4 weeks before conception and throughout pregnancy was undertaken with a validated caffeine assessment tool. Caffeine half life (proxy for clearance) was determined by measuring caffeine in saliva after a caffeine challenge. Smoking and alcohol were assessed by self reported status and by measuring salivary cotinine concentrations.

Main Outcome Measures.—Fetal growth restriction, as defined by customised birth weight centile, adjusted for alcohol intake and salivary cotinine concentrations.

Results.—Caffeine consumption throughout pregnancy was associated with an increased risk of fetal growth restriction (odds ratios 1.2 (95% CI 0.9 to 1.6) for 100-199 mg/day, 1.5 (1.1 to 2.1) for 200-299 mg/day, and 1.4 (1.0 to 2.0) for >300 mg/day compared with <100 mg/day; test fortrend P<0.001). Mean caffeine consumption decreased in the first trimester and increased in the third. The association between caffeine and fetal growth restriction was stronger in women with a faster compared to a slower caffeine clearance (test for interaction, P=0.06).

Conclusions.—Caffeine consumption during pregnancy was associated with an increased risk of fetal growth restriction and this association continued throughout pregnancy. Sensible advice would be to reduce caffeine intake before conception and throughout pregnancy.

▶ Coffee and tea contain a variety of chemical compounds, but the one of greatest significance to health is caffeine. A cup of coffee contains about 100 milligrams of caffeine and a cup of tea about half this amount. Obviously, this varies with cup size and brewing methods. Caffeine is not restricted to presence in coffee and tea, of course. It is present in most cola drinks, chocolate, cocoa, and in some drugs. Most of the caffeine that adults ingest comes from coffee. Although the word has gotten out that coffee is not good for you when you are pregnant, the message has not gotten out that tea is also not good for you. In pregnant women, as we see in this report, 60% of ingested caffeine comes from tea.

In the CARE Study Group report, we learn that consuming caffeine during pregnancy, whether it is from coffee or tea, is associated with an increased risk of fetal growth restriction. The risk of this is increased for those drinking 1 to 2 cups of coffee or the equivalent amount of caffeine in tea (100-199 milligrams caffeine a day). The odds ratio increases to 1.4 for those ingesting 200 to 299 milligrams of caffeine a day and for 300 milligrams of caffeine a day it is 1.15. Who would have imagined that drinking 3 cups of coffee a day would increase your risk of fetal growth restriction by 50%?

Caffeine easily crosses the fetoplacental unit. Its metabolism depends on genetic and environmental factors. Caffeine is metabolized in the liver primarily by cytochrome P450 1A2 (CYP1A2) and NAT2. Some people are fast metabolizers and others are slow metabolizers. It has been shown that the fetuses of women who are slow metabolizers are exposed to more caffeine than are fetuses of fast metabolizers when there is an equivalent amount of caffeine intake in the mother.

The findings in this report are truly important from the public health perspective. Every effort should be made to see that pregnant women either not consume caffeine or reduce their intake of caffeine greatly. It seems like sensible advice for those contemplating pregnancy. It would be easier to wean one's self off of caffeine before becoming pregnant than once one is already pregnant. It is the safest way to minimize the risk of fetal growth restriction.

J. A. Stockman III, MD

Epidemiology and Treatment of Painful Procedures in Neonates in Intensive Care Units

Carbajal R, Rousset A, Danan C, et al (Centre National de Ressources de lutte contre la Douleur, Paris, France; Unité de réanimation néonatale, CHI André Grégoire, Paris, France; Centre hospitalier général intercommunal de Créteil, Paris, France; et al)
JAMA 300:60-70, 2008

Context.—Effective strategies to improve pain management in neonates require a clear understanding of the epidemiology and management of procedural pain.

Objective.—To report epidemiological data on neonatal pain collected from a geographically defined region, based on direct bedside observation of neonates.

Design, Setting, and Patients.—Between September 2005 and January 2006, data on all painful and stressful procedures and corresponding analgesic therapy from the first 14 days of admission were prospectively collected within a 6-week period from 430 neonates admitted to tertiary care centers in the Paris region of France (11.3 millions inhabitants) for the Epidemiology of Procedural Pain in Neonates (EPIPPAIN) study.

Main Outcome Measure.—Number of procedures considered painful or stressful by health personnel and corresponding analgesic therapy.

Results.—The mean (SD) gestational age and intensive care unit stay were 33.0 (4.6) weeks and 8.4 (4.6) calendar days, respectively. Neonates experienced 60 969 first-attempt procedures, with 42 413 (69.6%) painful and 18 556 (30.4%) stressful procedures; 11 546 supplemental attempts were performed during procedures including 10 366 (89.8%) for painful and 1180 (10.2%) for stressful procedures. Each neonate experienced a median of 115 (range, 4-613) procedures during the study period and 16 (range, 0-62) procedures per day of hospitalization. Of these, each neonate experienced a median of 75 (range, 3-364) painful procedures during the study period and 10 (range, 0-51) painful procedures per day of hospitalization. Of the 42 413 painful procedures, 2.1% were performed with pharmacological-only therapy; 18.2% with nonpharmacological-only interventions, 20.8% with pharmacological, nonpharmacological, or both types of therapy; and 79.2% without specific analgesia, and 34.2% were performed while the neonate was receiving concurrent analgesic or anesthetic infusions for other reasons. Prematurity, category of procedure, parental presence, surgery, daytime, and day of procedure after the first day of admission were associated with greater use of specific preprocedural analgesia, whereas mechanical ventilation, noninvasive ventilation and administration of nonspecific concurrent analgesia were associated with lower use of specific preprocedural analgesia.

Conclusion.—During neonatal intensive care in the Paris region, large numbers of painful and stressful procedures were performed, the majority of which were not accompanied by analgesia.

▶ There are a wealth of background data to document that pain is not good for the neonate. In fact, it has been shown that newborns are more sensitive to pain than older infants, children, and adults. Furthermore, multiple lines of evidence suggest that repeated and prolonged pain exposure affects how an infant will later process pain in life. Infants experiencing pain in the newborn period may also show long-term developmental and behavioral issues. Despite the fact that we know a lot about the consequences of newborns experiencing pain, until the report of Carbajal et al appeared, we had very little knowledge about the epidemiology of neonatal pain and stressful procedures.

The Carbajal et al study examined neonates in a tertiary care setting serving a population of over 10 million people in the largest region of France. The study shows that newborns undergo numerous procedures that have been associated with pain and stress during the first 14 days of intensive care and that the frequency of painful procedures does not markedly decrease during an ICU stay. The investigators note that some procedures require 4 or more attempts to be successful in almost one-fifth of newborns and that many of the documented painful procedures were not performed with analgesia. The 430 newborns requiring intensive care experienced procedures causing pain, stress, or discomfort very frequently, with over 60 000 first-attempt procedures and over 11 000 repeat-attempt procedures occurring in a mean duration of just 8.4 days. One neonate had more than 350 painful procedures performed. The mean number of painful and painful plus stressful procedures per day were 12 and 16 respectively with some newborns experiencing as many as 62 procedures per day. The table shows the number of attempts to terminate some of the most common painful procedures (Table 6).

TABLE 6.—Number of Attempts to Terminate Some of the Most Common Painful Procedures Performed in 430 Neonates[a]

	Total Number of Procedures	No. of Attempts to Terminate the Procedure, %				Maximum No. of Attempts
		1	2	3	≥4	
Nasal aspiration	12 269	75.1	20.3	2.7	1.9	8
Tracheal suctioning	9883	75.3	21.2	2.8	0.7	10
Heel stick	8396	97.4	2.3	0.3	0.0	3
Gastric tube	1037	97.0	2.8	0.2	0.0	3
Venipuncture	757	70.2	18.5	7.8	3.5	10
Arterial puncture	755	62.1	21.6	9.9	6.4	10
Intravenous cannula insertion	576	45.9	22.5	13.1	18.5	14
Central catheter insertion[b]	240	40.8	14.2	15.4	29.6	12
Finger stick	238	98.3	1.3	0.4	0.0	3
Tracheal intubation	101	72.3	17.8	7.9	2.0	15
Peripheral arterial line insertion	43	39.5	27.9	11.6	21.0	9
Lumbar puncture	38	65.8	26.3	7.9	0.0	3
Urethral bladder catheter	36	77.8	11.1	5.6	5.5	10
All painful procedures	42 413	82.3	13.7	2.4	1.6	15

[a]Data are proportions of procedures unless otherwise specified.
[b]Peripherally inserted central catheter.
(Reprinted from Carbajal R, Rousset A, Danan C et al. Epidemiology and treatment of painful procedures in neonates in intensive care units. *JAMA.* 2008;300:60-70.)

This report should be read in detail. It provides some significant advice to minimize the pain associated with the types of procedures described. For example, for minor procedures, the combination of oral glucose/sucrose with other nonpharmacological pain reduction methods (eg, nonnutritive sucking) should be sufficient. For major procedures, while general nonpharmacological measures still apply, systemic analgesia with a rapidly acting opiate such as fentanyl would be typically necessary. Topical anesthetics can be used to reduce pain associated with needle punctures, but are ineffective for heel-stick pain. It should be noted in this report that virtually no baby undergoing a stressful but nonpainful procedure received sedation.

The data from this report are quite chilling. It would be to everyone's advantage to see this study repeated in the United States. It is clear that the number of painful procedures performed in our nurseries is quite high and possibly so high that the first step to improve procedural pain management would be to think twice about the absolute need for a painful procedure. The knowledge that some vulnerable neonates underwent 153 tracheal aspirations or 95 heel-sticks in a 2-week period should trigger a thoughtful and relevant analysis on the necessity and the risk-benefit ratio of the way we practice neonatal medicine.

J. A. Stockman III, MD

Traumatic lumbar punctures in neonates: test performance of the cerebrospinal fluid white blood cell count

Greenberg RG, Smith PB, Cotten CM, et al (Duke Univ, Durham, NC)
Pediatr Infect Dis J 27:1047-1051, 2008

Background.—Cerebrospinal fluid (CSF) findings are often used to diagnose meningitis in neonates given antibiotics before the lumbar puncture is performed. Traumatic lumbar punctures are common and complicate interpretation of CSF white blood cell counts. The purpose of this study is to evaluate the diagnostic utility of adjusting CSF white blood cell counts based on CSF and peripheral red blood cell counts.

Methods.—Cohort study of lumbar punctures performed between 1997 and 2004 at 150 neonatal intensive care units managed by the Pediatrix Medical group. Traumatic lumbar punctures were defined as CSF specimens with ≥500 red blood cells/mm. CSF white blood cell counts were adjusted downward for traumatic lumbar punctures using several commonly used methods. We calculated sensitivity, specificity, likelihood ratios, and area under the receiver operating characteristic curve of unadjusted and adjusted CSF white blood cell counts for predicting meningitis in neonates with traumatic lumbar punctures.

Results.—Of 6374 lumbar punctures, 2519 (39.5%) were traumatic. 114/6374 (1.8%) were positive for meningitis; 50 neonates with traumatic lumbar punctures had meningitis. The areas under the receiver operating characteristic curve for white blood cell count unadjusted and adjusted by all methods were similar.

Conclusions.—Adjustment of CSF white blood cell counts to account for increased red cells does not improve diagnostic utility. Adjustment can result in loss of sensitivity with marginal gain in specificity. Adjustment of WBC counts in the setting of a traumatic lumbar puncture does not aid in the diagnosis of bacterial and fungal meningitis in neonates.

▶ No one wants to miss a case of meningitis at any age, much less in the newborn period. The latter is the time, however, when lumbar punctures tend to be somewhat more difficult to perform and often are traumatic. We see in the Greenberg et al study that the prevalence of traumatic lumbar punctures was almost 40%, a value consistent with other reports. Relying on the cerebrospinal fluid (CSF) white blood cell (WBC) count to make a diagnosis of meningitis has significant limitations in view of the high prevalence of traumatic taps. The CSF WBC count can be altered by the presence of peripheral blood in CSF after a traumatic lumbar puncture (LP). In older pediatric patients and adults we have devised methods to attempt to correct the WBC in the CSF following a traumatic LP by adjusting the WBC based on the number of red blood cells (RBCs) in the CSF. Some authors have suggested using an average ratio of 500 or 1000 RBCs to 1 WBC in the CSF in making a correction for a bloody tap. One can also determine the ratio of RBCs to WBCs based on the peripheral blood count and then use a "more precise" correction for the CSF determination of WBCs. In doing this, the number of WBCs that be accounted for by the number of RBCs in a CSF specimen by simply subtracting the appropriate number of WBCs.

Although literature exists describing methods for interpreting CSF WBC count after traumatic LPs in adults and pediatric populations, previous reports in newborns are scarce. This is why the report from Duke University and the Pediatrix-Obstetrix Center for Research and Education is so helpful to those who work in the nursery setting. The investigators at these institutions designed a study to look at lumbar puncture results between 1997 and 2004 at 150 neonatal intensive care units managed by the Pediatrix Medical Group. A calculation was performed to determine sensitivity, specificity, likelihood ratios, and the area under the receiver operating characteristic curve of unadjusted and adjusted CSF WBC counts for predicting meningitis in neonates with traumatic lumbar punctures. Of 6374 lumbar punctures, 50 neonates were found to have meningitis. Adjustment of the CSF WBC counts to account for increased RBCs did not improve diagnostic utility and unfortunately did result in a loss of sensitivity while producing only a marginal gain in specificity of identifying these babies.

This report also documents a finding observed in earlier reports and that is that correction of the CSF WBC count by the peripheral RBC:WBC ratio overestimates the WBCs in the peripheral blood, leading to an underestimation of the true number of WBCs in the CSF. Thus, using a WBC value corrected by this method could result in the masking of a true increase in the number of WBCs in the CSF and consequently, in missed cases of meningitis.

We should be grateful to these investigators for publishing this report. Although normal values for CSF WBC count vary according to postnatal age and gestational age, most of us use a CSF WBC cutoff of 20 cells/mm^3 in accordance with reference values for term infants. What we learn from the Greenberg et al report is that should we attempt to correct down the CSF WBC count when a traumatic LP is performed based on the number of RBCs in the CSF, we do this with some significant risk of missing some cases of meningitis. We are all now forewarned of this problem.

J. A. Stockman III, MD

Maternal and paternal contribution to intergenerational recurrence of breech delivery: population based cohort study
Nordtveit TI, Melve KK, Albrechtsen S, et al (Univ of Bergen, Norway; Univ Hosp, Bergen, Norway; et al)
BMJ 336:872-876, 2008

Objective.—To investigate intergenerational recurrence of breech delivery, with a hypothesis that both women and men delivered in breech presentation contribute to increased risk of breech delivery in their offspring.

Design.—Population based cohort study for two generations.

Setting.—Data from the medical birth registry of Norway, based on all births in Norway 1967-2004 (2.2 million births).

Participants.—Generational data were provided through linkage by national identification numbers, forming 451 393 mother-offspring units and 295 253 father-offspring units. We included units where both parents and offspring were singletons and offspring were first born, forming 232 704 mother-offspring units and 154 851 father-offspring units for our analyses.

Main Outcome Measure.—Breech delivery in the second generation.

Results.—Men and women who themselves were delivered in breech presentation had more than twice the risk of breech delivery in their own first pregnancies compared with men and women who had been cephalic presentations (odds ratios 2.2, 95% confidence interval 1.8 to 2.7, and 2.2, 1.9 to 2.5, for men and women, respectively). The strongest risks of recurrence were found for vaginally delivered offspring and were equally strong for men and women. Increased risk of recurrence of breech delivery in offspring was present only for parents delivered at term.

Conclusion.—Intergenerational recurrence risk of breech delivery in offspring was equally high when transmitted through fathers and mothers. It seems reasonable to attribute the observed pattern of familial predisposition to term breech delivery to genetic inheritance, predominantly through the fetus.

▶ I have followed the literature on breech delivery with a special interest over the years. Our first-born, one of twins, was born breech. Just 3% to 4% of babies at term are born breech as opposed to those born preterm. Breech presentation runs 25% at 28 weeks gestation.[1] There are a number of known factors that increase the risk of breech presentation, such as first baby, older mother, low gestational age, and low birth weight. Mechanical factors such as uterine malformations, site of placental attachment, and low volume of amniotic fluid also increase the risk of breech presentation. Babies with congenital anomalies present more often breech at the time of delivery. Add to this list multifetal gestation and neuromuscular dysfunction, and you can see that the list of factors favoring breech presentation is quite long.

The high recurrence of breech presentation between siblings seems to be attributable to maternal uterine environment issues.[2] Nonetheless, recurrence between generations suggests that one or more genetic factors may be passed from the parent to the developing fetus. Nordtveit et al investigate this possibility by using the medical birth registry of Norway. This registry is a population-based compensatory registry of all live births and stillbirths of 16 weeks or more gestation. It contains the records of more than 2 million births since 1967 and is a respected source for medical and public health research. Using registry data, the authors linked mothers and fathers birth records to the records of their offspring. The authors' main conclusion is that an increased risk of breech delivery in first-born offspring is associated with both a maternal and a paternal history of breech delivery at term. The paternal effect is as strong as the maternal effect (odds ratio maternal 2.2; paternal 2.2). What is unclear is whether this could be a genetic-related issue or an environmental one. In any event, it seems that offspring are like apples; they do not fall far from the tree.

For now, it is difficult to understand what we should do with the information provided from this Norwegian study. Should we advise mothers of a higher risk of breech delivery, if their parents had a breech delivery? At best, the increase in risk is only a little over 2-fold. It will be interesting to see what obstetricians do with this information because an anticipated breech presentation does trigger thoughts about a planned externally cephalic version or a possible cesarean section delivery.

J. A. Stockman III, MD

References

1. Hill L. Prevalence of breech presentation by gestational age. *Am J Perinatol*. 1990; 7:92-93.
2. Albrechtsen S, Rasmussen S, Dalaker K, et al. Perinatal mortality in breech presentation sibships. *Obstet Gynecol*. 1998;92:775-780.

Increasing Prevalence of Gastroschisis: Population-based Study in California

Vu LT, Nobuhara KK, Laurent C, et al (Univ of California, San Francisco; California Birth Defects Monitoring Program, Berkeley)

J Pediatr 152:807-811, 2008

Objective.—To evaluate time trend of gastroschisis and examine the epidemiological risk factors for gastroschisis.

Study Design.—This population-based study analyzed the active surveillance data from the California Birth Defects Monitoring Program from 1987 to 2003.

Results.—The overall birth prevalence of gastroschisis was 2.6 cases per 10,000 births (908 cases in >3.5 million births). In the adjusted analysis, by using the age of 25 to 29 years as the reference, mothers aged 12 to 15 years had a 4.2-times greater birth prevalence (95% CI, 2.5-7.0), and fathers aged 16 to 19 years and 20 to 24 years had 1.6- and 1.5-times greater birth prevalence (95% CI, 1.1-2.1 and 1.2-1.8), respectively. Compared with non-Hispanic whites and US-born Hispanic, both foreign-born Hispanics and blacks had adjusted prevalence ratio of 0.6 (95% CI, 0.5-0.7 and 0.4-0.9, respectively). In addition, nulliparity was also associated with gastroschisis. Independent of maternal age, paternal age, and maternal ethnicity, the birth prevalence increased 3.2-fold (95% CI, 2.3-4.3) during the 17-year study period.

Conclusions.—The birth prevalence of gastroschisis continues to increase in California, and young, nulliparous women are at the greatest risk of having a child with gastroschisis (Fig).

▶ For reasons that are largely unknown, the prevalence of gastroschisis at birth has been increasing over the last several decades. Some have suggested that worldwide the increase has been 2-to 4-fold. Why this defect occurs is also largely unknown, but many have theorized that it is a result of an ischemic

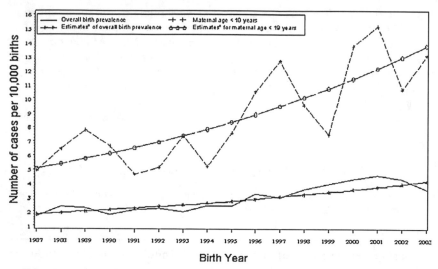

FIGURE.—Birth prevalence of gastroschisis from 1987 to 2003. *Estimates were calculated from the Poisson regression model that controlled for maternal age, maternal ethnicity, and paternal age. (Reprinted from Vu LT, Nobuhara KK, Laurent C, et al. Increasing prevalence of gastroschisis: population-based study in California. *J Pediatr.* 2008;152:807-811, with permission from Elsevier.)

event that disrupts the development of right omphalomesenteric artery. In addition, several studies have examined other factors associated with a higher risk of gastroschisis, including young maternal age. Women under 20 years of age have 16 times greater risk of having pregnancy complicated with this disorder. A whole potpourri of other risk factors have also been implicated including low socioeconomic status, poor maternal nutrition, tobacco smoking and the prenatal use of illicit drugs, aspirin, and vasoconstrictive medications, including pseudoephedrine.

The California Birth Defect Monitoring Program has provided us with excellent information about trends in the incidence of gastroschisis, at least. This program is a population-based active surveillance for collecting information on births with congenital malformation. Over a recent 15-year period, some 900 cases of gastroschisis were diagnosed in 3.5 million live births and stillbirths in that state, resulting in a birth prevalence of 2.57 per 10 000 births. If one follows the longitudinal trend, the birth prevalence of gastroschisis has been rising (Fig). Young maternal age was demonstrated to be a strong risk factor, consistent with several epidemiologic studies that have supported the theory that young, nulliparous, and socially disadvantaged women are at the highest risk of having a child with gastroschisis. In the California study, maternal education served as a very potent surrogate marker for socioeconomic status. This increased secular trend of gastroschisis has also been reported in Canada, Norway, the United Kingdom, and Western Australia. The explanation for this remains unknown. The authors of this report suggest that the increase could be related to a change in a putative exposure or maternal behavior that has yet to be elucidated. It is also speculated that the increasing prevalence could be a consequence of either increasing numbers of fetuses with this malformation surviving to the point of live birth because of improved maternal nutrition or a secular change in environmental exposures.

Needless to say, it is important to make an early diagnosis of gastroschisis by prenatal ultrasound with referral to a tertiary care center to help minimize postnatal morbidity associated with sepsis and poor nutrition. Given the increasing prevalence of gastroschisis, these recommendations seem extremely wise. Although the mortality rate with gastroschisis is currently low, it does carry a number of associated morbidities. The most expensive average neonatal hospital charges for noncardiac birth defects are for gastroschisis and congenital diaphragmatic hernia (> $150 000).[1]

J. A. Stockman III, MD

Reference

1. Centers for Disease Control and Prevention (CDC). Hospital stays, hospital charges and in-hospital deaths among infants with selected birth defects – United States, 2003. *MMWR.* 2007;56:25-29.

Newborn weight charts underestimate the incidence of low birthweight in preterm infants

Burkhardt T, Schäffer L, Zimmermann R, et al (Univ Hosp of Zurich, Switzerland)
Am J Obstet Gynecol 199:139.e1-139.e6, 2008

Objective.—The objective of the study was to compare sonographic fetal weight estimates with newborn weight charts and analyze the predictive accuracy of the ponderal index (PI) in preterm infants.

Study Design.—We generated sonographic reference curves for fetal weight and PI estimates from a database of fetal biometric records from 12,589 term deliveries. We then plotted sonographic and newborn weight and PI of 2406 preterm newborns on these curves and compared them with published newborn weight charts.

Results.—The third centiles of sonographic and newborn weights diverged markedly between 25 and 36 weeks of gestation and by more than 400 g at 32-33 weeks. In contrast, sonographic and newborn PI values were similar despite uncertainties as to fetal length.

Conclusion.—We suggest using sonographic reference fetal weights to screen preterm newborns for low birthweight. Uncertainties in fetal length threaten the reliability of the PI.

▶ This is an important report looking at intrauterine growth of more than 12 000 infants born at term and over 2400 infants born preterm. In utero assessment of growth was determined by Doppler ultrasound permitting in addition to an estimate of weight, the ponderal index (PI) that combines both body weight and length.[1] A study of this magnitude allowed the investigators to see whether there was a difference in in utero growth for babies who would ultimately be born at term versus those born preterm.

So what did the data from this study show? It clearly documented that fetuses subsequently delivered preterm are sonographically already significantly smaller at 32 weeks than those proceeding to term. When comparing the sonographic growth charts of 12 589 term children with the sonographic growth in 2406 preterm newborns, one saw a marked drop in weight beginning at about 25 weeks in the latter group. The fact that preterm newborns have markedly lower birth weights than expected from the estimated weights of intrauterine fetuses of the same gestational age proceeding to term means that newborn growth charts that we have been using are inappropriate for identifying low birthweight preterm infants.

The PI is a well-established parameter widely used by neonatologists for discriminating between growth-retarded and genetically small-for-gestational age fetuses. It has also been proposed as a prenatal diagnostic tool although a number of authors have questioned its ability to predict true intrauterine growth retardation in term and preterm newborns. That is largely because most neonatologists agree that neonatal length tends to be somewhat underestimated in routine sonographic clinical examination. Nonetheless, this study does suggest that infants born preterm by and large are smaller than what their gestational age would predict.

If there is a lesson to be learned from this study emanating from Zurich, Switzerland, it is that reference sonographic fetal weights might best be used for the early identification of low birth weight and that we should not rely on "normal" birthweight curve information to estimate gestational age given that the data from this report suggest that many preterm babies in fact are smaller for gestational age than might otherwise have been predicted.

J. A. Stockman III, MD

Reference

1. Vik T, Markestad T, Uhlsten G, et al. Body proportions and early neonatal morbidity in small for gestational age infants of successive births. *Acta Obstet Gynecol Scand Suppl.* 1997;165:76-81.

Duration of meconium passage in preterm and term infants

Bekkali N, Hamers SL, Schipperus MR, et al (Academic Med Ctr, AZ Amsterdam; The Netherlands)
Arch Dis Child Fetal Neonatal Ed 93:376-379, 2008

Background.—First passage of stool after birth, meconium, is delayed in preterm infants compared to term infants. The difference in duration of meconium passage until transition to normal stools has however never been assessed in preterm and term infants. Hypothesis: Preterm infants have prolonged duration of passage of meconium (PoM) compared to term infants.

Methods.—Between August and November 2006, all infants born in an academic and non-academic hospital with gestational age (GA) 25-42 weeks and without metabolical, congenital diseases or gastrointestinal disorders, were included. Infants were divided into four groups: (A) GA ≤ 30 weeks; (B) GA between 31 and 34 weeks; (C) GA between 35 and 36 weeks; (D) GA ≥ 37 weeks (term born).

Results.—A total of 198 infants (102 males); 32, 62, 33 and 71 infants in groups A, B, C and D, respectively, were included. With decreasing gestation a trend was found for delayed first PoM (p < 0.001). Compared to term infants 79% (56/71), less preterm infants passed their first stool within 24 h after birth–group A: 44% (14/32); group B: 68% (42/62); and group C: 73% (24/33). With decreasing gestation a trend for prolonged PoM was found (p < 0.001). The mean (SD) PoM duration was prolonged in group A: 7.8 days (2.5); group B: 4.3 days (2.4); and group C: 2.9 days (1.3) compared to term infants. Furthermore, PoM was associated with birth weights ≤2500 g (p = 0.03) and morphine therapy (p = 0.03). Duration of PoM was not associated with type of feeding, small for gestational age, large for gestational age or need for respiratory support.

Conclusion.—PoM was not only delayed but also prolonged in preterm infants. Duration of PoM was associated with GA, birth weight and morphine therapy.

▶ It has been known for some time that preterm babies have delayed passage of meconium, presumably from intestinal hypomotility, secondary to ongoing developmental maturation of bowel function. What is not known is what the precise parameters are that would define delayed passage of meconium in terms of outer limits of normal based on gestational age. This is what the article of Bekkali et al is all about. These investigators engaged in a study of premature infants who were divided into 4 groups based on gestational age: (a) gestational age ≤ 30 weeks; (b) between 31 and 34 weeks; (c) between 35 and 36 weeks; and (d) gestational age ≥ 37 weeks (born term). Small for gestational age babies and large for gestational age babies were excluded. Some 91 infants were followed to determine when the first bowel movement occurred and for how long a meconium stool was passed.

The results of this study underscored the known fact that prematurity is associated with prolonged passage of meconium as well as a delayed initial passage. While it is expected that more than 98% of term babies will pass their first meconium stool within 48 hours of birth, only 44% of newborns with a gestational age ≤ 30 weeks had a passage of a first bowel movement within 24 hours and just 75% did so within 48 hours. Thus, our normal time to worry about passage of a first stool (48 hours) would create undue anxiety if one applied this rule of thumb to preterm babies. It should also be noted that the smallest of preterm babies in this report took almost 8 days on average to clear meconium. Indeed, it took almost 13 days for 97% of these tiny infants to clear meconium from their stool. As expected, morphine therapy, given for whatever reason, was associated with prolonged duration of passage of meconium stools.

Now we have good data at hand from this report to tell us what is normal when it comes to the passage of meconium stools. One wonders if part of the exacerbated hyperbilirubinemia that is seen in preterms might relate to the "sluggish" bowel that these babies have, a topic of some suspicion for a long time.

J. A. Stockman III, MD

Spousal violence and potentially preventable single and recurrent spontaneous fetal loss in an African setting: cross-sectional study

Alio AP, Nana PN, Salihu HM (Univ of South Florida, Tampa; Univ of Yaoundé, Cameroon)
Lancet 373:318-324, 2009

Background.—Spousal violence is a global issue, with ramifications for the reproductive health of women. We aimed to investigate the effect of physical, sexual, and emotional violence on potentially preventable single and recurrent spontaneous fetal loss.

Methods.—We analysed data from the Cameroon Demographic Health Survey. In the violence module of this survey, women were questioned about their experience of physical, emotional, and sexual violence inflicted by their spouses. Respondents were also asked about any stillbirths and spontaneous abortions. We measured risk for single and recurrent fetal loss with odds ratios, with adjustment for intracluster correlations as appropriate. We also estimated the proportion of preventable excess fetal loss at various levels of violence reduction.

Findings.—2562 women responded to the violence module. Those exposed to spousal violence (n = 1307) were 50% more likely to experience at least one episode of fetal loss compared with women not exposed to abuse (odds ratio 1·5; 95% CI 1·3–1·8). Recurrent fetal mortality was associated with all forms of spousal violence, but emotional violence had the strongest association (1·7; 1·2–2·3). If the prevalence of spousal abuse could be reduced to 50%, 25%, or entirely eliminated, preventable excess recurrent fetal demise would be 17%, 25%, and 33%, respectively.

Interpretation.—Spousal violence increases the likelihood of single and repeated fetal loss. A large proportion of risk for recurrent fetal mortality is attributable to spousal violence and, therefore, is potentially preventable. Our findings support the idea of routine prenatal screening for spousal violence in the African setting, a region with the highest rate of fetal death in the world.

▶ It seems a shame that we have to look to colleagues in Cameroon to find information about the consequences to a pregnancy of intimate partner violence. There is very little, if anything, that you will find in the medical literature in the United States that tells us much about this problem. What Alio et al do is to summarize a study from the Cameroon Demographic and Health Survey. The investigators found a significant association between fetal loss and recurrent fetal loss in women who had ever experienced intimate partner violence, compared with women who reported no such violence. The study is an important contribution to the field, because it is 1 of the first to document this association and 1 of the first in Africa, where the rate of fetal loss happens to be high.

In this study, it was observed that recurrent fetal loss was associated with all forms of intimate partner violence. The strongest association was with emotional, not physical, abuse. Until recently, most studies of intimate partner violence have measured physical and often sexual violence, few have included anything to do with emotional abuse. There is now a growing understanding that emotional abuse are central elements in intimate partner violence and might indeed be most strongly associated with some of the poor health outcomes, particularly for mental health. These findings support the need to look at the impact of physical, sexual, and emotional intimate partner violence separately and the cumulative effect of these. It should be noted that Alio et al did not look specifically at violence during pregnancy. One can assume that the association with fetal loss would be even stronger had they done this.

Beyond the borders of Cameroon, the World Health Organization is engaged in a multicountry study on violence against women. That study currently reports violence rates for physical abuse during pregnancy of somewhere between 4% and 12% for most study sites.[1] The violence often involves blows or kicks to the abdomen. Of all abused women who reported abuse during their lifetime by a partner, between 11% and 44% were abused during pregnancy.

The findings from this report are clear. Spousal violence does increase the likelihood of single and repeated fetal loss. While the focus on fetal outcomes is important, it should not detract from the impact of violence on a woman's health. Violence against women is a violation of human rights. It affects health, well being, and the ability to exercise such rights, including a woman's reproductive rights. Policy makers at all levels should read this report in detail. It is a chilling reminder that we have a long way to go in protecting the rights of women and the unborn child.

J. A. Stockman III, MD

Reference

1. Garcia-Moreno C, Jansen HAFM, Ellsberg M, et al. *WHO Multi-Country Study on Women's Health and Domestic Violence Against Women: Initial Results on Prevalence, Health Outcomes, and Women's Responses.* Geneva: World Health Organization; 2005.

Granulocyte-macrophage colony stimulating factor administered as prophylaxis for reduction of sepsis in extremely preterm, small for gestational age neonates (the PROGRAMS trial): a single-blind, multicentre, randomised controlled trial

Carr R, Brocklehurst P, Doré CJ, et al (Guy's and St Thomas' Hosp, London, UK; Univ of Oxford, UK; Med Res Council Clinical Trials Unit, London, UK; et al)

Lancet 373:226-233, 2009

Background.—Systemic sepsis is a major cause of death in preterm neonates. There are compelling theoretical reasons why treatment with haemopoietic colony-stimulating factors might reduce sepsis and improve outcomes, and as a consequence these agents have entered into use in neonatal medicine without adequate evidence. We assessed whether granulocyte-macrophage colony stimulating factor (GM-CSF) administered as prophylaxis to preterm neonates at high risk of neutropenia would reduce sepsis, mortality, and morbidity.

Methods.—We undertook a single-blind, multicentre, randomised controlled trial in 26 centres between June, 2000, and June, 2006. 280 neonates of below or equal to 31 weeks' gestation and below the 10th centile for birthweight were randomised within 72 h of birth to receive GM-CSF 10 μg/kg per day subcutaneously for 5 days or standard management. From recruitment to day 28 a detailed daily clinical record form was completed by the treating clinicians. Primary outcome was sepsis-free survival to 14 days from trial entry. Analysis was by intention to treat. This study is registered as an International Standard Randomised Controlled Trial, number ISRCTN42553489.

Findings.—Neutrophil counts after trial entry rose significantly more rapidly in infants treated with GM-CSF than in control infants during the first 11 days (difference between neutrophil count slopes 0.34×10^9/L/day; 95% CI $0.12-0.56$). There was no significant difference in sepsis-free survival for all infants (93 of 139 treated infants, 105 of 141 control infants; difference -8%, 95% CI -18 to 3). A meta-analysis of this trial and previous published prophylactic trials showed no survival benefit.

Interpretation.—Early postnatal prophylactic GM-CSF corrects neutropenia but does not reduce sepsis or improve survival and short-term outcomes in extremely preterm neonates.

▶ We all know that sepsis remains a leading cause of death in the immediate newborn period. Much of this sepsis occurs in association with neutropenia. Indeed, neutropenia, which occurs frequently in the preterm and intrauterine growth-restricted infant, is believed to increase the risk of sepsis significantly. Since the hematopoietic growth factors, granulocyte colony stimulating factor (G-CSF), and granulocyte-macrophage colony stimulating factor (GM-CSF) became available and were shown to be effective for neutropenia-related infection in patients with cancer after chemotherapy, their potential use to reduce sepsis in other situations seems quite attractive. One strategy could be to use either G-CSF or GM-CSF to help manage sepsis in the newborn period. Both agents are being used in many neonatal units for the prophylaxis and treatment of sepsis, but their use is being undertaken without adequate evidence that they actually improve morbidity or mortality. That is what the report of Carr et al is all about.

Carr et al report a randomized trial (PROGRAMS) of GM-CSF for prevention of sepsis in small-for-gestational age preterm neonates. We see that GM-CSF increases the neutrophil count, but has no effect on the primary endpoint of sepsis-free survival to 14 days from trial entry. It should be noted that the trial was not designed to have adequate power to assess the effects of GM-CSF in newborns who were neutropenic at trial entry, but there was no suggestion that these babies had less sepsis or lower mortality. Indeed, 43% of babies given GM-CSF died before discharge compared with only 33% in the control group.

Needless to say, the trial reported by Carr et al was an extraordinarily complex one to design and carry out. Almost 300 small for gestational preterm babies entered the trial in some 26 centers that were widely scattered about. It must have been bitterly disappointing for the investigators that the promising treatments were not in fact beneficial. It should be noted that GM-CSF was used in this study. Compared with G-CSF, GM-CSF releases a wider range of cells and stimulates a stronger inflammatory response. It should be noted that not only both GM-CSF and G-CSF have reduced mortality in some animal studies of infection, but also have increased mortality in others, the latter presumably because of the exuberant inflammatory response that these agents are capable of inducing.

It is hard to say what nurseries will do with the information from this report. G-CSF and GM-CSF are quite expensive. As of now, there is no evidence of clear benefit for either agent. An unresolved question is whether these colony-stimulating factors might best work in combination with the administration of immunoglobulin in neonates with neutropenia. It should also be noted that the trial reported by Carr et al was a study of the prophylactic use of colony-stimulating factors. We do not have good data on treatment of established sepsis in neonates.

In an editorial that accompanied this report, Shann concluded that "G-CSF and GM-CSF should no longer be used routinely in neonatal intensive care without further evidence from randomized trials."[1] Whether this recommendation will be accepted or not remains to be seen. Most will probably feel that we need additional studies of G-CSF and GM-CSF, not only for the purposes of prophylaxis, but also as treatment modalities in neonates with established sepsis. As of now, unfortunately the news thus far is not exactly good.

J. A. Stockman III, MD

Reference

1. Shann F. Sepsis in babies: should we stimulate the phagocytes? *Lancet.* 2009;373: 188-190.

Timing of Elective Repeat Cesarean Delivery at Term and Neonatal Outcomes

Tita ATN, Landon MB, Spong CY, et al (Univ of Alabama at Birmingham; Ohio State Univ, Columbus; Eunice Kennedy Shriver Natl Inst of Child Health and Human Development, Bethesda; et al)
N Engl J Med 360:111-120, 2009

Background.—Because of increased rates of respiratory complications, elective cesarean delivery is discouraged before 39 weeks of gestation unless there is evidence of fetal lung maturity. We assessed associations between elective cesarean delivery at term (37 weeks of gestation or longer) but before 39 weeks of gestation and neonatal outcomes.

Methods.—We studied a cohort of consecutive patients undergoing repeat cesarean sections performed at 19 centers of the Eunice Kennedy Shriver National Institute of Child Health and Human Development Maternal–Fetal Medicine Units Network from 1999 through 2002. Women with viable singleton pregnancies delivered electively (i.e., before the onset of labor and without any recognized indications for delivery before 39 weeks of gestation) were included. The primary outcome was the composite of neonatal death and any of several adverse events, including respiratory complications, treated hypoglycemia, newborn sepsis, and admission to the neonatal intensive care unit (ICU).

Results.—Of 24,077 repeat cesarean deliveries at term, 13,258 were performed electively; of these, 35.8% were performed before 39 completed weeks of gestation (6.3% at 37 weeks and 29.5% at 38 weeks) and 49.1% at 39 weeks of gestation. One neonatal death occurred. As compared with births at 39 weeks, births at 37 weeks and at 38 weeks were associated with an increased risk of the primary outcome (adjusted odds ratio for births at 37 weeks, 2.1; 95% confidence interval [CI], 1.7 to 2.5; adjusted odds ratio for births at 38 weeks, 1.5; 95% CI, 1.3 to 1.7; P for trend <0.001). The rates of adverse respiratory outcomes, mechanical ventilation, newborn sepsis, hypoglycemia, admission to the neonatal ICU, and hospitalization for 5 days or more were increased by a factor of 1.8 to 4.2 for births at 37 weeks and 1.3 to 2.1 for births at 38 weeks.

Conclusions.—Elective repeat cesarean delivery before 39 weeks of gestation is common and is associated with respiratory and other adverse neonatal outcomes.

▶ This report is one of the most important of 2009. There has been an almost 50% increase in the rate of cesarean delivery here in the United States. Between 1996 and 2006, the rate jumped from just under 21% to over 31%.[1] The major reason for this increase in the United States is the decline in the rate of attempted vaginal birth after previous cesarean delivery. Unfortunately, all too often, elective cesarean delivery is scheduled to accommodate patient and physician convenience, and there is a risk that it may be performed earlier than is appropriate. Because 40% of the 1.3 million cesarean deliveries performed annually in the United States are repeat procedures and the number of cesarean deliveries continues to rise, the timing of elective cesarean delivery has increasingly important public implications. It is well known that delivery before term, even by a week, 2 or 3, can be associated with increased morbidity, the magnitude of which has not been clearly defined, at least until the report of Tita et al appeared.

The study abstracted contains data from the cesarean registry of the Eunice Kennedy Shriver National Institute of Child Health and Human Development Maternal-Fetal Medicine Units Network. The registry contains detailed, prospectively collected information on consecutive repeat cesarean deliveries performed at 19 academic centers here in the United States. This database has allowed the analysis of neonatal outcomes such as death, adverse respiratory outcomes (respiratory distress syndrome or transient tachypnea of the newborn), hypoglycemia, newborn sepsis, confirmed seizures, necrotizing enterocolitis, hypoxic-ischemic encephalopathy, cardiopulmonary resuscitation or ventilator support within 24 hours after birth, umbilical-cord-blood arterial pH below 7.0, a 5-minute Apgar score of 3 or below, admission to the neonatal intensive care unit (ICU), and prolonged hospitalization (5 days or longer).

What we learn from this report is that more than one-third of elective repeat cesarean deliveries are performed before 39 weeks of gestation. These early deliveries are associated with a significantly increased risk of adverse outcomes, particularly related to respiratory complications resulting in admission to the neonatal ICU. The risks of individual adverse neonatal outcomes were higher for delivery at 37 weeks (by a factor of 1.8-4.2) than for delivery at 38 weeks and by a factor of 1.3 to 2.1 relative to delivery at 39 weeks. It should be noted that delaying delivery beyond 40 weeks was also associated with increased rates of neonatal adverse outcomes. The data from this report did not include information about testing for fetal lung maturity. Delivery before 39 weeks of gestation in the presence of a documented mature lung is not considered a standard of care. Further study is warranted to assess whether an increased rate of adverse outcomes in deliveries occurring before 39 weeks is explained entirely by failure to test for fetal lung maturity before delivery, or whether testing indicating "maturity" does not fully protect against an increased rate of adverse outcomes in these early births. The latter is a study yet to be done.

Because (1) the vast majority of women with a previous cesarean delivery elect repeat cesarean delivery; (2) more than 25% of primary cesarean deliveries are performed before onset of labor; and (3) there may be increasing enthusiasm for cesarean delivery on maternal request, the timing of cesarean delivery and its effect on infant outcomes have substantial public health implications. Early deliveries (before 39 weeks) are associated with a preventable increase in neonatal morbidity and admissions to the neonatal ICU, both of which carry a high economic cost. We should be doing everything possible to delay elective cesarean section until 39 weeks of gestation. If performed before this, fetal lung maturity should be documented in all elective situations.

J. A. Stockman III, MD

Reference

1. Hamilton BE, Martin JA, Ventura SJ. Births: preliminary data for 2006. *Natl Vital Stat Rep*. 2007;56:1-18.

15 Nutrition and Metabolism

Misperceptions and misuse of Bear Brand coffee creamer as infant food: national cross sectional survey of consumers and paediatricians in Laos
Barennes H, Andriatahina T, Latthaphasavang V, et al (Institut de la Francophonie Pour la Médecine Tropicale, Vientiane, Lao Popular Democratic Republic; et al)
BMJ 337:670-681, 2008

Objective.—To investigate the use of Bear Brand coffee creamer as a food for infants and the impact on consumers of the logo of a cartoon baby bear held by its mother in the breastfeeding position.

Design.—Interviews with paediatricians throughout the country and a national survey of potential consumers regarding their perceptions and use of the Bear Brand coffee creamer.

Setting.—84 randomised villages in south, central, and northern Laos.

Participants.—26 Lao paediatricians and 1098 adults in households in a cluster sampling.

Results.—Of the 26 paediatricians, 24 said that parents "often" or "sometimes" fed this product to infants as a substitute for breast milk. In the capital city, paediatricians said that mothers used the product when they returned to work. In the countryside, they reported that poor families used it when the mother was ill or had died. Of 1098 adults surveyed, 96% believed that the can contains milk; 46% believed the Bear Brand logo indicates that the product is formulated for feeding to infants or to replace breast milk; 80% had not read the written warning on the can; and over 18% reported giving the product to their infant at a mean age of 4.7 months (95% confidence interval 4.1 to 5.3).

Conclusion.—The Bear Brand coffee creamer is used as a breast milk substitute in Laos. The cartoon logo influences people's perception of the product that belies the written warning "This product is not to be used as a breast milk substitute." Use of this logo on coffee creamer is misleading to the local population and places the health of infants at risk.

▶ A number of years ago when this editor was a resident in training, he had occasion to evaluate an infant for failure to thrive. On taking a careful history, it became quickly apparent what the source of the problem was. The mother had been using an inexpensive dairy creamer as a substitute for formula, thinking that it was all right to do so. Apparently, things are not very different in this decade, at least in Laos, where a popular coffee creamer is marketed with an illustration of a mother bear holding a baby bear in the breastfeeding position. The wording on the creamer can states: "This product is not to be used as breast milk substitute" written in English, Thai, and Lao. There is also an illustration of a feeding bottle with a cross through it. Unfortunately, physicians in Laos are seeing infants with failure to thrive with protein calorie malnutrition who were fed this product exclusively. The report of Barennes et al demonstrates that nearly half of adults surveyed believed that the cartoon logo on the can meant that the product is "good for infants" or "a replacement for breast milk." Nearly one-fifth of parents had given the product to their young infant.

It does not take a rocket scientist to recognize that an advertisement for something that looks like milk that has a bear holding a cub in the breast-feeding position would imply that the product is suitable for young infants, written warnings to the contrary. The company that brands Bear Brand, Nestle, better get on the stick. Also, even in the United States, we need to be aware of the chance that some parents unknowingly, particularly in tight financial situations, might be using an artificial dairy creamer as a substitute for an infant formula.

J. A. Stockman III, MD

High Body Mass Index for Age Among US Children and Adolescents, 2003-2006
Ogden CL, Carroll MD, Flegal KM (Ctrs for Disease Control and Prevention, Hyattsville, MD)
JAMA 299:2401-2405, 2008

Context.—The prevalence of overweight among US children and adolescents increased between 1980 and 2004.

Objectives.—To estimate the prevalence of 3 measures of high body mass index (BMI) for age (calculated as weight in kilograms divided by height in meters squared) and to examine recent trends for US children and adolescents using national data with measured heights and weights.

Design, Setting, and Participants.—Height and weight measurements were obtained from 8165 children and adolescents as part of the 2003-2004 and 2005-2006 National Health and Nutrition Examination Survey (NHANES), nationally representative surveys of the US civilian, noninstitutionalized population.

Main Outcome Measures.—Prevalence of BMI for age at or above the 97th percentile, at or above the 95th percentile, and at or above the 85th percentile of the 2000 sex-specific Centers for Disease Control and Prevention (CDC) BMI-for-age growth charts among US children by age, sex, and racial/ethnic group.

Results.—Because no statistically significant differences in the prevalence of high BMI for age were found between estimates for 2003-2004 and 2005-2006, data for the 4 years were combined to provide more stable estimates for the most recent time period. Overall, in 2003-2006, 11.3% (95% confidence interval [CI], 9.7%-12.9%) of children and adolescents aged 2 through 19 years were at or above the 97th percentile of the 2000 BMI-for-age growth charts, 16.3% (95% CI, 14.5%-18.1%) were at or above the 95th percentile, and 31.9% (95% CI, 29.4%-34.4%) were at or above the 85th percentile. Prevalence estimates varied by age and by racial/ethnic group. Analyses of the trends in high BMI for age showed no statistically significant trend over the 4 time periods (1999-2000, 2001-2002, 2003-2004, and 2005-2006) for either boys or girls (*P* values between .07 and .41).

Conclusion.—The prevalence of high BMI for age among children and adolescents showed no significant changes between 2003-2004 and 2005-2006 and no significant trends between 1999 and 2006.

▶ Most now accept that BMI is the best available clinical tool to screen for childhood obesity and to monitor progress with treatment. Recently, a consensus statement prepared by an expert committee, described BMI as the best tool for these purposes.[1] This consensus statement encourages primary care clinicians to assess obesity risk at all well-child visits using BMI-for-age percentiles. This same assessment approach has extended into schools and several states now mandate use of BMI to identify overweight or obese children and to evaluate the effectiveness of healthful lifestyle initiatives.

Despite all that has been written about BMI and its utility, there has been resistance on the part of some practitioners to use BMI as a tool. The reasons for this are several-fold. First, if pediatric obesity is defined as a BMI for age exceeding the 95th percentile, why do prevalence estimates differ from 5%? In 2000, the CDC released sex-specific BMI for age growth charts that established the basis for defining pediatric obesity. Aiming to develop nationally representative references, demographers calculated percentiles for boys and girls aged 2 to 20 years using data from several national surveys, including 2 cycles of the National Health Examination Survey (NHES). Because of the rapid increase in body weight beginning in the 1980s, data from the NHES study, which has been repeated several times now, have produced differing findings. During the last 3 decades, mean BMI in the pediatric age range has increased markedly and this increase is greatest among the heaviest individuals. The conundrum is how we can say the 95th percentile for BMI defines obesity when clearly so many more kids are obese than this.

The CDC tracks changes in the national prevalence of obesity based on BMI. The report of Ogden et al presents the latest data involving children. For 2003 to 2006, 11.3% of children and adolescents were at or above the 97th percentile of BMI for age using the 2000 CDC growth chart. For the same period, 16.3% of children and adolescents had a BMI for age at or above the 95th percentile, and 31.9% were at or above the 85th percentile. Current definitions are that children between the 85th and 95th percentile are considered overweight and those between the 95th and 99th percentile are considered obese. Those above the 99th percentile are defined as having severe obesity. For children, BMI does vary considerably with age and thus the BMI of a child must be compared with the BMI of a reference population of children of the same sex and age.

The 2000 CDC BMI-for-age growth charts are the most commonly used reference in the United States to screen for overweight. These charts were constructed from a reference population sample of United States children dating back to the 1960s, 1970s, and 1980s before the epidemic of current obesity became obvious. This is why when one deals with the 95th percentile, for example, of BMI a much larger percentage than 5% of current children are likely to be considered as obese. If there is any good news in all this it is that the prevalence of high BMI-for-age among children and adolescents seems to have reached some sort of plateau because there have been no significant changes between 2003 to 2004, and 2005, and 2006 in the prevalence of overweight and obesity.

This commentary closes with a *Clinical Fact/Curio* about nutrition. A new term has entered the medical lexicon. It is "xenohormesis." Xenohormesis is the adaptive remodeling of the body in response to ecological signals embedded in the diet. Two researchers now propose that taste preferences have evolved to serve a secondary function, that of xenohormesis.[2] The theory states that stress causes plants (such as ripening fruit) and animals (when being hunted, for example) to convert complex sugars to simple sugars and echoes of this stress experience are picked up along the food chain. As successive consumers incorporate, through dietary intake, the stress phenotypes of their prey, cues for stress may accumulate, giving new meaning to the phrase "you are what you eat."

If one takes to its logical conclusion the theory of xenohormesis, vegetarians who are sedentary will soon become potted plants.

J. A. Stockman III, MD

References

1. Barlow SE. Expert committee recommendations regarding the prevention, assessment, and treatment of childhood and adolescent overweight and obesity: summary report. *Pediatrics*. 2007;120:S164-S192.
2. Yun AJ, Doux JD. Unhappy meal: how our need to detect stress may have shaped our preferences for taste. *Med Hypotheses*. 2007;69:746-751.

Comparison of the Prevalence of Shortness, Underweight, and Overweight among US Children Aged 0 to 59 Months by Using the CDC 2000 and the WHO 2006 Growth Charts

Mei Z, Ogden CL, Flegal KM, et al (Natl Ctr for Chronic Disease Prevention and Health Promotion, CDC, Atlanta, GA; Centers for Disease Control and Prevention, Hyattsville, MD)

J Pediatr 153:622-628, 2008

Objective.—To compare the prevalence of shortness, underweight, and overweight by using the Centers for Disease Control and Prevention (CDC) 2000 and the World Health Organization (WHO) 2006 growth charts. These comparisons are undertaken with 2 sets of cutoff values.

Study Design.—Data from the National Health and Nutrition Examination Survey 1999-2004 were used to calculate the prevalence estimates in US children aged 0 to 59 months (n = 3920). Cutoff values commonly used in the United States, on the basis of the 5th percentile of height-for-age to define shortness, the 5th percentile of weight-for-height or weight-for-age to define underweight, and the 95th percentile of weight-for-height or body mass index-for-age to define overweight were compared with the cutoff values recommended by WHO, which use ≤2 z-score (equivalent to 2.3rd percentile) to define shortness and underweight and ≥2 z-score (equivalent to 97.7th percentile) to define overweight. A comparison with the same cutoff values (5th and 95th) in the 2 charts was also performed.

Results.—Applying the 5th or 95th percentile, we observed a higher prevalence of shortness and overweight for all the age groups when the WHO 2006 growth charts were used than when the CDC 2000 growth charts were used. Applying the 5th percentile to the WHO 2006 charts produced lower rates of underweight than did the CDC 2000 charts. However, applying the 5th or 95th percentiles to the CDC 2000 charts and the WHO-recommended cutoff values of −2 or +2 z-score to the WHO charts produced smaller differences in the prevalence of shortness and overweight than were seen when the 5th and 95th percentiles were applied to both the CDC and WHO charts.

Conclusions.—Estimates of the prevalence of key descriptors of growth in children aged 0 to 59 months vary by the chart used and the cutoff values applied. The use of the 5th and 95th percentiles for the CDC growth charts and the 2.3rd and 97.7th percentiles for the WHO growth charts appear comparable in the prevalence of shortness and overweight, but not underweight. If practitioners were to use the WHO growth charts, it might be more appropriate to adopt the WHO recommended cutoff values as well, but this would be a change for office practice.

▶ To understand the implications of this report, it is important to tell the story of how the growth curves that we currently use have evolved. It was back in 1977 that the National Center for Health Statistics (NCHS) developed growth charts for infants and older children that have been used widely in pediatric practice in the United States to assess the nutritional and health status of children and to monitor individual growth. In 1978, the Centers for Disease Control and Prevention (CDC) produced a normalized version of the 1977 NCHS percentile charts. The World Health Organization (WHO) subsequently adopted these normalized curves as an international growth chart (CDC-WHO growth charts) for monitoring the growth of individual children and assessing the nutritional status of populations. Both the NCHS and the CDC-WHO International Growth Charts, while serving valuable roles, have had a number of technical limitations and in May 2000, taking advantage of the availability of more recent comprehensive data and approved statistical smoothing procedures, these charts were revised by the CDC for use in the United States. The current charts are based primarily on nationally representative survey data, supplemented with limited data from other sources and use a descriptive approach to describe the distribution of size-for-age here in the United States. In 2006, the WHO released new global growth charts for infants and children as old as 5 years to replace the existing CDC-WHO International Growth Charts.[1] These charts were developed with the concept that all children, given a good start in life with optimal feeding and no economic constraints, have the same potential with respect to height and weight. In creating the WHO 2006 growth charts, data from sites in 6 countries were used (Brazil, Ghana, India, Norway, Oman, and the United States). Both the CDC 2000 and the WHO 2006 growth charts are widely available to health care providers and are now the growth charts of choice.

The article by Mei et al summarizes the data presented at a meeting held in 2006 where representatives of the CDC, National Institutes of Health, and the American Academy of Pediatrics discussed how the WHO curves might be used by clinicians in the United States and how these curves interface with the CDC 2000 growth curves for infants, children, and adolescents. The importance of this article is that it is the first direct comparison in a United States population of the prevalence of shortness, underweight, and overweight using the CDC 2000 curves and the WHO 2006 curves for age 0 to 59 months. It is clear from this article that the differences between these curves for the prevalence of overweight and shortness are minimized if the recommended (but different) CDC and WHO cut points for overweight (> 95th percentile for CDC 2000; > 97.7th percentile for WHO 2006) and shortness (< 5th percentile for CDC 2000; < 2.3rd percentile for WHO 2006) are used. For the prevalence of shortness, there are virtually no differences between 0 and 59 months, and for the prevalence of overweight, there are no real differences by 12 to 17 months. What is of some concern, however, are the differences using the CDC 2000 and WHO 2006 curves using the recommended cut points of < 5th percentile for CDC 2000 and < 2.3rd percentile WHO 2006. The prevalence of underweight is notably lower when using the WHO 2006 curves. Specifically, using low weight for age as the definition for underweight, the prevalence of underweight at age 12 to 17 months would be approximately 11% when using the CDC 2000 curves, but only 2% when using the WHO 2006 curve. These differences are significant, but it is not tenable that 11% of toddlers in the United States are underweight. This large difference probably reflects a problem in the generation of the CDC 2000 curves, which overestimate underweight.

The upside of using the WHO 2006 curves, in which fewer children are characterized as underweight, would be a decrease in the number of children referred to pediatric endocrinologists for growth hormone therapy and a decrease in the number of mothers overfeeding their children who have been labeled as "underweight." Obviously, whether all of these children defined as underweight on the CDC 2000 curves but not on the WHO 2006 curves are truly at a healthy weight remains to be determined. If one accepts the WHO curves as a growth standard for infants and children who are predominantly breast-fed early in life and whose diet and environment are optimal, then the likelihood that infants no longer categorized as underweight are actually unhealthy is low.

Many thanks to the people at the World Health Organization, the CDC, and the American Academy of Pediatrics for their strong advocacy in the development of these growth curves. We should all be grateful to them for their efforts.

As this commentary closes, another *Clinical Fact/Curio*, this having to do with nutrition. It appears that the Irish are not immune from the ballooning in size of its population. Epidemiologists I.J. Perry et al at University College Cork in Ireland compared data on the height and weight of Irish children from surveys conducted in 1948, 1970, and 2002. The gain in weight has been impressive: 14-year-old boys grew from an average of 146 cm in 1948 to 169 cm in 2002. The weight gain, on the other hand, has been quite staggering. These 14-year-old boys weighed 37 kg in 1948, but by 2002, the 14-year-old population was up to 61 kg. Girls gained 19 kg, going from 40 kg to 59 kg.[2] It would be interesting to see a comparison of similar data in the United States. One can bet that things are not much different on this side of the pond.

J. A. Stockman III, MD

References

1. Greer F. Time to step up to the plate: adopting the WHO 2006 growth curve for US infants. *J Pediatr.* 2008;153:592-594.
2. Irish expansion [editorial comment]. *Science.* 2009;323:789.

An Obesity-Associated *FTO* Gene Variant and Increased Energy Intake in Children

Cecil JE, Tavendale R, Watt P, et al (Univ of St Andrews, UK; Univ of Dundee, UK; Univ of Brighton, UK; et al)

N Engl J Med 359:2558-2566, 2008

Background.—Variation in the fat mass and obesity–associated (*FTO*) gene has provided the most robust associations with common obesity to date. However, the role of *FTO* variants in modulating specific components of energy balance is unknown.

Methods.—We studied 2726 Scottish children, 4 to 10 years of age, who underwent genotyping for *FTO* variant rs9939609 and were measured for height and weight. A subsample of 97 children was examined for possible association of the *FTO* variant with adiposity, energy expenditure, and food intake.

Results.—In the total study group and the subsample, the A allele of rs9939609 was associated with increased weight (P = 0.003 and P = 0.049, respectively) and body-mass index (P = 0.003 and P = 0.03, respectively). In the intensively phenotyped subsample, the A allele was also associated with increased fat mass (P = 0.01) but not with lean mass. Although total and resting energy expenditures were increased in children with the A allele (P = 0.009 and P = 0.03, respectively), resting energy expenditure was identical to that predicted for the age and weight of the child, indicating that there is no defect in metabolic adaptation to obesity in persons bearing the risk-associated allele. The A allele was associated with increased energy intake (P = 0.006) independently of body weight. In contrast, the weight of food ingested by children who had the allele was similar to that in children who did not have the allele (P = 0.82).

Conclusions.—The *FTO* variant that confers a predisposition to obesity does not appear to be involved in the regulation of energy expenditure but may have a role in the control of food intake and food choice, suggesting a link to a hyperphagic phenotype or a preference for energy-dense foods.

▶ This report reminds us not only that childhood obesity is a major public health problem, but that variation in the fat mass and obesity-associated (*FTO*) gene has been linked with obesity in a number of genome-wide associated studies. Currently, more than 100 genes have been implicated in the determination of body weight. These genes, acting in or through the central nervous system (primarily the hypothalamus and brain stem), affect conscious and unconscious aspects of food intake and energy expenditure. The genes mediate brain sensing of fat stores, calorie movement in the gut, hedonic responses to specific foods, rates of energy expenditure, and even the inclination to engage in physical activity. Mutations in one of these genes—the melanocortin 4 receptor (MC4R), which conveys hypothalamic signals suppressing food intake and increasing energy exposure—account for 3% to 5% of severe obesity. Other significant single genes have been somewhat hard to identify. It is likely that obesity is so physiologically complex that no single gene or even handful of genes has a significant or large part in the overall determination of who is obese and who is not obese. In a commentary by Leibel, it is postulated that examining gene-gene interactions is difficult without large numbers of subjects, and that variations among current gene candidates are not the most important contributors to human adiposity.[1]

This is where the genome-wide association study, which uses large numbers of common single-nucleotide polymorphisms (SNPs) in DNA spaced more or less evenly across the human genome can identify genetic variations associated with certain types of body phenotypes. Unlike the candidate-gene approach, the genome-wide association study is genetically blind: it looks for genetic intervals associated with the phenotype or phenotypes; the constituent genes are discovered after the fact by examining those in the implicated interval on a gene. The *FTO* gene examined in the article by Cecil et al was previously identified as a new obesity candidate by a genome-wide association study. Cecil et al studied the effects of genetic variations in the region around SNP rs9939609 in children. This specific region appears to be affecting energy intake and preference for foods of high caloric density. The magnitude of the increase in energy intake correlates with the A allele of this SNP and is high enough to account for some or all of the differences in adiposity. No effect of this genotype on resting energy expenditure was able to be detected, and physical activity was actually estimated to be increased in these children. Given the finding of these and other studies of the molecular physiology of weight regulation, excess intake (rather than reduced basal energy expenditure) is probably the major mechanism for obesity in humans.

Other studies by Frayling et al have shown that the frequency of the rs9939609 A allele is 0.45 in Europeans, 0.52 in West Africans, and 0.14 in Chinese.[2] These same investigators have shown that the odds ratio for the A allele is 1.31 for obesity and 1.18 for overweight. The attributable risk among all populations for overweight and obesity are 12.7% and 20.4% respectively. Hence, this locus accounts for only a small portion of differences in the body mass index (BMI) in the entire population, but it plays a substantial role in conveying the risk of actually becoming overweight or obese in these people. For example, in affected children, this genome will increase the relative risk of obesity by 35% and overweight by 16%. The effect is not seen at birth, but is apparent by 7 years of age.

The bottom line here is that variation in the FTO locus appears to confer a significant risk of obesity through a desire for an increased energy intake. Those with this gene pattern can exercise all day long, but if they do not decrease their energy intake, they will not lose weight. It is also obvious that the more we learn about obesity, the more we learn that some youngsters are preordained to have a problem and if we do not recognize the origins of this problem, it is less likely that we can do a lot for them.

This commentary closes with a query related to a *Clinical Fact/Curio* about heart healthy eating. Having a bar of chocolate a day is not thought to be a typically healthy way to protect your heart, but investigators have shown that it may be. The flavonoids in cocoa reduce risk factors for heart disease, but are usually destroyed when chocolate is made. Researchers, however, asked a Belgium chocolatier to formulate a type of chocolate with higher concentrations than usual of flavonoids. The investigators are now undertaking a study that seems to show significant benefit to the imbibition of chocolate. If you want to volunteer for this study or to find out more about it, e-mail: flavo@use.ac.uk.

J. A. Stockman III, MD

References

1. Leibel RL. Energy in, energy out, and the effects of obesity-related genes. *N Engl J Med.* 2008;359:2603-2604.
2. Frayling TM, Timpson NJ, Weedon NM, et al. A common variant in the *FTO* gene is associated with body mass index and predisposes to childhood and adult obesity. *Science.* 2007;316:889-894.

Maternal Overweight and Obesity and the Risk of Congenital Anomalies: A Systematic Review and Meta-Analysis
Stothard KJ, Tennant PWG, Bell R, et al (Newcastle Univ, UK)
JAMA 301:636-650, 2009

Context.—Evidence suggests an association between maternal obesity and some congenital anomalies.

Objective.—To assess current evidence of the association between maternal overweight, maternal obesity, and congenital anomaly.

Data Sources.—MEDLINE, EMBASE, CINAHL, and Scopus (January 1966 through May 2008) were searched for English-language studies using a list of keywords. Reference lists from relevant review articles were also searched.

Study Selection.—Observational studies with an estimate of prepregnancy or early pregnancy weight or body mass index (BMI) and data on congenital anomalies were considered. Of 1944 potential articles, 39 were included in the systematic review and 18 in the meta-analysis.

Data Extraction and Synthesis.—Information was extracted on study design, quality, participants, congenital anomaly groups and subtypes, and risk estimates. Pooled odds ratios (ORs) comparing risk among overweight, obese, and recommended-weight mothers (defined by BMI) were determined for congenital anomaly groups and subtypes for which at least 150 cases had been reported in the literature.

Results.—Pooled ORs for overweight and obesity were calculated for 16 and 15 anomaly groups or subtypes, respectively. Compared with mothers of recommended BMI, obese mothers were at increased odds of pregnancies affected by neural tube defects (OR, 1.87; 95% confidence interval [CI], 1.62-2.15), spina bifida (OR, 2.24; 95% CI, 1.86-2.69), cardiovascular anomalies (OR, 1.30; 95% CI, 1.12-1.51), septal anomalies (OR, 1.20; 95% CI, 1.09-1.31), cleft palate (OR, 1.23; 95% CI, 1.03-1.47), cleft lip and palate (OR, 1.20; 95% CI, 1.03-1.40), anorectal atresia (OR, 1.48; 95% CI, 1.12-1.97), hydrocephaly (OR, 1.68; 95% CI, 1.19-2.36), and limb reduction anomalies (OR, 1.34; 95% CI, 1.03-1.73). The risk of gastroschisis among obese mothers was significantly reduced (OR, 0.17; 95% CI, 0.10-0.30).

Conclusions.—Maternal obesity is associated with an increased risk of a range of structural anomalies, although the absolute increase is likely to be small. Further studies are needed to confirm whether maternal overweight is also implicated.

▶ This systematic review and meta-analysis remind us just how pervasive the problem is of obesity and also of an increased risk of a range of structural abnormalities in the offspring of obese mothers. By 2015, it is estimated that there will be 2.3 billion overweight and more than 700 million obese adults worldwide. Here in the United States, one-third of women aged 15 years and older are known to be obese. For a long time, we have known that infants of obese mothers are at increased risk of birth difficulties, macrosomia, and perinatal death. Maternal obesity may also be associated with the development of congenital anomalies. These are the leading cause of stillbirth and infant mortality, accounting for 1 in 5 infant deaths in the United States. The report of Stothard et al confirms that in women who are obese at the start of pregnancy, the literature clearly demonstrates a significantly increased risk of a pregnancy that can be affected by neural tube defects, including spina bifida; cardiovascular anomalies, including septal anomaly; cleft palate and cleft lip and palate; anorectal atresia; hydrocephaly; and a limb reduction anomaly. The data also suggest a potential increased risk of anencephaly.

What this report does not do is tell us what the link is between obesity and congenital malformations. A number of potential explanations for the association have been suggested. Obesity and diabetes share similar metabolic abnormalities, including insulin resistance and hyperglycemia, and obesity is a strong risk factor for type 2 diabetes. It is well known that maternal diabetes is an established risk factor for congenital anomalies, especially of the central nervous system, and for cardiovascular anomalies. Thus, undiagnosed diabetes and hyperglycemia in obese pregnant women is one potential explanation for the increased risk of congenital anomalies. Maternal obesity has also been associated with nutritional deficiencies, specifically, reduced folate levels. One can hypothesize that obese women may, to some extent, lack the protective effect of folic acid, increasing the risk of neural tube defects.

Whatever the mechanism is that links obesity with an increased risk of congenital anomalies, we should pay attention to the association. An estimated 3% of all live births in this country are affected by a structural anomaly with 0.68 per 1000 births being affected by a neural tube defect and 2.25 per 1000 births being affected by a serious heart anomaly.[1] The data from this report show us that a fair percentage of these anomalies may be attributable to maternal overweight, a largely preventable entity.

J. A. Stockman III, MD

Reference

1. California Birth Defects Monitoring Program registry data 1999-2003: live births and still births over 20 weeks. http://www.cbdmp.org/ddc_conditions.htm. Accessed January 7, 2009.

Childhood Sleep Time and Long-Term Risk for Obesity: A 32-Year Prospective Birth Cohort Study

Landhuis CE, Poulton R, Welch D, et al (Univ of Otago, Dunedin, New Zealand)
Pediatrics 122:955-960, 2008

Objective.—Associations between short sleep duration and increased BMI have been found in children and adults. However, it is not known whether short sleep time during childhood has long-term consequences. We assessed the association between sleep time in childhood and adult BMI in a birth cohort.

Methods.—Study members were a general-population birth cohort of 1037 participants (502 female) who were born in Dunedin, New Zealand, between April 1972 and March 1973. Parental reports of bedtimes and rising times collected at ages 5, 7, 9, and 11 years were used to estimate childhood sleep time. Linear regression analysis was used to analyze the association between childhood sleep time and BMI measured at 32 years of age.

Results.—Shorter childhood sleep times were significantly associated with higher adult BMI values. This association remained after adjustment for adult sleep time and the potential confounding effects of early childhood BMI, childhood socioeconomic status, parental BMIs, child and adult television viewing, adult physical activity, and adult smoking. In logistic regression analyses, more sleep time during childhood was associated with lower odds of obesity at 32 years of age. This association was significant after adjustment for multiple potential confounding factors.

Conclusions.—These findings suggest that sleep restriction in childhood increases the long-term risk for obesity. Ensuring that children get adequate sleep may be a useful strategy for stemming the current obesity epidemic.

▶ This report emanates from Dunedin, New Zealand where the Dunedin Multidisciplinary Health and Development Study has been undertaken. This is a longitudinal study of health and behavior in an unselected birth cohort. In that study, infants born in Queen Mary Hospital (the only maternity hospital in the city of Dunedin, New Zealand) between April 1972 and March 1973 have been followed throughout their lifespan with much information collected over the years having to do with health and personal traits, including assessments of sleep time reported at ages 5, 7, 9, and 11 years. With this information, comparisons were able to be drawn between sleep time in childhood and body mass index (BMI) assessed at 32 years of age. The results were quite striking. In this population-based birth cohort, it was readily shown that short sleep time in childhood was associated with increased adult BMI. This association was independent of other predictors of adult BMI such as early childhood BMI, parent BMI, physical activity, television viewing, and smoking.

This report from New Zealand does not offer up a mechanism for the association between short sleep time and the risk for adult obesity. Given the fact that the relationship exists independently of other factors that seem to influence adult BMI, the findings suggest that the association between sleep time and obesity is unlikely to be explained by the possibility that the families who have relaxed rules regarding bed times also have relaxed rules with respect to other health-related behaviors.

So what is the possible reason for the association between short sleep times and obesity? Some studies have suggested that shorter sleep times will cause an elevated level of ghrelin, the known appetite-stimulating hormone, and decreased levels of leptin, the appetite-suppressing hormone. This would imply that sleep deficiency may disrupt hunger and appetite regulation. Another explanation may be that tiredness, resulting from short sleep times, alters behavior causing a reduction in physical activity. Tiredness might also affect dietary habits. Folks who are tired may seek fast release, high-energy foods to compensate for perceived low energy levels. These are all interesting speculations, but a naïve individual such as this editor would simply suggest that the more time one spends sleeping, the less time one has the opportunity to eat.

Whatever the etiology is of the relationship between childhood sleep time and adult obesity, the relationship appears to be a real one. For kids, at least, it is best to follow the golden rule of "early to bed" and to get one's adequate number of Z's.

J. A. Stockman III, MD

Obesity and Excessive Daytime Sleepiness in Prepubertal Children With Obstructive Sleep Apnea

Gozal D, Kheirandish-Gozal L (Univ of Louisville, KY)
Pediatrics 123:13-18, 2009

Introduction.—The epidemic of childhood obesity has prompted remarkable changes in the relative proportions of symptomatic overweight or obese children being referred for evaluation of habitual snoring. However, it remains unclear whether obesity modifies the relative frequency of daytime symptoms such as excessive daytime sleepiness.

Methods.—Fifty consecutive, nonobese, habitually snoring, otherwise-healthy children (age range: 6–9 years) and 50 age-, gender-, and ethnicity-matched obese children (BMI z score: >1.67) underwent an overnight polysomnographic evaluation, followed by a multiple sleep latency test the following day.

Results.—The mean obstructive apnea/hypopnea index values for the 2 groups were similar (nonobese: 12.0 ± 1.7 episodes per hour of total sleep time; obese: 10.9 + 1.5 episodes per hour of total sleep time). However, the mean sleep latency for obese children was significantly shorter (12.9 ± 0.9 minutes) than that for nonobese children (17.9 ± 0.7 minutes). Furthermore, 21 obese children had mean sleep latencies of <12.0 minutes, compared with only 5 nonobese children. Although significant associations emerged between mean sleep latency, obstructive apnea/hypopnea index, proportion of total sleep time with oxygen saturation of <95%, and respiratory arousal index for the whole cohort, the slopes and intersects of the linear correlation of mean sleep latency with any of these polygraphic measures were consistently greater in the obese cohort.

Conclusions.—The likelihood of excessive daytime sleepiness for obese children is greater than that for nonobese children at any given level of obstructive sleep apnea severity and is strikingly reminiscent of excessive daytime sleepiness patterns in adults with obstructive sleep apnea.

▶ We can think of obstructive sleep apnea (OSA) as having short- and long-term effects. The short-term effect, as we see here, is excessive daytime sleepiness beginning as early as childhood. The long-term effects, which have their seeds planted in childhood if OSA is the result of obesity is a more complex affair. By the time one gets to adulthood, the consequences of OSA can be quite dramatic in terms of its effects on longevity.

OSA is a common disorder in which repetitive apneas expose the cardiovascular system to cycles of hypoxia, exaggerated negative intrathoracic pressure, and arousals. These noxious stimuli can, in turn, depress myocardial contractility, activate the sympathetic nervous system, raise blood pressure, heart rate, and myocardial wall stress, depress parasympathetic activity, provoke oxidative stress and systemic inflammation, activate platelets, and impair cardiovascular endothelial function. Epidemiological studies have shown significant independent associations between OSA and hypertension, coronary artery disease in adults, arrhythmias, heart failure and stroke. In randomized trials treating OSA with continuous positive airway pressure lowered blood pressure, attenuated signs of early atherosclerosis, and, in patients with heart failure, improved cardiac function. These are the truly long-term consequences of OSA seen usually well beyond childhood, but again the seeds of the problem are sown in childhood. Current data, therefore, do suggest that OSA increases the risk of developing cardiovascular disease and that its treatment has the potential to diminish such risk.

What we see in the report of Gozal et al is something that all of us probably have intuitively believed in and that is that OSA puts obese children at greater risk for developing excessive daytime sleepiness. Presumably it is the obesity that is the culprit behind OSA and the snoring that we so commonly observe in obese children. The authors of this report speculate that obesity is a low-grade systemic inflammatory disorder (a generally held view). Therefore, the authors suggest that it is plausible that the coexistence of obesity and OSA magnifies the inflammatory response associated with each of these conditions, thereby resulting in increased release of sleepiness-promoting compounds or other compounds yet to be identified. In some respects this makes sense because significant improvements in daytime sleepiness have been observed in adults with OSA after treatment with a synthetic tumor necrosis factor receptor acting as a decoy for inflammatory mediators. To say this differently, inflammation can make you sluggish during the day, a well-observed phenomenon. One of the causes of inflammation is obesity, which also causes obstructive sleep apnea, a double whammy on the cardiovascular system. The lesson here is that it is not just the disturbance in sleep itself that causes one to be sleepy during the day. Daytime sleepiness as a result of either obesity or OSA is a much more complex affair than simply not getting enough shut-eye at night.

For more on the adult consequences of obstructive sleep apnea, see the superb review by Bradley and Floras.[1]

J. A. Stockman III, MD

Reference

1. Bradley TD, Floras JS. Obstructive sleep apnea and its cardiovascular consequences. *Lancet.* 2009;373:82-93.

Prevalence and Predictors of Abnormal Liver Enzymes in Young Women with Anorexia Nervosa
Fong H-F, DiVasta AD, DiFabio D, et al (Harvard Medical School, Boston, MA; Children's, Hosp, Boston, MA)
J Pediatr 153:247-253, 2008

Objective.—To determine the prevalence and predictors of abnormal liver enzyme levels in ambulatory young women with anorexia nervosa (AN).

Study Design.—In this cross-sectional study of 53 females with AN, serum concentrations of liver enzymes and hormones were measured.

Anthropometric, dietary, and body composition information was collected. Correlational analyses were performed between liver enzyme concentrations and these variables.

Results.—Elevated alanine aminotransferase (ALT) and gamma-glutamyl transpeptidase (GGT) levels were found in 14 subjects (26%) and 5 subjects (9%), respectively. ALT and GGT were inversely correlated with body mass index (r = −0.27 to −0.30, P < .049) and percentage body fat (r = −0.36 to −0.47, P < .007) but showed no relationship with lean body mass. Subjects with percentage body fat < 18% had higher ALT levels than those above this threshold (median 26.5 vs 18.0 U/L, P = .01). Liver enzyme concentrations did not correlate with dietary variables, except for GGT and percentage of calories from protein (r = 0.28, P = .04).

Conclusions.—Serum ALT and GGT concentrations are inversely related to adiposity in young women with AN. Future studies are needed to determine whether these liver enzyme elevations signify unrecognized, clinically relevant liver disease.

▶ Most pediatricians have been involved with the care of teens with anorexia nervosa. Many of us, however, may not be aware that elevated liver enzymes are quite common in such patients and can be a sign of significant organ dysfunction. The cause and risk factors for elevated liver enzymes remain unclear. Some have suspected that hepatocellular injury from nonalcoholic fatty liver disease is one of the potential causes of enzyme elevations in anorexia nervosa and other disorders of nutrition. Nonalcoholic fatty liver disease is an entity that represents a spectrum of liver disease ranging from steatosis to cirrhosis and is characterized by the accumulation of excess lipid within hepatocytes. This problem in patients with anorexia nervosa may be linked to insulin resistance, which is occasionally seen in the disorder. Insulin resistance increases peripheral fatty acid mobilization and decreases hepatic oxidation of fatty acids.

What Fong et al have done is to look at several dozen young women with anorexia nervosa measuring serum concentration of liver enzymes and various hormone levels. Measures of insulin resistance and cortisol do not appear to correlate with elevated alanine aminotransferase (ALT) levels. An inverse trend, however, was noted between gamma-glutamyl transpeptidase (GGT) levels and both insulin and measures of insulin resistance. Age, duration of illness, and duration of amenorrhea are not associated with liver enzyme concentrations. There was a significant inverse relationship between body mass index (BMI) and ALT. Subjects with a percent body fat less than 18% have the highest levels of ALT.

All in all, this study confirms a relationship between elevated liver enzymes and the diagnosis of anorexia nervosa with more than 1-quarter of patients having elevated ALT concentrations. The lower the percentage of body fat, the higher the ALT, and GGT levels. This liver enzyme elevation may reflect nonalcoholic fatty liver disease-induced hepatocellular injury. This is true although none of the subjects studied exhibited particularly strong evidence of insulin resistance.

As of now, no one knows what the long-term consequences are of the liver abnormalities observed during periods of severe malnutrition associated with anorexia nervosa. Only time and careful study will determine whether the findings described have long-term consequences. In the meantime, elevated liver enzymes are just one more marker of what these young ladies are doing to their bodies.

This commentary closes with a *Clinical Fact/Curio* regarding nutrition. The Bill and Melinda Gates Foundation has given $16 million to an international network led by the University of California, Davis for studies in Malawi, Burkina Faso, and Ghana to develop and test a peanut butter-like food supplement that prevents malnutrition. Fat-based peanut butter paste has revolutionized the treatment of malnutrition in many poor countries thus far, but its use in the prevention of malnutrition is hotly debated.[1]

Another report shows just how useful a peanut butter product can be in treating malnutrition. In underdeveloped countries a product called Plumpy'nut is being distributed. Plumpy'nut comes in a foil-wrapped package containing 92 grams of a brown paste that looks like dark peanut butter. Each packet contains 500 calories and plenty of proteins, vitamins, and minerals. Aid organizations say the paste, a so-called ready-to-use therapeutic food (RUTF), has revolutionized the care of children who are malnourished. Plumpy'nut has a long shelf-life and does not need to be mixed with water, a major risk with standard RUTF products based on milk powder. Plumpy'nut is also easy for mothers to give their children at home and perhaps best of all, children love the sweet, sticky stuff.[2]

J. A. Stockman III, MD

References

1. Enserink M. Big push for peanut butter. *Science*. 2008;332:1313.
2. Enserink M. The peanut butter debate. *Science*. 2008;322:36.

Intra-abdominal Adiposity and Individual Components of the Metabolic Syndrome in Adolescence: Sex Differences and Underlying Mechanisms
Syme C, Abrahamowicz M, Leonard GT, et al (Univ Nottingham, England; McGill Univ, Montreal, Quebec, Canada; et al)
Arch Pediatr Adolesc Med 162:453-461, 2008

Objective.—To investigate the association between intra-abdominal adiposity and individual components of the metabolic syndrome (MS) in adolescent males and females.

Design.—Cross-sectional study of a population-based cohort.

Setting.—Saguenay Youth Study, Quebec, Canada.

Participants.—A total of 324 adolescents, aged 12 to 18 years.

Intervention.—Measures were compared between males and females with "high" or "low" intra-abdominal fat (IAF).

Main Outcome Measures.—Intra-abdominal fat was quantified with magnetic resonance imaging. Primary outcome measures were blood pressure (BP) and fasting serum glucose, insulin, lipids, and C-reactive protein levels. Secondary mechanistic measures were cardiovascular variability indexes of autonomic nervous system function, pubertal development, and serum levels of cortisol, leptin, and sex hormones.

Results.—The MS was completely absent in adolescents with low IAF and was present in 13.8% of males and 8.3% of females with high IAF. Excess IAF was associated with a higher homeostasis model assessment index (0.5 [95% confidence interval (CI), 0.3 to 0.8]; $P < .001$) and triglycerides level (17.7 mg/dL [to convert to millimoles per liter, multiply by 0.0113] [95% CI, 9.7 to 25.7 mg/dL]; $P < .001$), lower high-density lipoprotein cholesterol level (-3.9 mg/dL [to convert to millimoles per liter, multiply by 0.0259] [95% CI, -6.2 to -1.5 mg/dL]; $P = .003$), and higher C-reactive protein level (0.03 mg/L [to convert to nanomoles per liter, multiply by 9.524] [95% CI, 0.01 to 0.05 mg/L]; $P = .003$). High IAF was associated with elevations of BP and sympathetic activity in males only (higher systolic BP, 6 mm Hg [95% CI, 1 to 11 mm Hg]; $P = .02$ and low-frequency power of diastolic BP, 629 mm Hg^2 [95% CI, 37 to 1222 mm Hg^2]; $P = .04$).

Conclusions.—Our results suggest that, already in adolescence, accumulation of IAF may promote development of the MS, affecting the metabolic and inflammatory components similarly in both sexes but influencing BP adversely only in males. The latter may be attributed, in part, to the augmentation of sympathetic activity also seen only in males.

▶ If there is anything unique about this interesting report, it is that it is the first to examine the relationship between intra-abdominal obesity and the metabolic syndrome by using MRI of the abdomen. Using MRI, it was determined that the metabolic syndrome was completely absent in adolescents with low intra-abdominal amounts of fat while it was present in some 14% of males and 8% of females with high intra-abdominal quantities of fat. The information provided from this report fills an important void that has existed in our understanding of the relationship between fat in the tummy and the metabolic syndrome. Most of us have used body mass index (BMI) as the surrogate for the major risk factor for the metabolic syndrome. It is true that body mass index is a reasonable proxy for body fatness, but it certainly does not tell you where that fat is. The article by Syme et al tells us about the metabolic risk of high versus low visceral fat, even after controlling for BMI. We now know for sure that body fat distribution is more predictive of risk than total fat and certainly more predictive than more whole body measures, such as BMI, particularly among youth already defined as overweight according to standard BMI percentile cut points for overweight/obesity.

As interesting as this study is, it is a research study and there is no way that anyone in practice is going to use MRI to assess intra-abdominal fat as a risk factor for the metabolic syndrome. Investigators have been trying for some time to find more inexpensive alternatives to costly measurements such as this. Waist circumference has been proposed as one strategy for measuring abdominal fat distribution, but unfortunately waist circumference measurements are not satisfactory proxies of children's visceral fat or even change in children's visceral fat. More specifically, in a longitudinal natural history study of visceral fat among children that simultaneously examined changes in proxy measures of visceral fat, some 70% and 50% increases in visceral fat for boys and girls, respectively, were accompanied by a mere 9.7% and 7.5% increases in waist circumference, respectively.[1]

We should not conclude from this report that we should not continue to measure BMI. We should. It is probably also worth measuring waist circumference and triceps/subscapular skinfold thickness to identify children meeting criteria for health risks, but we need to understand that at best these are only rough measures of the greatest risk factor for the development of metabolic syndrome, that being the amount of excess intra-abdominal fat that kids and adults carry around with them. Until someone finds a cheap surrogate for an MRI and its precision, the simple office tools we have at hand are the best there is.

J. A. Stockman III, MD

Reference

1. Fox KR, Peters DM, Sharpe P, Bell M. Assessment of abdominal fat development in young adolescents using magnetic resonance imaging. *Int J Obes Relat Metab Disord.* 2000;24:1653-1659.

Aliskiren Combined with Losartan in Type 2 Diabetes and Nephropathy

Parving H-H, for the AVOID Study Investigators (Rigshospitalet, Copenhagen, Denmark; et al)
N Engl J Med 358:2433-2446, 2008

Background.—Diabetic nephropathy is the leading cause of end-stage renal disease in developed countries. We evaluated the renoprotective effects of dual blockade of the renin–angiotensin–aldosterone system by adding treatment with aliskiren, an oral direct renin inhibitor, to treatment with the maximal recommended dose of losartan (100 mg daily) and optimal antihypertensive therapy in patients who had hypertension and type 2 diabetes with nephropathy.

Methods.—We enrolled 599 patients in this multinational, randomized, double-blind study. After a 3-month, open-label, run-in period during which patients received 100 mg of losartan daily, patients were randomly assigned to receive 6 months of treatment with aliskiren (150 mg daily for 3 months, followed by an increase in dosage to 300 mg daily for another 3 months) or placebo, in addition to losartan. The primary outcome was a reduction in the ratio of albumin to creatinine, as measured in an early-morning urine sample, at 6 months.

Results.—The baseline characteristics of the two groups were similar. Treatment with 300 mg of aliskiren daily, as compared with placebo, reduced the mean urinary albumin-to-creatinine ratio by 20% (95% confidence interval, 9 to 30; P<0.001), with a reduction of 50% or more in 24.7% of the patients who received aliskiren as compared with 12.5% of those who received placebo (P<0.001). A small difference in blood pressure was seen between the treatment groups by the end of the study period (systolic, 2 mm Hg lower [P = 0.07] and diastolic, 1 mm Hg lower [P = 0.08] in the aliskiren group). The total numbers of adverse and serious adverse events were similar in the groups.

Conclusions.—Aliskiren may have renoprotective effects that are independent of its blood-pressure–lowering effect in patients with hypertension, type 2 diabetes, and nephropathy who are receiving the recommended renoprotective treatment. (ClinicalTrials.gov number, NCT00097955.)

▶ This is another report dealing with the management of type 2 diabetes in adults. Once again, there are few data that tell us much about the long-term outcomes of management of type 2 diabetes during childhood. We must pay attention to the adult literature in order to give us some direction in terms of our thinking about the care of children who generally do not develop evidence of macrovascular disease or microvascular disease on our watch in pediatrics. Needless to say, these findings are important because diabetic nephropathy, a consequence of type 2 diabetes, is the leading cause of end stage renal disease in developed countries. Parving et al report the results of the Aliskiren in the Evaluation Proteinuria in Diabetes (AVOID) trial, a double-blind, randomized, placebo-controlled trial in which patients with type 2 diabetes, hypertension, and proteinuria who were already receiving losartan and other antihypertensive therapy to reach an optimal blood-pressure goal were randomly assigned to additionally receive aliskiren or placebo. The primary outcome of the trial was a reduction in albuminuria, a goal that was achieved. By way of background, patients who are treated with angiotensin-converting-enzyme (ACE) inhibitors or angiotensin-receptor blockers have an increase in activity of renin. In the renin-angiotensin-aldosterone system, renin cleaves a leucine-valine bond in the angiotensinogen molecule to release angiotensin I, which in turn is cleaved to angiotensin II by ACE. It has been anticipated that the ability to control renin directly would actually improve blood pressure control and might modify the other actions of this important vasoactive system. The recent approval of aliskiren, an oral renin inhibitor, by the Food and Drug Administration is permitting new clinical questions to be examined. At least in the AVOID trial, the addition of a renin inhibitor in patients with type 2 diabetes did help to improve their renal status.

There are no studies of the use of renin inhibitors in children either to control hypertension or to prevent the complications of diabetes that involve the kidneys. There are concerns about dual-agent blockade of the renin-angiotensin-aldosterone system. The concern is the potential increase in the incidence of hyperkalemia and decrease in the glomerular filtration rate. Only long-term studies will tell us whether there is additional value of adding new agents such as aliskiren as part of the management of type 2 diabetes.

J. A. Stockman III, MD

Effects of Intensive Glucose Lowering in Type 2 Diabetes

The Action to Control Cardiovascular Risk in Diabetes Study Group (McMaster Univ and Hamilton Health Sciences, ON, Canada; Wake Forest Univ School of Medicine, Winston-Salem, NC; et al)
N Engl J Med 358:2545-2559, 2008

Background.—Epidemiologic studies have shown a relationship between glycated hemoglobin levels and cardiovascular events in patients with type 2 diabetes. We investigated whether intensive therapy to target normal glycated hemoglobin levels would reduce cardiovascular events in patients with type 2 diabetes who had either established cardiovascular disease or additional cardiovascular risk factors.

Methods.—In this randomized study, 10,251 patients (mean age, 62.2 years) with a median glycated hemoglobin level of 8.1% were assigned to receive intensive therapy (targeting a glycated hemoglobin level below 6.0%) or standard therapy (targeting a level from 7.0 to 7.9%). Of these patients, 38% were women, and 35% had had a previous cardiovascular event. The primary outcome was a composite of nonfatal myocardial infarction, nonfatal stroke, or death from cardiovascular causes. The finding of higher mortality in the intensive-therapy group led to a discontinuation of intensive therapy after a mean of 3.5 years of follow-up.

Results.—At 1 year, stable median glycated hemoglobin levels of 6.4% and 7.5% were achieved in the intensive-therapy group and the standard-therapy group, respectively. During follow-up, the primary outcome occurred in 352 patients in the intensive-therapy group, as compared with 371 in the standard-therapy group (hazard ratio, 0.90; 95% confidence interval [CI], 0.78 to 1.04; $P = 0.16$). At the same time, 257 patients in the intensive-therapy group died, as compared with 203 patients in the standard-therapy group (hazard ratio, 1.22; 95% CI, 1.01 to 1.46; $P = 0.04$). Hypoglycemia requiring assistance and weight gain of more than 10 kg were more frequent in the intensive-therapy group ($P<0.001$).

Conclusions.—As compared with standard therapy, the use of intensive therapy to target normal glycated hemoglobin levels for 3.5 years increased mortality and did not significantly reduce major cardiovascular events. These findings identify a previously unrecognized harm of intensive glucose lowering in high-risk patients with type 2 diabetes. (ClinicalTrials.gov number, NCT00000620.)

▶ Interestingly, there are little data in pediatrics to tell us exactly how "tight" the control of type 2 diabetes should be. In some respects this is not surprising since the controversy about this topic rages in adult medicine. If there were an answer to the controversy, it should come from the care of adults because in that population evidence of morbidity resulting from type 2 diabetes is more obvious and also, many more adults have the disorder than do children, although the "epidemic" in childhood is quite apparent to all. Recently, several studies have appeared in the adult literature telling us a little bit about the value, or lack of value, of intensive glycemic control. Absent data from the pediatric literature, we should pay careful attention to these adult studies because they may ultimately provide some insight into what we should be doing in our care of youngsters.

Although there is a link between hyperglycemia and cardiovascular risk, there is less evidence that glucose lowering is associated with a reduction in risk. For example, adult patients with type 2 diabetes whose glycated hemoglobin levels were reduced from 8% to 7% (the United Kingdom prospective diabetes study), did not exhibit a reduction in cardiovascular events, although a subset of patients treated with metformin had a lower risk of cardiovascular events.[1] On the other hand, among patients with type 1 diabetes, glucose lowering was associated with a long-term benefit with regard to cardiovascular complications, a benefit that became apparent only after years of treatment. The ACCORD (Action to Control Cardiovascular Risk in Diabetes) trial compared intensive and standard glucose-lowering targets in type 2 diabetes. In this study, there was no restriction on glucose-lowering treatments to reach glycemic targets. Participants were randomly assigned to undergo intensive therapy or standard therapy for lowering of blood pressure or to receive fenofibrate or placebo.

The primary outcome in the ADVANCE trial was a composite endpoint of macrovascular and microvascular events. The most compelling message from this study is that the near-normal glycemic control for an average of 3.5 to 5 years does not reduce cardiovascular events, at least within that timeframe. A troubling finding from the ACCORD trial is that near-normal glucose control achieved with combination chemotherapy including oral hypoglycemics and insulin is associated with significantly increased risk of death from any cause and death from cardiovascular causes, the very outcomes the trial was designed to prevent.

The cause of these unexpected excess deaths in the ACCORD trial obviously is of great interest. One wonders if some of the "unexpected or presumed cardiovascular disease events" might have been precipitated by episodes of hypoglycemia and therefore misclassified as having a cardiovascular cause. Combination therapy with oral hypoglycemics and insulin are known to be associated with a significant increased risk for hypoglycemia.

The conclusion from adult studies appears to be that the most appropriate target for glycated hemoglobin should remain at 7%, although lower individualized targets may be appropriate when the focus is primary prevention of this macrovascular disease. Internists now recognize that when glycated hemoglobin values under 7% are the goal, needs to balance the incremental benefit of a reduction in microvascular events with the increased risk of adverse events, a very delicate balance indeed.

One can honestly say that the adult literature, although cautioning against too rigid control, does clearly tell us the importance of glycemic control in general. It is not possible at this point to translate these data in any meaningful way into childhood, but we should be aware of the long-term consequences of "loose" versus "tight" diabetic control.

For more on intensive blood glucose control and vascular outcomes in patients with type 2 diabetes, see the data from the ADVANCE collaborative group.[2]

J. A. Stockman III, MD

References

1. Effect of intensive glucose-control with metformin on complications in overweight patients with type 2 diabetes (UKPDS 34): UK Prospective Diabetes Study (UKPDS) Group. *Lancet*. 1998;352:854-865.
2. The ADVANCE collaborative group. Intensive blood glucose control and cardiovascular outcomes in patients with type 2 diabetes. *N Engl J Med*. 2008;358: 2560-2572.

Risk of microalbuminuria and progression to macroalbuminuria in a cohort with childhood onset type 1 diabetes: prospective observational study
Amin R, Widmer B, Prevost AT, et al (Addenbrooke's Hosp, Cambridge; Univ of Cambridge, MA et al)
BMJ 336:697-701, 2008

Objectives.—To describe independent predictors for the development of microalbuminuria and progression to macroalbuminuria in those with childhood onset type 1 diabetes.

Design.—Prospective observational study with follow-up for 9.8 (SD 3.8) years.

Setting.—Oxford regional prospective study.

Participants.—527 participants with a diagnosis of type 1 diabetes at mean age 8.8 (SD 4.0) years.

Main outcome measures.—Annual measurement of glycated haemoglobin (HbA_{1c}) and assessment of urinary albumin:creatinine ratio.

Results.—Cumulative prevalence of microalbuminuria was 25.7% (95% confidence interval 21.3% to 30.1%) after 10 years of diabetes and 50.7% (40.5% to 60.9%) after 19 years of diabetes and 5182 patient years of follow-up. The only modifiable adjusted predictor for microalbuminuria was high HbA_{1c} concentrations (hazard ratio per 1% rise in HbA_{1c} 1.39, 1.27 to 1.52). Blood pressure and history of smoking were not predictors. Microalbuminuria was persistent in 48% of patients. Cumulative prevalence of progression from microalbuminuria to macroalbuminuria was 13.9% (12.9% to 14.9%); progression occurred at a mean age of 18.5 (5.8) years. Although the sample size was small, modifiable predictors of macroalbuminuria were higher HbA_{1c} levels and both persistent and intermittent microalbuminuria (hazard ratios 1.42 (1.22 to 1.78), 27.72 (7.99 to 96.12), and 8.76 (2.44 to 31.44), respectively).

Conclusion.—In childhood onset type 1 diabetes, the only modifiable predictors were poor glycaemic control for the development of microalbuminuria and poor control and microalbuminuria (both persistent and intermittent) for progression to macroalbuminuria. Risk for macroalbuminuria is similar to that observed in cohorts with adult onset disease but as it occurs in young adult life early intervention in normotensive adolescents might be needed to improve prognosis.

▶ Unfortunately, the knowledge we have of the relation between control of childhood type 1 diabetes and the risk of renal complications of this disease comes from data in adults and adolescents. The primary goal of managing childhood type 1 diabetes is to prevent or delay retinal and renal microvascular complications. Amin et al report on the risk of diabetic renal disease in the Oxford Regional Prospective Study, a population-based cohort study of children with type 1 diabetes. The prevalence of microalbuminuria was about 25% and 50% after 10 and 20 years of diabetes, respectively. The natural course of microalbuminuria was such that about half the patients reverted at least transiently to normoalbuminuria and 13% progressed to macroalbuminuria. This study does answer some important questions for those pediatricians who care for children with diabetes.

The main result of the study is that mean HbA1c is a strong predictor - and the only modifiable one able to be identified—of microalbuminuria. The risk ratio for having microalbuminuria is 1.39 for each 1% increase in HbA1c. There seemed to be no lower threshold for HbA1c, because the lowest seen population here (≤ 8.5%) was not fully protective. The latter patients had around a 15% risk of microalbuminuria at age 20 years.

Some of the other interesting and important findings in this report are that after 15 years of disease the prevalence of microalbuminuria was not influenced by the age of onset of diabetes, indicating that the deleterious effect of hyperglycemia is similar in childhood and later in life. This is in contradiction to a Finne et al study that found a lower risk of endstage renal disease after 30 years of diabetes in patients who were diagnosed before the age of 5 years.[1]

While this study was performed in Europe, the data probably equally apply to the situation here in the United States. The data remind us that, in practice, we are far from the HbA1c threshold of less than 7.5% in teenagers, 8% in children, and 8.5% in toddlers recommended by the American Diabetes Association because even the best controlled group of patients in the Oxford study did not reach these thresholds. Another finding in this report was that the use of antihypertensives, specifically angiotensin-converting enzyme inhibitors and angiotensin II receptor antagonists, did not prevent the onset of microalbuminuria in adolescents. These antihypertensives have been thought to be somewhat protective against microvascular disease.

The bottom line here is that data from overseas suggest that the future is dim for children with diabetes unless their disease is absolutely rigorously controlled throughout childhood and adolescence by diet, education, adequate delivery of insulin, and control of blood glucose while avoiding hypoglycemia. All too often parents are tempted to cut corners on sophisticated but demanding treatments such as multiple injections, insulin pumps and, more recently, continuous glucose monitoring. Such cutting of corners has the potential for long-term, irreversible consequences.

J. A. Stockman III, MD

Reference

1. Finne P, Reunanen A, Stenman S, et al. Incidence of end-stage renal disease in patients with type 1 diabetes. *JAMA.* 2005;294:1782-1787.

Nasal insulin to prevent type 1 diabetes in children with HLA genotypes and autoantibodies conferring increased risk of disease: a double-blind, randomized controlled trial

Näntö-Salonen K, Kupila A, Simell S, et al (Univ of Turku, Finland, et al)
Lancet 372:1746-1755, 2008

Background.—In mouse models of diabetes, prophylactic administration of insulin reduced incidence of the disease. We investigated whether administration of nasal insulin decreased the incidence of type 1 diabetes, in children with HLA genotypes and autoantibodies increasing the risk of the disease.

Methods.—At three university hospitals in Turku, Oulu, and Tampere (Finland), we analysed cord blood samples of 116 720 consecutively born infants, and 3430 of their siblings, for the HLA-DQB1 susceptibility alleles for type 1 diabetes. 17 397 infants and 1613 siblings had increased genetic risk, of whom 11 225 and 1574, respectively, consented to screening of diabetes-associated autoantibodies at every 3–12 months. In a double-blind trial, we randomly assigned 224 infants and 40 siblings positive for two or more autoantibodies, in consecutive samples, to receive short-acting human insulin (1 unit/kg; n = 115 and n = 22) or placebo (n = 109 and n = 18) once a day intranasally. We used a restricted randomisation, stratified by site, with permuted blocks of size two. Primary endpoint was diagnosis of diabetes. Analysis was by intention to treat. The study was terminated early because insulin had no beneficial effect. This study is registered with ClinicalTrials.gov, number NCT00223613.

Findings.—Median duration of the intervention was 1·8 years (range 0–9·7). Diabetes was diagnosed in 49 index children randomised to receive insulin, and in 47 randomised to placebo (hazard ratio [HR] 1·14; 95% CI 0.·73–1·77). 42 and 38 of these children, respectively, continued treatment until diagnosis, with yearly rates of diabetes onset of 16·8% (95% CI 11·7–21.·9) and 15.·3% (10·5–20·2). Seven siblings were diagnosed with diabetes in the insulin group, versus six in the placebo group (HR 1·93; 0·56–6·77). In all randomised children, diabetes was diagnosed in 56 in the insulin group, and 53 in the placebo group (HR 0·98; 0·67–1·43, p = 0·91).

Interpretation.—In children with HLA-conferred susceptibility to diabetes, administration of nasal insulin, started soon after detection of autoantibodies, could not be shown to prevent or delay type 1 diabetes.

▶ There is a good basis for the hypothesis that administration of insulin in advance of the onset of type 1 diabetes in children would help prevent the disease in those who are a genetic setup for it. The genetic risk for diabetes mellitus is well described and is mainly confirmed by HLA-DR and HLA-DQ haplotypes, although environmental factors are needed to induce islet-related autoimmunity in individuals who carry the genetic risk. Early intervention is warranted because this immune-mediated disorder is associated with antibodies against β-cell components, antibodies that often appear in very young children well before the onset of clinical disease. The question has existed as to whether exogenous insulin might prevent the development of type 1 diabetes, allowing β cells to rest, implying that low metabolic activity in islet cells is associated with reduced autoantigen expression. Insulin administration before clinical onset of disease might also induce tolerance to insulin, a key antigen. Insulin might have a direct effect on lymphocytes. Early human pilot studies administering insulin before or early in the course of the disease were in fact encouraging, but a larger diabetes prevention trial showed no protective effect of subcutaneous or oral insulin in antibody-positive first-degree relatives of those with diabetes. There was a suggestion, however, that in a subset of patients oral insulin might have delayed the onset of clinical disease.

The Type 1 Diabetes Prediction and Prevention Study investigated whether nasal insulin reduces the incidence of type 1 diabetes in children from the general population, who have genotypes and autoantibodies that increase the risk of developing the disease. The study reported is a randomized, double-blind, placebo-controlled study in 3 Finnish university hospitals where newborn babies from the general population and their older siblings were screened for HLA-DQB1 associated susceptibility to type 1 diabetes. Children older than 1 year of age with at least 2 types of islet cell autoantibodies in 2 consecutive serum samples drawn 3 to 6 months apart were invited to participate in the intervention trial. Children with clinical diabetes, any significant chronic disease, or a family history of maturity-onset diabetes were excluded. Treated children were given nasal sprays containing insulin that was administered once daily. The patients then were followed up every 3 months with extensive monitoring of blood glucose and insulin. Intravenous glucose tolerance tests were also performed. The study results demonstrated that nasal insulin did not delay or prevent type 1 diabetes in children with HLA-conferred risk of disease, even when started soon after seroconversion to antibody positivity.

It should be noted that the administration of insulin in this study via the nasal route was not to "rest" the islet cells by the provision of circulating insulin. The concept was to give insulin as an antigen to induce tolerance against the development of autoantibodies. While insulin did not work for this purpose, it also did not result in any accelerated production of diabetes autoantibodies. This report is not the first and will not be the last in the struggle to prevent the onset of type 1 diabetes in children.

J. A. Stockman III, MD

Vitamin D supplementation in early childhood and risk of type 1 diabetes: a systematic review and meta-analysis
Zipitis CS, Akobeng AK (Stockport NHS Foundation Trust, Stockport, UK; Central Manchester and Manchester Children's Univ Hosps, UK)
Arch Dis Child 93:512-517, 2008

Objectives.—To assess whether vitamin D supplementation in infancy reduces the risk of type 1 diabetes in later life.

Methods.—This was a systematic review and meta-analysis using Medline, Embase, Cinahl, Cochrane Central Register of Controlled Trials and reference lists of retrieved articles. The main outcome measure was development of type 1 diabetes. Controlled trials and observational studies that had assessed the effect of vitamin D supplementation on risk of developing type 1 diabetes were included in the analysis.

Results.—Five observational studies (four case-control studies and one cohort study) met the inclusion criteria; no randomised controlled trials were found. Meta-analysis of data from the case-control studies showed that the risk of type 1 diabetes was significantly reduced in infants who were supplemented with vitamin D compared to those who were not supplemented (pooled odds ratio 0.71, 95% CI 0.60 to 0.84). The result of the cohort study was in agreement with that of the meta-analysis. There was also some evidence of a dose-response effect, with those using higher amounts of vitamin D being at lower risk of developing type 1 diabetes. Finally, there was a suggestion that the timing of supplementation might also be important for the subsequent development of type 1 diabetes.

Conclusion.—Vitamin D supplementation in early childhood may offer protection against the development of type 1 diabetes. The evidence for this is based on observational studies. Adequately powered, randomised controlled trials with long periods of follow-up are needed to establish causality and the best formulation, dose, duration and period of supplementation.

▶ Studies reported elsewhere in this work have documented the extraordinarily high prevalence of vitamin D deficiency, at least biochemical evidence thereof, in the United States in early childhood. Confusing, however, is what the implications of hypovitaminosis really are on the growing child. Very few who have biochemical evidence of vitamin D deficiency have bone problems as a consequence. Most infants outgrow the latter difficulty. Even less clear, however, are the possible other consequences of vitamin D deficiency, specifically the potential for an increased risk of cancer, diabetes, cardiovascular disease, depression, and schizophrenia.[1] The report of Zipitis et al, from the United Kingdom, should give us pause, in this regard. The report represents a meta-analysis of data from case-controlled studies attempting to establish a potential link between type 1 diabetes and low levels of vitamin D in early childhood. Infants supplemented with higher amounts of vitamin D seem to be clearly at a lower risk of developing type 1 diabetes. Specifically, meta-analysis of data from the case-controlled studies showed that the risk of type 1 diabetes in infants who were supplemented with vitamin D compared with those who are not supplemented was just 71% of the risk seen in nonsupplemented infants. The findings from the Zipitis et al report do underscore the relationship between vitamin D and the incidence of certain autoimmune diseases including type 1 diabetes, rheumatoid arthritis, and multiple sclerosis.[2,3]

It is fairly obvious that we are still in the very early stages of understanding the relationship between low levels of vitamin D and a greater risk of autoimmune diseases. Randomized controlled trials with long periods of follow-up are clearly needed to establish causality and the best formulation, dose, duration, and period of supplementation of vitamin D during childhood and even during adulthood. There would seem to be no harm from being sure that a youngster gets adequate amounts of vitamin D and perhaps there would be much good to come of this later in life.

J. A. Stockman III, MD

References

1. Holick MF. Vitamin D deficiency. *N Engl J Med*. 2007;357:266-281.
2. Merlino LA, Curtis J, Mikuls TR, et al. Vitamin D intake is inversely associated with rheumatoid arthritis: results from the Iowa Women's Health Study. *Arthritis Rheum*. 2004;50:72-77.
3. Hayes CE. Vitamin D: a natural inhibitor of multiple sclerosis. *Proc Nutr Soc*. 2000;59:531-535.

Hypovitaminosis D among healthy children in the United States: a review of the current evidence

Rovner AJ, O'Brien KO (Eunice Kennedy Shriver Natl Inst of Child Health and Human Development, Rockville, MD)
Arch Pediatr Adolesc Med 162:513-519, 2008

Objective.—To review the published literature on serum 25-hydroxyvitamin D concentrations in US children.

Data Sources.—Articles were identified by searching MEDLINE using 25-hydroxyvitamin D, vitamin D, hypovitaminosis D, vitamin D insufficiency, vitamin D deficiency, children, and adolescents as key words and by screening references from original studies.

Study Selection.—Studies were included if they fulfilled the following a priori criteria: contained a well-defined sample of children, included only healthy children, presented data on serum 25-hydroxyvitamin D concentrations, were published in the past 10 years, and were conducted in the United States.

Data Extraction.—Serum 25-hydroxyvitamin D concentrations and prevalence of low vitamin D status (hypovitaminosis D).

Data Synthesis.—Fourteen articles fulfilled the criteria. There were no consistent definitions of hypovitaminosis D; values corresponding to vitamin D deficiency ranged from less than 5 ng/mL to less than 12 ng/mL, and those for vitamin D insufficiency ranged from less than 10 ng/mL to less than 32 ng/mL (to convert 25-hydroxyvitamin D concentrations to nanomoles per liter, multiply by 2.496). The following assays were used: radioimmunoassay (7 studies), competitive binding protein assay (3 studies), automated chemiluminescence protein-binding assay (3 studies), and enzyme-linked immunosorbent assay (1 study). Breastfed infants in winter who did not receive vitamin D supplementation were the most severely vitamin D deficient (78%). Estimates of the prevalence of hypovitaminosis D ranged from 1% to 78%. Older age, winter season, higher body mass index, black race/ethnicity, and elevated parathyroid hormone concentrations were associated with lower 25-hydroxyvitamin D concentrations.

Conclusion.—Although overt vitamin D deficiency is no longer common in US children, lesser degrees of vitamin D insufficiency are widespread.

▶ The mountain of evidence has been emerging now in recent years that cause us to recognize the importance of vitamin D for various aspects of health. Rovner et al found that there were no significant definitions of vitamin D deficiency or of tests used to measure serum levels of vitamin D in a meta-analysis of the literature. Despite these deficiencies, the meta-analysis does clearly show that vitamin D deficiency remains prevalent, affecting healthy children of all ages and races. As one might suspect, breast-fed infants, especially during the winter months, who do not receive vitamin D supplementation, are the group most commonly affected with some degree of vitamin D deficiency. Other risk factors included being black, and having a higher body mass index. The risk is especially high in babies who are continuously swaddled with clothing as part of religious custom.

If you believe the literature, it has been estimated that 1 million people worldwide have hypovitaminosis D. In addition to the deficiency causing bone problems, the literature indicates effects of vitamin D on asthma, cancer, cardiovascular disease, diabetes, depression, and schizophrenia rates.[1]

Accompanying the Rovner et al report was one by Gordon et al.[2] The latter report attempted to calculate the prevalence of vitamin D deficiency in healthy infants and toddlers. These investigators found that 12.1% of 365 healthy infants and toddlers in the Boston, Massachusetts area had vitamin D deficiency, while 40.0% had suboptimal levels. In this report, some 90% of those who showed biochemical evidence of vitamin D deficiency also had knee and wrist radiographs. These showed "rachitic changes" in 7.5% of the children while another 33% had evidence of bone demineralization. There seems to be little doubt that the findings of the Gordon et al report are valid, but what remains is the uncertainty about what the results actually mean because the significant majority of infants with biochemical evidence of vitamin D deficiency show no bone abnormalities.

If there is anything to be learned from what we are now understanding about vitamin D deficiency in infants and toddlers, it is that a vitamin D level is not a good screening test for rickets in asymptomatic children. More than 90% of those with hypovitaminosis D (as defined by vitamin D levels) have no evidence of rickets on radiographic study. The only way out of this conundrum is to be sure that all at-risk babies must be supplemented with vitamin D.

For more on the topic of vitamin D deficiency in infants and toddlers, see the excellent summary of this topic by Taylor.[3]

J. A. Stockman III, MD

References

1. Holick MF. Vitamin D deficiency. *N Engl J Med.* 2007;357:266-281.
2. Gordon CM, Feldman HA, Sinclair L, et al. Prevalence of vitamin D deficiency among healthy infants and toddlers. *Arch Pediatr Adolesc Med.* 2008;162: 505-512.
3. Taylor JA. Defining vitamin D deficiency in infants and toddlers. *Arch Pediatr Adolesc Med.* 2008;162:583-584.

Diagnosis, symptoms, frequency and mortality of 260 patients with urea cycle disorders from a 21-year, multicentre study of acute hyperammonaemic episodes

Summar ML, Dobbelaere D, Brusilow S, et al (Vanderbilt Univ Med Ctr, Nashville, TN; Hosp Univ Med Ctr of Lille, Lille Cedex, France; Johns Hopkins Med Ctr, Baltimore, MD; et al)

Acta Pædiatr 97:1420-1425, 2008

Aim.—A large longitudinal interventional study of patients with a urea cycle disorder (UCD) in hyperammonaemic crisis was undertaken to amass a significant body of data on their presenting symptoms and survival.

Methods.—Between 1982 and 2003, as part of the FDA approval process, data were collected on patients receiving an intravenous combination of nitrogen scavenging drugs (Ammonul® sodium phenylacetate and sodium benzoate (10%, 10%)) for the treatment of hyperammonaemic crises caused by urea cycle disorders.

Results.—A final diagnosis of a UCD was made for 260 patients, representing 975 episodes of hospitalization. Only 34% of these patients presented within the first 30 days of life and had a mortality rate of 32%. The most common presenting symptoms were neurological (80%), or gastrointestinal (33%). This cohort is the largest collection of patients reported for these diseases and the first large cohort in the United States.

Conclusion.—Surprisingly, the majority (66%) of patients with heritable causes of hyperammonaemia present beyond the neonatal period

(>30 days). Patients with late-onset presenting disorders exhibited prolonged survival compared to the neonatal-presenting group.

▶ 2009 seemed to be the year in which people reflected back on urea cycle disorders. No sooner had the report of Summar et al appeared in the literature than a similar review of urea cycle diseases emanated from Finland. Most of us learned in medical school that the urea cycle was first described in 1932 by Krebs et al.[1] In Finland, the overall incidence of urea cycle disorders runs 1:39 000, a figure that is comparable to that reported in other European

TABLE 1.—Frequency of Presenting Signs and Symptoms

Symptom	First Episode n = 260	No. of Episodes Subsequent Episode n = 715	Any Episode n = 975
Any	240 (92.3%)	670 (93.7%)	910 (93.3%)
Neurological	208 (80.0%)	532 (74.4%)	740 (75.9%)
Decreased level of consciousness	164 (63.1%)	365 (51.0%)	529 (54.3%)
Altered mental status	83 (31.9%)	268 (37.5%)	351 (36.0%)
Abnormal motor function	78 (30.0%)	155 (21.7%)	233 (23.9%)
Seizures	25 (9.6%)	34 (4.8%)	59 (6.1%)
Other*	17 (6.5%)	65 (9.1%)	82 (8.4%)
Gastrointestinal	85 (32.7%)	340 (47.6%)	425 (43.6%)
Vomiting	50 (19.2%)	242 (33.8%)	292 (29.9%)
Poor feeding	24 (9.2%)	75 (10.5%)	99 (10.2%)
Diarrhoea	9 (3.5%)	58 (8.1%)	67 (6.9%)
Nausea	9 (3.5%)	31 (4.3%)	40 (4.1%)
Constipation	0	9 (1.3%)	9 (0.9%)
Other†	13 (5.0%)	73 (10.2%)	86 (8.8%)
Co-morbid conditions	118 (45.4%)	299 (41.8%)	417 (42.8%)
Infection	75 (30.0%)	252 (35.2%)	330 (33.8%)
Respiratory	16 (6.2%)	57 (8.0%)	73 (7.5%)
Renal	17 (6.5%)	12 (1.7%)	29 (3.0%)
Cardiovascular	10 (3.8%)	3 (0.4%)	13 (1.3%)
Haematological	7 (2.7%)	6 (0.8%)	13 (1.3%)
Hepatic	3 (1.2%)	1 (0.1%)	4 (0.4%)
Other‡	15 (5.8%)	27 (3.8%)	42 (4.3%)
General/constitutional	35 (13.5%)	84 (11.7%)	119 (12.2%)
Fever	17 (3.5%)	56 (7.8%)	73 (7.5%)
Dehydration	11 (4.2%)	26 (3.6%)	37 (3.8%)
Hypothermia	5 (1.9%)	1 (0.1%)	6 (0.6%)
Weight loss	2 (0.8%)	2 (0.3%)	4 (0.4%)
Failure to thrive	0	1 (0.1%)	1 (0.1%)
Other§	2 (0.8%)	3 (0.4%)	5 (0.5%)
Routine check-up	0	18 (2.5%)	18 (1.8%)

*Includes headache, stroke, cerebral oedema, cerebral haemorrhage, cortical blindness, hemianopsia with scotoma and burning eyes.
†Includes abdominal pain, gastritis, duodenitis, ileus, gastro-oesophageal reflux, gastrointestinal (GI) dysmotility, intestinal obstruction, irritable bowel syndrome, pancreatitis, GI bleed, duodenal atresia, gastroparesis, pyloric ulcer and pyloric stenosis.
‡Includes rash, fracture, burn, surgery, cholelithiasis, ovarian cyst, hernia and necrosis of femoral heads.
§Includes hypovolaemia, paleness, puffiness and oedema.
(Reprinted from Summar ML, Dobbelaere D, Brusilow S, et al. Diagnosis, symptoms, frequency and mortality of 260 patients with urea cycle disorders from a 21-year, multicentre study of acute hyperammonaemic episodes. *Acta Pædiatr.* 2008;97:1420-1425.)

countries.[2] In the United States, the incidence of these disorders is roughly estimated to be at least 1:25 000 births, but partial defects may mean that the number is much higher. Urea cycle deficiencies basically are made up of 4 types: carbamyl phosphate synthetase I (CPS-I); ornithine transcarbamylase (OTC); argininosuccinate synthetase (AS); argininosuccinate lyase (AL); or the cofactor producer N-acetyl glutamate synthetase (NAGS). These disorders result in the accumulation of ammonia or other metabolites during the first few days of life in those who have severe deficiencies. In milder or partial urea cycle enzyme deficiencies, high blood ammonia levels may be triggered by illness or stress at almost any time of life resulting in multiple mild elevations of plasma ammonia concentration. In such cases, the hyperammonaemias are less severe and the symptoms more subtle than in patients with early-onset disease. The report of Summar et al is important because it is the largest summary of urea cycle defects in terms of patient numbers than has ever been reported. The data are somewhat revealing in that they contradict the commonly held belief that urea cycle defects are primarily disorders of the newborn period. Even when female carriers are excluded, the most common presentation period for all diseases seems to be now outside the newborn period. Two-thirds of all patients showed late onset disease, and childhood (age 2 to 12 years) appears to be another vulnerable time period for the first hyperammonemic episode. Thus, all of us caring for children, including older children, and those taking care of adults, should strongly consider a diagnosis of a urea cycle defect when confronted with the relevant signs and symptoms. Diagnosis is important since the data of Summar et al show that the highest mortality peaks for all disorders roughly close to the time of initial presentation.

The survival data from this study are somewhat more encouraging than the commonly held belief that these are fatal disorders. In all disease groups, at least 50% of patients were alive at 5 years with mortality correlating closely with age of presentation, with the newborn group having the lowest survival statistics. The data also justify the consideration of alternative therapies such as liver transplantation in those enzyme deficiencies such as OTC and CPS-I that present in the neonatal period. As was suspected, the clinical presentation of most patients was associated with neurological signs (Table 1). Almost 65% of patients showed decreased level of consciousness at the first episode. Just 20% presented with vomiting. In addition to fatigue, lethargy, drowsiness, unresponsiveness, coma or obtundation, many patients presented with abnormal motor function such as slurred speech, tremors, weakness, decreased or increased muscle tone, and ataxia. Altered mental status presenting with irritability, tantrums, strange behavior, dizziness, confusion, agitation, and combativeness was slightly more frequent at subsequent episodes than at the first episode.

J. A. Stockman III, MD

References

1. Krebs HA, Henseleit K. Untersuchungen uber die harnstoffbildung im tierkorper. *Hoppe-Seyler's Z Physiol Chem.* 1932;210:325-332.
2. Keskinen P, Siitonen A, Salo M. Hereditary urea cycle diseases in Finland. *Acta Paediatr.* 2008;97:1412-1419.

16 Oncology

Childhood cancer in the offspring born in 1921–1984 to US radiologic technologists

Johnson KJ, Alexander BH, Doody MM, et al (Univ of Minnesota, Minneapolis; Nat Insts of Health, Bethesda, MD; et al)

Br J Cancer 99:545-550, 2008

We examined the risk of childhood cancer (< 20 years) among 105 950 offspring born in 1921–1984 to US radiologic technologist (USRT) cohort members. Parental occupational *in utero* and preconception ionising radiation (IR) testis or ovary doses were estimated from work history data, badge dose data, and literature doses (the latter doses before 1960). Female and male RTs reported a total of 111 and 34 haematopoietic malignancies and 115 and 34 solid tumours, respectively, in their offspring. Hazard ratios (HRs) and 95% confidence intervals (CIs) were calculated using Cox proportional hazards regression. Leukaemia ($n = 63$) and solid tumours ($n = 115$) in offspring were not associated with maternal *in utero* or preconception radiation exposure. Risks for lymphoma ($n = 44$) in those with estimated doses of <0.2, 0.2–1.0, and >1.0 mGy *vs* no exposure were non-significantly elevated with HRs of 2.3, 1.8, and 2.7. Paternal preconception exposure to estimated cumulative doses above the 95th percentile (≥ 82 mGy, $n = 6$ cases) was associated with a non-significant risk of childhood cancer of 1.8 (95% CI 0.7–4.6). In conclusion, we found no convincing evidence of an increased risk of childhood cancer in the offspring of RTs in association with parental occupational radiation exposure.

▶ It is actually not too terribly difficult to study childhood cancer incidence in the offspring of radiology technologists. Both preconception and in utero occupational radiation exposure effects on offspring cancer risk can be readily studied. Studies of medical radiation workers have reported increases in the incidence and mortality of skin cancer, breast cancer, and leukemia, especially in individuals who started working before 1950, when both radiation doses and permitted levels of exposure were higher. The only study of childhood cancer incidence in the offspring of medical radiology workers found no excess risk.[1]

This report from Minnesota looked at the incidence of childhood cancer in over 100 000 offspring born from 1929 through 1984 to radiology technicians here in the United States. Both men and women radiology technicians were included in the report. Given the several decades long observational period, as one would suspect, the occupational dose of radiation decreased fairly markedly from the 1930s through the 1980s, by almost 6-fold. No significant increase in risk or dose-response was found for leukemia, lymphoma, solid tumors, or childhood cancer overall in association with in utero radiation exposure. No appreciable increased risk or dose-response was observed between maternal preconception exposure and childhood cancer. Paternal exposure doses above the 95th percentile were associated with a nonstatistically significant increased risk of 1.8 relative to a reference group on the basis of 6 offspring who developed cancer (2 leukemias, 2 lymphomas, 1 sarcoma, and 1 oral cancer).

Overall, the data from this report do not indicate that there is an increased risk of childhood cancer in the offspring of radiation technicians who are exposed to occupational radiation either in utero or as the result of preconception exposure. Consistent with these results, most previous studies have not provided strong support for an association between childhood cancer and parental preconception exposures to either low or high doses of atomic bomb radiation, medical or nuclear occupational radiation, or therapeutic or diagnostic medical radiation. Please recognize, however, that this study has some limitations. Electronic files of film-badge doses were not routinely available until the late 1970s. To estimate the exposure doses going back some decades, the investigators undertook a comprehensive dose reconstruction that used hundreds of thousands of badge doses from electronic files from 1977 onward, thousands of badge doses from hard copy records for the period 1960-1976, and literature-based dose data for the period before 1960. These dose reconstructions are somewhat imperfect, although they are likely to be adequate for the purposes of this study.

The bottom line here is that while this report does not have data that are sufficient to detect very small increases in cancer risk, one can conclude with reasonable certainty that the risk of cancer is not remarkably increased, if at all, in the offspring of radiology technologists. The findings have important implications in many other situations and therefore the data from this report are useful.

J. A. Stockman III, MD

Reference

1. Roman E, Doyle P, Ansell P, Bull D, Beral V. Health of children born to medical radiographers. *Occup Environ Med.* 1996;53:73-79.

Computed tomography before transfer to a level I pediatric trauma center risks duplication with associated increased radiation exposure
Chwals WJ, Robinson AV, Sivit CJ, et al (Case Western Reserve Univ School of Med, Cleveland, OH)
J Pediatr Surg 43:2268-2272, 2008

Introduction.—Community hospitals commonly obtain computed tomographic (CT) imaging of pediatric trauma patients before triaging to a level I pediatric trauma center (PTC). This practice potentially increases radiation exposure when imaging must be duplicated after transfer.

Methods.—A retrospective review of our level 1 PTC registry from January 1, 2004, to December 31, 2006, was conducted. Level I and II trauma patients were grouped based on whether they had undergone outside CT examination (head and/or abdomen) at a referring hospital (group 1) or received initial CT examination at our institution (group 2). Subgroups were analyzed based on whether duplicate CT examination was required at our PTC (Fischer's Exact test).

Results.—A duplicate CT scan (within 4 hours of transfer) was required in 91% (30/33) of group 1 transfer patients, whereas no group 2 patient required a duplicate scan (0/55; $P < .0001$). There was no significant difference within the groups for weight, age, or intensive care unit length of stay.

Conclusion.—A significant number of pediatric trauma patients who receive CT scans at referring hospitals before transfer to our level I PTC require duplicate scans of the same anatomical field(s) after transfer, exposing them to increased potential clinical risk and cost.

▶ The data are mounting suggesting that we are using CT scans far more often than may be needed. One example of this is the fact that so many children with a common problem, acute appendicitis, are undergoing CT scans for diagnostic purposes when the clinical examination, in and of itself, or supporting laboratory data would seem to be sufficient for the diagnosis.[1] The CT scanner has replaced ultrasound in most instances as a diagnostic procedure for acute appendicitis. What we see in the report of Chwals et al is that all too many pediatric patients with trauma are undergoing CT imaging before transfer to a trauma center. Advanced Trauma Life Support guidelines for the evaluation of level I and II trauma specifically do not include CT examinations before transfer of the patient to a trauma center for definitive care. This use of CT imaging for triage has a number of unfortunate consequences including a delay in the time associated with the CT examination. Such testing also increases radiation exposure and adds cost since invariably the CT scans will be repeated. While an abdominal CT with contrast, for example, can take only 10 minutes to perform, the actual time from ordering to transfer it back to the emergency room can take the better part of an hour in most instances. This is all too long a time for a potentially seriously injured child.

The best available estimate of the lifetime cancer mortality risk attributable to the radiation exposure from a single abdominal CT scan in a one-year-old child is approximately 1 in 550 to 1 in 1500 for a head CT examination. These estimated risks are in order of magnitude higher than for a similar study done in adults. In the United States, at least 600 000 abdominal and head CT examinations are performed per year on children younger than 15 years of age. If one runs the math, approximately 500 of these youngsters will ultimately develop cancer attributable to the radiation from a CT scan. Some of this risk can be minimized by use of equipment that appropriately restricts radiation exposure based on body mass. The risk described obviously doubles if a CT scan is repeated because of one that was unnecessarily performed before transport to a regional trauma center.

J. A. Stockman III, MD

Reference

1. Wong KKY, Cheung TWY, Tam PKH. Diagnosing acute otitis media: are we over-using radiologic investigations? *J Pediatr Surg.* 2008;43:2239-2241.

Breast Cancer Surveillance Practices Among Women Previously Treated With Chest Radiation for a Childhood Cancer

Oeffinger KC, Ford JS, Moskowitz CS, et al (Memorial Sloan-Kettering Cancer Ctr, NY; et al)
JAMA 301:404-414, 2009

Context.—Women treated with chest radiation for a pediatric malignancy have a significantly increased risk of breast cancer at a young age and are recommended to have an annual screening mammogram starting at age 25 years or 8 years after radiation, whichever occurs last.

Objective.—To characterize the breast cancer surveillance practices among female pediatric cancer survivors who were treated with chest radiation and identify correlates of screening.

Design, Setting, and Participants.—Between June 2005 and August 2006, a 114-item questionnaire was administered to a random sample of 625 women aged 25 through 50 years who had survived pediatric cancer, who had been treated with chest radiation, and who were participating in the Childhood Cancer Survivor Study (CCSS), a North American cohort of long-term survivors diagnosed from 1970-1986. Comparisons were made with similarly aged pediatric cancer survivors not treated with chest radiation (n = 639) and the CCSS siblings cohort (n = 712).

Main Outcome Measure.—Screening mammogram within the previous 2 years.

Results.—Of 1976 cancer survivors and siblings who were contacted, 87.9% participated. Among the 551 women with a history of chest radiation, 55% reported a screening mammogram in the past 2 years (ages 25-39 years, 36.5%; 95% confidence interval [CI], 31.0%-42.0%; ages 40-50 years, 76.5%; 95% CI, 71.3%-81.7%). In comparison, 40.5% of survivors without chest radiation and 37.0% of CCSS siblings reported a screening mammogram in the same time interval. Notably, among women with a history of chest radiation, 47.3% (95% CI; 41.6%-53.0%) of those younger than 40 years had never had a mammogram and only 52.6% (95% CI; 46.4%-58.8%) of women aged 40 through 50 years were being regularly screened (2 mammograms within 4 years). Screening rates were higher among women who reported a physician recommendation than those who did not (ages 25-39 years, 76.0% vs 17.6%; ages 40-50 years, 87.3% vs 58.3%). In multivariate models, the association was particularly strong for younger women (ages 25-39 years, prevalence ratio [PR], 3.0; 95% CI, 2.0-4.0; ages 40-50 years, PR, 1.3; 95% CI, 1.1-1.6).

Conclusions.—In this cohort of women who had childhood cancer treated with chest radiation, 63.5% of those aged 25 through 39 years and 23.5% of those aged 40 through 50 years had not had mammography screening for breast cancer within the previous 2 years despite a guideline recommendation that survivors of childhood cancer who were treated with chest radiation should undergo annual screening mammography.

▶ Breast cancer is a well-known complication of chest irradiation for childhood cancer. Current recommendations for surveillance of this problem include the need for regular clinical examination and annual screening mammography beginning just 8 years after the radiation therapy is completed or starting at age 25 years, whichever is appropriate depending on the initial age of the child at the time of irradiation. The median age of the onset of breast cancer for those who have been treated with chest irradiation in childhood ranges from 32 to 35 years depending on what study one reads. This risk is greatest among women who have been treated with high-dose mantle radiation for Hodgkin lymphoma. By 45 years of age, it is estimated that from 12% to 20% of women treated with moderate-to-high dose chest radiation will be diagnosed with breast cancer. These numbers are as high as nonirradiated women who carry the *BRCA* gene mutation, illustrating just how problematic postirradiation breast cancer is.

What we see in the report of Oeffinger et al is that we are not doing a very good job of surveillance of pediatric cancer survivors who have received chest irradiation. The investigators found that just a little over half of women in the chest irradiation therapy group reported having a screening mammogram within the previous 2 years. The rates of screening mammography varied by age at the time of delivery, with less than 25% of women aged 25 through 39 years and 53.6% of women 40 to 50 years reporting a screening mammogram in the previous year.

The most current Childhood Oncology Group (COG) guidelines for breast cancer surveillance after pediatric cancer in the United States recommend yearly clinical breast examination from the age of puberty until 25 years, and then every 6 months if the survivor was treated with irradiation of at least 20 Gy to mantle, minimantle, mediastinal, chest (thoracic), or axillary fields. In addition, it is recommended that these survivors have annual mammography and adjunct breast magnetic resonance imaging (MRI) starting at age 25 years or 8 years after radiation, whichever is last. The effectiveness of the standard mammogram in detecting preinvasive and invasive breast cancer is relatively poor in young women due to the density of breast tissue in this age group, increasing the importance of MRI in the detection and diagnosis of breast cancer in young women. This approach, of course, raises the issue of whether there is a risk from getting frequent mammograms. The estimated dose of radiation from a standard 2-view screening mammogram is approximately 3.85 mGy per mammogram. Although it is accepted that the additional dose is small compared with the higher therapeutic dose already received, it is not known to what extent repeated exposure to small doses of breast irradiation in women already at increased risk of breast cancer may result in an increased risk of second primary breast cancer. This is an important question that needs further investigation.

The increased risk of breast cancer experienced by survivors of childhood cancer constitutes just one long-term health risk. Other effects of radiation include impaired bone growth, endocrine deficiencies, and potential long-term cardiac effects, particularly of anthracycline chemotherapy. As the number of adult survivors of childhood cancer increases, attention will need to be given to these "survivorship issues." Appropriate transition of care from the pediatric oncology team to adult providers is critical so that none of these youngsters as they grow up fall between the cracks of our health care system. It is fairly clear from the data of Oeffinger et al that only about half of women at risk for breast cancer are being adequately and carefully followed for the risk they carry with them throughout the remainder of their lives.

J. A. Stockman III, MD

Male reproductive health after childhood cancer

Lähteenmäki PM, Arola M, Suominen J, et al (Turku Univ Central Hosp, Finland)
Acta Paediatr 97:935-942, 2008

Aim.—Twenty-five male patients were investigated to elucidate the correlation of semen parameters and other related parameters in the assessment of spermatogenesis after childhood cancer treatment.

Methods.—Evaluation of given cancer treatment, anthropometric and testicular size measurements, semen analysis, and measurement of gonadotrophins, testosterone, sex hormone-binding globulin (SHBG), and inhibin B were performed according to a protocol.

Results.—Median (range) sperm concentration (SC) was 35.5 (0-273)×10(6)/mL, and percentage of motile sperm 56 (0-86)%. Testicular size (r = 0.73, p < 0.001) and the level of inhibin B (r = 0.66, p < 0.001) correlated strongly to SC. SC correlated negatively to FSH (r = 0.46, p = 0.03). Only testicular size predicted SC significantly (p = 0.03). Inhibin B showed highest area under ROC curve (0.83, 95% CI 0.67-0.99) in showing SC<20×10(6)/mL. Body mass index (BMI) did not correlate with SC, but negative correlation between BMI and SHBG was found (r = −0.41, p = 0.04).

Conclusion.—Although semen analysis is a useful instrument for fertility assessment in men, it is often difficult to get these samples from childhood cancer survivors. Thus, indirect methods are needed in prediction of possible sperm count impairment in postpubertal adolescents after cancer treatment. When combined with the data on testicular size and follicle-stimulating hormone (FSH) level, inhibin B gives valuable addition to the estimations of spermatogenesis.

▶ The authors of this report do us a great favor by reminding us about a common, but often not addressed, long-term sequela of cancer therapy, that of infertility/sterility in boys. About 15% of male survivors of childhood acute lymphoblastic leukemia have been shown to have reduced fertility when determined either directly with semen samples or indirectly with increased levels of gonadotropins and reduced testicular volume. While this may be the result of the administration of chemotherapy, cranial irradiation also plays a role. Also, there are studies suggesting impaired fertility in up to two-thirds of survivors of childhood solid tumors. Survivors of childhood Hodgkin lymphoma, depending on the stage of the disease and the intensity of the chemotherapy, have anywhere from a 30% to 60% likelihood of having elevated follicle-stimulating hormone (FSH) levels, suggesting an organ testicular failure. Irreversible azoospermia or oligozoospermia have been reported in 63% and 32% of survivors of childhood Hodgkin's disease, respectively.[1]

In this report from Finland, adult survivors of childhood cancer were evaluated to see if they had evidence of reduced fertility. In addition to measuring sperm count and sperm mobility, the study also included serum samples that measured levels of inhibin B. Not all men are willing to give a sperm sample, thus the reason for measuring inhibin B. The latter has been considered as a serum marker of spermatogenesis.[2] Serum levels of inhibin B correlate with FSH and possibly with sperm density, offering the hope that inhibin B may be a direct marker of seminiferous tubular damage and may aid in the prediction of normospermia. In this study, the median values for inhibin B were clearly less in cancer survivors than in controls. Measuring inhibin B provided valuable additional information on the likelihood of an individual being infertile.

If there is one take-home message from this report, it is that we should be thinking about assessing the consequences of our cancer therapies while our patients are still on our watch. There are ways of doing this, shy of having to get semen samples from boys. Measurement of serum inhibin B may tell us a lot because the damaging effects of radiation and/or chemotherapy on seminiferous tubules occur early in disease management.

J. A. Stockman III, MD

References

1. Heikens J, Behrandt H, Adriaanse R, Berghout A. Irreversible gonadal damage in male survivors of pediatric Hodgkin's disease. *Cancer.* 1996;78:2020-2024.
2. Wallace EM, Groome NP, Riley SC, Parker AC, Wu FC. The effects of chemotherapy-induced testicular damage on Inhibin B, gonadotropin, and testosterone secretion: a prospective longitudinal study. *J Clin Endocrinol Metab.* 1997;82:3111-3115.

Do doctors discuss fertility issues before they treat young patients with cancer?

Anderson RA, Weddell A, Spoudeas HA, et al (Univ of Edinburgh, UK; Great Ormond Street Hosp and Univ College Hosps, London, UK; et al)
Hum Reprod 23:2246-2251, 2008

Background.—Many children treated for cancer are at risk of infertility, but for girls and prepubertal boys, all fertility preservation techniques remain experimental. We have assessed UK practice relating to information provision about the effects of cancer treatment on fertility and options for fertility preservation.

Methods.—Paediatric oncologists prospectively completed a data form for each new patient registered over a 12 month period.

Results.—Data were available on 1030 patients (68% of total registered). The effect of cancer treatment on fertility was discussed with 63% of patients. Of these, 61% were judged to be at high or medium risk of fertility problems. Discussions took place more commonly with boys than girls; the commonest reason for discussion not occurring was young age. The majority (83%) of post-pubertal boys assessed as high/medium risk of infertility were referred for semen cryopreservation. This rate fell to 39% of those in early puberty. Only 1% ($n = 4$) of girls were referred to an assisted conception unit.

Conclusions.—These data indicate a high awareness of the potential adverse effects of therapy on fertility among UK paediatric oncologists. High referral rates for older boys indicate that current guidelines are followed, but there is a need for fertility preservation techniques for girls and younger boys.

▶ The prospect of infertility associated with the therapies we provide to children with cancer should always be on our minds as therapy is initiated. Chemotherapy and radiation therapy reduce the number of germ cells within the ovary and decrease testicular spermatogenesis. This reduction is related to the dose, agent use, and age at treatment. In addition, patients are at risk of permanent gonadal failure. It should also be recognized that the persistence of menstrual cycles after treatment in no way precludes the presence of ovarian damage, and the preservation of testosterone production does not confirm the preservation of spermatogenesis.

There are options available for children with cancer in order to maximally preserve fertility. Adolescent boys preparing for chemotherapy can be offered semen cryostorage, which has been shown to be effective in many small observational studies and is recommended by the American Society for Clinical Oncology. Large studies have found no increase in abnormalities in children born after semen cryopreservation, although sperm that have been frozen may be less effective in assisted reproduction. The situation for girls is substantially less varied in terms of option. If there truly is a high risk of infertility related to a particular therapy, one could consider the harvesting of oocytes and the freezing of these, although this is infrequently done.

Children pose a particularly difficult ethical problem when it comes to pres-ervation of fertility because while they may have some insight into the potential effect of their cancer treatment on their fertility, it is usually their parents who are more worried about preserving reproductive functioning. There are many ethical considerations that have to be taken into account if one were to consider something like surgery for testicular extraction of sperm in an adolescent male unable to masturbate or in a prepubertal or early adolescent girl if one were to consider ovarian tissue harvesting. In most cases, the secondary consequence of chemotherapy and/or radiation therapy are not paramount considerations when the primary goal is to achieve a lifelong cure of the disease. Adoption is always a possibility.

J. A. Stockman III, MD

Deletion of *IKZF1* and Prognosis in Acute Lymphoblastic Leukemia
Mullighan CG, the Children's Oncology Group (St. Jude Children's Research Hosp, Memphis, TN; et al)
N Engl J Med 360:470-480, 2009

Background.—Despite best current therapy, up to 20% of pediatric patients with acute lymphoblastic leukemia (ALL) have a relapse. Recent genomewide analyses have identified a high frequency of DNA copy-number abnormalities in ALL, but the prognostic implications of these abnormalities have not been defined.

Methods.—We studied a cohort of 221 children with high-risk B-cell-progenitor ALL with the use of single-nucleotide–polymorphism microar-rays, transcriptional profiling, and resequencing of samples obtained at diagnosis. Children with known very-high-risk ALL subtypes (i.e., BCR-ABL1–positive ALL, hypodiploid ALL, and ALL in infants) were excluded from this cohort. A copy-number abnormality was identified as a predictor of poor outcome, and it was then tested in an independent validation cohort of 258 patients with B-cell-progenitor ALL.

Results.—More than 50 recurring copy-number abnormalities were identified, most commonly involving genes that encode regulators of B-cell development (in 66.8% of patients in the original cohort); *PAX5* was involved in 31.7% and *IKZF1* in 28.6% of patients. Using copy-number abnormalities, we identified a predictor of poor outcome that was validated in the independent validation cohort. This predictor was strongly associated with alteration of *IKZF1*, a gene that encodes the lymphoid transcription factor IKAROS. The gene-expression signature of the group of patients with a poor outcome revealed increased expres-sion of hematopoietic stem-cell genes and reduced expression of B-cell-lineage genes, and it was similar to the signature of BCR-ABL1–positive ALL, another high-risk subtype of ALL with a high frequency of *IKZF1* deletion.

Conclusions.—Genetic alteration of *IKZF1* is associated with a very poor outcome in B-cell-progenitor ALL.

▶ This report reminds us that we still have a bit of a way to go in curing all cases of childhood acute lymphoblastic leukemia (ALL). There are a number of risk factors for poor survivorship with ALL. One of these, of course, is age at diagnosis. If there is a "good" age to have leukemia, it is somewhere between 2 and 7 years. Older youngsters generally do not do quite as well with ALL. A recent report, for example, tells us that historically ALL, while an uncommon disease in adults, has been highly fatal.[1] Nonetheless, in the last 30 years major improvements in survival have been observed for adult patients less than 60 years of age, an improvement in survival that is greater for women than for men. The greatest improvement in adult ALL survival is now seen in patients aged 15 to 19, in whom 5-year relative survival has improved over a couple of decade period from 41% to 61%. Lesser but significant improvements have been seen in all other adult age groups except for those over age 60. In the latter age group, survivorship with ALL has remained unchanged at levels at or below 10%.

The report of Mulligan et al gives us new insights into risk stratification in B-cell-progenitor ALL. Recent genome-wide analyses of DNA copy-number abnormalities have identified numerous recurring genetic alterations in ALL. The report of Mullighan et al tells us about a study of copy-number abnormalities in 221 children with high-risk ALL. The investigators identified a predictor of poor outcome based on copy-number abnormalities that was driven by the deletion or mutation of *IKZF1*, which is associated with an extraordinarily high risk of relapse. The data from this investigation and several others that have appeared in recent years tell us how critical accurate risk stratification is for ensuring that patients with high-risk ALL receive treatment of appropriate intensity and that low-risk patients are spared unnecessary toxic chemotherapy.

When this editor was a resident and fellow, all we had to look at was a bone marrow to make a diagnosis of ALL and risk was largely dependent on age and level of white blood cell count at the time of diagnosis. Risk stratification currently is based primarily on clinical variables, immunophenotype, detection of sentinel cytogenetic or molecular lesions, and early response to therapy. To this we now have to add genome-wide copy-number analysis for the detection of genetic lesions known to be associated with clinical outcomes. Most striking is the strong association between the mutations of *IKZF1* and poor outcomes. IKAROS is a transcription factor with well-established roles in lymphopoiesis and cancer. The gene related to this transcription factor (*IKZF1*) is a common target of retroviruses that are mutagenetic.

There is no such thing as the "Lone Oncologist" any more than there ever really was a "Lone Ranger." By that is meant that the cure of childhood cancer is a team activity. That team includes a robust molecular genetic laboratory that is capable of underpinning the clinician's work. A CBC, bone marrow slide, and a clinical examination no longer cut it when it comes to establishing an accurate diagnosis or prognosis.

J. A. Stockman III, MD

Reference

1. Pulte D, Gondos A, Brenner H. Improvement in survival in younger patients with acute lymphoblastic leukemia from the 1980s to the early 21st century. *Blood.* 2009;113:1408-1411.

Clinical significance of minimal residual disease in childhood acute lymphoblastic leukemia and its relationship to other prognostic factors: a Children's Oncology Group study

Borowitz MJ, Devidas M, Hunger SP, et al (Johns Hopkins Med Insts, Daltimore, MD; Univ of Florida, Gainesville; Univ of Colorado Denver; et al)
Blood 111:5477-5485, 2008

Minimal residual disease (MRD) is an important predictor of relapse in acute lymphoblastic leukemia (ALL), but its relationship to other prognostic variables has not been fully assessed. The Children's Oncology Group studied the prognostic impact of MRD measured by flow cytometry in the peripheral blood at day 8, and in end-induction (day 29) and end-consolidation marrows in 2143 children with precursor B-cell ALL (B-ALL). The presence of MRD in day-8 blood and day-29 marrow MRD was associated with shorter event-free survival (EFS) in all risk groups; even patients with 0.01% to 0.1% day-29 MRD had poor outcome compared with patients negative for MRD patients (59% ± 5% vs 88% ± 1% 5 year EFS). Presence of good prognostic markers TEL-AML1 or trisomies of chromosomes 4 and 10 still provided additional prognostic information, but not in National Cancer Institute high-risk (NCI HR) patients who were MRD⁺. The few patients with detectable MRD at end of consolidation fared especially poorly, with only a 43% plus or minus 7% 5-year EFS. Day-29 marrow MRD was the most important prognostic variable in multi-variate analysis. The 12% of patients with all favorable risk factors, including NCI risk group, genetics, and absence of days 8 and 29 MRD, had a 97% plus or minus 1% 5-year EFS with nonintensive therapy. These studies are registered at www.clinicaltrials.gov as NCT00005585, NCT00005596, and NCT00005603.

▶ When this editor was a fellow in pediatric hematology, more years ago than one would like to recall, the only way to know whether a patient had minimal residual disease following induction therapy was to do a bone marrow examination to see if you could find any blasts less than 5% when the patient was in remission. That was the best we could do. Since that time, it has been recognized that the presence of minimal residual disease following therapy for acute lymphoblastic leukemia (ALL) is an important prognostic marker in numerous studies. Minimal residual disease is now detected either by polymerase chain reaction (PCR) amplification of clonotypic immunoglobulin or by flow cytometry, the latter based on the principle that leukemic cells express combinations of antigens that are different from those present on normal bone marrow cells. The former technique can be more sensitive, though to achieve adequate sensitivity, it is necessary to synthesize optimized clone-specific reagents. As a consequence, it is often difficult to use the information provided by this technique in real time to make clinical decisions. Although less well standardized, flow cytometry is faster, generally less expensive, and provides informative results in a higher percentage of patients and does so quite quickly. For this reason, flow cytometry is the technique most often used to detect residual disease and it has the potential for rapidly identifying patients at increased risk of relapse, allowing for prompt changes in therapy, including earlier intensification.

Although minimal residual disease has been shown to retain prognostic significance even adjusting for some other common risk factors (eg, age, white blood cell count, cytogenetic features of blasts, etc), the relationship between minimal residual disease and other prognostic factors has been incompletely explored. It is not clear if minimal residual disease by itself is all that is needed to predict outcome, if other risk factors add additional information, or whether there are complex interactions between these factors and the presence of minimal residual disease.

Back in 1999, the Pediatric Oncology Group began a prospective study of minimal residual disease to sort out some of these issues. The report of Borowitz et al describes the relationship of minimal residual disease to outcomes taking into account various other risk factors. The results demonstrate that the single most powerful prognostic marker of poor outcome is the presence of minimal residual disease at the end of the induction therapy. This statement applies in all clinical- and laboratory-defined risk groups. It was also clear in this report that flow cytometry, although lacking in sensitivity compared with certain molecular techniques such as PCR, does provide results very early in therapy allowing changes to be made shortly after, or conceivably even during induction. Early intensification of therapy has been shown to help patients with slow response to therapy. Measurement of minimal residual disease in the peripheral blood at day 8 provides additional useful information, especially to identify patients at low risk for relapse. In fact, measurement of minimal residual disease at day 8 in peripheral blood followed by examination for minimal residual disease at the end of induction therapy eliminates the need for earlier bone marrow examination. By combining all favorable good risk features, the addition of studies of minimal residual disease makes it possible to identify a group of patients that account for about 12% of all children with precursor (B)-ALL who are almost certain to be cured with limited therapy, avoiding the need for high toxicity drugs such as anthracycline or alkylating agents.

J. A. Stockman III, MD

Genome-wide Interrogation of Germline Genetic Variation Associated with Treatment Response in Childhood Acute Lymphoblastic Leukemia

Yang JJ, Cheng C, Yang W, et al (St Jude Children's Res Hosp, Memphis, TN; et al)

JAMA 301:393-403, 2009

Context.—Pediatric acute lymphoblastic leukemia (ALL) is the proto-type for a drug-responsive malignancy. Although cure rates exceed 80%, considerable unexplained interindividual variability exists in treatment response.

Objectives.—To assess the contribution of inherited genetic variation to therapy response and to identify germline single-nucleotide polymor-phisms (SNPs) associated with risk of minimal residual disease (MRD) after remission induction chemotherapy.

Design, Setting, and Patients.—Genome wide interrogation of 176 796 germline SNPs to identify genotypes that were associated with MRD in 2 independent cohorts of children with newly diagnosed ALL: 318 patients in St Jude Total Therapy protocols XIIIB and XV and 169 patients in Children's Oncology Group trial P9906. Patients were enrolled between 1994 and 2006 and last follow-up was in 2006.

Main Outcome Measures.—Minimal residual disease at the end of induction therapy, measured by flow cytometry.

Results.—There were 102 SNPs associated with MRD in both cohorts (median odds ratio, 2.18; $P \leq .0125$), including 5 SNPs in the interleukin 15 (*IL15*) gene. Of these 102 SNPs, 21 were also associated with hemato-logic relapse ($P < .05$). Of 102 SNPs, 21 were also associated with antileu-kemic drug disposition, generally linking MRD eradication with greater drug exposure. In total, 63 of 102 SNPs were associated with early response, relapse, or drug disposition.

Conclusion.—Host genetic variations are associated with treatment response for childhood ALL, with polymorphisms related to leukemia cell biology and host drug disposition associated with lower risk of residual disease.

▶ Childhood acute lymphoblastic leukemia (ALL) has long served as a proto-type for a malignancy that is curable by drugs. Early minimal residual disease measures are strongly associated with cure rates and are used to modify therapy. One likes to see the lowest burden of disease after initial go-rounds with anticancer drugs used to treat ALL. Eradication of minimal residual disease is affected by genetic characteristics of the blast cells (eg, the Philadelphia chromosome) and by host characteristics such as age. A few germline genetic variations have also been shown to affect the level of minimal residual disease, but this has not been previously assessed on a genome-wide level. The inves-tigators in the report abstracted used a genome-wide interrogation to identify 102 germline genetic variations associated with the level of residual leukemia and found that a high proportion of those discovered also affected early response, relapse risk, or antileukemic drug disposition. Specifically, these investigators identified germline single-nucleotide polymorphisms (SNPs) that were likely to produce adverse outcomes.

Because genome-wide interrogations for pharmacogenetics are still in their infancy, there are no published whole-genome data linking polymorphisms with anticancer drug response. The authors of this report did look for SNPs that affected the clearance of 2 antileukemic agents (etoposide and methotrexate) and the intracellular disposition of the latter. More than 20 SNPs were significantly associated with the disposition of these 2 antileukemic agents.

Now that we know a great deal more about the human genome, we are learning how what otherwise we might have considered subtle variations in our genes in fact do affect the outcome of many disease states, including childhood leukemia. The authors of this report remark that although the acquired genetic variations of tumor cells play a critical role in drug responsiveness, the results of their studies show that inherited genetic variation also influences the effectiveness of anticancer therapy, and that genome-wide approaches can identify novel and yet plausible pharmacogenetic variations. It will not be too far down the line that such variations will be factored into treatment decisions allowing additional emphasis on optimizing drug delivery to overcome host genetic variations, in addition to the current emphasis on tumor genetic variation.

There once was a time that when a child with ALL presented and you did a bone marrow examination, you simply started induction therapy and hoped for the best. Now and forever after, we will be assessing a great deal more about the nature of the malignant cell and the host that is carrying that cell as we embark on our treatment protocols.

J. A. Stockman III, MD

Twenty-five–year follow-up among survivors of childhood acute lymphoblastic leukemia: a report from the Childhood Cancer Survivor Study
Mody R, Li S, Dover DC, et al (Univ of Michigan, Ann Arbor; Univ of Alberta, Edmonton; et al)
Blood 111:5515-5523, 2008

Survivors of childhood acute lymphoblastic leukemia (ALL) are at risk for late effects of cancer therapy. Five-year ALL survivors (< 21 years at diagnosis; n = 5760 eligible, 4151 participants), diagnosed from 1970 to 1986 were compared with the general population and a sibling cohort (n = 3899). Cumulative mortality of 5760 5-year survivors was 13% at 25 years from diagnosis. Recurrent ALL (n = 483) and second neoplasms (SNs; n = 89) were the major causes of death. Among 185 survivors, 199 SNs occurred, 53% in the CNS. Survivors reported more multiple chronic medical conditions (CMCs; odds ratio [OR], 2.8; 95% CI, 2.4-3.2) and severe or life-threatening CMCs (OR, 3.6; 95% CI, 3.0-4.5) than siblings. Cumulative incidence of severe CMCs, including death, 25 years from diagnosis was 21.3% (95% CI, 18.2-24.4; 23.3% [95% CI, 19.4-27.2] and 13.4% [95% CI, 8.4-18.4] for irradiated and nonirradiated survivors, respectively). Survivors reported more adverse general and mental health, functional impairment, and activity limitations compared with siblings ($P < .001$). Rates of marriage, college graduation, employment, and health insurance were all lower compared with sibling controls ($P < .001$). Long-term survivors of childhood ALL exhibit excess mortality and morbidity. Survivors who received radiation therapy as part of their treatment or had a leukemia relapse are at greatest risk for adverse outcomes.

▶ Everyone knows that we have come a long way in the treatment of patients with acute lymphoblastic leukemia (ALL). The outcome of youngsters newly diagnosed in this decade is far better than years ago. Approximately 3000 new cases will be diagnosed each year with a 5-year overall survival approaching 90% in comparison with a 30% 5-year survival 35 to 40 years ago. As good as this news is, at the present time, many of the earliest survivors of childhood ALL, now well into adulthood, are being lost to follow up. These patients have had considerable exposure to chemotherapy and radiotherapy as children, and it is clear that many of the late effects of these therapies will not be manifested until many years later. The Childhood Cancer Survivor Study is attempting to follow these patients. It is the largest and most comprehensively characterized research study of long-term childhood cancer survivorship. This study has produced many reports dealing with late mortality, second neoplasms, chronic health conditions, and health status in survivors of childhood cancers, including ALL. This report of Mody et al from the Childhood Cancer Survivor Study provides results of a more in-depth and detailed analysis of ALL survivors.

So what do we learn from this, the largest and most comprehensive assessment of the health of childhood ALL survivors to date? It is clear from the analysis of the study data that more than 20 years from diagnosis, adult survivors of childhood ALL continue to have medical and psychosocial sequelae of their original diagnosis and therapy. All groups, including nonirradiated, nonrelapsed survivors report late effects. This latter category of patients constitute the large majority of future children who will be treated with contemporary therapies, by analogy. Second neoplasms are one of the most serious and devastating morbidities associated with cancer therapy and have been strongly associated with the use of therapeutic radiation for the treatment of the original cancer. The study data show that the central nervous system is the most common site of the second malignancy, a finding consistent with many other investigations. Regrettably, the cumulative incidence of second neoplasms is continuing to rise, even 25 years after diagnosis. Those who did not receive radiation also have a higher rate of secondary neoplasms than would be expected compared with the general population, albeit at a lower rate than cancer survivors who had received radiation therapy. Although there is a much higher risk of the development of chronic diseases among survivors of childhood leukemia, some 92% of survivors who did not relapse or receive radiation therapy are experiencing no clinical evidence of a chronic disease.

In summary, the findings from this report demonstrate that survivors of childhood ALL experience excess mortality, chronic morbidity, and poor socioeconomic outcomes for many years following completion of therapy. These late effects are greatest among survivors who had received radiation therapy or who have survived a relapse. At the same time, nonirradiated and nonrelapsed survivors also report excessive chronic health issues and poor health status, although their socioeconomic outcomes are similar to their siblings. These data demonstrate that the least therapy, including the elimination of radiotherapy if appropriate, necessary to produce good outcomes is the way to go. For this reason, it is critically important to continue to define risk factors for relapse such as the presence of minimal residual disease. If a patient presents with all favorable prognostic factors, and at the end of induction therapy has no evidence of minimal residual disease, nonaggressive therapy is in order to minimize the long-term consequences of treatment.

J. A. Stockman III, MD

Mutations of *JAK2* in acute lymphoblastic leukaemias associated with Down's syndrome

Bercovich D, Ganmore I, Scott LM, et al (Migal-Galilee Biotechnology Centre, Kiryat Shmona, and Tel-Hai Academic College, Israel; Sheba Med Centre, Tel-Hashomer, Ramat Gan, Israel; Cambridge Inst for Med Res, UK; et al)
Lancet 372:1484-1492, 2008

Background.—Children with Down's syndrome have a greatly increased risk of acute megakaryoblastic and acute lymphoblastic leukaemias. Acute megakaryoblastic leukaemia in Down's syndrome is characterised by a somatic mutation in *GATA1*. Constitutive activation of the JAK/STAT (Janus kinase and signal transducer and activator of transcription) pathway occurs in several haematopoietic malignant diseases. We tested the hypothesis that mutations in *JAK2* might be a common molecular event in acute lymphoblastic leukaemia associated with Down's syndrome.

Methods.—*JAK2* DNA mutational analysis was done on diagnostic bone marrow samples obtained from 88 patients with Down's syndrome-associated acute lymphoblastic leukaemia; and 216 patients with sporadic acute lymphoblastic leukaemia, Down's syndrome-associated acute megakaryoblastic leukaemia, and essential thrombocythaemia. Functional consequences of identified mutations were studied in mouse haematopoietic progenitor cells.

Findings.—Somatically acquired *JAK2* mutations were identified in 16 (18%) patients with Down's syndrome-associated acute lymphoblastic leukaemia. The only patient with non-Down's syndrome-associated leukaemia but with a *JAK2* mutation had an isochromosome 21q. Children with a *JAK2* mutation were younger (mean [SE] age 4·5 years [0·86] vs 8·6 years [0·59], p<0.0001) at diagnosis. Five mutant alleles were identified, each affecting a highly conserved arginine residue (R683). These mutations immortalised primary mouse haematopoietic progenitor cells in vitro, and caused constitutive Jak/Stat activation and cytokine-independent growth of BaF3 cells, which was sensitive to pharmacological inhibition with JAK inhibitor I. In modelling studies of the JAK2 pseudokinase domain, R683 was situated in an exposed conserved region separated from the one implicated in myeloproliferative disorders.

Interpretation.—A specific genotype-phenotype association exists between the type of somatic mutation within the *JAK2* pseudokinase domain and the development of B-lymphoid or myeloid neoplasms. Somatically acquired R683 *JAK2* mutations define a distinct acute lymphoblastic leukaemia subgroup that is uniquely associated with trisomy 21. JAK2 inhibitors could be useful for treatment of this leukaemia.

Funding.—Israel Trade Ministry, Israel Science Ministry, Jewish National Fund UK, Sam Waxman Cancer Research Foundation, Israel Science Foundation, Israel Cancer Association, Curtis Katz, Constantiner Institute for Molecular Genetics, German-Israel Foundation, and European Commission FP6 Integrated Project EUROHEAR.

▶ All of us know that children with Down syndrome have a remarkably increased risk for the development of leukemia, particularly acute myeloid leukemia, which is often of the megakaryocytic lineage, a form of leukemia that is highly sensitive to cytotoxic chemotherapy. If one calculates this risk, it is a 40-fold one in comparison with children not having Down syndrome. Down syndrome children are also at increased risk of acute lymphoblastic leukemia. Unlike myeloid leukemia cells associated with Down syndrome, the leukemic cells in lymphoblastic leukemia associated with Down syndrome are not more sensitive to chemotherapy and the outcome is often quite poor. The nature of the genetic abnormalities underlying acute lymphoblastic leukemia in Down syndrome is poorly understood. Bercovich et al's finding that Janus kinase (*JAK2*) is mutated in a substantial portion of acute lymphoblastic leukemia cases is quite notable. *JAK2* is now implicated in the pathogenesis of a lymphoid rather than a myeloid malignancy.

Mutations of the *JAK2* gene on chromosome 9p24 are common in the myeloproliferative diseases polycythemia vera, essential thrombocytopenia, and primary myelofibrosis, but these mutations are not generally found in acute lymphoblastic leukemia. The *JAK2* gene is a kinase that activates many signaling pathways leading to transformation of hematopoietic cells. Bercovich et al found mutations in *JAK2* to be 20 times more common in cases of acute lymphoblastic leukemia in non-Down syndrome children. These findings suggest that *JAK2* mutations define a distinct acute lymphoblastic leukemia subgroup that arises exclusively in the context of trisomy 21. The study also suggests that the one non-Down syndrome child with acute lymphoblastic leukemia who had the *JAK2* mutation in this report most likely was a Down syndrome mosaic.

If all this talk about genetic mutations and leukemia is a bit too dense for you, the bottom line here is that the more we learn about leukemia in children related to genetic mutations, the greater the possibility that targeted therapies can be applied to specific forms of leukemia. For example, *JAK2* has a signaling function for pro-B cells that can be modified pharmacologically in normal people. Perhaps, some specific target for leukemic cells will be able to be found with this new information in the report of Bercovich et al.

J. A. Stockman III, MD

SFCE (Société Française de Lutte contre les Cancers et Leucémies de l'Enfant et de l'Adolescent) Recommendations for the Management of Tumor Lysis Syndrome (TLS) With Rasburicase: An Observational Survey
Bertrand Y, Mechinaud F, Brethon B, et al (Hôpital Debrousse, Lyon; Hôtel Dieu, Nantes; Hôpital Saint Louis; et al)
J Pediatr Hematol Oncol 30:267-271, 2008

Rasburicase (Fasturtec), a recombinant urate oxidase, is highly effective in preventing and treating hyperuricemia in children with hematologic malignancies. We conducted a prospective, multicenter observational study in 174 patients at 8 pediatric hemato-oncology centers to establish whether the SFCE (Société Française de Lutte contre les Cancers et Leucémies de l'Enfant et de l'Adolescent) recommendations for the use of rasburicase in the management of pediatric patients at risk of tumor lysis syndrome (TLS) are valid in routine clinical practice. Patients were classified as being at high or low risk of TLS according to the Children's Oncology Group criteria and were treated in accordance with the SFCE recommendations. The primary end point was the number of patients requiring a higher dose of rasburicase or a longer duration of treatment than advised in the SFCE recommendations. Of the 135 patients at high risk of TLS, 27 patients received a higher dose and 35 patients received a longer duration of treatment. Some patients received treatment with rasburicase for less than the recommended duration (median 4 d for high-risk patients). One patient required hemodialysis. Only minor adjustments to the SFCE recommendations were required to ensure the optimal use of rasburicase in pediatric patients at risk of TLS.

▶ The tumor lysis syndrome (TLS), if not properly prevented or managed can be more life threatening than the malignancies with which it is associated. Allopurinol, hydration, alkalinization, and diuresis are the usual ways that are used to prevent or treat the hyperuricemia, which is the cause of TLS. Unfortunately, allopurinol frequently fails to do its job and some believe that urinary alkalinization carries with it an unacceptably high risk of calcium phosphate precipitation in patients who have high serum phosphate levels. This is where a new agent comes into play. This agent is rasburicase, a recombinant urate oxidase. Rasburicase acts at the end of the purine catabolic pathway and therefore does not induce accumulation of xanthine or hypoxanthine, which when using allopurinol frequently precipitate in the kidneys and lead to impaired renal function. Rasburicase merely converts uric acid into a soluble compound allantoin, which is 5 to 10 times more soluble than uric acid, thereby enhancing urinary excretion. If you have not tried this interesting agent, it rapidly and dramatically reduces uric acid levels, improves a patient's electrolyte status, and reverses renal insufficiency, thus allowing a more rapid initiation of chemotherapy. In a previous randomized trial on pediatric patients, rasburicase was more effective than allopurinol in controlling hyperuricemia and had a quicker onset of action.[1] Evidence from this trial and others has shown that rasburicase seems to be well tolerated and effective in preventing and treating hyperuricemia and TLS. While this drug has been approved in certain parts of the world, there have been no treatment guidelines for its use in clinical practice and the optimal use of rasburicase to prevent or TLS in children has been unclear. The aim of the prospective study reported was to evaluate the feasibility and effectiveness of certain recommendations for the use of rasburicase.

You will have to read this report in some detail to see the specific guidelines on the use of rasburicase, but the results of this study show that treatment according to these guidelines is effective in preventing or controlling hyperuricemia and TLS in children with hematologic malignancies. Just one child out of 174 developed any evidence of renal impairment while on rasburicase. This single patient had severe TLS requiring hemodialysis. The youngster had an underlying diagnosis of Burkitt lymphoma, pre-existing renal insufficiency, and severe TLS even before treatment was begun. The bottom line is that no, or very few, patients at high risk for TLS will be expected to require dialysis after prophylaxis or treatment with rasburicase.

As many as 1 in 4 or 5 at extremely high risk for TLS, such as those with Burkitt lymphoma or mature B-cell leukemia might be expected to develop TLS, despite prophylaxis, thus showing how good rasburicase can be. Best yet, a single dose of rasburicase may be all that is necessary in terms of drug therapy, but in this report the drug was continued well into the chemotherapy treatment just to be sure there would be no complications related to TLS. Anyone who has been involved with the care of children with malignancy knows how problematic TLS can be and how it can delay the initiation of the all-important chemotherapy necessary to treat a malignancy. Perhaps, we now have a better pharmacologic agent to deal with this than ever before.[1]

J. A. Stockman III, MD

Reference

1. Goldman SC, Holcenberg JS, Finkelstein JZ, et al. A randomized comparison between rasburicase and allopurinol in children with lymphoma or leukemia at high risk for tumor lysis. *Blood.* 2001;97:2998-3003.

Retrospective Study of Childhood Ganglioneuroma
De Bernardi B, Gambini C, Haupt R, et al (Natl Inst for Cancer Res, Genova, Italy; Univ of Napoli, Italy; Natl Cancer Inst, Milano, Italy; et al)
J Clin Oncol 26:1710-1716, 2008

Purpose.—To review a historical cohort of childhood ganglioneuroma (GN), the benign representative of the peripheral neuroblastic tumor (PNT) family.

Patients and Methods.—Of 2,286 PNTs enrolled between 1979 and 2005, 146 (6.4%) were registered as GN. Histological revision was carried out on 76 tumors. Diagnosis was confirmed in 45, while 27 were reclassified as ganglioneuroblastoma intermixed (GNBI) and four were reclassified as other PNT subtypes.

Results.—GNs differed from other PNTs for sex, age, tumor site, stage, tumor markers, and scintigraphic results. Characteristics of 76 reviewed and 70 nonreviewed patients were comparable. Reviewed GN and GNBI patients were comparable except for homovanillic acid excretion, metaiodobenzylguanidine scintigraphy, and DNA content. Seven patients were only biopsied and 139 underwent surgery. Twenty-two patients suffered surgery-related complications, of which two were fatal and seven were severe. Radical tumor resection and surgery-related complication rates were comparable for GN, GNBI, and nonreviewed instances. Six patients developed tumor progression but survived. Two patients developed a late malignancy but survived. None of the 146 patients received chemotherapy. Of 146 patients, two died of surgery-related complications and 144 survived.

Conclusion.—Diagnosis was changed to GNBI for approximately one third of 76 reviewed tumors. Patients with confirmed GN, reclassified as GNBI, and nonreviewed histology presented with comparable clinical, biochemical, and biologic features. Surgical results, complication rate, number of progressions, and outcome were similar for the three groups. Surgery was associated with significant risk of complications. Survival was not influenced by extent of tumor resection. Aggressive surgical approach should not be recommended for childhood GN and GNBI.

▶ The histologic diagnosis of ganglioneuroma (GN) has always been controversial, especially for its distinction from ganglioneuroblastoma. In general, GN is the uncommon, benign representative of the neuroblastic tumors that include neuroblastoma and ganglioneuroblastoma.

Symptoms resulting from GN usually result from the compressive effect of the tumor on neighboring tissues. Surgical resection is the therapy of choice, although such resection can sometimes be challenging if not down right risky. Sometimes a tumor is better left alone in such circumstances. The report of De Bernardi et al represents a useful review of GN in that the literature regarding childhood GN is quite scarce.

So what do we learn about GN? We learn that there are few occurrences of late malignant changes that have been reported with GN. In general, it is considered a benign tumor. It is critically important that GN be able to be histologically differentiated from ganglioneuroblastoma, which has a much less favorable prognosis. We also learn the risk of attempting to remove GNs. Because GN can tightly adhere to, or encase major vascular structures, attempting resection may lead to severe and even life-threatening complications. Indeed, patients have died as a result of profuse bleeding in or following surgery. Overall, the literature tells us that surgery-related complications occur in as many as 1 in 5 cases of surgical resection of GN. In this series, no case of malignant transformation was observed in residual tumors left after incomplete resection.

The bottom line here is that the benign nature of GN requires a more cautious surgical approach when surgical risk factors are identified. In such cases, a watchful waiting period should be established with debulking surgery becoming justified when excessive growth has occurred. Two sets of experts are critically important when evaluating the possibility of a diagnosis of GN. One is a pathologist who knows their way around the differentiation between GN and ganglioneuroblastoma. The other is the pediatric surgeon who knows his way around the human body and its vascular and nervous components.

J. A. Stockman III, MD

Effectiveness of screening for neuroblastoma at 6 months of age: a retrospective population-based cohort study

Hiyama E, Iehara T, Sugimoto T, et al (Hiroshima Univ, Japan; Kyoto Prefectural Univ of Medicine, Japan; et al)
Lancet 371:1173-1180, 2008

Background.—In Japan, a nationwide programme between 1984 and 2003 screened all infants for urinary catecholamine metabolites as a marker for neuroblastoma. Before 1989, this was done by qualitative spot tests for vanillylmandelic acid in urine, and subsequently by quantitative assay with high-performance liquid chromatography (HPLC). However, the Japanese government stopped the mass-screening programme in 2003, after reports that it did not reduce mortality due to neuroblastoma. We aimed to assess the effectiveness of the programme, by comparing the rates of incidence and mortality from neuroblastomas diagnosed before 6 years of age in three cohorts.

Methods.—We did a retrospective population-based cohort study on all children born between 1980 and 1998, except for a 2-year period from 1984. We divided these 22 289 695 children into three cohorts: children born before screening in 1980–83 (n=6 130 423); those born during qualitative screening in 1986–89 (n=5 290 412); and those born during quantitative screening 1990–98 (n=10 868 860). We used databases from hospitals, screening centres, and national cancer registries. Cases of neuroblastoma were followed up for a mean of 78·7 months.

Findings.—21·56 cases of neuroblastoma per 100 000 births over 72 months were identified in the qualitatively screened group (relative risk [RR] 1·87, 95% CI 1·66–2·10), and 29·80 cases per 100 000 births over 72 months in the quantitatively screened group (RR 2·58, 2·33–2·86). The cumulative incidence of neuroblastoma in the prescreening cohort (11·56 cases per 100 000 births over 72 months) was lower than that in other cohorts (p<0·0001 for all comparisons), but more neuroblastomas were diagnosed after 24 months of age in this cohort (p=0·0002 for qualitative screening vs prescreening, p<0·0001 for quantitative screening vs prescreening). Cumulative mortality was lower in the qualititative screening (3·90 cases per 100 000 livebirths over 72 months) and quantitative screening cohorts (2·83 cases) than in the prescreening cohort (5·38 cases). Compared with the prescreening cohort, the relative risk of mortality was 0·73 (95% CI 0·58–0·90) for qualitative screening, and 0·53 (0·42–0·63) for quantitative screening. Mortality rates for both the qualitative and quantitative screening groups were lower than were those for the prescreening cohort (p=0·0041 for prescreening vs qualitative screening, p<0·0001 for prescreening vs quantitative screening).

Interpretation.—More infantile neuroblastomas were recorded in children who were screened for neuroblastoma at 6 months of age than in those who were not. The mortality rate from neuroblastoma in children who were screened at 6 months was lower than that in the prescreening cohort, especially in children screened by quantitative HPLC. Any new screening programme should aim to decrease mortality, but also to minimise overdiagnosis of tumours with favourable prognoses (eg, by screening children at 18 months).

▶ There has been little that has been more controversial than screening for neuroblastoma in the newborn period. It is the only solid tumor of early childhood that has been a focus of large-scale screening. Screening in this case involves urinary assay of catecholamine metabolites from tumor cells. In theory, there should be no controversy about screening for neuroblastoma in early infancy except for the fact it is not biologically a uniform disease. Much of neuroblastoma that starts in infancy is biologically quite favorable and typically stays a benign disease regressing spontaneously in many patients. Unfortunately, about half the cases develop beyond a year and a half or so of age and frequently present with metastatic disease. These patients do poorly, despite aggressive treatment. If one looks at survival data, there have not been remarkable improvements in the latter circumstances in over a quarter of a century. There are prognostic features that involve pathology and molecular markers that do determine prognosis at the time of initial diagnosis.

It was back in the early 1980s that the Japanese began to screen for neuroblastoma, this at about 6 months of age. Initial reports seemed to show an increased survivorship with this disease in pilot programs as the result of this early screening. It was in 1984, then, that nationwide screening in Japan began. There was some skepticism throughout the rest of the world about the approach the Japanese were using. For example, the decision to nationalize screening in that country were initially based on survival data, which can be easily artificially raised if screening increases the incidence of detecting benign disease, rather than reducing mortality. Another criticism was that these early studies lacked concurrent controls and was inconsistent in their way of determining the numbers of cases in death related to the disease.

Later studies throughout the world cast some doubt on the value of early screening for neuroblastoma. In Quebec, Canada, a study looked at over 500 000 infants followed for 5 years. This was concurrent with a United States study where over 4 million infants were followed with rigorous documentation.

The incidence of neuroblastoma did in fact double in Quebec compared with control populations, but with no lowering of the incidence of unfavorable disease. Total mortality at 8 years into the study was no different than that observed in concurrent or retrospective controls. An even larger study investigated screening at a year of age in Germany. The German results were similar to those found in North America.

So what do we learn from the most recent study performed in Japan, that of Hiyama et al? These investigators provide data on a retrospective review of over 13 million infants offered screening in Japan. Children were divided into 3 groups—prescreening, qualitative screening, and quantitative screening. The results again showed a higher incidence of benign neuroblastomas diagnosed during infancy in screened patients, an almost 3-fold difference compared with nonscreened infants. Importantly, from the authors' viewpoint, mortality decreased from 5.4 deaths per 100 000 births in the prescreening era to 2.8 in the quantitative-screening era, which might seem to validate the idea that screening saves lives. The incidence of advanced stage disease decreased between ages of 2 years and 6 years, in a comparison of screened and pre-screened groups. Unfortunately, major methodological issues remain. The study was retrospective with no concurrent population-based controls. While the investigators argue that neuroblastoma survival did increase over 20 years in a subset, one cannot assess whether these results would reflect all patients with neuroblastoma in Japan. Also, the 3 time-based groupings of children are not precise. Some prefectures were already screening during the prescreening era, and the transition from qualitative to quantitative screening was not black and white in time.

So what is the bottom line here? It is pretty simple, the results of the North American and German trials are fairly bulletproof and widely accepted. There are just too many pitfalls in retrospective reviews. Add to that the low positive-predictive value of urine screening for catecholamine metabolites, and you see the problem. False-positive results or diagnosis of disorders in asymptomatic children that would have never come to clinical attention can lead to physician-induced morbidity through diagnostic testing and certainly psychological harm to patients.

Even in Japan, there is a very cautious approach being taken before possibly reopening nationwide screening. Japan has at least 5 or more years of experience now of births with no screening, so it should be easy to determine whether there has been any increase in mortality as a consequence of the cessation of mandatory screening. For more on the topic of neuroblastoma screening, see the excellent editorial on this topic by Maris and Woods.[1]

You can bet that the information provided from this report from Japan will be viewed very cautiously here in the United States. It would take someone moving a mountain to make anyone believe that screening is of value in the reduction of morbidity and mortality for neuroblastoma. We will leave it to our Japanese colleagues to carry out the needed studies to see if they can convince us that this would be a worthwhile effort.

J. A. Stockman III, MD

Reference

1. Maris JM, Woods WG. Screening for neuroblastoma: a resurrected idea? *Lancet.* 2008;371:1142-1143.

Chromosome 6p22 Locus Associated with Clinically Aggressive Neuroblastoma

Maris JM, Mosse YP, Bradfield JP, et al (Children's Hosp of Philadelphia, PA; et al)

N Engl J Med 358:2585-2593, 2008

Background.—Neuroblastoma is a malignant condition of the developing sympathetic nervous system that most commonly affects young children and is often lethal. Its cause is not known.

Methods.—We performed a genomewide association study by first genotyping blood DNA samples from 1032 patients with neuroblastoma and 2043 control subjects of European descent using the Illumina Human-Hap550 BeadChip. Samples from three independent groups of patients with neuroblastoma (a total of 720 patients) and 2128 control subjects were then genotyped to replicate significant associations.

Results.—We observed a significant association between neuroblastoma and the common minor alleles of three consecutive single-nucleotide polymorphisms (SNPs) at chromosome band 6p22 and containing the predicted genes *FLJ22536* and *FLJ44180* ($P = 1.71 \times 10^{-9}$ to 7.01×10^{-10}; allelic odds ratio, 1.39 to 1.40). Homozygosity for the at-risk G allele of the most significantly associated SNP, rs6939340, resulted in an increased likelihood of the development of neuroblastoma (odds ratio, 1.97; 95% confidence interval, 1.58 to 2.45). Subsequent genotyping of the three 6p22 SNPs in three independent case series confirmed our observation of an association ($P = 9.33 \times 10^{-15}$ at rs6939340 for joint analysis). Patients with neuroblastoma who were homozygous for the risk alleles at 6p22 were more likely to have metastatic (stage 4) disease ($P = 0.02$), amplification of the *MYCN* oncogene in the tumor cells ($P = 0.006$), and disease relapse ($P = 0.01$).

Conclusions.—A common genetic variation at chromosome band 6p22 is associated with susceptibility to neuroblastoma.

▶ Many are not aware that stage for stage, neuroblastoma has become the most curable of the pediatric solid tumors. More than 90% of patients with localized neuroblastoma, including those with spread to regional lymph nodes will survive, often with little or no cytotoxic therapy. Rates of cure of metastatic neuroblastoma exceed 90% among infants (who are usually treated with low-dose chemotherapy) and are approximately 25% among toddlers; in contrast, osteomedullary metastases associated with other pediatric solid tumor confer less than a 5% chance of cure. The long-held view that many cases of neuroblastoma actually spontaneously regress or mature into asymptomatic ganglioneuroma has been confirmed by the results of urine cate-cholamine screening programs in infants. Such programs yielded as many as twice the numbers of neuroblastoma as the natural history of the disease pre-senting otherwise could account for in unscreened populations. These programs did not reduce the incidence of high-risk disease indicating a fair number of neuroblastomas disappeared on their own.

We now know that many neuroblastomas can be categorized into a high-risk subset based on chromosomal and genetic findings. The presence of these chromosomal abnormalities—including involvement of the *MYCN* proto-onco-gene, 1p2 p, 11q14q or 17q—conveys prognostic insights that aid in risk-based care. Findings actually suggest that that there may be an inborn susceptibility to neuroblastoma.

Maris et al report on a study that is noteworthy for several reasons. First, it implicates 3 closely linked single-nucleotide polymorphisms at chromosome band 6p22 in the initiation of neuroblastoma. Second, the study involves sizable cohorts of patients (a total of almost 1800) with a representative distri-bution of clinical and biological characteristics. The size of this study is truly impressive given the rarity of neuroblastoma (just 700 cases per year here in the United States). Findings, for example, show that patients with neuroblas-toma have more than a two-fold likelihood of having an at-risk chromosome CP22 allele. Given the fact that neuroblastoma is so rare and the 6p22 allele is so common, the absolute risk conferred by the susceptibility allele is extremely small.

Although the chromosome 6p22 status has little clinical use for preventative measures, it may have a role in prognostication. Variants on chromosome 6p22 are linked to clinically aggressive forms of neuroblastoma and the powerful adverse biological prognostic marker, *MYCN* amplification.

This study points out that the likelihood for malignant transformation of developing neuroblasts is significantly influenced by chromosome 6p22 vari-ants. This report provides a strong underpinning for a genome approach to neuroblastoma and the relationship to the risk of malignant transformation in this disease.

J. A. Stockman III, MD

Stool DNA and Occult Blood Testing for Screen Detection of Colorectal Neoplasia

Ahlquist DA, Sargent DJ, Loprinzi CL, et al (Mayo Clinic, Rochester, MN; et al)
Ann Intern Med 149:441-450, 2008

Background.—Stool DNA testing is a new approach to colorectal cancer detection. Few data are available from the screening setting.

Objective.—To compare stool DNA and fecal blood testing for detec-tion of screen-relevant neoplasia (curable-stage cancer, high-grade dysplasia, or adenomas >1 cm).

Design.—Blinded, multicenter, cross-sectional study.

Setting.—Communities surrounding 22 participating academic and regional health care systems in the United States.

Participants.—4482 average-risk adults.

Measurements.—Fecal blood and DNA markers. Participants collected 3 stools, smeared fecal blood test cards and used same-day shipment to a central facility. Fecal blood cards (Hemoccult and HemoccultSensa, Beckman Coulter, Fullerton, California) were tested on 3 stools and DNA assays on 1 stool per patient. Stool DNA test 1 (SDT-1) was a pre-commercial 23-marker assay, and a novel test (SDT-2) targeted 3 broadly informative markers. The criterion standard was colonoscopy.

Results.—Sensitivity for screen-relevant neoplasms was 20% by SDT-1, 11% by Hemoccult ($P = 0.020$), 21% by HemoccultSensa ($P = 0.80$); sensitivity for cancer plus high-grade dysplasia did not differ among tests. Specificity was 96% by SDT-1, compared with 98% by Hemoccult ($P < 0.001$) and 97% by HemoccultSensa ($P = 0.20$). Stool DNA test 2 detected 46% of screen-relevant neoplasms, compared with 16% by Hemoccult ($P < 0.001$) and 24% by HemoccultSensa ($P < 0.001$). Stool DNA test 2 detected 46% of adenomas 1 cm or larger, compared with 10% by Hemoccult ($P < 0.001$) and 17% by HemoccultSensa ($P < 0.001$). Among colonoscopically normal patients, the positivity rate was 16% with SDT-2, compared with 4% with Hemoccult ($P = 0.010$) and 5% with HemoccultSensa ($P = 0.030$).

Limitations.—Stool DNA test 2 was not performed on all subsets of patients without screen-relevant neoplasms. Stools were collected without preservative, which reduced detection of some DNA markers.

Conclusion.—Stool DNA test 1 provides no improvement over HemoccultSensa for detection of screen-relevant neoplasms. Stool DNA test 2 detects significantly more neoplasms than does Hemoccult or Hemoccult-Sensa, but with more positive results in colonoscopically normal patients. Higher sensitivity of SDT-2 was particularly apparent for adenomas.

▶ Obviously the report of Ahlquist et al deals with screening for the detection of colorectal neoplasia in adults. While colon cancer is rare in children, there is a lot to be learned from this report about cancer detection in general, including cancer of the GI tract. It has been known for some time that testing for occult blood in stool is notoriously insensitive for detecting adenomas. Adenomas, of course, are part of the progression to malignancy. The adenoma-to-carcinoma sequence in colon cancer is based on the stepwise accumulation of specific genetic alterations that parallel the histopathologic progression from preneoplasia to neoplasia. Researchers have cleverly translated these insights into molecular diagnostic assays that detect gene mutations in tumor cells sloughed into stool. It was back in 1992 that the first report of a K-ras mutations in the stool of patients with colon cancer were reported, a finding that ushered in the era of stool DNA testing for colon cancer. Since then, advances have taken place in the specific genes analyzed, techniques to separate and preserve tumor DNA from the vast quantities of bacterial DNA, and mutation detection methods accumulated in the introduction of commercial stool DNA tests for

23 genetic markers. These markers currently are capable of detecting more than 50% of colon cancers by a simple stool DNA analysis.

Ahlquist et al have evaluated a new variety of stool DNA tests in screening a population of over 4000 adults and compared their sensitivity and specificity of that of occult blood tests for the diagnosis of colon cancer, including precancerous adenomas. The newer stool DNA test showed sensitivity over twice that of a Hemoccult test for blood in the stool. The flip side of this is that even the best of the DNA tests still miss almost half of colon cancers.

Surely DNA testing of the stool for cancer will improve over time. Currently, the cost of such DNA testing runs in excess of $200 per sample. While far less expensive than a colonoscopy, these DNA tests are still too insensitive to provide any true assurance that someone does not have colon cancer, in contradistinction to a colonoscopy. A noninvasive test that preselects individuals who are likely to have an advanced adenoma or cancer for a subsequent colonoscopy is a truly worthy goal. Anyone who has reached the ripe age of 50-something knows how unpleasant a colonoscopy is, particularly if one has to do it on a somewhat regular basis. The development of a test based on the early molecular genetic changes in precancerous adenomas is quite logical. It is critical to remember that the adenoma is the real target of a screening program whose goal is to prevent colon cancer. The report of Ahlquist et al provides exciting evidence of a noninvasive approach that indeed may be plausible. While there are not many children around who are at risk of dying from colon cancer because of a genetic increased risk of having adenomas, such kids do in fact exist and therefore it is worthy of us to follow this adult literature carefully. Perhaps in time, a few strands of DNA will be all it takes to deliver an ounce of prevention for both children and adults.

J. A. Stockman III, MD

The Gist of literature on pediatric GIST: review of clinical presentation
Kaemmer DA, Otto J, Lassay L, et al (Rheinish-Westphalian Technical Univ, Aachen, Germany)
J Pediatr Hematol Oncol 31:108-112, 2009

Aim/Background.—To provide a review of existing literature on pediatric GIST with focus on clinical presentation.

Methods.—A MEDLINE search was conducted in July 2007 to give an overview on literature concerning pediatric gastrointestinal stromal tumors (GISTs) with a focus on clinical presentation, using keywords "gastrointestinal stromal tumor" and one of the following "young/boy/girl/child/children/pediatric." Two of the authors sorted the resulting abstracts by relevance for a review on clinical aspects of pediatric GIST if they were in English language, not explicitly only reporting of adults and describing clinical features of patients.

Results.—One hundred and six articles were found, 43 of which were excluded because they did not match the criteria mentioned above. We found 97 patients in the articles meeting our criteria, of which 38 cases had to be excluded, because of lacking clinical data, negative staining for CD117 or syndromal occurrence. This left 59 patients for analysis of clinical symptoms in the presentation of nonsyndromal CD117-positive GIST in children.

Discussion.—Clinical feature most frequent was anemia in 86.4% (n = 51) symptomatic either through acute or subacute bleeding. There was no palpable tumor in 88.1% (n = 52), no abdominal pain in 84.7% (n = 50), and no vomiting in 88.1% (n = 52). Girls tend to show more high-grade tumors and existing case reports show a 2.7-fold higher incidence in females. Altogether epithelioid cell tumors are most frequent, although in boys spindle-cell tumors are reported more often. On the basis of National Institute of Health criteria (6) tumors were low grade in 22% (n = 13), medium grade in 37.3% (n = 22), and high grade in 35.6% (n = 21). There were more high-grade tumors in girls than in boys (40.5% vs. 28.6%). Local excision was the operation most often performed, but details of surgery were missing in most cases.

Conclusions.—Pediatric GIST is a rare but considerable diagnosis in chronic anemia, which is the most frequent clinical finding with this tumor entity. Recent review articles focus on histopathologic criteria but omit clinical features and course of disease. In nonsyndromal CD117-positive GIST, girls tend to show more high-grade tumors and existing literature on pediatric GIST shows a 2.7-fold higher incidence in females. Altogether epithelioid cell tumors are most frequent, although in boys spindle-cell tumors are reported more often. Together with known differences in molecular changes and local as well as systemic tumor behavior this strongly suggests that pediatric GIST represents a different entity than adult GIST. After establishment of clear-cut pathologic features in the past, reports on preoperative diagnostic findings, long-term follow-up, and therapy have to be emphasized to clarify the relationship of these entities.

▶ It is not often that we include reports of rare entities, but gastrointestinal stromal tumors (GIST) is a quite interesting problem. Despite being the most common mesenchymal tumors, GISTs represent rare neoplasms of the gastrointestinal tract. Of all GISTs, 1.4% to 2.7% occur in children and adolescents in large reported series and only sporadic cases have been reported in neonates. Histologic features show epithelioid, spindle-cell, or mixed-type tumors. Most of the literature published heretofore has not included much in the way of the clinical presentation of GISTs, thus the value of the report of Kaemmer et al, which gives insights to the clinical presentations related to this tumor. The report was based on a MedLine search of the literature on GISTs.

What this report tells us is quite interesting and that is that the most frequent clinical feature of GISTs is anemia. This occurs in slightly over 85% of pediatric-age patients with this diagnosis. This is an important marker of the tumor because no palpable tumor was observed in almost 90% of patients. The anemia appears to be due to occult gastrointestinal bleeding.

The review of the literature performed by Kaemmer et al provides us with some other useful information about GISTs. The incidence of GISTs peaks about the sixth to seventh decade of life and typical onset is at an age over 40 years. Prognosis is largely based on tumor size and the mitotic rate of the tumor as determined histologically. Complete resection without lymph node dissection is accepted as first-line treatment. In a case series reported, there appears to be an almost 3-fold higher incidence of GIST in girls than in boys.

Although most of us are unlikely to see a child with GIST, we should be grateful to the authors of this report for assembling what little information can be gleaned from the literature about the clinical presentation of this rare disorder. Put GIST into the back of your mind and pull out any knowledge you retain from this report the next time you see a child with GI bleeding and anemia. Chances are the latter will be due to a polyp, but you never know.

J. A. Stockman III, MD

17 Ophthalmology

Outdoor Activity Reduces the Prevalence of Myopia in Children
Rose KA, Morgan IG, Ip J, et al (Univ of Sydney, Australia; Australian Natl Univ, Canberra; Westmead Millennium Inst, Sydney, Australia; et al)
Ophthalmology 115:1279-1285, 2008

Objective.—To assess the relationship of near, midworking distance, and outdoor activities with prevalence of myopia in school-aged children.

Design.—Cross-sectional study of 2 age samples from 51 Sydney schools, selected using a random cluster design.

Participants.—One thousand seven hundred sixty-five 6-year-olds (year 1) and 2367 12-year-olds (year 7) participated in the Sydney Myopia Study from 2003 to 2005.

Methods —Children had a comprehensive eye examination, including cycloplegic refraction. Parents and children completed detailed questionnaires on activity.

Main Outcome Measures.—Myopia prevalence and mean spherical equivalent (SE) in relation to patterns of near, midworking distance, and outdoor activities. Myopia was defined as SE refraction ≤ -0.5 diopters (D).

Results.—Higher levels of outdoor activity (sport and leisure activities) were associated with more hyperopic refractions and lower myopia prevalence in the 12-year-old students. Students who combined high levels of near work with low levels of outdoor activity had the least hyperopic mean refraction (+0.27 D; 95% confidence interval [CI], 0.02–0.52), whereas students who combined low levels of near work with high levels of outdoor activity had the most hyperopic mean refraction (+0.56 D; 95% CI, 0.38–0.75). Significant protective associations with increased outdoor activity were seen for the lowest ($P = 0.04$) and middle ($P = 0.02$) tertiles of near-work activity. The lowest odds ratios for myopia, after adjusting for confounders, were found in groups reporting the highest levels of outdoor activity. There were no associations between indoor sport and myopia. No consistent associations between refraction and measures of activity were seen in the 6-year-old sample.

Conclusions.—Higher levels of total time spent outdoors, rather than sport per se, were associated with less myopia and a more hyperopic mean refraction, after adjusting for near work, parental myopia, and ethnicity.

▶ Most studies show that myopia is appearing with greater prevalence in young children, which places these children at greater risk of developing high myopia (≤-6 diopters). Why this increase is occurring has remained unexplained to date. We do know that if parents have myopia, a child has a greater probability of developing myopia. East Asian ethnicity has also been proposed as a risk factor. Aside from these 2 likely genetic predispositions, myopia is also considered to have a multifactorial etiology. Thus, the rapid rise in the prevalence of myopia indicates that it's possible that some rapidly evolving environmental factors are playing a significant role in the occurrence of this increasing problem. When this editor was growing up, it was pretty common for kids to be told by their parents that if they sat too close to the television they would go blind. In fact, there has been a suspicion that excessive reading or close work might lead to a risk of myopia, but the contribution of these factors obviously is quite small, if the contribution exists at all.

A myopia study has been going on for some time in Sydney, Australia. This study allows an analysis of time spent on outdoor activities and engagement in near work at indoor activities in order to assess any possible relationship with the occurrence of myopia. The findings from Australia suggest that being outdoors, rather than sport per se, may be a crucial factor in reducing the prevalence of myopia. Sporting activities were excluded because time spent outdoors absent sporting activity still seemed to be protective against the development of myopia. The study also showed that the most myopia was indeed seen in students who combined high levels of near work and low levels of outdoor activity.

Needless to say, the impact of outdoor activity and its effects on vision need to be explained. One possibility is that being outside simply means you are not inside involved in near-work activity. It is also possible that outdoor activities require low accommodative demand in distance vision, essentially allowing the eyes to remain at rest. It is also conceivable that light intensity may be an important factor. Light intensity is obviously higher outdoors than indoors (light constricting the pupils). This would result in a greater depth of field and less image blur. Alternatively, release of dopamine from the retina is known to be stimulated by light. Dopamine has been shown to be an inhibitor of eye growth. Excessive eye growth (front to back) can cause myopia.

Well worth your reading is an interesting editorial by Wallace discussing whether comprehensive eye examinations should be mandated before entry into school.[1] Wallace points out that a 1-time mandated eye examination does not solve the problem of lack of follow-up after an abnormal vision screening. A properly done screening would cost about $100 per examination (in a state like North Carolina this would add up to about a $10 million tab for this screening). The real cost of such screening comes with the prescription writing for glasses. One recent study from Tennessee found that after examining children without any risk of vision problems, ophthalmologists and optometrists prescribed glasses in 6% and 35% of cases, respectively.[2] In most cases, the prescription for glasses is unnecessary for the common problem of hyperopia, because children have a tremendous capacity to accommodate (14 diopters for an average 8-year-old). Some argue for preschool screening for visual difficulties suggesting that it will detect amblyopia and that this is a worthy effort. Unfortunately, the optimal time to detect and treat amblyopia is well before the age of entering school. Wallace concludes that evidence is lacking to mandate comprehensive eye examinations for all children before school entry and that such screening would be poorly timed, has a low yield, and would likely result in glasses being prescribed unnecessarily for many children. Instead of a comprehensive eye examination, it would be better to identify other appropriate screening tools to detect visual problems and then select only those children who need it for a full examination.

J. A. Stockman III, MD

References

1. Wallace DK. Mandating comprehensive eye examinations for children: where is the evidence? *Ophthalmology.* 2008;115:1271-1272.
2. Donahue SP. How often are spectacles prescribed to "normal" preschool children? *AAPOS.* 2004;8:224-229.

Mental Illness in Young Adults Who Had Strabismus as Children

Mohney BG, McKenzie JA, Capo JA, et al (Mayo Clinic and Mayo Foundation, Rochester, MN)
Pediatrics 122:1033-1038, 2008

Objective.—We investigated the prevalence and types of psychiatric disorders diagnosed by early adulthood among patients who had common forms of strabismus as children.

Methods.—The medical records of children (<19 years) who were diagnosed as having esotropia ($N = 266$) or exotropia ($N = 141$) while residents of Olmsted County, Minnesota, between January 1, 1985, and December 31, 1994, were reviewed retrospectively for psychiatric disease diagnoses. Each case subject was compared with a randomly selected, individually birth- and gender-matched, control subject from the same population.

Results.—A mental health disorder was diagnosed for 168 (41.3%) of the 407 patients with a history of childhood strabismus, who were monitored to a mean age of 17.4 years, compared with 125 control subjects (30.7%). Children with exotropia were 3.1 times more likely to develop a psychiatric disorder than were control subjects when monitored to a mean age of 20.3 years. Children with esotropia were no more likely to develop mental illness than were control subjects when monitored for similar periods. Patients with intermittent exotropia also were significantly more likely to have greater numbers of mental health disorders, mental health emergency department visits, and mental health hospitalizations and to have suicidal or homicidal ideation.

Conclusions.—Children diagnosed as having strabismus in this population, especially those with exotropia, were at increased risk for developing mental illness by early adulthood. Patients with intermittent exotropia seemed to be particularly prone to developing significant psychiatric diseases by the third decade of life.

▶ Kids with crossed eyes or outgoing eyes have often been stigmatized by their peers or even adults over many centuries. These kids have frequently been treated as being "unusual." Unfortunately, it turns out that there actually is an association, albeit a small one, between strabismus and psychiatric illness. Investigators have looked at the medical records of subjects in Olmsted County, Minnesota who were diagnosed by an ophthalmologist as having esotropia or exotropia. Children with exotropia were 3.1 times more likely to develop a psychiatric disorder when followed up to a mean age of 20 years. Youngsters with esotropia were no more likely to develop mental illness than were control subjects. Youngsters with exotropia were also more likely to have suicidal ideation.

Why exotropia would be associated with the development of mental illness by early adulthood is unclear. Ocular misalignment would seem to have similar effects on individuals with strabismus regardless of whether it is esotropic or exotropic. There are no studies to suggest that exotropia is associated with greater psychosocial stress or other precipitating factors for psychiatric disorders. Heredity is more likely to be the basis for any association between exotropia and mental illness. The more prevalent forms of strabismus and most childhood mental illnesses are thought to be the result of interactions between a number of susceptibility genes. Such interactions make it unlikely for any single gene to have a large effect on the onset of strabismus or childhood mental disorders. However, this provides a potential hypothesis for how an individual gene may be associated with 2 distinct illnesses. An adult has been described with a specific but rare form of strabismus (constant exotropia) and schizophrenia.[1]

It is difficult to tell what we should do with the information provided by this report. The data seem fairly clear that children with esotropia are no more likely than control subjects to develop mental illness. Those with intermittent exotropia, the most prevalent form of exotropia, however are more likely to have a greater number of mental health disorders, a greater number of mental health emergency department visits and hospitalizations for mental health problems, including suicidal or homicidal ideation. Pack away in your minds this information for future use. Hopefully at some point in time we will learn more about the nature of these associations.

This commentary closes with a *Clinical Fact/Curio* regarding the eyes. An ophthalmologist in the United States examined the issue of whether the wearing of glasses makes you look brainy. Eighty children ranging in age from 6 to 10 years were shown pictures of 24 pairs of children, one with and one without glasses, of both sexes and varying ethnicity. The children were asked questions including which member of the pair looked smarter. The study results indicate that although gender has a strong influence on some impressions—boys were perceived as better athletes regardless of whether they wore glasses, for example—glasses trumped other characteristics when it comes to brains. Female glasses-wearers, in particular, had a 72% likelihood of being seen as smarter than the non-bespeckled children with whom they were paired. Ethnicity had no effect on choices.

By the way, if you were not aware, there is a well-known correlation between higher IQ and myopia, so maybe there is some basis for the subtle and psychological thinking that those of us who wear spectacles are smarter.[2]

J. A. Stockman III, MD

References

1. Toyota T, Yoshitsugu K, Ebihara M, et al. Association between schizophrenia and ocular misalignment and polyalanine length variation in PXM2B. *Hum Mol Genet.* 2004;13:551-561.
2. High eye-Q [editorial comment]. *Science.* 2008;320:993.

Pediatric Golf-Related Ophthalmic Injuries
Hink EM, Oliver SCN, Drack AV, et al (Univ of Colorado School of Medicine, Denver; et al)
Arch Ophthalmol 126:1252-1256, 2008

Objectives.—To document ophthalmic morbidity of golf-related injuries in children and to report specific injury patterns.

Design.—A noncomparative, interventional, retrospective case series of 11 pediatric patients treated at 2 institutions for ophthalmic trauma resulting from golf-related injuries during 15 years.

Results.—Eleven eyes of 11 patients were injured. There were 6 boys and 5 girls, with a mean age of 10.2 years (age range, 7-14 years). Ten patients were injured by golf clubs and 1 patient by a golf ball. One injury occurred on a golf course. At the initial ophthalmic examination, visual acuity was 20/20 in 4 eyes (36%), 20/25 to 20/80 in 3 eyes (27%), no light perception in 3 eyes (27%), and undeterminable in 1 eye (9%). Nine of 11 patients required surgery. Follow-up ranged from 0 to 66 months (mean follow-up, 12 months). Three of 11 subjects had permanent deficits, including blindness, decreased vision, and anophthalmia. Final visual acuity was no light perception in 2 eyes (18%), 20/70 in 1 eye (9%), and 20/20 or better in 8 eyes (73%).

Conclusions.—The findings from this series reveal that pediatric ophthalmic golf injuries, although rare, may be devastating to the eye, periocular adnexa, and visual system. Among our cases, most injuries occurred off the golf course, many required surgery, and some resulted in permanent loss of vision.

▶ Before reading this report, this editor had not realized that almost 1 million people in the United States are visually impaired as the result of ocular trauma with the majority of these individuals having monocular blindness. Obviously only a small percentage of these injuries are the result of sports-related activity, but among all traumatic injuries resulting in enucleation, sports-specific cases account for more cases than caused by motor vehicle crashes, occupational accidents, violent attacks, and gunshot wounds. Data suggest that some 42 000 individuals per year in the United States are treated for eye injuries from sports-related trauma. Among these are injuries related to golf. The report of Hink et al summarizes data from 2 institutions revealing information about golfing-related eye injuries.

Golf is a popular sport. As many as 2 million youngsters under the age of 17 are golfers in the United States. This number seems to be increasing, and it has been suggested that the popularity of young golf professionals, especially Tiger Woods, may have sparked an interest in golf among the older pediatric population resulting in a higher rate of associated injuries. The potential severity of sports-related ophthalmic injuries in younger populations has led the American Academy of Pediatrics and the American Academy of Ophthalmology to issue a joint policy statement recommending appropriate eye protection for certain sports. The joint policy statement categorizes sports as high-risk, moderate-risk, low-risk, or safe with respect to eye injury. Golf shows as a moderate-risk sport by these organizations along with tennis, badminton, soccer, volleyball, water polo, football, and fishing, and as such, there is not a necessary recommendation for eye protection. In fact, there are no product performance specifications by the American Society of Testing and Materials or the Protective Eyewear Certification Counsel regarding protective eyewear for golf participants of any age. It is hard to say based on data from this report whether such eye gear would do any good because most children with eye injuries resulting from exposure to golf equipment do not happen in the setting of a golf course or under supervised play. Most children are injured by other children wielding a golf club while at play away from the golf course. One should potentially consider a golf club as a lethal weapon since more than a dozen pediatric deaths have been reported as caused by golf clubs.

The bottom line here is that children should be taught that golf equipment should never be used without supervision. While we pay a great deal of attention to the prevention of hockey- and baseball-related eye injuries, similar degrees of injuries can occur, albeit less frequently, with other sporting activities, including the use of golf equipment. Golf is not just a good walk spoiled; it is a good walk spoiled that next time might require the assistance of a white cane.

This commentary closes with a *Clinical Fact/Curio* about an injury to the eye. How would you handle the following situation? You are covering a pediatric emergency room and have been called to see a 5-year-old Hispanic boy complaining of eye pain after handling a bag of "cal" in a neighborhood grocery store, causing some of the material to get into his eyes. The nurses have already irrigated the eye extensively. When you examine the youngster, the eye is slightly inflamed. The question is should you let this youngster go home, or is there more that you should be doing?

"Cal" is a calcium hydroxide powder well known in the Hispanic and Native American communities. It is a cooking additive used to make limewater. The limewater is needed to process dried corn into masa dough used for making tortillas and tamales. This powder is packaged in bags and is sold in grocery stores and is present in many Spanish-speaking and Native American family homes. If not properly secured, this product can be a hazard. Calcium hydroxide is also called slaked or hydrated lime. It is made from the hydroxylation of calcium oxide (quicklime). Calcium hydroxide is available as a white powder or an aqueous solution and is a strong alkali with a pH of 12. Calcium hydroxide is less damaging than lye, potassium, or ammonium hydroxide because it forms calcium soaps that precipitate and limit ocular penetration. However, these particles may collect in the fornices of the eye and can serve as a reservoir for ongoing alkali injury if not properly identified and removed. In addition to being the component of "cal," calcium hydroxide is found in commercial and household plaster and cement compounds and is the most common cause of alkali ocular burns in adults.

Recently a 5-year-old Hispanic male presented to the emergency room at Children's Memorial Hospital in Chicago after handling a bag of "cal" in a grocery store after some of the material got into his eyes. His mother noticed irritation of the skin on his nose as well as eye redness and pain. She attempted to wash his face and eyes with water before coming to the emergency room. At the time of examination, the pH of his eyes was 8 to 9, and particulate matter was visualized in both eyes. The eyes were irrigated with normal saline for approximately 90 minutes. Pediatric ophthalmologic evaluation approximately 4½ hours after the injury found retained particulate matter in the fornices of the patient's eyes requiring further irrigation with 6 liters of normal saline and direct removal of the particles using a cotton-tipped applicator under the direction of the pediatric emergency medicine team and a pediatric ophthalmologist. Fluorescein and portable slit lamp examination subsequently revealed significant ocular burns in both eyes. The left eye had a diffuse stromal haze and loss of 90% of the corneal epithelium while the right eye had a loss of 60% of the corneal epithelium. With intensive follow-up, his uncorrected visual acuity was 20/20 in both eyes some 3 months later.

Needless to say, you cannot easily flush out "cal" from an eye. The cal crystals hang around in the niches and corners of the eye and may need to be manually removed. Remember this case.[1]

J. A. Stockman III, MD

Reference

1. Schmidt SM, Schmidt CJ, Adler M. Corneal injury due to calcium hydroxide-containing food preparation product ("cal"). *Pediatr Emerg Care.* 2008;24: 468-470.

A survey of ophthalmology residents' attitudes toward pediatric ophthalmology

Hasan SJ, Castanes MS, Coats DK (Cullen Eye Inst, Houston, TX)
J Pediatr Ophthalmol Strabismus 46:25-29, 2009

Purpose.—To assess the level of ophthalmology resident interest in pediatric ophthalmology.

Methods.—An 18-item 5-point Likert scale was used to determine interest in pediatric ophthalmology among ophthalmology residents in the United States.

Results.—The response rate was 23% (316 of 1,341). Of the respondents, 74% agreed they had a clinical role model in pediatric ophthalmology, 66% perceived a good job market for this field, and 67% cited liking strabismus surgery. The majority of residents (56%) found pediatric patients difficult to examine and 50% stated income levels for pediatric ophthalmologists are low.

Conclusions.—Although most residents have an overall positive view about pediatric ophthalmology, few indicate interest in pursuing a fellowship. Specifically, most residents reported having a clinical role model in pediatric ophthalmology, perceiving a good job market, and liking strabismus surgery, whereas few residents had interest in further pediatric training and many found pediatric patients difficult to examine and income levels low.

► It is important for us to keep up on what is going on with the workforce of our non-medical pediatric care providers. The report of Hasan et al tells us about the workforce in pediatric ophthalmology. There are about 850 pediatric ophthalmologists in practice in the United States. This means there are about 2.84 pediatric ophthalmologists for every 1 million folks in the United States. Most of these ophthalmologists tend to live and work in highly urban environments. Unfortunately, a problem has emerged in recent years with the workforce in this discipline.

In 1994, 42 of 43 pediatric ophthalmology fellowship positions were filled. In 1997, only 2 fellowship positions were not filled. However, by 1999, the match rate slipped to the current level of approximately 11 of 38 existing fellowships remaining vacant. Clearly, pediatric ophthalmology currently is not as popular with residents seeking further training as other specialties of ophthalmology.

The report of Hasan et al attempts to outline the reasons why there are fewer residents going into pediatric ophthalmology and what might be able to be done to reverse the trend. The report suggests that ophthalmology residents may be finding pediatric patients too difficult to examine. This hardly seems like the likely reason explaining the decline in the pipeline, however. Children are no more difficult to examine today, presumably, than they were 10 and 20 years ago. What does stand out as a potential viable explanation is the lower financial compensation associated with being a pediatric ophthalmologist. It takes more training to be a pediatric ophthalmologist than a general ophthalmologist, and the reimbursement rates are lower. In an editorial accompanying this report, Dr Leonard Nelson, Editor of the *Journal of Pediatric Ophthalmology & Strabismus* asks the question: "Why does strabismus surgery get reimbursed less than cataract surgery when it takes the same amount of time, if not more?" That is a very legitimate question and actually applies to a number of different procedures related to the care of children and adults.

The pediatric population census is on the move upward, once again, at a time when the workforce of some of our non-medical subspecialists is not keeping up. While there is a free market economy in the United States, it is important to figure out exactly why this problem is occurring.

This chapter closes with a *Clinical Fact/Curio* about the cornea. See how you would handle the following situation. You are seeing a teenager who is referred to you for a corneal ulcer. She had been using a steroid and antibiotic drop prescribed by her family doctor for 2 weeks because of onset of pain and phobia. When the symptoms did not resolve, the family physician stained the cornea with fluorescein, which caused the entire cornea to light up, suggesting a diffuse corneal ulcer. The question is, what otherwise normal condition might cause such fluorescein staining? The answer to this question comes from a short report by Lockington and Gupta.[1] The individual in question was finally seen by an ophthalmologist who did a slit lab examination that merely showed that the patient had contact lenses, which will readily stain green with fluorescein. Unfortunately, soft contact lenses are known to take up fluorescein avidly but also irreversibly. It is useful to be aware of this fact because many contact lenses are not all that apparent to the casual medical examiner.

J. A. Stockman III, MD

Reference

1. Lockington DA, Gupta S. Corneal staining mimicking a corneal ulcer. *BMJ.* 2008; 336:622.

18 Respiratory Tract

Oral Prednisolone for Preschool Children with Acute Virus-Induced Wheezing

Panickar J, Lakhanpaul M, Lambert PC, et al (Univ of Leicester, UK; et al)
N Engl J Med 360:329-338, 2009

Background.—Attacks of wheezing induced by upper respiratory viral infections are common in preschool children between the ages of 10 months and 6 years. A short course of oral prednisolone is widely used to treat preschool children with wheezing who present to a hospital, but there is conflicting evidence regarding its efficacy in this age group.

Methods.—We conducted a randomized, double-blind, placebo-controlled trial comparing a 5-day course of oral prednisolone (10 mg once a day for children 10 to 24 months of age and 20 mg once a day for older children) with placebo in 700 children between the ages of 10 months and 60 months. The children presented to three hospitals in England with an attack of wheezing associated with a viral infection; 687 children were included in the intention-to-treat analysis (343 in the prednisolone group and 344 in the placebo group). The primary outcome was the duration of hospitalization. Secondary outcomes were the score on the Preschool Respiratory Assessment Measure, albuterol use, and a 7-day symptom score.

Results.—There was no significant difference in the duration of hospitalization between the placebo group and the prednisolone group (13.9 hours vs. 11.0 hours; ratio of geometric means, 0.90; 95% confidence interval, 0.77 to 1.05) or in the interval between hospital admission and signoff for discharge by a physician. In addition, there was no significant difference between the two study groups for any of the secondary outcomes or for the number of adverse events.

Conclusions.—In preschool children presenting to a hospital with mild-to-moderate wheezing associated with a viral infection, oral prednisolone was not superior to placebo. (Current Controlled Trials number, ISRCTN58363576.)

▶ This report and one other that appeared simultaneously in the same issue of the *New England Journal of Medicine* tell us the role of steroids as part of the management for wheezing in preschoolers.[1] Anyone who has been in pediatric practice for more than a few days knows about this problem because about one-third of preschool children 4 years of age or younger will have intermittent wheezing, and the most common trigger of this is a respiratory viral infection.

Wheezing with viral colds may persist into adult life or may disappear before school age. Some children, particularly those with atopy, have a different clinical phenotype known as "multitrigger" wheezing. This condition is characterized by wheezing after exposure to multiple triggers, such as exercise and exposure to smoke, allergens, or cold air as well as viral infections.

Although the basis for the treatment of preschool wheezing is pitifully small in terms of evidence in the literature, what studies there are have suggested that the early use of inhaled corticosteroids (either intermittently for viral symptoms or continuously) does not prevent the progression of any type of preschool wheezing to established asthma in childhood. Recognizing this, most believe that treatment should be based solely on relief of symptoms. The current approach to the treatment of acute virus-associated wheezing among preschoolers has been based on the treatment for asthma in school-aged children. Oral corticosteroids are the bedrock of therapy. However, the report of Panickar et al describes an extension of their earlier work on the role of oral corticosteroids in acute virus-induced wheezing. The authors previously reported that in preschool children with an episode of wheezing that was sufficiently severe for admission to a hospital, a parent-initiated course of oral prednisolone made no difference in the outcome.[2] In this report, we see the results of a double-blind randomized, placebo-controlled trial showing no benefit of oral prednisolone in preschool children hospitalized with acute virus-associated wheezing (Fig 2). However, Ducharme et al had described the intermittent use of a very high-dose inhaled fluticasone (1.5 mg per day) in preschool children with episodic wheezing.[1] Although the treatment showed modest benefits in terms of a shorter duration of symptoms and less use of rescue β2-agonists, the safety data are worrisome. Because approximately 10% of children have more than 10 viral colds per year and symptoms may last 2 weeks or more,

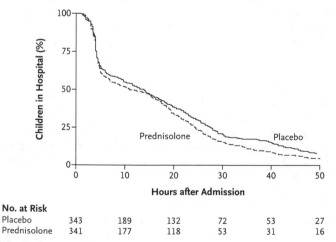

FIGURE 2.—Kaplan–Meier Estimates of the Proportion of Children Remaining in the Hospital. (Reprinted from Panickar J, Lakhanpaul M, Lambert PC, et al. Oral prednisolone for preschool children with acute virus-induced wheezing. *N Engl J Med.* 2009;360:329-338. Copyright 2009 Massachusetts Medical Society. All rights reserved.)

some children could receive large cumulative doses of fluticasone if the same steroid protocol were to be used. This is a very real possibility. In the study by Ducharme et al, the investigators documented a small reduction in linear growth in children receiving high-dose inhaled fluticasone, and there are probably other adverse effects of such therapy. Given the fact that the clinical benefit of fluticasone was fleeting, not likely to be disease modifying, and produced only a relatively minor effect on symptoms, one would think that the use of such steroids is not the way to go unless additional studies document better outcomes than reported to date.

There are a few take-home messages from the reports by Panickar et al and Ducharme et al. One is that there can no longer be justification for the administration of prednisolone to preschoolers without atopy who have episodic (viral) wheezing in either a community or hospital setting unless a severe clinical course is anticipated. It is possible that prednisolone might have a role in the treatment of preschool children with atopy who have acute exacerbations, particularly in patients with multitrigger wheezing. The use of steroids in such cases is a study waiting to be done. In a commentary that accompanied this report, it was remarked that it is disturbing to contemplate how many unnecessary courses of prednisolone have been given over the years, in good faith, because we all assume that preschool children are little adults.[3] A wise statement indeed. This same commentary also suggests that on the basis of these new data, we should be rethinking our management of viral-associated wheezing. β2-agonists that are inhaled through an appropriate spacer, with a mask if age appropriate, should be given. Prophylactic or intermittent use of leukotriene receptor antagonists may be beneficial, but comparisons with intermittent inhaled corticosteroids are needed. Prednisolone should be administered to preschoolers only when they are severely ill in the hospital. Intermittent, high-dose inhaled corticosteroids should not be used according to the commentary.

Needless to say, any child enrolled in one of these therapeutic trials should be followed well into adulthood to see if they have persistent, atopic, multitrigger wheezing (true asthma). Perhaps, we will learn more about whether those who ultimately develop true asthma fared any better, or worse, with the use of episodic steroids during episodes of viral-associated wheezing early in life.

This commentary closes with a *Clinical Fact/Curio* about our environment and air pollution, another cause of wheezing. Many of us complain about the amount of time we have to spend on airplanes traveling to and from meetings, conferences, etc. Recently, a commentary appeared in the *British Medical Journal* suggesting just how much such travel results in air pollution. The next time we get on a plane to go to a medical conference, we should think about the environmental consequences and ask ourselves whether abandoning such travel might make a material difference in terms of impact on global warming. Look at the facts. Take for example the American Thoracic Society meetings, a relatively small slice of big conferences. Every year, over 15 000 physicians and scientists, of whom about 3500 are from Europe, trek to some location in the United States for a meeting. It has recently been calculated that the carbon burden of flying delegates to and from the 2006 conference in San Diego was about 10 800 tons of carbon production. For the American Cardiac Society meeting, attended by more than 45 000 individuals, the total was over 300 million person air miles. If there are, say, 20 major medical conferences per year in the United States and if we add in conferences in Europe, Asia, and Australasia, the impact from travel to medical conferences would be at least 6 billion person air miles, equating to the sustainable carbon emissions for about half a million people in India or the carbon dioxide absorbed by 120 million mature trees covering 120 thousand acres of rain forest. To all this you can add the energy cost of operating huge hotels and enormous conference centers with all the attendant activities. The environmental impact cumulatively becomes mind boggling.

Let's commit to attending virtual conferences. If teens can communicate with each other all over the world by VOIP (voice over internet protocol) or via Skype® or video links using only their home computers, surely we could follow their example. The excitement of a foreign visit might be lacking, but the practicalities of a trip to London or even a regional hub are hardly all that enticing these days. There would be no jet lag, no interminable waits at airports, no lost luggage, and no weekends away from home. Make the need for large conferences as irrelevant as carbon paper and the horse drawn carriage.

J. A. Stockman III, MD

References

1. Ducharme FM, Lemire C, Noya FJD, et al. Presumptive use of high-dose fluticasone for virus-induced wheezing in young children. N Engl J Med. 2009;360: 39-53.
2. Oommen A, Lambert P, Grigg J. Efficacy of a short course of parent-initiated oral prednisolone for viral wheeze in children aged 1-5 years: randomized controlled trial. Lancet. 2003;362:1433-1438.
3. Bush A. Practice imperfect – treatment for wheezing in preschoolers. N Engl J Med. 2009;360:409-410.

Effectiveness of PTC124 treatment of cystic fibrosis caused by nonsense mutations: a prospective phase II trial
Kerem E, Hirawat S, Armoni S, et al (Hadassah Hebrew Univ Hosp, Jerusalem, Israel; PTC Therapeutics, South Plainfield, NJ; et al)
Lancet 372:719-727, 2008

Background.—In about 10% of patients worldwide and more than 50% of patients in Israel, cystic fibrosis results from nonsense mutations (premature stop codons) in the messenger RNA (mRNA) for the cystic fibrosis transmembrane conductance regulator (CFTR). PTC124 is an orally bioavailable small molecule that is designed to induce ribosomes to selectively read through premature stop codons during mRNA translation, to produce functional CFTR.

Methods.—This phase II prospective trial recruited adults with cystic fibrosis who had at least one nonsense mutation in the *CFTR* gene. Patients were assessed in two 28-day cycles. During the first cycle, patients received PTC124 at 16 mg/kg per day in three doses every day for 14 days, followed by 14 days without treatment; in the second cycle, patients received 40 mg/kg of PTC124 in three doses every day for 14 days, followed by 14 days without treatment. The primary outcome had three components: change in CFTR-mediated total chloride transport; proportion of patients who responded to treatment; and normalisation of chloride transport, as assessed by transepithelial nasal potential difference (PD) at baseline, at the end of each 14-day treatment course, and after 14 days without treatment. The trial was registered with who.int/ictrp, and with clinicaltrials.gov, number NCT00237380.

Findings.—Transepithelial nasal PD was evaluated in 23 patients in the first cycle and in 21 patients in the second cycle. Mean total chloride transport increased in the first treatment phase, with a change of -7.1 (SD 7.0) mV (p<0.0001), and in the second, with a change of -3.7 (SD 7.3) mV (p=0.032). We recorded a response in total chloride transport (defined as a change in nasal PD of -5 mV or more) in 16 of the 23 patients in the first cycle's treatment phase (p<0.0001) and in eight of the 21 patients in the second cycle (p<0.0001). Total chloride transport entered the normal range for 13 of 23 patients in the first cycle's treatment phase (p=0.0003) and for nine of 21 in the second cycle (p=0.02). Two patients given PTC124 had constipation without intestinal obstruction, and four had mild dysuria. No drug-related serious adverse events were recorded.

Interpretation.—In patients with cystic fibrosis who have a premature stop codon in the *CFTR* gene, oral administration of PTC124 to suppress nonsense mutations reduces the epithelial electrophysiological abnormalities caused by CFTR dysfunction.

Funding.—PTC Therapeutics, Cystic Fibrosis Foundation Therapeutics.

▶ By now, everyone in the medical field should know that cystic fibrosis results from mutations in the gene that encodes the cystic fibrosis transmembrane conductance regulator (CFTR), a chloride channel that promotes chloride efflux and secondarily inhibits sodium influx via the epithelial sodium channel. Dysfunction of this regulator leads to epithelial mucus dehydration and viscous secretions, resulting in chronic inflammation and occlusion of respiratory airways and obstruction of pancreatic ducts, biliary tract ducts, and the passage of fluid in the vas deferens. Nonsense mutations are responsible for about 10% of cystic fibrosis cases worldwide. A nonsense mutation is a single point alteration in DNA causing a stop-codon resulting in premature cessation of translation, resulting in a shortened protein leading to loss of function and consequent disease. In some parts of the world, nonsense mutations are the primary cause of cystic fibrosis in the majority of patients with the disease.

So what do nonsense mutations, stop-codons, and aminoglycosides have to do with one another? It has been known for some time that certain aminoglycoside antibiotics such as gentamicin will induce ribosomes to read through a premature stop-codon in messenger RNA, resulting in incorporation of an amino acid and continuation of translation to produce a complete protein.

For example, it has been demonstrated that topical application of gentamicin drops to the nasal mucosa can cause a local increase in CFTR-mediated chloride transport in cystic fibrosis patients who have sufficient CFTR that contain a nonsense mutation.

So why can't we give gentamicin to everybody with cystic fibrosis to see if it might help? Obviously, this is not possible since this antibiotic would have to be given parenterally and its toxic effects would preclude long-term systemic use for the suppression of nonsense mutations. On the other hand, PTC124 might be able to be used. PTC124 is an orally bioavailable, nonaminoglycoside compound that has been specifically developed to induce ribosomes to read through premature stop-codons, but not normal stop-codons. It has been tested in mice and does generate full production of functional CFTR in a mouse model of cystic fibrosis.

In this phase II report of Kerem et al, 23 adults with cystic fibrosis in whom the disease was caused by nonsense mutations (premature stop-codons) in messenger RNA encoding the CFTR, received the new drug. Marked improvements in nasal epithelial cell membrane function were observed in the majority of patients. Researchers also saw modest improvements in lung function but no correction with improvements in the sweat chloride channel defect. Treatment with PTC124 did cause small increases in FEV1, FVC, and body weight in most patients as well as a reduction in neutrophil counts. Some patients also reported a decrease in pulmonary symptoms such as cough. The drug was generally well tolerated and secondary clinical events and laboratory abnormalities were quite infrequent. Compliance with treatment was excellent.

Obviously not all patients with cystic fibrosis will benefit from agents such as PTC124 since not all patients have nonsense mutations, and it is not clear what the real benefit of PTC124 might be in those who do have nonsense mutations. Additional trials are under way to assess longer-term efficacy and safety and use of this agent and similar agents. Given the fact that stop-codon mutations have also been found in other entities such as Duchenne muscular dystrophy, the drug is also being studied in additional disorders. These studies must be carried out with great care since the development of agents that suppress premature stop-codons is not without theoretical risk. Such agents might lead to erroneous suppression of normal stop-codons. PTC124 could also disrupt nonsense-mediated messenger RNA decay—the major machinery that has evolved to protect against harmful products of nonsense mutations. As noted, to date, PTC124 seems to be remarkably selective for premature, rather than normal, stop-codons and its effects also appear to restrict its action to those ribosomes that are involved in productive translation of proteins rather than those that are involved in nonsense-mediated messenger RNA decay. By the way, similar stop-codon abnormalities have been reported not just in cystic fibrosis and Duchenne muscular dystrophy, but also Hurler's syndrome, polycystic renal disease, and several types of cancers.[1]

J. A. Stockman III, MD

Reference

1. Holbrook JA, New-Yilik G, Hentze MW, Kulozik AE. Nonsense-mediated decay approaches the clinic. *Nat Genet.* 2004;36:801-808.

Sweat Chloride Testing in Infants Identified as Heterozygote Carriers by Newborn Screening

Soultan ZN, Foster MM, Newman NB, et al (Upstate Med Univ, Syracuse, NY)
J Pediatr 153:857-859, 2008

The reference ranges for sweat [Cl⁻] were reevaluated in 300 infants referred to our Center as carriers of at least 1 cystic fibrosis mutation identified through newborn screening. The recommended borderline range of 30 to 59 mmol/L failed to identify all individuals who were compound heterozygotes. Our data support using a borderline range of 24 to 59 mmol/L.

▶ This report appeared along with another one in the *Journal of Pediatrics* by Mishra et al that also attempted to define better age-specific reference values for normal sweat chloride test results.[1] Out of nearly 300 children tested, Soultan et al identified 3 with sweat chloride values between 24 mmol/L and 30 mmol/L. In most centers, these children would have been deemed unaffected carriers. These children underwent extensive genetic testing and were found to be heterozygous for the ΔF508 mutation and the 5T-12TG variant. Soultan et al argue that we should consider lowering the accepted upper limit of normal for screened infants from 30 mmol/L to 24 mmol/L. This suggestion that we should lower the reference range for infants was the subject of a commentary by O'Sullivan and Zwerdling.[2] O'Sullivan and Zwerdling feel that the proposed change in the sweat test reference range for infants is not warranted and indeed could be harmful for a number of reasons. It is not known whether youngsters in this questionable lower range of values of sweat chloride (24 mmol/L-30 mmol/L) might even develop clinical disease consistent with cystic fibrosis. O'Sullivan and Zwerdling note that the proposed change in the sweat test reference range for children is not warranted and could be harmful for the following reasons: (1) possible development of the "vulnerable child syndrome"; (2) performance of unnecessary, costly, and anxiety-producing genetic testing; (3) impact on future reproductive decisions; (4) potential unnecessary diagnostic evaluations possibly, including high resolution computed tomography scans with their attendant radiation risk; and (5) exposure to possible adverse events from therapeutic interventions that have not yet been tested in infants with classical cystic fibrosis, never mind in children with forme fruste cystic fibrosis. It is suggested that adopting new lower reference ranges and identifying children who may not have disease as part of a newborn screening algorithm is inappropriate.

Bet you were not aware that Frederic Chopin may have had cystic fibrosis. Chopin died in France in 1849 at the age of 39 of what his death certificate recorded as "tuberculosis of the lungs and larynx." After his death, friends had the composer's heart removed, submerged in a jar of cognac, and placed in a Warsaw church in his native Poland in accordance with his wishes. Now, Polish scientists want to reopen the jar to see whether Chopin actually died of cystic fibrosis. It has been argued that Chopin had childhood symptoms matching a mild form of the genetic illness, including respiratory infections, weakness, and delayed puberty. As an adult, Chopin was slight of stature, had a hard time climbing stairs, and occasionally had to be carried off stage after concerts. Investigators hope to have the answer by 2010, which is the 200th anniversary of his birth. Needless to say, the diagnosis will be made on the basis of DNA analysis.[3]

J. A. Stockman III, MD

References

1. Mishra A, Greaves R, Smith K, et al. Diagnosis of cystic fibrosis by sweat testing: age-specific reference intervals. *J Pediatr.* 2008;153:758-763.
2. O'Sullivan BP, Zwerdling RG. By the sweat of our brows: how salty should a person be? *J Pediatr.* 2008;153:735-736.
3. Editorial comment. Chopin's heart. *Science.* 2008;321;181.

Diagnosis of Cystic Fibrosis by Sweat Testing: Age-Specific Reference Intervals

Mishra A, Greaves R, Smith K, et al (The Royal Children's Hosp, Parkville, Victoria, Australia; et al)
J Pediatr 153:758-763, 2008

Objective.—To develop reference intervals (RIs) for sweat chloride and sodium in healthy children, adolescents, and adults.

Study Design.—Healthy, unrelated subjects aged from 5 to >50 years and subjects who were pancreatic insufficient with cystic fibrosis (CF) were recruited. Sweat collection was performed on all subjects with the Wescor Macroduct system. Sweat electrolytes were analyzed with direct ion selective electrodes. $\Delta F508$ mutation analysis was performed on the healthy subjects ≥ 15 years old.

Results.—A total of 282 healthy and 40 subjects with CF were included for analysis. There was no overlap of sweat chloride between the group with CF and the group without CF, but there was some overlap of sweat sodium. Sweat chloride increased with age, with the rate of increase slowing progressively to zero after the age of 19 years. The estimated median (95% RI) for sweat chloride were: 5 to 9 years, 13 mmol/L (1-39 mmol/L); 10 to 14 years, 18 mmol/L (3-47 mmol/L); 15 to 19 years, 20 mmol/L (3-51 mmol/L); and 20+ years 23 mmol/L (5-56 mmol/L).

Conclusions.—We have successfully developed the age-related RI for sweat electrolytes, which will be useful for clinicians interpreting sweat test results from children, adolescents, and adults.

▶ Who would have thought after all these years that we would still be seeing studies of what is a normal or abnormal sweat chloride level? Traditionally, a sweat chloride value greater than 60 mmol/L has been considered to be diagnostic of cystic fibrosis, while a value of less than 40 mmol/L is negative, with values between 40 mmol/L and 60 mmol/L being borderline. The report of Mishra et al gives information on a study that tracked a large number of individuals screened for cystic fibrosis over many years. This allows careful tracking by age category. Excluded from the normative data were carriers of cystic fibrosis, relatives of known patients with cystic fibrosis, and individuals with chronic respiratory problems, thus minimizing to the extent possible the likelihood of including in the results subjects with milder forms of cystic fibrosis in the reference data. The study unequivocally documents that the traditional cutoff value for normal sweat chloride value in a child is 40 mmol/L. It should be noted that the study also found a gradual but significant rise in normal sweat chloride values with age. For example, by young adulthood, the median sweat chloride value in unaffected individuals is 22.7 mmol/L with a 95th percentile value of 59.6 mmol/L. Again, this value is consistent with the accepted belief that a sweat test value greater than 60 mmol/L is diagnostic of cystic fibrosis, but many unaffected adults were observed to have sweat chloride values in the range of 40 mmol/L to 60 mmol/L showing that there are adults who are otherwise normal who have borderline values of sweat chloride concentrations.

See the related article by Soultan et al[1] that addresses the other end of the age spectrum, the infancy period.

J. A. Stockman III, MD

Reference

1. Soultan ZN, Foster MM, Newman NB, et al. Sweat chloride testing in infants identified as heterozygote carriers by newborn screening. *J Pediatr.* 2008;153: 857-859.

Sweat test in patients with glucose-6-phosphate-1-dehydrogenase deficiency

Casaulta C, Stirnimann A, Schoeni MH, et al (Univ of Berne, Switzerland; et al)
Arch Dis Child 93:878-879, 2008

Background.—A false-positive sweat test in patients with deficiency of glucose-6-phosphate-1-dehydrogenase (EC 1.1.1.49; G6PD) is repeatedly reported.

Methods.—Sweat chloride or conductivity was measured in 11 patients with G6PD deficiency.

Results.—Mean (SD) chloride level (n = 8, median age 9.2 years, range 1.9–48.5) was 18.8 (9.6 mmol/l) and, mean (SD) sodium level was 26.0 (10.0 mmol/l), respectively, and mean (SD) conductivity (n = 3, median age 6.6 years, range 1.9–40.5) was 34.3 (6.5 mmol/l).

Conclusion.—In sweat of 11 patients with G6PD deficiency we did not find any abnormality. The reason for alleged false-positive sweat test in patients with G6PD deficiency is not known and we were unable to identify any original reference. It appears that tables of putative false-positive sweat tests in several disease states have been directly "copied and pasted" from one paper or textbook to another without verifying the original literature, a phenomenon one can call "chain citation".

▶ All of us are aware of the fact that there are false negatives associated with sweat tests as well as false positives. The most common cause of a false-negative sweat test is the inadequate securing of appropriate amounts of sweat for testing purposes. However, there is no single predominant cause of a false-positive sweat test. There are many causes that occur on an infrequent basis (Table 1). The table lists those causes that we have come to accept over the years. On this list is glucose-6-phosphate-1-dehydrogenase (G6PD) deficiency.

How G6PD deficiency made the list of conditions that raise sweat electrolyte levels has remained a mystery because no one has been able to find the original source of this observation in the literature. This led Casaulta et al to carry out sweat testing by classic pilocarpine iontophoresis in a group of youngsters with G6PD deficiency. In every case, these patients had normal sweat chloride studies.

The authors of this report searched back through references in the literature for the source of the report on elevated sweat chlorides in patients with G6PD deficiency and showed that over the years, various tables of putative false-positive sweat tests in several disease states appeared to have been directly copied and pasted from one article or textbook to another. Aficionados of the literature know that this phenomenon is called "chain citation."

TABLE 1.—Conditions Other than CF Associated with Raised Sweat Electrolytes

---

With accurate references:
▶ Glucose-6-phosphatase[3]
▶ Adrenal insufficiency[9]
▶ Familial hypoparathyroidism[10]
▶ Nephrogenic diabetes insipidus[11]
▶ Mauriac's syndrome[12]
▶ Familial cholestatic syndrome[13]
▶ Anorexia nervosa[14]
▶ Severe malnutrition[15]
▶ Atopic dermatitis[16]
▶ KID syndrome[17]
▶ Fucosidose[18]
▶ Pseudohypoaldosteronism[19]
▶ Patients undergoing prostaglandin infusions[20]

Accurate references lacking:
▶ Glucose-6-phosphate-1-dehydrogenase deficiency
▶ Ectodermal sdyplasia
▶ Hypothyroidism
▶ Nephrosis

Editor's Note: Please refer to original journal article for full references.
(Reprinted from Casaulta C, Stirnimann A, Schoeni MH, et al. Sweat test in patients with glucose-6-phosphate-1-dehydrogenase deficiency. *Arch Dis Child.* 2008;93:878-879.)

Thus it is that you will have to take with a grain of salt the accuracy of tables purporting to show causes of false-positive sweat tests. Given the phenomenon of "chain citation," nothing can be taken at face value unless you are willing to research the origins of things that appear in the literature. Needless to say, it is highly unlikely that G6PD deficiency is a cause of a raised sweat chloride concentration.

J. A. Stockman III, MD

Silver-Coated Endotracheal Tubes and Incidence of Ventilator-Associated Pneumonia: The NASCENT Randomized Trial

Kollef MH, Afessa B, Anzueto A, et al (Washington Univ School of Medicine, St Louis, MO; Mayo Clinic College of Medicine, Rochester, MN; South Texas Veterans Health Care System Audie L. Murphy Division, San Antonio, et al)
JAMA 300:806 813, 2008

Context.—Ventilator-associated pneumonia (VAP) causes substantial morbidity. A silver-coated endotracheal tube has been designed to reduce VAP incidence by preventing bacterial colonization and biofilm formation.

Objective.—To determine whether a silver-coated endotracheal tube would reduce the incidence of microbiologically confirmed VAP.

Design, Setting, and Participants.—Prospective, randomized, single-blind, controlled study conducted in 54 centers in North America. A total of 9417 adult patients ($\geq$18 years) were screened between 2002 and 2006. A total of 2003 patients expected to require mechanical ventilation for 24 hours or longer were randomized.

Intervention.—Patients were assigned to undergo intubation with 1 of 2 high-volume, low-pressure endotracheal tubes, similar except for a silver coating on the experimental tube.

Main Outcome Measures.—Primary outcome was VAP incidence based on quantitative bronchoalveolar lavage fluid culture with 10^4 colony-forming units/mL or greater in patients intubated for 24 hours or longer. Other outcomes were VAP incidence in all intubated patients, time to VAP onset, length of intubation and duration of intensive care unit and hospital stay, mortality, and adverse events.

Results.—Among patients intubated for 24 hours or longer, rates of microbiologically confirmed VAP were 4.8% (37/766 patients; 95% confidence interval [CI], 3.4%-6.6%) in the group receiving the silver-coated tube and 7.5% (56/743; 95% CI, 5.7%-9.7%) ($P = .03$) in the group receiving the uncoated tube (all intubated patients, 3.8% [37/968; 95% CI, 2.7%-5.2%] and 5.8% [56/964; 95% CI, 4.4%-7.5%] [$P = .04$]), with a relative risk reduction of 35.9% (95% CI, 3.6%-69.0%; all intubated patients, 34.2% [95% CI, 1.2%-67.9%]). The silver-coated endotracheal tube was associated with delayed occurrence of VAP ($P = .005$). No statistically significant between-group differences were observed in durations of intubation, intensive care unit stay, and hospital stay; mortality; and frequency and severity of adverse events.

Conclusion.—Patients receiving a silver-coated endotracheal tube had a statistically significant reduction in the incidence of VAP and delayed time to VAP occurrence compared with those receiving a similar, uncoated tube.

Trial Registration.—clinicaltrials.gov Identifier: NCT00148642.

▶ Kollef et al report the results of the North American Silver-Coated Endotracheal Tube Study, which examined the potential efficacy of a new endotracheal tube for preventing ventilator-associated pneumonia. It is not only adults who get into problems with being mechanically ventilated. Kids also develop ventilator-associated pneumonias when on a ventilator for extended periods of time. What Kollef et al have done is to see whether a silver-coated endotracheal tube which is otherwise similar to standard endotracheal tubes would help reduce ventilator-associated pneumonia rates by preventing biofilm formation at its surface, thus hampering respiratory tract bacterial colonization. These tubes have a coating of silver ions, which are microdispersed in a proprietary polymer. The presence of an endotracheal tube not only compromises the natural barrier between the oropharynx and trachea, but also facilitates the entry of bacteria into the lung by pooling and leaking of contaminated secretions around the cuff. Moreover, biofilm formation on the inner and outer surfaces of the endotracheal tube provides a protected environment for pathogens to grow. These bacterial aggregates and biofilm can become easily dislodged during suctioning. Previous data have suggested that in animal models, an endotracheal tube coated externally and internally with a potent antiseptic product such as silver could exert a sustained antimicrobial effect, including the blocking of biofilm formation.

What Kollef et al observed in 1509 patients intubated for more than 24 hours was that silver-coated endotracheal tubes lower the frequency of ventilator-associated pneumonia from 7.5% in a control group to just 4.8%. This represents a relative risk reduction of almost 36% and an absolute risk reduction of 2.7%, suggesting that 37 patients had to be treated with the silver-coated tube to prevent one case of ventilator-associated pneumonia. Use of the silver-coated tube did not reduce mortality rates, duration of intubation, duration of ICU or hospital length of stay, or the frequency or severity of adverse effects.

It is worthwhile reading the editorial that accompanied the Kollef et al report. Chastre notes that silver-coated tubes should not be viewed as the definitive answer for ventilator-associated pneumonia prevention and that their use should be restricted to high-risk patients treated in ICUs.[1] High-risk patients, for example, would include the neurologically impaired individual or the trauma patient. These statements are made because many uncertainties exist regarding the exact benefit of silver-coated endotracheal tubes. Needless to say, the use of such tubes in children has been totally unexplored, a study waiting to happen.

J. A. Stockman III, MD

Reference

1. Chastre J. Preventing ventilator-associated pneumonia. could silver-coated endotracheal tubes be the answer? *N Engl J Med*. 2008;300:842-844.

Prevalence and Time Course of Acute Mountain Sickness in Older Children and Adolescents After Rapid Ascent to 3450 Meters

Bloch J, Duplain H, Rimoldi SF, et al (Univ Hosp, Lausanne, Switzerland; Univ Hosp, Bern, Switzerland, et al)
Pediatrics 123:1-5, 2009

Objective.—Acute mountain sickness is a frequent and debilitating complication of high-altitude exposure, but there is little information on the prevalence and time course of acute mountain sickness in children and adolescents after rapid ascent by mechanical transportation to 3500 m, an altitude at which major tourist destinations are located throughout the world.

Methods.—We performed serial assessments of acute mountain sickness (Lake Louise scores) in 48 healthy nonacclimatized children and adolescents (mean ± SD age: 13.7 ± 0.3 years; 20 girls and 28 boys), with no previous high-altitude experience, 6, 18, and 42 hours after arrival at the Jungfraujoch high-altitude research station (3450 m), which was reached through a 2.5-hour train ascent.

Results.—We found that the overall prevalence of acute mountain sickness during the first 3 days at high altitude was 37.5%. Rates were similar for the 2 genders and decreased progressively during the stay (25% at 6 hours, 21% at 18 hours, and 8% at 42 hours). None of the subjects needed to be evacuated to lower altitude. Five subjects needed symptomatic treatment and responded well.

Conclusion.—After rapid ascent to high altitude, the prevalence of acute mountain sickness in children and adolescents was relatively low; the clinical manifestations were benign and resolved rapidly. These findings suggest that, for the majority of healthy nonacclimatized children and adolescents, travel to 3500 m is safe and pharmacologic prophylaxis for acute mountain sickness is not needed.

▶ You don't have to be a mountaineer to find yourself at high altitudes these days. Ask anyone who has driven in Colorado. Trips by car to high altitude can take very little time. Unfortunately, there is little information on the prevalence of acute mountain sickness in children and teens after rapid ascent by mechanical transportation to altitudes that may be problematic. The report of Bloch et al studied this issue by looking at a group of 48 healthy Swiss children and adolescents (mean age 13.7 ± 0.3 years; range 10 to 17 years). All except 2 of these youngsters normally lived at altitudes of < 800 m. The participants ascended to the high altitude research station on a mountainside in Switzerland having gotten there on a 2.5 hour train ride. They then spent 2 days and 2 nights in a laboratory at 3450 m and symptoms of acute mountain sickness were assessed (headache, gastrointestinal symptoms, fatigue, dizziness, and sleep disturbance).

The study reported that on the evening of the day of arrival, 25% of the children and adolescents suffered from headache of a significant degree. The majority of the headaches resolved by the next morning, but 10% of the youngsters had persistent headache and another 10% had developed new onset headache by that time. All in all, 1 out of the 5 youngsters met the criteria for acute mountain sickness. None of the subjects needed to be evacuated to a lower altitude or experienced progression of acute mountain sickness to high altitude cerebral edema, the most dangerous complication of acute mountain sickness. None of the subjects developed high altitude pulmonary edema. The trend for higher numbers of acute mountain sickness on day 2 than on day 1 most likely related to the fact that insomnia contributed to the symptom scores of these youngsters.

If one looks at the adult literature, one sees that many more adults will develop acute mountain sickness at altitudes of 3450 m than we see in the children and adolescents in the Swiss study. It should be noted that the prevalence of acute mountain sickness did not differ between girls and boys in this report.

For adults planning rapid ascent to high altitudes, current guidelines propose prophylaxis with drugs that may have significant side effects. When it comes to children, if the data from this report hold up, it would seem that for children and adolescents with no history of moderate/severe acute mountain sickness who plan to ascend rapidly to the altitudes reported in this study, pharmacologic prophylaxis may not be needed with the use of such agents being restricted for actual treatment of symptoms (mainly headache) if they appear. All too often we do not think about acute mountain sickness in the casual tourist, but we should realize it can be a problem for even the youngest among us.

As this commentary closes, another *Clinical Fact/Curio*, this having to do with high altitude conditions. Where in the world might you go to study the effects of altitude on travelers? The answer to this question could be as simple as examining those who take a train ride from Golmud in the Shanghai Qinghai Province of China to Lhasa, Tibet. This relatively new train route is a breakthrough in high-altitude transportation. The trip takes slightly over 14 hours on a track that is 1142 km long at an average altitude of 4500 m. Eighty-five percent of the track is above 4000 m, and the highest altitude reached is 5074 m, with a rapid initial ascent from Golmud, altitude of 2808 m, to Mount Kunlun, altitude of 4768 m, in only 1.5 hours. Each train carries more than 900 people, and the total number of passengers by 2008 had exceeded 3 million. Because many passengers who live near sea level reach these very high altitudes in less than 2 days, the potential exposure to severe hypoxia represents a significant challenge. Other studies done at these altitudes show that at 5000 m, one will see an alveolar Po_2 of about 40 mm Hg. With full acclimatization, the Po_2 increases by about 8 mm Hg, but little acclimatization will occur during an exposure of just 14 hours. The arterial Po_2 will be less than 40 mm Hg with an arterial oxygen saturation falling to near 75% at the highest point on the railroad train traveling from Golmud to Lhasa. This would be true were there no intervention taken, an intervention that is unequivocally necessary because people of all ages and physical conditions travel on this train despite recommendations that those with lung or heart disease not make the journey, because it has been shown that a substantial proportion of acclimatized people exposed to an altitude of 4500 m for 14 hours will develop symptoms of acute mountain sickness.

So how are the trains engineered in China to mitigate this problem? The Po_2 of inhaled air is determined by 2 factors: barometric pressure and oxygen concentration. The only way to alleviate hypoxia is to increase one of these. In an airplane, this is accomplished by increasing cabin pressure such that the cabin altitude does not exceed 2440 m. Unfortunately, it is impractical to pressurize an entire train. The alternative solution is to increase the oxygen concentration of the air inside the train, not an easy engineering feat, but it can be done. For example, in the United States, home builders in high-altitude ski resorts in Colorado and New Mexico are installing oxygen enrichment equipment in bedrooms because many people have difficulty sleeping at high altitude. In each of these situations, generators extract oxygen from the air. For every 1% increase in oxygen concentration (for example, from 21%-22% oxygen), the equivalent altitude is reduced by about 300 m (the equivalent altitude is that which provides the same inhaled Po_2 for ambient air breathing). For example, astronomers at the California Institute of Technology operate a radio telescope at an altitude of 5080 m in north Chile, living in an oxygen concentration of 27%. Those breathing 27% oxygen will have their equivalent altitude reduced by 1800 to 3200 m, an altitude that is tolerable in people with some altitude acclimatization. Oxygen enrichment of room air at high altitude has been shown to improve neuropsychological function, sleep quality, and daily working efficiency.

So exactly how does the Qinghai-Tibet railway pull off the feat of defeating high altitude symptoms? This railway, commonly known as the Lhasa train, was designed by the Bombardier Corporation of Montreal, which also makes airplanes that are commonly flown in the United States. The train has 16 cars. Four of these are "hard seat" coaches, each containing 96 passengers who are seated for the 48-hour journey from Beijing to Lhasa. Next there are 7 "hard sleepers," each carrying 60 passengers; 2 "soft sleepers," each with 32 passengers; a dining car; a generating car; and 2 diesel electric locomotives. Cigarette smoking is strictly prohibited throughout the train. Each passenger car has a special compartment with an oxygen generator that uses the membrane separation technique. The principle is that nitrogen diffuses faster through a thin membrane than oxygen under high pressure, allowing partial separation of these 2 gases. The generator typically produces 40% to 50% oxygen, which is added to the ventilation in each car to achieve 24% to 25% oxygen concentration in the car. Although this may seem a rather small degree of oxygen enrichment, an oxygen concentration of 25% yields a reduction in equivalent altitude of 1200 m. Therefore, at the train's highest altitude, about 5000 m, the cabin altitude is reduced to about 3800 m. Given the fact that train passengers are relatively sedentary, they do not need further oxygen enrichment. The train terminates at Lhasa, an altitude of 3658 m, which is lower than the train route, but still high enough to cause acute mountain sickness in some tourists, and oxygen is therefore available in many hotel rooms. Oxygen and carbon dioxide levels in the train cars are monitored and automatically regulated to keep the oxygen-enriched airflow appropriate as the altitude changes. Passengers can actually see the indicators showing the oxygen concentration of the air in their coaches. Although oxygen enrichment of room air introduces a fire hazard, the oxygen concentration at an altitude of 5000 m has to be increased above 31% before the burning rate of common materials exceeds that of sea level. Although oxygen enrichment increases the Po_2 in the train air, it is still far below the Po_2 at sea level. Each coach has its own generator, and parallel systems on attached cars can be engaged to serve as backups in case of failure of any one system on a single car. Needless to say, at train stops, doors are opened only for as short a time as necessary to discharge or take on passengers. The train typically stops at only 3 stations between Golmud and Lhasa, and all doors are opened at only 1 of these stations. The gangways between the carriages are gas tight. The passenger cars have automatic plug sliding doors that fit tightly when they are closed. The train has a vacuum system for disposal of waste with large wastewater tanks so that nothing is released into the environment. Windows are tightly sealed, and the exhaust system maintains a slight positive pressure so that any air leak is outbound, not inbound.

J. A. Stockman III, MD

When should oxygen be given to children at high altitude? A systematic review to define altitude-specific hypoxaemia
Subhi R, Smith K, Duke T (Univ of Melbourne, Victoria, Australia; Royal Children's Hosp, Victoria, Australia)
Arch Dis Child 94:6-10, 2009

Background.—Acute respiratory infections (ARI) cause 3 million deaths in children worldwide each year. Most of these deaths occur from pneumonia in developing countries, and hypoxaemia is the most common fatal complication. Simple and adaptable indications for oxygen therapy are important in the management of ARI. The current WHO definition of hypoxaemia as any arterial oxygen saturation (SpO_2) <90% does not take into account the variation in normal oxygen saturation with altitude. This study aimed to define normal oxygen saturation and to estimate the threshold of hypoxaemia for children permanently living at different altitudes.

Methods.—We carried out a systematic review of the literature addressing normal values of oxygen saturation in children aged 1 week to 12 years. Hypoxaemia was defined as any SpO_2 at or below the 2.5th centile for a population of healthy children at a given altitude. Metaregression analysis was performed to estimate the change in mean SpO_2 and the hypoxaemia threshold with increasing altitude.

Results.—14 studies were reviewed and analysed to produce prediction equations for estimating the expected mean SpO_2 in normal children, and the threshold SpO_2 indicating hypoxaemia at various altitudes. An SpO_2 of 90% is the 2.5th centile for a population of healthy children living at an altitude of ~2500 m above sea level. This decreases to 85% at an altitude of ~3200 m.

Conclusions.—For health facilities at very high altitudes, giving oxygen to all children with an SpO_2 <90% may be too liberal if oxygen supplies are limited. In such settings, SpO_2 <85% may be more appropriate to identify children most in need of oxygen supplementation.

▶ A study by Bloch et al looked at the prevalence and time course of acute mountain sickness in older children and adolescents after rapid ascent to 3450 meters.[1] The Bloch et al report suggested that children and adolescents who quickly ascend to such altitudes by mechanical transportation have about a 1 in 5 chance of developing symptoms consistent with acute mountain sickness. The report of Subhi et al looks at the role of oxygen supplementation and when it should be given at high altitude as part of the management of children with respiratory problems.

Subhi et al give us an analysis of normal oxygen saturation levels in children up to 5 years of age living in regions with altitudes as high as approximately 4000 m. Their work is an essential part of a program looking at how oxygen concentrators and pulse oximetry might help to improve the outcome of childhood pneumonia in Papua, New Guinea. The intent was to provide a solution to the question of when oxygen should be given to sick children at altitude. The findings are intended to inform health policy and clinical decision-making. The conclusion of the report is that above altitudes of 2500 m, giving oxygen for saturation less than 90% may be too liberal for facilities with limited oxygen supplies. There is evidence that at altitudes greater than 2500 m, a threshold of oxygen saturation of 85% can be used to identify children who are most in need of oxygen supplementation.

For those who are interested in the topic of living at high altitude, it may be worthwhile to read the commentary that accompanied this report.[2] Depending on one's racial/ethnic background, the adaptation to living at high altitudes can be very different. For example, endogenous Andeans at 4000 m have a hemoglobin concentration and oxygen saturation more than 1 standard deviation higher than endogenous Tibetans at the same altitude. These changes are equivalent to an arterial oxygen content 16% higher and 10% lower than at sea level reference values in Andeans and Tibetans, respectively. The high altitude threshold for increasing red cell mass is also different in these 2 populations. It appears to be approximately 1600 m in Andeans and above 4000 m in Tibetans, despite their profoundly low oxygen saturations. In the study of Subhi et al, the threshold for change in oxygen saturation seemed to occur at 1600 m. This is consistent with multiple other studies in children that show that children living below 1600 m would be expected to have normal hematologic values and normal oxygen saturations. This has direct relevance to similar altitudes here in the United States when determining normative hemoglobin values.

While on the topic of acute mountain sickness, were you aware that the mortality rate among mountaineers attempting a climb on Mount Everest runs 1.3%? Mount Everest is the highest point on earth at 8850 m above sea level.

Firth et al examined patterns of mortality among climbers on Mount Everest over an 86-year period (1921-2006).[3] The death rate during all descents was higher for climbers than for Sherpas (2.7% vs 0.4%). Of all mountaineers who died after climbing above 8000 m, 56% died during descent from the summit, 17% after turning back, and 10% during ascent. For the remainder, the stage of the summit bid was not known at the time of demise. The median time to reach the summit was earlier for survivors than for nonsurvivors.

The data from Mount Everest document that when you are climbing high, high mountains, reaching the summit is only half the battle. Chances are if you are going to die it will be on the way down.

This comment closes with a miscellaneous *Clinical Fact/Curio* about a particularly serious problem related to the respiratory tract, namely drowning, related to recreational boating. Approximately 70 million persons in the United States participate in recreational boating and paddle sports (ie, using vessels such as canoes, kayaks, and inflatable rafts). They make up the fastest growing segment of the boating market. For example, from 2005-2006, canoe sales in the United States increased by 23%, kayak sales increased by 11%, while powerboat sales decreased by 5%. Given the price of biofuels these days, one can only guess that sail boating and paddle sports will continue to increase in popularity.

The state that has the most data on paddle sports fatalities is Maine. During the period 2000-2007, a total of 38 paddle sport fatalities were identified in Maine. Twenty-nine (76%) of those who died were Maine residents; 8 were residents of other states; and one was a resident of another country. Paddle sports fatalities accounted for 40% of the 82 total boating deaths during this period in Maine. Fifty-eight percent of the deaths were associated with canoes, 32% with kayaks, and 10% with rafts. The primary cause of death in 61% was drowning after capsizing. Twenty-one percent resulted from drowning after falling overboard, 5% from drowning after entrapment, 5% from drowning in persons who had a history of seizure, 5% from cardiac arrest while boating, and 3% from hypothermia. No deaths were directly attributed to trauma. Almost 70% of those who died in a paddle sport activity were not wearing personal flotation devices (PFDs). Ninety-five percent of canoeists who died did so not wearing a PFD, although almost 40% actually had a PFD in their canoes. About 1 in 5 who had a blood alcohol test performed as part of a postmortem had a blood alcohol that was above the legal limit for driving and boating in the state of Maine. In fact, in those with an elevated blood alcohol, the average level was twice the legal limit. The median water temperature at the time of the fatal incidents was just 54°F.

There are several messages to take home from the experience of Maine. The first is the most obvious: do not paddle and drink. The second is to always wear a PFD, even if you think you are a good swimmer. Last, while there is nothing you can do to avoid paddling in 54°F water, there is a lot you can do to learn about boat safety, particularly when it comes to rafting, canoeing, and kayaking. The United States Power Squadrons, a non-profit educational organization dedicated to promoting boating safety, offers a Paddle Smart[TM] seminar with safety information specific to paddle sports.[4] This seminar and other prevention strategies that promote PFD use, discourage alcohol use before and during boating, and support boating safety education, might indeed help reduce paddle sports fatalities.

J. A. Stockman III, MD

References

1. Bloch J, Duplain H, Rimoldi SF, et al. Prevalence and time course of acute mountain sickness in older children and adolescents after rapid ascent to 3450 meters. *Pediatrics.* 2009;123:1-5.
2. Tasker RC. Oxygen and living at altitude. *Arch Dis Child.* 2009;94:1-2.
3. Firth PG, Zheng H, Windsor JS, et al. Mortality on Mount Everest, 1921-2006: descriptive study. *BMJ.* 2008;337:1430-1433.
4. United States Power Squadrons. Paddle Smart^TM Boating Seminar. Raleigh, NC: United States Power Squadrons; 2008, http://www.usps.org/e_stuff/seminars/paddlesmart_sem.htm; 2008. Accessed July 27, 2009.

19 Therapeutics and Toxicology

Adverse Events From Cough and Cold Medications in Children

Schaefer MK, Shehab N, Cohen AL, et al (Natl Ctr for Preparedness, Detection and Control of Infectious Diseases; Ctrs for Disease Control and Prevention, Atlanta, GA)
Pediatrics 121:783-787, 2008

Background.—Adverse drug events in children from cough and cold medications have been identified as a public health issue with clinical and policy implications. Nationally representative morbidity data could be useful for targeting age-appropriate safety interventions.

Objective.—To describe emergency department visits for adverse drug events from cough and cold medications in children.

Methods.—Emergency department visits for adverse drug events attributed to cough and cold medications among children aged <12 years were identified from a nationally representative stratified probability sample of 63 US emergency departments from January 1, 2004, through December 31, 2005.

Results.—Annually, an estimated 7091 patients aged <12 years were treated in emergency departments for adverse drug events from cough and cold medications, accounting for 5.7% of emergency department visits for all medications in this age group. Most visits were for children aged 2 to 5 years (64%). Unsupervised ingestions accounted for 66% of estimated emergency department visits, which was significantly higher than unsupervised ingestions of other medications (47%), and most of these ingestions involved children aged 2 to 5 years (77%). Most children did not require admission or extended observation (93%).

Conclusions.—Timely national surveillance data can help target education, enforcement, and engineering strategies for reducing adverse events from cough and cold medications among children. Engineering innovations could be particularly helpful in addressing unsupervised ingestions, which is the most frequent cause of adverse events. These innovations could be applicable to other children's medications.

▶ It was in 2007 that national experts petitioned the United States Food and Drug Administration (FDA) to advise that cough and cold medications not be used in children under the age of 6 years. The FDA's Nonprescription

Drugs Committee and Pediatric Advisory Committee have since unanimously recommended that these drugs not be used in children ages 2 years and under by majority vote and that they not be used in children under the age of 6 based on lack of evidence of effectiveness and increased risk of harm. The Consumer Healthcare Products Association, which represents manufacturers of over-the-counter medications, has issued a voluntary market recall of over-the-counter cough and cold medications labeled for use in infants, but has also issued a positive statement that cautioned against the recommendation to make cold and cough medications unavailable to children aged to 6 years. Despite this widespread attention, questions remain regarding the relative contribution of adverse effects from recommended use, unsupervised ingestions, and inadvertent overdoses, as well as the relative burden of adverse events according to age. The study of Schaefer et al addresses the latter set of issues.

By assessing the National Electronic Injury Surveillance System-Cooperative Adverse Drug Events Surveillance, these investigators found that two-thirds of the estimated emergency department visits for adverse drug events attributable to cough and cold medications resulted from children accessing these medications without adult supervision, a significantly higher proportion than for adverse drug events attributable to all other medications. As one might suspect, children aged 2 to 5 years accounted for most of the unsupervised ingestions. A smaller subset of youngsters came to the emergency room as the result of a medication error on the part of a parent. In fact, medication errors were more common with cough and cold medications than with all other medications with most of these errors occurring in children under 2 years of age. In most of the latter instances, the cough and cold medication labels did not specify dosages, but, instead, directed caregivers to consult a pediatrician.

A number of national pediatric experts have continued to cite lack of evidence demonstrating the efficacy of cold and cough medications in children over the age of 2 years, and some have called for the removal of these products pending additional pediatric studies. Manufacturers have stated that they will continue to market these products for children but would work with the FDA to design efficacy studies. As long as these products continue to be marketed for use in children, additional safety interventions must be in place to address a common cause of injuries from these products, which is unsupervised ingestions, particularly in 2 to 5 year olds.

The United States is not the only country that has placed restrictions on the sale of cold and cough medications intended for use in children. In March 2008, the United Kingdom Medicine and Healthcare Products Regulatory Agency announced that over-the-counter cough medicines are no longer suitable for children younger than 2 years. This followed by some months the FDA's similar decision. Those in England looked at data for the United States, which showed 3 infant deaths in 2005 in the treatment of an estimated 1519 children in United States emergency departments in 2004 and 2005 related to cough and cold medicines.

It should be noted that a January 2008 Cochrane review of randomized controlled trials spanning the last 40 years concluded that there is no good evidence for or against the effectiveness of over-the-counter medicines in acute cough.[1] Stated otherwise, until there is evidence that cough medicines are actually effective in children, they should be removed from sale.

J. A. Stockman III, MD

Reference

1. Smith SM, Schroeder K, Fahey T. Over-the-counter medications for acute cough in children and adults in ambulatory settings. *Cochrane Database Syst Rev.* 2008;1:CD001831. http://www.mrw.interscience.wiley.com/cochrane/clsysrev/articles/CD001831/pdf_ts.html. Accessed June 11, 2009.

Pseudoephedrine Use Among US Children, 1999–2006: Results From the Slone Survey

Vernacchio L, Kelly JP, Kaufman DW, et al (Boston Univ, MA)
Pediatrics 122:1299-1304, 2008

Objective.—Pseudoephedrine, a decongestant found in many cough-and-cold and allergy medications, has been associated with deaths and adverse events in young children; however, the absolute risks of pediatric pseudoephedrine use are difficult to assess because the number of children exposed on a population basis and typical patterns of use are unknown. In addition, use may be changing because of the Combat Methamphetamine Epidemic Act of 2005, which limited pseudoephedrine availability. We sought to describe the prevalence and patterns of pseudoephedrine use among US children and to assess any change since the 2005 law took effect.

Methods.—We analyzed data on pseudoephedrine use among 4267 children who were aged 0 to 17 years and enrolled from 1999 to 2006 in the Slone Survey, a national random-digit-dial telephone survey of medication use in the US population.

Results.—Overall, 214 children took pseudoephedrine in a given week. Use was highest for children who were younger than 2 years. Sixteen children (7.5% of users) took > 1 pseudoephedrine-containing product within the same week, including 6 children who were younger than 2 years. Of the pseudoephedrine products used, most were multiple-ingredient liquids (58.9%) and multiple-ingredient tablets (24.7%). Fifty-two children (25.0% of users) took pseudoephedrine for >1 week, including 7 children who were younger than 2 years. Use in 2006 (2.9%) was significantly lower than in 1999–2005 (5.2%).

Conclusions.—Pseudoephedrine exposure, mostly in the form of multiple-ingredient products, is common among US children, especially children who are younger than 2 years, who are at the highest risk for toxicity and for whom safe dosing recommendations are lacking. Concerning patterns of use include taking > 1 pseudoephedrine-containing product concurrently and using pseudoephedrine for extended periods. Pediatric pseudoephedrine use seems to be declining since the institution of the 2005 Combat Methamphetamine Epidemic Act.

▶ This report tells us how quickly bad news influences the sales of certain pharmaceuticals. All of us are aware of the recent report from the Centers for Disease Control and Prevention that highlighted the link between pseudo-ephedrine overdose and the deaths of 3 infants back in 2005.[1] 2005 also saw legislation being passed that may have affected pediatric pseudoephedrine use. This was the "Combat Methamphetamine Epidemic Act." This Federal law was designed to reduce illicit methamphetamine production from pseudoephe-drine by requiring all pseudoephedrine-containing products to be kept behind pharmacy counters and sold to individuals in limited quantities. The law took full effect in September 2006, but many large pharmacy chains began to move pseudoephedrine-containing products behind the counter in mid 2005. The report of Vernacchio et al tells us what impact these 2 events have had on the prevalence and pattern of pseudoephedrine use in United States children.

What we learn from this report is that pseudoephedrine use is still quite common, with the highest use still occurring in children who are younger than 2 years. Well over half a million United States children younger than age 2 are being exposed to pseudoephedrine weekly despite evidence of little or no efficacy and absence of safe dosing recommendations for this age group. The data from this report demonstrate a monumental failure on our part to get the message through that these are products that should not be used in young children.

In 2008, Rimsza and Newberry reported a large number of unexpected infant deaths associated with the use of cough and cold medications.[2] Chamberlain recently ran the math in this regard.[3] If you extrapolate the 10 infant deaths associated with cough and cold medication from Arizona's population of 6 million, to the combined United States and Canadian population of 337 million, the estimated deaths associated with cough and cold medications would be over 500 per year. While this may sound like an exaggerated number, and it could be, every one of whatever deaths do occur should be on all of our consciences for allowing this situation to continue. These types of medications need to be pulled from pharmacy shelves.

J. A. Stockman III, MD

References

1. Infant deaths associated with cough and cold medications: two states, 2005. *MMWR Morb Mortal Wkly Rep.* 2007;56:1-4.
2. Rimsza ME, Newberry S. Unexpected infant deaths associated with the use of cough and cold medications. *Pediatrics.* 2008;122:e318-e322.
3. Chamberlain JL. Unexpected infant deaths associated with the use of cough and cold medications. *Pediatrics.* 2008;122:1413.

Medicines for Children: A Matter of Taste

Davies EH, Tuleu C (Great Ormond Street Hosp for Children NHS Trust, London, UK; Univ of London, UK)
J Pediatr 153:599-604, 2008

The aim of this paper was to systematically search the peer-reviewed literature on palatability testing of medicines in children to give a deeper insight into how such studies have been performed to date. The methods used were screened and reviewed to evaluate them to highlight key issues to be considered when performing such studies and provide practical help to design reliable age-appropriate sensory tests.

▶ Until this article appeared, this editor had very little understanding of how complex it is to actually measure the palatability of a medication that is used to treat medical conditions in children.[1] Currently, the European Union requires the submission of pharmaceutical development plans for medicines used for children. There is a requirement to evaluate taste and palatability of medicines used for children. Obviously an acceptable taste is critical with pediatric patients. Were you aware that compounds are now tested by 5 basic tests? These are sweetness, saltiness, sourness, bitterness, and umami (protein, "meaty" taste). In addition, touch, temperature, appearance, and especially smell are also important.

The report of Davies et al was undertaken to summarize the world's literature that describes the assessment of medicinal product taste in children. One can see how little there is in the literature that is of high quality. One could argue that adults could be used to test acceptability because they are more capable of making a full analysis of the palatability of certain formulations (taste, smell, texture, aftertaste) and to assess taste-masking strategies. They could also be seen as appropriate to taste medication to be given to children on a short-term basis. Thus far there are very little data to tell us that extrapolation of adult data for palatability assessment of children's medicines is of any value. On the other hand, you can imagine all the problems associated with trying to standardize a group of young children and their ratings of the palatability of oral medications.

Read this article in detail and you will learn a lot about taste testing in children, its triumphs and failures. If nothing else, young children, you will learn, do not like unusual flavors such as that of pineapples and peaches. When in doubt, strawberries always win out.

This commentary closes with another *Clinical Fact/Curio*, regarding medical toxicology. Recently, a major health concern took place in Nigeria when a pain killer was identified as a cause of a number of children's deaths. The National Agency for Food and Drug Administration and Control in Nigeria announced in 2009 that 84 children had died and a further 27 had fallen ill between November 2008 and January 2009 after taking a pain relief syrup called My Pikin. It was determined that the product contained the chemical diethylene glycol, an industrial solvent found in antifreeze that is sometimes used as a cheap alternative to glycerin, a base compound often used in pharmaceuticals. Blame for the problem was not placed as of the end of 2009.[2]

J. A. Stockman III, MD

References

1. Regulation (EC) No 1901/2006 of the European Parliament and the council of December 12, 2006 on medicinal products for pediatric use. http://ec.europa.eu/enterprise/pharmaceuticals/eudralex/vol1/reg_2006_1901/reg_2006_1901_en.pdf. Accessed July 1, 2009.
2. Pain killer blamed for childrens deaths in Nigeria. [Editorial comment]. *BMJ.* 2009;338:374.

News Media Coverage of Medication Research: Reporting Pharmaceutical Company Funding and Use of Generic Medication Names
Hochman M, Hochman S, Bor D, et al (Cambridge Health Alliance, and Harvard Med School, Cambridge, MA)
JAMA 300:1544-1550, 2008

Context.—The news media are an important source of information about medical research for patients and even some physicians. Little is known about how frequently news articles report when medication research has received funding from pharmaceutical companies or how frequently news articles use generic vs brand medication names.

Objectives.—To assess the reporting of pharmaceutical company funding and generic medication name use in news articles about medication studies and to determine the views of newspaper editors about these issues.

Design, Setting, and Participants.—We reviewed US news articles from newspaper and online sources about all pharmaceutical company–funded medication studies published in the 5 most prominent general medical journals between April 1, 2004, and April 30, 2008. We also surveyed editors at the 100 most widely circulated newspapers in the United States.

Main Outcome Measures.—The percentage of news articles indicating when studies have been pharmaceutical company–funded and the percentage that refer to medications by their generic vs brand names. Also the percentage of newspaper editors who indicate that their articles report pharmaceutical company funding; the percentage of editors who indicate that their articles refer to medications by generic names; and the percentage of newspapers with policies about these issues.

Results.—Of the 306 news articles about medication research identified, 130 (42%; 95% confidence interval [CI], 37%-48%) did not report that the research had received company funding. Of the 277 of these articles reporting on medications with both generic and brand names, 186 (67%; 95% CI, 61%-73%) referred to the study medications by their brand names in at least half of the medication references. Eighty-two of the 93 (88%) newspaper editors who responded to our survey reported that articles from their publications always or often indicated when studies had received company funding (95% CI, 80%-94%), and 71 of 92 (77%) responding editors also reported that articles from their publications always or often referred to medications by the generic names (95% CI, 67%-85%). However, only 3 of 92 newspapers (3%) had written policies stating that company funding sources of medical studies be reported (95% CI 1%-9%), and 2 of 93 (2%) newspapers had written policies stating that medications should be referred to by their generic names (95% CI 1%-8%).

Conclusion.—News articles reporting on medication studies often fail to report pharmaceutical company funding and frequently refer to medications by their brand names despite newspaper editors' contention that this is not the case.

▶ While this report does not specifically deal with pediatric medication research and the reporting of this in the news media, clearly the data from this report apply to such research. This study is the most comprehensive analysis that has examined the reporting of pharmaceutical company funding in medical research by the United States media and builds on previous research including a substantially larger number of news articles, a broader array of news sources (including online sources), and survey data from journalists. It is also the first study that examines the use of generic versus brand medication names by United States news media. News articles do in fact represent an important source of information for pharmaceuticals for the lay public, including patients and families. Thus it is that the information from this report is important because it tells us whether or not journalists acknowledge any potential commercial bias in medical research by indicating in their news coverage whether the research is supported by the pharmaceutical industry. This is especially true of research that involves medications that the public may be taking. Another way the news media may reduce commercial bias in medical information they present is by using nonproprietary medication names. Generic names may also be preferable because many medications come in multiple brands, and the use of generic names may reduce confusion in even potentially dangerous medication errors. Indeed, failure to use generic names may be one of the reasons why there may be as much as a $9 billion wasteful expenditure related to the use of brand name drugs instead of generic drugs, which are totally equivalent. For these reasons, most medical journals require the use of generic names and the Institute for Safe Medication Practices recommends that generic medication names be used as the primary nomenclature in electronic ordering systems, and the United States Food and Drug Administration mandates the use of generic names in advertising and on labels and brochures.

We see in the report of Hochman et al that news articles from United States newspapers and online sources frequently fail to indicate when medication studies have received company funding. As often, they also tend to use brand names rather than generic names for the medications that are being reported on. The study also documents that the majority of major newspapers lack written policies on the reporting of pharmaceutical company funding and the use of generic medication names. These findings may partially explain why journalists so frequently neglect to report when research has received corporate funding and so frequently refer to medications by their brand names. One might speculate that the reason journalists frequently neglect to provide this information is because they are unaware of when a study has been company-sponsored. This information is frequently buried within the methods section or at the end of a journal article and finding this information could be a difficult task for those without a medical background. All too often, of course, journalists rely on derivative information rather than the original source and that derivative information may not provide the requisite statements about pharmaceutical funding.

The authors of this report indicate that for patients to evaluate new research findings, it is important that they know how the research was funded so that they can assess commercial biases that could affect the results. One wonders, however, whether the public would even be capable of making such an assessment even if the information were provided. This is where it is critical for journal editors to do their homework in being sure there is no conflict of interest before an article is accepted for publication. In the meantime, it does not hurt for a journalist to snoop around in an attempt to do the same thing. We would all be better off.

This commentary closes with a therapeutic *Clinical Fact/Curio*. Have you ever heard of the following pharmaceuticals: Indolebant and Strivor? What is their relationship to the entity MDD? In response, MDD is the abbreviation for "motivational deficiency disorder." In fact, MDD is a spoof illness that started life on the Internet 2 years ago as a satirical dig at drug industry marketing strategies. MDD has now emerged as the subject of a fake television story designated as an educational aid for the public and for health professionals to better understand how pharmaceutical companies sell their wares in terms of new drugs. Indolebant (trade name Strivor) is a fictitious drug used to treat MDD. What started out as a disturbingly successful April Fool's Day prank in the *British Medical Journal* back in 2006[1] has been relaunched in a series of video clips by Consumers International (www.consumersint ernational.org) as part of its Marketing Overdose campaign, a campaign aimed to immunize the public against the aggressive marketing strategies of some elements of the drug industry. The international consumer group wishes that there be established a ban on drug industry gifts to physicians, that the industries' funding of patient groups be made more transparent, and that there be substituted a genuinely independent health information review for direct advertising to consumers. Videos, available online at http://marketingoverdose.org, are called *Pharma TV, Pharma Confidential, and Pharma Facts*. *Pharma TV* is a one-minute spoof television story on Strivor. *Pharma Confidential* is a 10-minute behind-the-scenes mockumentary on a drug industry training session on how to market Strivor. A 24-minute version, titled *The New Epidemic*, has been produced separately for use as an educational tool in medical schools. *Pharma Facts* is a conventionally styled set of video interview clips of leading commentators talking about marketing strategies that have been used by Pharma to reach doctors, the general public, and patient groups.

When some of these video clips began to appear on You Tube, physicians throughout the world were getting calls from their patients to write prescriptions for Strivor. This is somewhat reminiscent of Orson Welles' broadcast of *War of the Worlds*, when fiction becomes reality.[2]

J. A. Stockman III, MD

References

1. Moynihan R. Scientists find new disease: motivational deficiency disorder. *BMJ*. 2006;332:745.
2. Burton B. The return of the spoof. *BMJ*. 2008;336:589.

Paracetamol plus ibuprofen for the treatment of fever in children (PITCH): randomised controlled trial

Hay AD, Costelloe C, Redmond NM, et al (Univ of Bristol; et al)

BMJ 337:a1302, 2008

Objective.—To investigate whether paracetamol (acetaminophen) plus ibuprofen are superior to either drug alone for increasing time without fever and the relief of fever associated discomfort in febrile children managed at home.

Design.—Individually randomised, blinded, three arm trial.

Setting.—Primary care and households in England.

Participants.—Children aged between 6 months and 6 years with axillary temperatures of at least 37.8°C and up to 41.0°C.

Intervention.—Advice on physical measures to reduce temperature and the provision of, and advice to give, paracetamol plus ibuprofen, paracetamol alone, or ibuprofen alone.

Main Outcome Measures.—Primary outcomes were the time without fever (<37.2°C) in the first four hours after the first dose was given and the proportion of children reported as being normal on the discomfort scale at 48 hours. Secondary outcomes were time to first occurrence of normal temperature (fever clearance), time without fever over 24 hours, fever associated symptoms, and adverse effects.

Results.—On an intention to treat basis, paracetamol plus ibuprofen were superior to paracetamol for less time with fever in the first four hours (adjusted difference 55 minutes, 95% confidence interval 33 to 77; P<0.001) and may have been as good as ibuprofen (16 minutes, −7 to 39; P=0.2). For less time with fever over 24 hours, paracetamol plus ibuprofen were superior to paracetamol (4.4 hours, 2.4 to 6.3; P<0.001) and to ibuprofen (2.5 hours, 0.6 to 4.4; P=0.008). Combined therapy cleared fever 23 minutes (2 to 45; P=0.025) faster than paracetamol alone but no faster than ibuprofen alone (−3 minutes, 18 to −24; P=0.8). No benefit was found for discomfort or other symptoms, although power was low for these outcomes. Adverse effects did not differ between groups.

Conclusion.—Parents, nurses, pharmacists and doctors wanting to use medicines to supplement physical measures to maximise the time that children spend without fever should use ibuprofen first and consider the relative benefits and risks of using paracetamol plus ibuprofen over 24 hours.

Trial Registration.—Current Controlled Trials ISRCTN26362730.

▶ Needless to say, fever is one of the most common presenting signs of illness in young children and also one that can put fear into the hearts of parents who have heard horror stories about high fever causing brain damage. For this reason, antipyretic agents are one of the most commonly employed pharmaceuticals throughout the world. A lot has been discussed about the potential of alternating different types of antipyretics to achieve a successful outcome of fever control while limiting the side effects of any one anti-fever medication.

In the study reported by Hay et al, one sees the results of a randomized controlled trial of acetaminophen, ibuprofen, and the combination of the 2 used to control fever in 156 children age 6 months to 6 years. The investigators were looking for 2 primary outcomes—time without fever in the first 4 hours and fever associated with discomfort after 48 hours. This study is important given the enormous use of antipyretics. In 2004, the expenditure in Europe alone on over-the-counter acetaminophen and ibuprofen for children exceeded $756 million.[1] I have previously discussed details regarding the implications of single or drug combination for management of fever. The study of Hay et al is an important one also because a National Institute for Health and Clinical Excellence review of fever-related illnesses in children found no evidence that reducing temperature would in any way shorten the duration of illness or reduces the occurrence of complications such as febrile convulsions.[2] The latter report suggested that reducing fever might actually prolong illness. This was shown in a trial of the use of acetaminophen in 50 children with malaria where the clearance time of the malarial parasite was 16 hours longer in children treated with antipyretics plus quinine in comparison with those treated with quinine alone.[3] Similarly, in a trial of acetaminophen in 72 children with chickenpox, the time to total scabbing was significantly longer in the acetaminophen-treated group.[4]

So what did the trial of Hay et al show? When advising parents to use antipyretics, we try to reduce the child's discomfort associated with fever and manage the parent's anxiety. Time without fever is arguably a proxy of parent concern, so the most important primary outcome examined in the Hay et al trial is the discomfort associated with fever at 48 hours. Recruiting large numbers of children with acute illness in primary care into research studies, as we all know, is quite difficult and Hay et al were unable to recruit enough children to give sufficient power to detect differences for this outcome. Nonetheless, their data suggest no additional improvement in fever associated with discomfort in the combined treatment group at 24 hours, 48 hours, and 5 days. A trial with much greater power would be needed to confirm this. The study did show that acetaminophen and ibuprofen are effective at reducing temperature and that ibuprofen acts longer than acetaminophen. The largest trial comparing acetaminophen, ibuprofen, and an alternating combination was conducted in Israel back in 2006. In total, 464 febrile children age 6 to 36 months were randomly allocated into 3 groups. The group that had received alternating combination had significantly lower mean fever over 3 days, a decline in a validated checklist of children's pain, and fewer drug doses. However, that particular study is difficult to interpret because investigators used a complicated design, which loaded each of the 3 groups of children with either acetaminophen or ibuprofen at study entry.[5]

The bottom line here is that no truly persuasive evidence exists for recommending a combination or an alternating regimen of acetaminophen and ibuprofen. One should use whatever one is comfortable with given the known toxicities of each of these agents. Needless to say, parents should be reassured that fever in and of itself is not harmful. Last, the longer action of ibuprofen makes this drug, for many, the most suitable antipyretic to use.

J. A. Stockman III, MD

References

1. Hollinghurst S, Redmond N, Costelloe C, et al. Paracetamol plus ibuprofen for the treatment of fever in children (PITCH): economic evaluation of the randomized controlled trial. *BMJ.* 2008;337:a1490.
2. National Institute for Health and Clinical Excellence: Feverish illness in young children. Assessment and initial management in children younger than 5 years. www.nice.org.uk/nicemedia/pdf/cg47niceguideline.pdf; 2007. Accessed July 30, 2009.
3. Brandts CH, Ndjave M, Graninger W, Kremsner PG. The effect of paracetamol on parasite clearance time in plasmodium falciparum malaria. *Lancet.* 1997;350:704-709.
4. Doran TF, DeAngelis C, Baumgardner RA, Mellits ED. Acetaminophen: more harm than good for chickenpox? *J Pediatr.* 1989;114:1045-1048.
5. Sarrell EM, Wielunsky E, Cohen HA. Antipyretic treatment in young children with fever: acetaminophen, ibuprofen, or alternating combinations in a randomized, double-blind study. *Arch Pediatr Adolesc Med.* 2006;160:197-202.

Paracetamol plus ibuprofen for the treatment of fever in children (PITCH): economic evaluation of a randomised controlled trial
Hollinghurst S, Redmond N, Costelloe C, et al (Univ of Bristol; et al)
BMJ 337:a1490, 2008

Objective.—To estimate the cost to the NHS and to parents and carers of treating febrile preschool children with paracetamol, ibuprofen, or both, and to compare these costs with the benefits of each treatment regimen.

Design.—Cost consequences analysis and cost effectiveness analysis conducted as part of a three arm, randomised controlled trial.

Participants.—Children between the ages of 6 months and 6 years recruited from primary care and the community with axillary temperatures ≥37.8°C and ≤41°C.

Interventions.—Paracetamol, ibuprofen, or both drugs.

Main Outcome Measures.—Costs to the NHS and to parents and carers. Cost consequences analysis at 48 hours and 5 days comparing cost with children's temperature, discomfort, activity, appetite, and sleep; cost effectiveness analysis at 48 hours comparing cost with percentage of children "recovered."

Results.—Difficulties in recruiting children to the trial lowered the precision of the estimates of cost and some outcomes. At 48 hours, cost to the NHS was £11.33 for paracetamol, £8.49 for ibuprofen, and £8.16 for both drugs. By day 5 these costs rose to £19.63, £18.36, and £13.92 respectively. For parents and carers, the 48 hour costs were £23.86 for paracetamol, £20.60 for ibuprofen, and £25.07 for both, and the day 5 costs were £26.35, £29.90, and £24.02 respectively. Outcomes measured at 48 hours and 5 days were inconclusive because of lack of power; the cost effectiveness analysis at 48 hours provided little evidence that one treatment choice was significantly more cost effective than another. At 4 hours ibuprofen and the combined treatment were superior to paracetamol in terms of the trial primary outcome of time without fever; at 24 hours the combined treatment performed best on this outcome.

Conclusions.—There is no strong evidence of a difference in cost between the treatments, but clinical and cost data indicate that using both drugs together may be most cost effective over the course of the illness. This treatment option performs best and is no more expensive because of less use of healthcare resources, resulting in lower costs to the NHS and to parents.

▶ This report accompanied the one of Hay et al, which looked at the responses to fever in children age 6 months to 6 years who were given acetaminophen, ibuprofen, or a combination of the 2.[1] The report of Hollinghurst et al represents an economic analysis and confirms that the cost associated with childhood fever is predominantly borne by parents and primary care providers. The authors constructed a cost consequences matrix of results at 48 hours and 5 days using cost to the National Health Service in Great Britain and to parents, and a combination of discomfort, activity, appetite, sleep, and resolution of fever to determine a variable "return to normal" for that child. Their data show no significant differences between these drug regimens.

Given that there are no unequivocal data showing which antipyretic given singly or in combination works best, the suggestion is that one should use whatever antipyretic one is comfortable with, recognizing, however, that ibuprofen-type antipyretics tend to reduce fever for a bit longer than acetaminophen. One should take into account the side effects of each of these agents. Both are safe for children when given at the recommended doses. Despite a commonly held view, no evidence exists that ibuprofen will exacerbate reactive airway disease in children. The rub with antipyretics is that many parents do not use them in a safe manner. The most worrying aspect of the study of Hay et al is that even when given under clinical trial conditions, one out of 5 children received a drug overdose.[1] The same study suggested that when combination antipyretics are used, it is more likely that a parent will have difficulty administering the correct safe doses of these agents.

J. A. Stockman III, MD

Reference

1. Hay AD, Costelloe C, Redmond NM, et al. Paracetamol plus ibuprofen for the treatment of fever in children (PITCH): randomised controlled trial. *BMJ*. 2008; 337:729-733.

Alternating Antipyretics: Antipyretic Efficacy of Acetaminophen Versus Acetaminophen Alternated With Ibuprofen in Children
Kramer LC, Richards PA, Thompson AM, et al (Madigan Army Med Ctr, Tacoma, WA; Weed Army Community Hosp, Fort Irwin, CA; et al)
Clin Pediatr 47:907-911, 2008

Methods.—A prospective, randomized double-blind placebo control study comparing the efficacy of acetaminophen to acetaminophen alternated with ibuprofen in 38 healthy outpatient children 6 months to 6 years presenting to the outpatient clinic with fever >38°C was conducted. Temperatures were recorded at 0, 3, 4, 5, and 6 hours. Side effect diaries and parental perception of efficacy were filled out hourly by parents.

Results.—There were no significant differences in temperature between the 2 groups at times 0, 3, and 6 hours. The alternating group had significantly lower mean temperatures at both 4 hours (38.0°C vs 37.4°C; $P = .05$) and 5 hours (37.1°C vs 37.9°C; $P = .0032$). Parents did not perceive any difference in fever control between the groups.

Conclusions.—An alternating regimen of acetaminophen with ibuprofen significantly decreased fever at 4 and 5 hours compared with acetaminophen alone. However, parents did not perceive a difference in efficacy.

▶ Half or more of pediatricians routinely advise parents to alternate acetaminophen with ibuprofen to manage fever in the pediatric population.[1] We do this despite the limited evidence on the safety or efficacy of such combined treatments. Safety relates to the combined toxicity and potential parent confusion in timing and dosing when one is using 2 different drugs for the same purpose. Although 2 recent studies have suggested that alternating acetaminophen and ibuprofen might be more effective in fever control than using a single medication, neither of these 2 studies considered the role for parent education about fever in fever management.[2,3] The report of Kramer et al is the first one of its type evaluating the antipyretic efficacy of alternating acetaminophen with ibuprofen versus acetaminophen alone in the United States. The study also assessed the safety of these 2 regimens and evaluated the parent's perception of efficacy of the regimens in the setting of preceding education about fever myths and fever facts.

The study of Kramer et al reports significant differences in fever reduction with the alternating antipyretic medication regimen compared with acetaminophen given alone. This is if one looks at fever at 4 hours and 5 hours after the start of antipyretic therapy. However, the difference of fever reduction was transient and of questionable clinical significance. This raises the issue of whether safety concerns should be taken into consideration when endorsing alternating antipyretic therapy. Even without the added complication of combination therapy, parents often overdose or underdose antipyretics. The addition of alternating schedules could increase the likelihood of errors. Pediatricians and family physicians also contribute to the potential for dosing errors. In one study, 47% of physicians instructed patients to give a complex schedule of acetaminophen every 4 hours alternating with ibuprofen every 6 hours, and 9% recommended alternating the medications every 2 hours, a practice that is clearly outside the standard dosing guidelines.[1]

One particularly interesting aspect of this report is that parents were given fever education previous to the beginning of antipyretic medication administration. Parents in this intervention group were less likely to have inappropriate physician visits and phone calls and inappropriate use of antipyretic medication.

Parents are concerned about fever and are largely unaware that the biological value of fever (ie, whether it is beneficial or harmful) is actually disputed. The negative views held about fever by many in society likely have historical roots. Throughout most of history, fever has been feared by ordinary people as a manifestation of punishment induced by evil spirits or as a marker of death.[4] In 1917 Wagner von Jauregg gave enormous credence to the idea of fever as a therapeutic agent by treating neurosyphilis with malarial fever.[5] Indeed, fever has been noted by some to have a beneficial effect in eradicating disease states. To learn more about the evidence regarding the practice of fever management, see the excellent commentary on this topic by El-Radhi.[6] It is fair to say that when we as providers focus upon "treating" fever, we are giving the impression to parents that fever in and of itself is harmful and that antipyresis is beneficial. If you look carefully, you will find no scientific evidence to support this practice and we might as well at least be honest about it. This is not to say that lowering a fever will not make someone more comfortable. Rather this means that in most instances, we do not have a clue about whether what we are doing in the management of fever really does make any other difference.

J. A. Stockman III, MD

References

1. Mayoral CE, Marino RV, Rosenfeld W, Greensher J. Alternating antipyretics: is this an alternative? *Pediatrics*. 2000;105:1009-1012.
2. Nabulsi MM, Tamim H, Mahfoud Z, et al. Alternating ibuprofen and acetaminophen in the treatment of febrile children: a pilot study. *BMC Med*. 2006;4:4.
3. Sarrell EM, Wielunsky E, Cohen HA. Antipyretic treatment in young children with fever: acetaminophen, ibuprofen or both alternating in a randomized double-blind study. *Arch Pediatr Adolesc Med*. 2006;160:197-202.
4. El-Radhi AS. Changing concepts of fever: BC to the present. *Proc R Coll Physicians Edinb*. 1995;25:267-278.
5. Solomon HC, Kopp I. Fever therapy. *N Engl J Med*. 1937;217:805-814.

6. El-Radhi ASM. Why is the evidence not affecting the practice of fever management? *Arch Dis Child.* 2008;93:918-920.

Association between paracetamol use in infancy and childhood, and risk of asthma, rhinoconjunctivitis, and eczema in children aged 6–7 years: analysis from Phase Three of the ISAAC programme

Beasley R, for the ISAAC Phase Three Study Group (Med Res Inst of New Zealand, Wellington; et al)

Lancet 372:1039-1048, 2008

Background.—Exposure to paracetamol during intrauterine life, childhood, and adult life may increase the risk of developing asthma. We studied 6–7-year-old children from Phase Three of the International Study of Asthma and Allergies in Childhood (ISAAC) programme to investigate the association between paracetamol consumption and asthma.

Methods.—As part of Phase Three of ISAAC, parents or guardians of children aged 6–7 years completed written questionnaires about symptoms of asthma, rhinoconjunctivitis, and eczema, and several risk factors, including the use of paracetamol for fever in the child's first year of life and the frequency of paracetamol use in the past 12 months. The primary outcome variable was the odds ratio (OR) of asthma symptoms in these children associated with the use of paracetamol for fever in the first year of life, as calculated by logistic regression.

Findings.—205 487 children aged 6–7 years from 73 centres in 31 countries were included in the analysis. In the multivariate analyses, use of paracetamol for fever in the first year of life was associated with an increased risk of asthma symptoms when aged 6–7 years (OR 1·46 [95% CI 1·36–1·56]). Current use of paracetamol was associated with a dose-dependent increased risk of asthma symptoms (1·61 [1·46–1·77] and 3·23 [2·91–3·60] for medium and high use vs no use, respectively). Use of paracetamol was similarly associated with the risk of severe asthma symptoms, with population-attributable risks between 22% and 38%. Paracetamol use, both in the first year of life and in children aged 6–7 years, was also associated with an increased risk of symptoms of rhinoconjunctivitis and eczema.

Interpretation.—Use of paracetamol in the first year of life and in later childhood; is associated with risk of asthma, rhinoconjunctivitis, and eczema at age 6 to 7 years. We suggest that exposure to paracetamol might be a risk factor for the development of asthma in childhood.

▶ Acetaminophen was first synthesized back in 1878. Marketing of acetaminophen began in the 1950s when the drug became popular as an analgesic replacement for phenacetin, which was known to have renal side effects. By the 1980s, acetaminophen use had become as common as aspirin for management of fever. When the linkage was described between an increased risk of

Reye syndrome and aspirin use in the 1980s, acetaminophen quickly became the drug of choice for fever control.

Beasley et al undertook a study to determine whether the increasing use of acetaminophen is associated with the rise in asthma, a prevalence that has been seen over the last several decades. Indeed, the increased use of acetaminophen over the past 50 years has occurred contemporaneously with the rise in prevalence of asthma worldwide. Several biological mechanisms have been proposed to explain a potential association between acetaminophen consumption and asthma, including development of oxidant-induced airway inflammation due to reduced concentrations of antioxidant glutathione in the lung and stimulation of the T-helper-cell-2 response, which increases the clinical expression of allergic disease. To investigate the hypothesis that there might be a link between acetaminophen use and a rise in prevalence of asthma, data from the International Study of Asthma and Allergies in Childhood (ISAAC) were reviewed. The data seem to show that the use of acetaminophen for fever in the first year of life is associated with symptoms of asthma later in childhood. The data also suggest a strong dose-dependent association between the use of acetaminophen and symptoms of asthma in children age 6 to 7 years with a 3-fold increased risk associated with frequent acetaminophen use, at least once per month.

The strengths of the study are its power, size, and multinational nature. A consistent association between acetaminophen use and asthma in populations with different lifestyles and medical practices appears to exist. Furthermore, the data from the study suggest that there is an increased risk of rhinoconjunctivitis and eczema in those receiving acetaminophen in higher doses.

This report from the ISAAC Phase 3 is the largest and most important contribution to date on the growing literature possibly linking acetaminophen use and childhood asthma. The report ends, appropriately, with a question rather than a conclusion, and that question is about causality. No one has found a specific reason why an association should exist between acetaminophen use and childhood asthma. Clearly, the studies done to date proposing such a linkage are suggestive but not definitive enough to recommend a wholesale change in antipyretic use in children. Beasley et al strongly recommend that a population-based randomized trial of adequate power and duration to examine childhood asthma incidence, with acetaminophen compared with an active control such as a nonsteroidal and placebo is warranted. If a linkage is found between asthma and acetaminophen use, the shot will be heard around the world. Stay tuned for the possible noise.

This commentary closes with a *Clinical Fact/Curio* related to pain therapeutics. Bet you were not aware that religious thoughts are capable of alleviating pain. Recently, brain researchers have explored what might be called faith-based analgesia. Stimulating a religious state of mind in devout Catholics apparently triggers brain processes associated with substantial relief from physical pain as reported recently by a neuroscientist.[1] Data from a study suggest that religious belief alters the brain in a way that changes how a person responds to pain. In the study, practicing Catholics perceived electrical pulses as less painful while viewing an image of the Virgin Mary than while viewing a non-religious picture. In alternating trials, 12 Catholics and 12 atheists or agnostics spent 30 seconds observing an image of either a painting of the Virgin Mary or of *Lady with an Ermine*, by Leonardo DaVinci. Functional MRI showed a change in the study subjects who were Catholic only during viewing of the religious icon. Pain relief for Catholics was accompanied by vigorous activity in the right ventrolateral prefrontal cortex, which has been linked to pain relief associated with emotional detachment and perceived control over pain. This response was not observed in non-religious volunteers.

J. A. Stockman III, MD

Reference

1. Pain you can believe in [editorial comment]. *Sci News*. October 11, 2008;9.

Antiemetic Medications in Children with Presumed Infectious Gastroenteritis—Pharmacoepidemiology in Europe and Northern America
Pfeil N, Uhlig U, Kostev K, et al (Univ of Leipzig, Germany; Inst of Med Statistics Health, Frankfurt am Main, Germany; et al)
J Pediatr 153:659-662, 2008

Objective.—To investigate the prescription pattern of antiemetic medications in 0- to 9-year-old children with infectious gastroenteritis in several industrialized countries during 2005.

Study Design.—We retrospectively retrieved data from 4 national and international databases (IMS MIDAS, IMS disease analyzer, WIdO databases).

Results.—Between 2% and 23% of children with gastroenteritis (*International Classification of Diseases code A08.X or A09*) received prescriptions for antiemetic medications (United States, 23%; 95% CI, 15-31; Germany, 17%; 95% CI, 15-20; France, 17%; 95% CI, 14-19; Spain, 15%; 95% CI, 10-19; Italy, 11%; 95% CI, 7-16; Canada, 3%; 95% CI, 0-16; United Kingdom, 2%; 95% CI, 1-2). The antihistamines dimenhydrinate and diphenhydramine were most frequently used in Germany and Canada, whereas promethazine was prescribed preferentially in the United States. In France, Spain, and Italy, the dopamine receptor antagonist domperidone was preferred as antiemetic treatment. Ondansetron was used in a minor proportion of antiemetic prescriptions (Germany, Canada, Spain, and Italy, 0%; United States, 3%; United Kingdom, 6%).

Conclusion.—Antiemetic drugs are frequently used in children with gastroenteritis. In different industrialized countries, prescription of antiemetic medication varies considerably. Ondansetron, the only drug with evidence-based antiemetic efficacy, plays a minor role among antiemetic prescriptions.

▶ The fact that pediatricians all too frequently use antiemetics to control vomiting in children has been our gorilla in the room. Although treatment guidelines clearly do not recommend antiemetic medications for use in children with acute gastroenteritis and vomiting, their application seems to be quite rather common in clinical practice in many developed countries. Thus the value of this report by Pfeil et al, which looked at antiemetic use both here in North America as well as in Europe.

This report showed that different antiemetics tend to be preferred in differing parts of the world. The antihistaminic drug dimenhydrinate is preferred in Germany and Canada, while in France and the United States this drug is much less commonly used. In the United States, promethazine is the most commonly prescribed antiemetic. The dopamine receptor antagonist, domperidone, is preferred in Spain, France, and Italy. It should be noted that this latter drug has recently been demonstrated to cause prolongation of the QT interval. The serotonin receptor antagonist, ondansetron, is occasionally used throughout North America and Europe.

This report reminds us that only ondansetron has been clearly demonstrated to reduce vomiting or to improve oral rehydration in children with gastroenteritis. This finding has been documented in several randomized controlled trials. All other prescribed antiemetic medications lack proof of efficacy in randomized controlled trials. The drug used most commonly in the United States, promethazine, was first classified as a neuroleptic agent that also has antihistaminic and anticholinergic activity. No therapeutic effect of promethazine on dehydration and vomiting during episodes of infectious gastroenteritis has been shown with clinical trials. Adverse effects of promethazine include drowsiness, sedation, extrapyramidal reactions, coordination disturbance, and blurred vision. An analysis of the United States prescription writing patterns in 1998 showed that as many as 10% of children with gastroenteritis received a prescription for antiemetic medications, usually promethazine.[1]

If you believe the data from this report, and you should, we are overusing antiemetics when managing children with acute gastroenteritis. The figure (Fig 2) shows that we very well may be among the worst offenders. Should

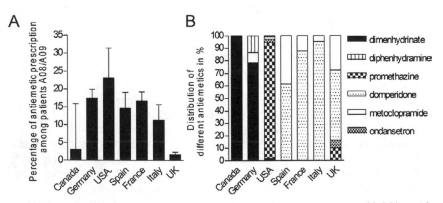

FIGURE 2.—Differential use of antiemetic medications in children. Zero- to 9-year old children with infectious gastroenteritis (ICD-10 code A08.x/A09) were considered for this analysis. Data were obtained from the IMS MIDAS database. 95% CIs are provided. **A,** Percentage of antiemetic drugs among the total prescriptions to children with gastroenteritis. **B,** Relative distribution of antiemetic medications. (Reprinted from Pfeil N, Uhlig U, Kostev K, et al. Antiemetic medications in children with presumed infectious gastroenteritis-pharmacoepidemiology in Europe and Northern America. *J Pediatr.* 2008;153:659-662, with permission from Elsevier.)

you truly feel that an antiemetic is needed, think about using ondansetron. While chances are it is not needed, at least there is evidence of some effectivity on this drug's part.

J. A. Stockman III, MD

Reference

1. Li ST, DiGiuseppe DL, Christakis DA. Antiemetic use for acute gastroenteritis in children. *Arch Pediatr Adolesc Med.* 2003;157:475-479.

Safety and efficacy of acupuncture in children: a review of the evidence
Jindal V, Ge A, Mansky PJ (Natl Insts of Health, Bethesda, MD)
J Pediatr Hematol Oncol 30:431-442, 2008

Acupuncture has been used therapeutically in China for thousands of years and is growing in prominence in Europe and the United States. In a recent review of complementary and alternative medicine use in the US population, an estimated 2.1 million people or 1.1% of the population sought acupuncture care during the past 12 months. Four percent of the US population used acupuncture at any time in their lives. We reviewed 31 different published journal articles, including 23 randomized controlled clinical trials and 8 meta-analysis/systematic reviews. We found evidence of some efficacy and low risk associated with acupuncture in pediatrics. From all the conditions we reviewed, the most extensive research has looked into acupuncture's role in managing postoperative and chemotherapy-induced nausea/vomiting. Postoperatively, there is far more evidence of acupuncture's efficacy for pediatrics than for children treated with chemotherapy. Acupuncture seems to be most effective in preventing postoperative induced nausea in children. For adults, research shows that acupuncture can inhibit chemotherapy-related acute vomiting, but conclusions about its effects in pediatrics cannot be made on the basis of the available published clinical trials data to date. Besides nausea and vomiting, research conducted in pain has yielded the most convincing results on acupuncture efficacy. Musculoskeletal and cancer-related pain commonly affects children and adults, but unfortunately, mostly adult studies have been conducted thus far. Because the manifestations of pain can be different in children than in adults, data cannot be extrapolated from adult research. Systematic reviews have shown that existing data often lack adequate control groups and sample sizes. Vas et al, Alimi et al, and Mehling et al demonstrated some relief for adults treated with acupuncture but we could not find any well-conducted randomized controlled studies that looked at pediatrics and acupuncture exclusively. Pain is often unresolved from drug therapy, thus there is a need for more studies in this setting. For seasonal allergic rhinitis, we reviewed studies conducted by Ng et al and Xue et al in children and adults, respectively. Both populations showed some relief of symptoms through acupuncture, but questions remain about treatment logistics. Additionally, there are limited indications that acupuncture may help cure children afflicted with nocturnal enuresis. Systematic reviews show that current published trials have suffered from low trial quality, including small sample sizes. Other areas of pediatric afflictions we reviewed that suffer from lack of research include asthma, other neurologic conditions, gastrointestinal disorders, and addiction. Acupuncture has become a dominant complementary and alternative modality in clinical practice today, but its associated risk has been questioned. The National Institutes of Health Consensus Statement states "one of the advantages of acupuncture is that the incidence of adverse effects is substantially lower than that of many drugs or other accepted procedures for the same conditions." A review of serious adverse events by White et al found the risk of a major complication occurring to have an incidence between 1:10,000 and 1:100,000, which is considered "very low." Another study found that the risk of a serious adverse event occurring from acupuncture therapy is the same as taking penicillin. The safety of acupuncture is a serious concern, particularly in pediatrics. Because acupuncture's mechanism is not known, the use of needles in children becomes questionable. For example, acupoints on the vertex of infants should not be needled when the fontanel is not closed. It is also advisable to apply few needles or delay treatment to the children who have overeaten, are overfatigued, or are very weak. Through our review of pediatric adverse events, we found a 1.55 risk of adverse events occurring in 100 treatments of acupuncture that coincides with the low risk detailed in the studies mentioned previously. The actual risk to an individual patient is hard to determine because certain patients, such as an immunosuppressed patient, can be predisposed to an increased risk, acupuncturist's qualifications differ, and practices vary in certain parts of the world. Nevertheless, it seems acupuncture is a safe complementary/alternative medicine modality for pediatric patients on the basis of the data we reviewed.

▶ The report of Jindal et al serves a purpose in providing us with some information on the value, or lack of value in many cases, of acupuncture when used in children. Most data now show that the significant majority of adults do treat themselves with some form of complementary and alternative medicine (CAM). Most of us have been scrambling to catch up with the exponential increase in CAM among our patients and their families. Limiting the indiscriminate use of costly or dangerous ineffective therapies—whether based on conventional or unconventional medicine—should be a priority for all of us. The trick is trying to figure out what works and does not work. The number of randomized controlled trials of CAM indexed in MEDLINE increased 6-fold in the 20-year period from 1982-2002 (from 200-1200 trials). In the last couple of years, however, more than 7500 CAM trials were indexed in MEDLINE with more than 1600 involving children aged 18 years or younger. In a study assessing the quality of 207 randomized controlled trials used for systematic reviews of homeopathy, acupuncture, and herbal extracts, Linde et al reported that less than half of the randomized controlled trials were in English or indexed in MEDLINE, and most failed to describe how the randomization sequence was generated, inadequately concealed the allocation sequence, did not catalog the number and reasons for postrandomization attrition, or did not use intent-to-treat data analyses.[1] Most studies of CAM efficacy in both adults and children are generally of poor quality. While the randomized controlled trials should remain the gold standard for providing evidence of treatment efficacy for both CAM and conventional therapies, many interventions pose unique challenges to rigorous randomized controlled trial methodology. Researchers may have difficulty defining precise and measurable outcomes for therapies for which the main effect is subjective or dependent on the skill of the practitioner.

What Jindal et al have done is to review the efficacy data from 32 articles that described acupuncture's effectiveness for specific indications when used in children. When employing Cochrane review analysis, 12 trials examining vomiting due to chemotherapy or postanesthesia showed some benefit of acupuncture. All in all, the review of 32 different published journal articles, including 23 randomized controlled trials and 8 meta-analysis/systematic reviews suggest some efficacy and low risk associated with acupuncture in pediatrics. For all the conditions reviewed, the most extensive research has looked into acupuncture's role in managing postoperative and chemotherapy-induced nausea and vomiting. There is far more evidence supporting acupuncture for postoperative vomiting control in pediatrics than for vomiting associated with chemotherapy. Acupuncture is commonly used for pain control in adults, but the data in children are inconclusive largely because of problems with study design. The manifestations of pain are very different in children than adults, and data from adults cannot be extrapolated to children however convincing the adult data are.

There is very little written about acupuncture safety in children. In adults, serious adverse effects have been examined. The risk of major complications has been found to be somewhere between 1:10 000 and 1:100 000 acupuncture sessions. Obviously, we need more multicenter, randomized, controlled trials that look at not only effectiveness but also safety of acupuncture when applied to children's illnesses.

J. A. Stockman III, MD

Reference

1. Linde K, Jonas WB, Melchart D, Willich S. The methodological quality of randomized controlled trials of homeopathy, herbal medicines and acupuncture. *Int J Epidemiol.* 2001;30:526-531.

Transdermal Patch Medication Delivery Systems and Pediatric Poisonings, 2002-2006

Parekh D, Miller MA, Borys D, et al (Darnall Army Med Ctr, Ft Hood; Central Texas Poison Control Ctr, Temple, TX; et al)
Clin Pediatr 47:659-663, 2008

Transdermal drug delivery systems are an increasingly popular method of medication delivery containing large quantities of medication and presenting new opportunities for toxicity. To provide a description of exposures to transdermal medications in a pediatric population, we studied exposures in individuals less than 12 years of age. This is a retrospective database study in which the Texas Poison Center Network database from 2002 to 2006 was reviewed. In all, 336 poison control center records of patch exposures over the 5-year period were identified. Of those, 110 cases involved children less than 12 years old. A majority of cases resulted in no significant clinical effects. One death resulted from opioid toxicity. Although a majority of patch exposures in children less than 12 years of age resulted in no significant clinical toxicity, practitioners and the public must be made aware of the available patch-based medications and their potential for toxicity in children.

▶ Most of us do not tend to think too much about transdermal patches in pediatrics, but this report reminds us that we should know a bit about these, especially when it comes to their potential to cause poisoning in the young set. Transdermal patches have become quite popular because they provide effective medication dosing over prolonged periods at even rates. The drugs that enter the body bypass many major organs involved with first-pass metabolism, decreasing metabolite concentrations, and improving the bioavailability of the drug compounds in the patches. This also decreases the risk for interactions with other medications. Because transdermal drug penetration relies heavily on drug gradients between the patch and tissues, patches contain high concentrations of drugs. Most transdermal systems contain 20-fold more drug than will be absorbed during application. Therefore, when the patches are removed, a very significant amount of drug is retained within the patches, and if left about, can become a hazard.

What we see in this report from the Texas Poison Center Network, a network consisting of 6 regional poison centers throughout Texas, is a summary of more than 300 patch exposures and the consequences of these exposures over the 5-year period that was under review. In this series, the average age of children reported was just 11.5 months with almost 90% of calls to the poison center involving unintentional exposures. About half of these exposures involved oral exposure only, where the child was found sucking or chewing on the medicated patch, whereas about 13% of cases involved the actual ingestion of the patch. In some kids, the exposure was by application of the patch to the skin. Readily available over-the-counter patch medications frequently used in children were most commonly involved, such as camphor or menthol patches, sold in a number of formulations, including the Triaminic Vapor Patch. The latter patch was recalled in 2006 after a child suffered seizures after chewing on a patch.

The table shows the evidence involved in pediatric patch accidental exposures. While some 40% of exposures had no side effects at all, about 1 in 7 children did have symptoms resulting from the exposures (Table 2).

As this report reminds us, although the majority of patch exposures in children result in no or minimal toxicity, there are inherent dangers and significant risk for a small subset of children. Be wary of these over-the-counter patches for children and certainly recommend that parents who use patches themselves dispose of them properly.

This commentary closes with a *Clinical Fact/Curio* about medical toxicology. Spiders and other insects living near a mercury contaminated river contain unusually high levels of the toxic metal, a recent study has shown. It is well known that certain bacteria can convert inorganic mercury in contaminated streams to methylmercury, the form that accumulates most easily in the tissues of living things. The metal then travels up the food chain. Investigators from William and Mary College have found surprisingly high mercury levels in the blood of 12 insect-eating bird species living along a tributary of the Shenandoah River in Virginia. The only link between the birds and the mercury came when the birds' diet was studied. That diet consisted of spiders. Birds living along the Shenandoah River have a diet that is made up of 20% to 30% spiders. These spiders have been observed to contain high quantities of methylmercury. The spiders themselves are predatory and apparently are just one more element of a food chain themselves. The spiders apparently eat mercury-laden insects, the bird eats the spider, and so on.[1]

TABLE 2.—Clinical Signs and Symptoms Possible From Medication Exposure

Medication	Signs and Symptoms
Anticholinergic	Dry mouth, inability to urinate, feeling hot or temperature elevation, altered mental status, mild-moderate pulse, and blood pressure elevation
Camphor or menthol or methyl salicylate	Seizures, drowsiness, altered mental status
Clonidine	Initial blood pressure elevations followed by lethargy, miosis, bradycardia, hypotension, and coma
Estrogen hormone	Minimal effects expected from single exposure
Lidocaine or topical anesthetics	Seizures, methemoglobinemia from some local anesthetics
Methylphenidate	Agitation, hyperactivity, sweating, elevated pulse, and blood pressure
Nicotine	Nausea, vomiting, autonomic instability, diaphoresis, altered mental status
Nitroglycerin	Hypotension
Opiate	Obtundation, miosis, respiratory depression, bradycardia
Salicylic acid	Salicylism: fevers, altered mental status, tinnitus, metabolic acidosis, hyperventilation
Testosterone hormone	Minimal effects expected from single exposure
Multiple classes or other	Various

(Reprinted from Parekh D, Miller MA, Borys D, et al. Transdermal patch medication delivery systems and pediatric poisonings, 2002-2006. *Clin Pediatr.* 2008;47:659-663.)

If there is a lesson in all this, it is that if you are into eating birds, eat the type that enjoy a diet of caterpillars, which eat plants, not spiders.

J. A. Stockman III, MD

Reference

1. Ehrenberg R. Spiders boost mercury levels: birds eating arachnids get high dose of toxic metal. *Sci News.* May 10, 2008;14.

Fetal alcohol syndrome: a prospective national surveillance study
Elliott EJ, Payne J, Morris A, et al (Univ of Sydney, Australia)
Arch Dis Child 93:732-737, 2008

Objective.—To describe the epidemiology of cases of fetal alcohol syndrome (FAS) seen by Australian paediatricians.

Methods.—Active, national case-finding using the Australian Paediatric Surveillance Unit (APSU). Monthly reporting of incident cases aged <15 years by paediatricians between January 2001 and December 2004.

Results.—Over 1150 paediatricians submitted reports each month to the APSU. Of 169 reported cases, 92 fulfilled the study criteria for FAS. There was a significant increase in the number of children reported each year from 2001 to 2004. Of 92 children, 53.3% were male, 35.7% were preterm (<37 weeks' gestation) and 64.6% were of low birth weight (<2.5 kg). Most (94.4%) had high risk exposure to alcohol in utero and 78.3% were exposed to one or more additional drugs. The median age at diagnosis was 3.3 years (range: newborn to 11.9 years): 6.5% were diagnosed at birth and 63% by 5 years of age. Of the 92 cases, 56% had growth deficiency, 53.2% had microcephaly, 85.9% had evidence of central nervous system dysfunction, 24% had additional birth defects, 5.4% had sensorineural deafness and 4.3% had visual impairment. Of children with FAS, 65% were Indigenous, 51% had a sibling with FAS, and only 40.2% lived with a biological parent.

Conclusion.—Our data are the only prospective national data available on FAS throughout the world. These findings highlight the severity, complexity and impact of FAS, the need for effective strategies for prevention, and the necessity for education to facilitate earlier diagnosis, referral and reporting of cases.

▶ This report reminds us of the extraordinary burden put upon children and families, and society, as the result of the fetal alcohol syndrome (FAS). Data going back 20 years show that FAS was costing the United States economy over $4 billion annually and the estimated lifetime cost per individual with FAS has been running $2.9 million in recent years.[1] The case-finding national surveillance study from Australia shows the very low rate of underreporting of this syndrome, at least in that country; presumably the situation is not very different here. This lack of detection of FAS most likely is based on deficient skills to make a diagnosis, lack of awareness and recognition of FAS, lack of reporting, lack of available expertise, and perhaps an unwillingness to seek out an FAS diagnosis. If you believe the data from this report and elsewhere, the average pediatric practice with 1500 children per pediatrician would be expected to have about 5 patients at any one time with FAS per pediatrician. Obviously, this rate of FAS will vary quite widely depending on the type of one's practice, but even in affluent communities, you can bet there is a lot of drinking going on, even during pregnancy. An editorial accompanying an article of Elliott et al by Albert Chudley reminds us that while rare diseases may be rare, some rare diseases are rare simply because they are rarely diagnosed.[2]

In the report of Elliott, more than 1000 pediatricians in Australia logged their newly diagnosed cases of FAS into a database. That database showed that the median age at diagnosis was 3.3 years with some children eluding diagnosis until almost 12 years of age. A solid third of children were diagnosed only after 5 years of age. Common problems included growth retardation, microcephaly, and cognitive dysfunction, with a scattering of deafness and visual impairments. Behavioral and emotional problems ran high.

If this situation is the same here in the United States as Australia (highly likely), we are not doing the patients we serve a great service. Early diagnosis has been shown to decrease morbidity in FAS, and it would be unconscionable to be making diagnoses as late as 12 years of age. Our task is to recognize FAS-affected children as soon as possible in order to provide them with a better chance to succeed in life despite the fact that the injury they have sustained is a permanent one.

This commentary closes with another *Clinical Fact/Curio* about medical toxicology. By the time almost 3 dozen patients had been diagnosed with lead poisoning in and about the city of Leipzig, Germany, it became clear that there was a common pattern in those affected. The patients were young, were unemployed or students, had a history of smoking, and had body piercings. On questioning, all the patients eventually conceded that they were regular users of marijuana smoked in a "joint" form or with the use of a water pipe. Investigators were able to retrieve half-used packages of home supplies of marijuana from some of these patients. Elemental lead was identified in the marijuana using atomic absorptiometry and high-pressure liquid chromatography. In fact, one package contained obvious lead particles, strongly indicating that the lead was likely to have been deliberately added to the package rather than inadvertently incorporated into the marijuana plants from contaminated soil.

A full criminal investigation ensued and anonymous screening of marijuana users for lead poisoning detected an additional 95 persons whose blood leads were sufficiently elevated (> 25 µg/deciliter) to require chelation therapy. Some of these individuals had quite dangerous levels of lead (> 80 µg/deciliter). It is highly likely that lead, in this situation, was used to increase the weight of street marijuana sold by the gram and therefore to maximize profits among dealers. Lead has a high specific gravity and an inconspicuous grayish color. In the material that was obtained, the lead content was on average 10% by weight, which translates into a profit increase of approximately United States $1500 per kilogram of marijuana. Lead particles smoked in a joint can reach a core temperature of 1200°C and are effectively absorbed via the respiratory tract.[3]

By the way, this interesting event did cause the German government to notify medical practitioners, including pediatricians, about the need to consider adulterated marijuana as a potential source of lead poisoning. Most of us do not think too terribly much about inhalation as a source of lead, but ask any plumber who uses a torch and he will tell you that it is an occupational hazard, even if you do not smoke from a bong.

J. A. Stockman III, MD

References

1. Lupton C, Burd L, Harwood RR. Cost of fetal alcohol spectrum disorders. *Am J Med Genet.* 2004;127C:42-50.
2. Chudley AE. Fetal alcohol spectrum disorder: counting the invisible? mission impossible. *Arch Dis Child.* 2008;208:721-722.
3. Busse F, Omidi L, Leichtle A, et al. Lead poisoning due to adulterated marijuana. *N Engl J Med.* 2008;358:1641-1642.

Association of Urinary Bisphenol A Concentration With Medical Disorders and Laboratory Abnormalities in Adults
Lang IA, Galloway TS, Scarlett A, et al (Peninsula Med School, Exeter, UK; Univ of Exeter; et al)
JAMA 300:1303-1310, 2008

Context.—Bisphenol A (BPA) is widely used in epoxy resins lining food and beverage containers. Evidence of effects in animals has generated concern over low-level chronic exposures in humans.

Objective.—To examine associations between urinary BPA concentrations and adult health status.

Design, Setting, and Participants.—Cross-sectional analysis of BPA concentrations and health status in the general adult population of the United States, using data from the National Health and Nutrition Examination Survey 2003-2004. Participants were 1455 adults aged 18 through 74 years with measured urinary BPA and urine creatinine concentrations. Regression models were adjusted for age, sex, race/ethnicity, education, income, smoking, body mass index, waist circumference, and urinary creatinine concentration. The sample provided 80% power to detect unadjusted odds ratios (ORs) of 1.4 for diagnoses of 5% prevalence per 1-SD change in BPA concentration, or standardized regression coefficients of 0.075 for liver enzyme concentrations, at a significance level of $P < .05$.

Main Outcome Measures.—Chronic disease diagnoses plus blood markers of liver function, glucose homeostasis, inflammation, and lipid changes.

Results.—Higher urinary BPA concentrations were associated with cardiovascular diagnoses in age-, sex-, and fully adjusted models (OR per 1-SD increase in BPA concentration, 1.39; 95% confidence interval

[CI], 1.18-1.63; $P = .001$ with full adjustment). Higher BPA concentrations were also associated with diabetes (OR per 1-SD increase in BPA concentration, 1.39; 95% confidence interval [CI], 1.21-1.60; $P < .001$) but not with other studied common diseases. In addition, higher BPA concentrations were associated with clinically abnormal concentrations of the liver enzymes γ-glutamyltransferase (OR per 1-SD increase in BPA concentration, 1.29; 95%CI, 1.14-1.46; $P < .001$) and alkaline phosphatase (OR per 1-SD increase in BPA concentration, 1.48; 95% CI, 1.18-1.85; $P = .002$).

Conclusion.—Higher BPA exposure, reflected in higher urinary concentrations of BPA, may be associated with avoidable morbidity in the community-dwelling adult population.

▶ Until this report appeared, this editor was not aware of how ubiquitous bisphenol A (BPA) is. It is, indeed, one of the world's highest production-volume chemicals. It is noted that more than 2 million metric tons of BPA are produced annually, and the demand continues to increase. We are continuously exposed to this chemical because it is used to make polycarbonate plastic food and beverage containers. It is in dental sealants. It is the resin lining cans in our food cupboards, and virtually all of us touch it every day because it is in the "carbonless" paper used for receipts. Remember that the next time you tear off your copy of a receipt at the gasoline pump.

So what is the problem with BPA? For some time it has been recognized that BPA does have estrogenic activity. Reports have also highlighted problems related to liver damage, abnormal pancreatic beta-cell function, thyroid hormone disruption, and obesity-promoting effects. The debate has been whether the health effects of BPA in humans are really all that important, a debate that has been hamstrung by the lack of epidemiologic data of sufficient statistical power to detect low-dose effect. Data from the United States National Health and Nutrition Examination Survey (NHANES) provide important clues to help tilt the debate. NHANES surveys were developed to assess the health and diet of the United States population. The study is administered by the National Center for Health Statistics. One-third of NHANES participants supplied urine samples that could be analyzed for BPA concentration thus allowing correlations with disease status.

Based on data from the NHANES 2003-2004, Lang et al now report a significant relationship between urine concentrations of BPA and cardiovascular disease, type 2 diabetes, and liver-enzyme abnormalities in adults. Presumably the genesis of these problems begins in childhood. The effects of BPA appear to occur at levels significantly less than the dose used by the United States Food and Drug Administration and the Environmental Protection Agency to estimate the current human acceptable daily intake deemed safe for humans for BPA.

Exactly how BPA does a job on the human body is not entirely clear. Rat studies suggest that BPA decreases the activities of antioxidant enzymes resulting in increased lipid peroxidation, thereby increasing oxidative stress.[1] At higher doses, in mice, BPA stimulates pancreatic beta cells to release insulin and at even higher doses, mice will develop insulin resistance similar to what is seen in adult humans with type 2 diabetes.

For a long time, the FDA has suggested that BPA is "safe," ignoring warnings from expert panels. The findings by Lang et al that BPA is significantly related to serum markers of liver damage (such as increased gamma-glutamyltransferase levels) that are predictive of metabolic disease, cardiovascular disease, and increased mortality go against the FDA's historic position on BPA.

Thus it is that adults with increased levels of BPA do seem to be at greater risk for metabolic diseases. Exposure to BPA during development poses the greatest risk for adverse effects. The fetus and infant are believed to be more susceptible to the estrogenic effects of BPA because of small body size and limited capacity to metabolize BPA. Interestingly, the exponential increase in the use of BPA products in the last 20 years parallels the dramatic increase in the incidence of obesity and type 2 diabetes in the pediatric population. This does not mean there is a direct cause and effect, but the association is so strong as to not be ignored. It has also been shown that BPA can alter the programming of genes during critical periods of cell differentiation in fetal and neonatal development.

The rub with BPA is that it does not go away. We can diminish the side effects of BPA on the human body by eliminating exposures to it in food and drink products. Recognize, however, that the 7 billion pounds of BPA produced each year will wind up in landfills. No one knows the consequences of BPA in these landfills a millennium away from now.

This commentary closes with a *Clinical Fact/Curio* posed in the form of a question about toxins. Why are our homebound pets similar to canaries in a coal mine? The answer is that while Spot and Puff not only lighten our lives, they may also act like canaries in a coal mine, giving early warning signs of toxicity from household chemicals. The Washington, DC-based Environmental Working Group examined blood and urine samples from 20 dogs and 37 cats in nearby Virginia and analyzed them for 70 industrial chemicals and pollutants, including heavy metals, fire retardants, stain removers, and plastic softeners. These were agents implicated in the causation of cancers, thyroid problems, neurological conditions, and other disorders. Among the findings were 35 chemicals in cats, including mercury levels 5 times as high as in humans and fire retardant levels 23 times as high. More than a dozen endocrine toxins may help to explain the thyroid disease frequently seen in cats, say the investigators.

The Environmental Working Group suggests that pets may well be serving as sentinels for the health of children. The Group even goes out on a limb to argue that the rising rates of diagnosis of problems such as attention deficit disorder mirror the increasing rates of behavioral problems in pets.[2]

J. A. Stockman III, MD

References

1. Bindhumol V, Chitra KC, Mathur BP. Bisphenol A induces reactive oxygen species generation in the liver of male rates. *Toxicol.* 2003;188:117-124.
2. Pets as toxin-catchers [editorial comment]. *Science.* 2008;320:429.

Caustic ingestion in children: is endoscopy always indicated? The results of an Italian multicenter observational study

Betalli P, Caustic Ingestion Italian Study Group (Univ of Padova, Italy; et al)
Gastrointest Endosc 68:434-439, 2008

Background.—The ingestion of caustic substances can represent a serious medical problem in children.

Objective.—Whether or not an urgent endoscopy should be performed is still a matter of debate, particularly in asymptomatic patients.

Design.—We conducted a multicenter observational study to investigate the predictive value of signs and symptoms in detecting severe esophageal lesions.

Setting and Patients.—The records of 162 children who presented with accidental caustic substance ingestion were analyzed.

Interventions.—Signs and symptoms were divided into minor (oral and/or oropharyngeal lesions and vomiting) and major (dyspnea, dysphagia, drooling, and hematemesis). An endoscopy was performed in all patients within 12 to 24 hours of the substance being ingested.

Main Outcome Measurements.—The types of substance ingested, signs and symptoms, age, sex, and severity of esophageal injury were correlated.

Results.—Mild esophageal lesions were identified in 143 of 162 patients (88.3%), and severe (third degree) esophageal lesions in 19 patients (11.7%). The risk of severe esophageal lesions without signs and/or symptoms was very low (odds ratio [OR] 0.13 [95% CI, 0.02-0.62], $P = .002$). Indeed, the presence of 3 or more symptoms is an important predictor of severe esophageal lesions (OR 11.97 [95% CI, 3.49-42.04], $P = .0001$). Multivariate analysis showed that the presence of symptoms is the most significant predictor of severe esophageal lesions (OR 2.3 [95% CI, 1.57-3.38], $P = .001$).

Conclusions.—The results demonstrated that the incidence of patients with third-degree lesions without any early symptoms and/or signs is very low, and an endoscopy could be avoided. The risk of severe damage increases proportionally with the number of signs and symptoms, and an endoscopy is always mandatory in symptomatic patients.

▶ This study from Italy asked a very relevant and contemporary question for those who work in pediatric emergency rooms. This question is whether completely asymptomatic patients who are seen after the unintentional ingestion of a caustic substance always must undergo urgent endoscopy. The literature on this topic has been quite confusing. A number of studies have attempted to correlate the initial signs and symptoms with the gravity of the lesions to avoid any unnecessary endoscopy, but the matter still remains unresolved. Most studies have suggested that the lack of lesions in the mouth and pharynx or related symptoms does not rule out the presence of esophageal or gastric injury. Other investigators have concluded that patients at risk of severe esophageal injury and subsequent stricture always show signs and symptoms after the ingestion of caustic substances. The major conundrum for those working in emergency rooms is whether to resist the temptation to perform an endoscopy in children with no visible lesions and no signs and symptoms, thus the question, do completely asymptomatic patients always require the performance of an endoscopic procedure?

In the reported study from Italy, 162 patients presenting with accidental caustic substance ingestion were evaluated with endoscopy. It was clear that the risk of severe damage to the esophagus does increase proportionately with the number of signs and symptoms a child presents with. Unfortunately, the presence of only "minor" symptoms such as oropharyngeal lesions and vomiting, does not rule out any presence of relevant injuries to the esophagus, clearly indicating that endoscopy is warranted in all symptomatic children. The results of the study additionally demonstrate that the incidence of patients with third-degree lesions without any early signs and symptoms is extremely low and that endoscopy could be possibly avoided in such circumstances. Important symptoms such as hematemesis, dyspnea, and stridor are the most obvious predictors of severe lesions.

If you work in an emergency room that cares for children, this report will be an important addition to the way in which you make decisions about children who have ingested caustic substances. The latter is a common problem, and one does not want to routinely do an endoscopy in everyone presenting with a history of a caustic ingestion. This is especially true given the fact that often one cannot be entirely sure that any ingestion at all has occurred. Although the recommendation from this report is that asymptomatic children need not undergo endoscopy, I, for one, would like to see more data emerge on this issue before totally accepting the conclusions.

J. A. Stockman III, MD

Arsenic Exposure and Prevalence of Type 2 Diabetes in US Adults

Navas-Acien A, Silbergeld EK, Pastor-Barriuso R, et al (Johns Hopkins Bloomberg School of Public Health, Baltimore, MD; Instituto de Salud Carlos III, Madrid, Spain; et al)
JAMA 300:814-822, 2008

Context.—High chronic exposure to inorganic arsenic in drinking water has been related to diabetes development, but the effect of exposure to low to moderate levels of inorganic arsenic on diabetes risk is unknown. In contrast, arsenobetaine, an organic arsenic compound derived from seafood intake, is considered nontoxic.

Objective.—To investigate the association of arsenic exposure, as measured in urine, with the prevalence of type 2 diabetes in a representative sample of US adults.

Design, Setting, and Participants.—Cross-sectional study in 788 adults aged 20 years or older who participated in the 2003-2004 National Health and Nutrition Examination Survey (NHANES) and had urine arsenic determinations.

Main Outcome Measure.—Prevalence of type 2 diabetes across intake of arsenic.

Results.—The median urine levels of total arsenic, dimethylarsinate, and arsenobetaine were 7.1, 3.0, and 0.9 µg/L, respectively. The prevalence of type 2 diabetes was 7.7%. After adjustment for diabetes risk factors and markers of seafood intake, participants with type 2 diabetes had a 26% higher level of total arsenic (95% confidence interval [CI], 2.0%-56.0%) and a nonsignificant 10% higher level of dimethylarsinate (95% CI, −8.0% to 33.0%) than participants without type 2 diabetes, and levels of arsenobetaine were similar to those of participants without type 2 diabetes. After similar adjustment, the odds ratios for type 2 diabetes comparing participants at the 80th vs the 20th percentiles were 3.58 for the level of total arsenic (95% CI, 1.18-10.83), 1.57 for dimethylarsinate (95% CI, 0.89-2.76), and 0.69 for arsenobetaine (95% CI, 0.33-1.48).

Conclusions.—After adjustment for biomarkers of seafood intake, total urine arsenic was associated with increased prevalence of type 2 diabetes. This finding supports the hypothesis that low levels of exposure to inorganic arsenic in drinking water, a widespread exposure worldwide, may play a role in diabetes prevalence. Prospective studies in populations exposed to a range of inorganic arsenic levels are needed to establish whether this association is causal.

▶ This report having to do with arsenic exposure and a risk of type 2 diabetes in adults actually has direct relevance to the care of children because they too are exposed to environmental toxins such as arsenic. The precise etiology of type 2 diabetes remains poorly understood and the role of environmental pollutants, specifically arsenic, in the cause of diabetes has received relatively little attention. In some ways this is quite remarkable in that a link between type 2 diabetes and arsenic was reported back in the 1950s. This was when a patient developed type 2 diabetes after receiving intravenous arsenicals as treatment for a sexually transmitted disease.[1] This link between type 2 diabetes and arsenic became much stronger when reports began to appear about 10 years ago from Southeast Asia showing that chronic high exposure to arsenic from drinking water would cause this form of diabetes. Most of these patients also showed frank signs of arsenic toxicity.

The report by Navas-Acien et al clearly shows a strongly positive association between low arsenic exposures and the prevalence of type 2 diabetes in the United States. Once again this was documented using information from the National Health and Nutrition Examination Survey, a population-based survey conducted by the Centers for Disease Control and Prevention that collects information on the health and nutrition of our population. The report abstracted shows a 3.6-fold increase in the odds of diabetes for participants with the highest total urinary arsenic concentrations as compared with participants with the lowest total urinary arsenic concentrations. It should also be noted that based on the information provided, the linkage between low-dose exposure to arsenic and diabetes is occurring at environmental exposures to arsenic that are 3 times lower than the United States Environmental Protection Agency reference dose. Animal studies have shown that arsenic disturbs glucose production in the liver and decreases insulin secretion and synthesis in pancreatic beta cells, while in rats arsenic exposure causes high blood sugars, high insulin levels, and decreased insulin sensitivity, all findings typical of type 2 diabetes.[2]

There is a lot of arsenic around these days. Inorganic arsenic is found in certain sources of drinking water. Arsenic exposures also can occur with the ingestion of seaweed, fish, and some types of shellfish. In other parts of the world, unfortunately, children are exposed to a wide variety of heavy metal poisons. One particular exposure is rising very quickly and that is exposure to heavy metals being released during the recycling of electronic equipment. Scrap dealers in India, for example, frequently hire children to dismantle old computers. Such child workers earn 2500 to 3000 rupees (about 60 dollars) a month doing this, which is good money for these kids. Unfortunately, electronic devices contain a mix of materials, many of which are toxic and create serious problems if not handled properly. These include heavy metals such as mercury, lead, cadmium, and chromium and flame-retardants such as polybrominate, biphenyls, and polybrominated diphenyl ethers. Dismantling usually involves breaking down old computers using pliers, screwdrivers, and hammers, separating parts from others. This process can cause injuries, but is not as hazardous as the next step because there is no toxic emission involved. Unfortunately, these kids are exposed to air in the environment when printed circuit boards are then burned using acid to extract copper. This process gives off a host of fumes containing heavy metals and which clearly are harmful.

If you want to read more about the hazards of recycling and its impact on children, see the interesting overview of this topic by Chatterjee.[3] Only time will tell whether chronic exposure to low levels of arsenic in children might be a setup for an increased risk of type 2 diabetes.

This commentary closes with a *Clinical Fact/Curio*, this having to do with another toxin, mercury poisoning. Bet you were not aware that there are species of animals that feed on flies and fly larvae. Those that have an appetite for the latter may well be killing themselves as a result of mercury poisoning. It was recently commented on that if an old lady were to swallow a blowfly, she may be better off ingesting an adult insect than an immature one. That is one implication of the discovery that blowflies, which absorb mercury from fish carcasses that they feed on as larvae, rid themselves of much of the toxic metal when they develop into adult flies. Canadian and French researchers documented this by raising blowflies on mercury-containing trout carcasses and then collecting some flies for testing at each developmental stage, from egg to adult. Average mercury concentrations in the flies rose steadily as development progressed, reaching a maximum value of about 160 ng/g in the pupal stage. It dropped to about 50 ng/g in adults. Nearly all methylmercury, the chemical form most toxic to people, disappeared from the flies in that transition.

Flies, unlike humans, seem to be able to readily excrete the metal once they reach maturity. Given the varying concentrations of mercury in the developmental stages of the fly, animals that feed on adult flies are at less risk of poisoning than are, for example, juvenile salmon and certain birds that eat larvae[4]...who would have thought!

J. A. Stockman III, MD

References

1. Stolzer BL, Miller G, White WA. Postarsenical obstructive jaundice complicated by xanthomatosis and diabetes mellitus. *Am J Med*. 1950;9:124-132.
2. Diaz-Villasenor A, Sanchez-Soto MC, Cerbrian ME, et al. Sodium arsenite impairs insulin secretion and transcription in pancreatic beta-cells. *Toxicol App Pharmacol*. 2006;214:30-34.
3. Chatterjee P. Health cost of recycling. *BMJ*. 2008;337:376-377.
4. Blowflies shed mercury at maturity [editorial comment]. *Sci News*. 2005;167:253.

Fine-Particulate Air Pollution and Life Expectancy in the United States

Pope CA III, Ezzati M, Dockery DW (Brigham Young Univ, Provo, UT; Harvard School of Public Health, Boston, MA)
N Engl J Med 360:376-386, 2009

Background.—Exposure to fine-particulate air pollution has been associated with increased morbidity and mortality, suggesting that sustained reductions in pollution exposure should result in improved life expectancy. This study directly evaluated the changes in life expectancy associated with differential changes in fine particulate air pollution that occurred in the United States during the 1980s and 1990s.

Methods.—We compiled data on life expectancy, socioeconomic status, and demographic characteristics for 211 county units in the 51 U.S. metropolitan areas with matching data on fine-particulate air pollution for the late 1970s and early 1980s and the late 1990s and early 2000s. Regression models were used to estimate the association between reductions in pollution and changes in life expectancy, with adjustment for changes in socioeconomic and demographic variables and in proxy indicators for the prevalence of cigarette smoking.

Results.—A decrease of 10 µg per cubic meter in the concentration of fine particulate matter was associated with an estimated increase in mean (±SE) life expectancy of 0.61±0.20 year (P = 0.004). The estimated effect of reduced exposure to pollution on life expectancy was not highly sensitive to adjustment for changes in socioeconomic, demographic, or proxy variables for the prevalence of smoking or to the restriction of observations to relatively large counties. Reductions in air pollution accounted for as much as 15% of the overall increase in life expectancy in the study areas.

Conclusions.—A reduction in exposure to ambient fine-particulate air pollution contributed to significant and measurable improvements in life expectancy in the United States.

▶ The last couple of years have seen much in the adult and pediatric literature about the impact of ambient air pollution. The report of Pope et al provides even more data in this regard. In an analysis that correlates reductions in fine particulate matter (ie, particles less than 2.5 µm in aerodynamic diameter or PM$_{2.5}$) in the air with life expectancies, the investigators found that a decrease in the

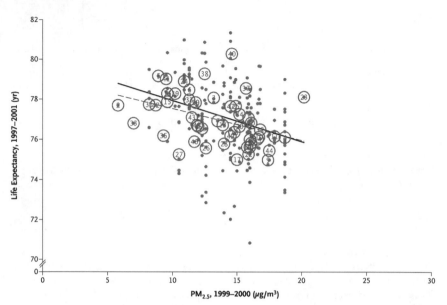

FIGURE 3.—Cross-Sectional Life Expectancies for 1997–2001, Plotted against PM$_{2.5}$ Concentrations for 1999–2000. Dots and circles labeled with numbers represent population-weighted mean life expectancies at the county level and the metropolitan-area–level, respectively. The solid and broken lines represent regression lines with the use of county-level and metropolitan-area–level observations, respectively. The metropolitan areas are coded by number as follows: 1 — Akron, Ohio; 2 — Albuquerque, New Mexico; 3 — Allentown, Pennsylvania; 4 — Atlanta; 5 — Boise, Idaho; 6 — Boston; 7 — Buffalo, New York; 8 — Charlotte, North Carolina; 9 — Charleston, West Virginia; 10 — Chicago; 11 — Cincinnati; 12 — Cleveland; 13 — Dallas; 14 — Dayton, Ohio; 15 — Denver; 16 — El Paso, Texas; 17 — Gary, Indiana; 18 — Houston; 19 — Indianapolis; 20 — Jersey City, New Jersey; 21 — Kansas City, Missouri; 22 — Little Rock, Arkansas; 23 — Los Angeles; 24 — Minneapolis; 25 — New York City; 26 — Norfolk, Virginia; 27 — Oklahoma City; 28 — Philadelphia; 29 — Phoenix, Arizona; 30 — Pittsburgh; 31 — Portland, Oregon; 32 — Providence, Rhode Island; 33 — Pueblo, Colorado; 34 — Raleigh, North Carolina; 35 — Reno, Nevada; 36 — St. Louis; 37 — San Diego, California; 38 — San Francisco; 39 — Salt Lake City; 40 — San Jose, California; 41 — Seattle; 42 — Spokane, Washington; 43 — Springfield, Massachusetts; 44 — Steubenville, Ohio; 45 — Tampa, Florida; 46 — Topeka, Kansas; 47 — Washington, D.C.; 48 — Wichita, Kansas; 49 — Wilmington, Delaware; 50 — Worcester, Massachusetts; 51 — Youngstown, Ohio. PM$_{2.5}$ denotes particulate matter with an aerodynamic diameter less than or equal to 2.5 μm. (Reprinted from Pope CA III, Ezzati M, Dockery DW. Fine-particulate air pollution and life expectancy in the United States. *N Engl J Med.* 2009;360:376-386. Copyright 2009 Massachusetts Medical Society. All rights reserved.)

concentration of PM$_{2.5}$ of 10 μg per cubic meter is associated with an increase in life expectancy of 0.77 years (Fig 3). These findings are based on data over the last several decades in 217 counties in 51 metropolitan areas in the United States. These findings seem to be valid in that they are compatible with previous reductions in life expectancy of 1.11 years in the Netherlands, 1.37 years in Finland, and 0.80 years in Canada resulting from increases in PM$_{2.5}$ concentrations of 10 μg per cubic meter.[1] The strength of the study by Pope et al lies in its ability to demonstrate an increase in life expectancy resulting from actual reductions in particulate air pollution. Previous studies have shown decreasing life expectancy with rising air pollution. The Pope et al findings provide direct confirmation of the population health benefits of actually reducing air pollution and greatly strengthens the foundations of the argument for air-quality management.

Pope et al probably go out on a limb suggesting that decreases in fine particulate air pollution could account for as much as 18% of the increase in life expectancy of about 2.74 years occurring in the United States in between 1980 and 1999, when other factors may also be partly responsible. Decreased tobacco use, improvement in socioeconomic status, dietary patterns, body mass index, physical activity, and access to health services all contribute to the improved longevity on our shores. This does not mean that we should not continue to strive for further gains in the reduction of air pollution. We should. This editor recently flew to Los Angeles and enjoyed the scenery all the way from the east coast to the west coast on a crystal clear day until nearing the LA basin, which was obscured by typical Southern California smog. How unfortunate it is that those living in such an environment may be losing a fraction, however small, of their life.

J. A. Stockman III, MD

Reference

1. Krewski D. Evaluating the effects of ambient air pollution on life expectancy. *N Engl J Med.* 2009;360:413-415.

Article Index

Chapter 1: Adolescent Medicine

Age at Menarche in the Canadian Population: Secular Trends and Relationship to Adulthood BMI   1

Age at Menarche and First Pregnancy Among Psychosocially At-Risk Adolescents   2

Reducing At-Risk Adolescents' Display of Risk Behavior on a Social Networking Web Site: A Randomized Controlled Pilot Intervention Trial   3

Display of Health Risk Behaviors on MySpace by Adolescents: Prevalence and Associations   5

The Availability and Portrayal of Stimulants Over the Internet   6

Noncoital Sexual Activities Among Adolescents   7

Why Do Young Women Continue to Have Sexual Intercourse Despite Pain?   9

Waterpipe Tobacco Smoking on a U.S. College Campus: Prevalence and Correlates   11

Longitudinal Risk Factors for Persistent Fatigue in Adolescents   12

Moderate-to-Vigorous Physical Activity From Ages 9 to 15 Years   14

Bone Metabolism in Adolescent Boys with Anorexia Nervosa   17

Chapter 2: Allergy and Dermatology

Good prognosis, clinical features, and circumstances of peanut and tree nut reactions in children treated by a specialist allergy center   19

Tolerance to extensively heated milk in children with cow's milk allergy   21

Birth by cesarean section, allergic rhinitis, and allergic sensitization among children with a parental history of atopy   22

Mediterranean Diet as a Protective Factor for Wheezing in Preschool Children   24

Wheezing and bronchial hyper-responsiveness in early childhood as predictors of newly diagnosed asthma in early adulthood: a longitudinal birth-cohort study   26

Childhood eczema and asthma incidence and persistence: A cohort study from childhood to middle age   28

MAS063DP is Effective Monotherapy for Mild to Moderate Atopic Dermatitis in Infants and Children: A Multicenter, Randomized, Vehicle-Controlled Study   30

Differences in Acne Treatment Prescribing Patterns of Pediatricians and Dermatologists: An Analysis of Nationally Representative Data   32

Infantile Acne: A Retrospective Study of 16 Cases   35

Growth characteristics of infantile hemangiomas: implications for management   37

Pediatric morphea (localized scleroderma): Review of 136 patients   39

Adjuvant therapy with pegylated interferon alfa-2b versus observation alone in resected stage III melanoma: final results of EORTC 18991, a randomised phase III trial   43

Outbreak of rash in children associated with recreational mud exposure   46

Chapter 3: Blood

Dyshemoglobinemias and pulse oximetry: a therapeutic challenge 49

An Economic Analysis of Anemia Prevention during Infancy 50

Reticulocyte hemoglobin content for the diagnosis of iron deficiency 53

Long-Term Outcome of Pediatric Patients with Severe Aplastic Anemia Treated with Antithymocyte Globulin and Cyclosporine 54

Systematic Review: Hydroxyurea for the Treatment of Adults with Sickle Cell Disease 56

Cell-Free Hemoglobin-Based Blood Substitutes and Risk of Myocardial Infarction and Death: A Meta-analysis 60

Adverse Reactions to Allogeneic Whole Blood Donation by 16- and 17-Year-Olds 61

A Syndrome with Congenital Neutropenia and Mutations in *G6PC3* 64

Severe hemorrhage in children with newly diagnosed immune thrombocytopenic purpura 66

Effect of eltrombopag on platelet counts and bleeding during treatment of chronic idiopathic thrombocytopenic purpura: a randomised, double-blind, placebo-controlled trial 67

Inflammation induces hemorrhage in thrombocytopenia 69

Chapter 4: Child Development

Predicting Stuttering Onset by the Age of 3 Years: A Prospective, Community Cohort Study 73

Prevalence of Autism Among Adolescents With Intellectual Disabilities 75

Autism prevalence and precipitation rates in California, Oregon, and Washington counties 77

A Functional Genetic Link between Distinct Developmental Language Disorders 79

Early head injury and attention-deficit/hyperactivity disorder: retrospective cohort study 81

Toilet training of healthy young toddlers: a randomized trial between a daytime wetting alarm and timed potty training 82

Like parent, like child: child food and beverage choices during role playing 84

Chapter 5: Dentistry and Otolaryngology (ENT)

Neonatal repair of cleft lip: a decision-making protocol 87

Sudden oronasal bleeding in a young child 90

Tooth Extraction Socket Healing in Pediatric Patients Treated with Intravenous Pamidronate 92

Dexamethasone and Risk of Nausea and Vomiting and Postoperative Bleeding After Tonsillectomy in Children: A Randomized Trial 93

Respiratory Viruses in Laryngeal Croup of Young Children   95

Pathogens Causing Recurrent and Difficult-to-Treat Acute Otitis Media, 2003-2006   96

Overuse of tympanostomy tubes in New York metropolitan area: evidence from five hospital cohort   98

Lateral Sinus Thrombosis as a Complication of Otitis Media: 10-Year Experience at the Children's Hospital of Philadelphia   100

Etiologic and Audiologic Evaluations After Universal Neonatal Hearing Screening: Analysis of 170 Referred Neonates   102

Chapter 6: Endocrinology

Etiology of Failure to Thrive in Infants and Toddlers Referred to a Pediatric Endocrinology Outpatient Clinic   105

Mutations in the Idotyrosine Deiodinase Gene and Hypothyroidism   107

Inaccurate hemoglobin A(1C) levels in patients with type 1 diabetes and hereditary persistence of hemoglobin F   109

Role of blood pressure in development of early retinopathy in adolescents with type 1 diabetes: prospective cohort study   110

Shared and Distinct Genetic Variants in Type 1 Diabetes and Celiac Disease   113

Birth Weight and Risk of Type 2 Diabetes: A Systematic Review   115

Chapter 7: Gastroenterology

Natural evolution of infantile regurgitation versus the efficacy of thickened formula   119

14 years of eosinophilic esophagitis: clinical features and prognosis   121

Effect of eradication of *Helicobacter pylori* on incidence of metachronous gastric carcinoma after endoscopic resection of early gastric cancer: an open-label, randomised controlled trial   122

The changing epidemiology of infantile hypertrophic pyloric stenosis in Scotland   124

Recovery after open versus laparoscopic pyloromyotomy for pyloric stenosis: a double-blind multicentre randomised controlled trial   126

Circumumbilical pyloromyotomy in the era of minimally invasive surgery   127

Minimally invasive closure of pediatric umbilical hernias   129

Post-Infectious Functional Gastrointestinal Disorders in Children   131

Increased Gastrointestinal Permeability and Gut Inflammation in Children with Functional Abdominal Pain and Irritable Bowel Syndrome   133

Effect of fibre, antispasmodics, and peppermint oil in the treatment of irritable bowel syndrome: systematic review and meta-analysis   135

Natural History of Paediatric Inflammatory Bowel Diseases Over a 5-Year Follow-up: A Retrospective Review of Data From the Register of Paediatric Inflammatory Bowel Diseases   136

Use of complementary medicine in pediatric patients with inflammatory bowel disease: results from a multicenter survey   138

Transition of adolescents with inflammatory bowel disease from pediatric to adult care: a survey of adult gastroenterologists   139

Quality of life in adolescents with treated coeliac disease: influence of compliance and age at diagnosis   141

Difference in Celiac Disease Risk Between Swedish Birth Cohorts Suggests an Opportunity for Primary Prevention   143

Fructose intolerance in children presenting with abdominal pain   146

Health Utilization and Cost Impact of Childhood Constipation in the United States   148

Waist circumference correlates with liver fibrosis in children with non-alcoholic steatohepatitis   150

Wilson disease in children: analysis of 57 cases   151

Chapter 8: Genitourinary Tract

Prevalence of Urinary Tract Infection in Childhood: A Meta-Analysis   155

Delay in Diagnosis in Poststreptococcal Glomerulonephritis   157

Risk Factors for End Stage Renal Disease in Children With Posterior Urethral Valves   159

Long-Term Consequences of Kidney Donation   160

Genetic Alterations Associated With Cryptorchidism   162

Transient Asynchronous Testicular Growth in Adolescent Males With a Varicocele   164

Chapter 9: Heart and Blood Vessels

Prevalence of Congenital Heart Defects in Metropolitan Atlanta, 1998-2005   167

Effectiveness of teaching cardiac auscultation to residents during an elective pediatric cardiology rotation   170

First Day of Life Pulse Oximetry Screening to Detect Congenital Heart Defects   173

Impact of pulse oximetry screening on the detection of duct dependent congenital heart disease: a Swedish prospective screening study in 39 821 newborns   176

Screening newborns for congenital heart disease with pulse oximetry: survey of pediatric cardiologists   178

Cardiac surgery in adults performed at children's hospitals: Trends and outcomes   180

Hospital mortality for Norwood and arterial switch operations as a function of institutional volume   182

Developmental and Functional Outcomes at School Entry in Children with Congenital Heart Defects   184

Outcomes in Adults With Bicuspid Aortic Valves   185

Shared Genetic Causes of Cardiac Hypertrophy in Children and Adults   188

Angiotensin II Blockade and Aortic-Root Dilation in Marfan's Syndrome   191

Left Ventricular Mass Index in Children with White Coat Hypertension — 193

Effect of Domperidone on QT Interval in Neonates — 195

Cardiovascular evaluation, including resting and exercise electrocardiography, before participation in competitive sports: cross sectional study — 197

Mandarin juice improves the antioxidant status of hypercholesterolemic children — 200

Spectrum and Management of Hypertriglyceridemia Among Children in Clinical Practice — 202

Chapter 10: Infectious Diseases and Immunology

The stethoscope as a vector of infectious diseases in the paediatric division — 205

Influenza-Associated Pediatric Mortality in the United States: Increase of *Staphylococcus aureus* Coinfection — 207

Effectiveness of Maternal Influenza Immunization in Mothers and Infants — 209

Influenza Vaccine Effectiveness Among Children 6 to 59 Months of Age During 2 Influenza Seasons: A Case-Cohort Study — 211

Prognostic Factors in Influenza-associated Encephalopathy — 213

Acute Childhood Encephalitis and Encephalopathy Associated With Influenza: A Prospective 11-Year Review — 214

Probable limited person-to-person transmission of highly pathogenic avian influenza A (H5N1) virus in China — 216

A Clinical Trial of a Whole-Virus H5N1 Vaccine Derived from Cell Culture — 219

The Burden of Respiratory Syncytial Virus Infection in Young Children — 221

Lack of antibody affinity maturation due to poor Toll-like receptor stimulation leads to enhanced respiratory syncytial virus disease — 223

Human bocavirus infection in children with respiratory tract disease — 225

Measles in Europe: an epidemiological assessment — 226

Factors associated with uptake of measles, mumps, and rubella vaccine (MMR) and use of single antigen vaccines in a contemporary UK cohort: prospective cohort study — 228

Human Papillomavirus Vaccination Coverage on YouTube — 230

Monovalent Type 1 Oral Poliovirus Vaccine in Newborns — 232

Effectiveness of Immunization against Paralytic Poliomyelitis in Nigeria — 234

Hepatitis B Virus Screening for Internationally Adopted Children — 235

Tenofovir Disoproxil Fumarate versus Adefovir Dipivoxil for Chronic Hepatitis B — 237

Estimation of HIV incidence in the United States — 239

CD4⁺/CD8⁺ T Cell Ratio for Diagnosis of HIV-1 Infection in Infants: Women and Infants Transmission Study — 242

Early Antiretroviral Therapy and Mortality among HIV-Infected Infants — 243

Extended Antiretroviral Prophylaxis to Reduce Breast-Milk HIV-1 Transmission — 245

Effects of Early, Abrupt Weaning on HIV-free Survival of Children in Zambia — 247

Circumcision Status and Risk of HIV and Sexually Transmitted Infections Among Men Who Have Sex With Men: A Meta-analysis   249

Extensively Drug-Resistant Tuberculosis in the United States, 1993-2007   251

Latent Tuberculosis Diagnosis in Children by Using the QuantiFERON-TB Gold In-Tube Test   253

Effect of Pneumococcal Conjugate Vaccine on Pneumococcal Meningitis   255

Performance of a Rapid Antigen-Detection Test and Throat Culture in Community Pediatric Offices: Implications for Management of Pharyngitis   258

Streptococcal Infection and Exacerbations of Childhood Tics and Obsessive-Compulsive Symptoms: A Prospective Blinded Cohort Study   260

Impact of rapid screening tests on acquisition of meticillin resistant *Staphylococcus aureus*: cluster randomised crossover trial   262

Methicillin-Resistant *Staphylococcus aureus* Central Line–Associated Bloodstream Infections in US Intensive Care Units, 1997-2007   264

Prevalence of and Risk Factors for Community-Acquired Methicillin-Resistant and Methicillin-Sensitive *Staphylococcus aureus* Colonization in Children Seen in a Practice-Based Research Network   266

Methods of Investigation and Management of Infections Causing Febrile Seizures   269

Utility of Lumbar Puncture for First Simple Febrile Seizure Among Children 6 to 18 Months of Age   270

Predictors of cerebrospinal fluid pleocytosis in febrile infants aged 0 to 90 days   272

Test Characteristics and Interpretation of Cerebrospinal Fluid Gram Stain in Children   276

Exposure to Nontraditional Pets at Home and to Animals in Public Settings: Risks to Children   277

Gene Therapy for Immunodeficiency Due to Adenosine Deaminase Deficiency   281

Chapter 11: Miscellaneous

Inequalities in healthy life years in the 25 countries of the European Union in 2005: a cross-national meta-regression analysis   287

Socioeconomic Inequalities in Health in 22 European Countries   289

Comfort of General Internists and General Pediatricians in Providing Care for Young Adults with Chronic Illnesses of Childhood   291

Awareness and Use of California's Paid Family Leave Insurance Among Parents of Chronically Ill Children   293

Staff-Only Pediatric Hospitalist Care of Patients With Medically Complex Subspecialty Conditions in a Major Teaching Hospital   296

Trends in Pediatric and Adult Bicycling Deaths Before and After Passage of a Bicycle Helmet Law   298

Recurrent Rearrangements of Chromosome 1q21.1 and Variable Pediatric Phenotypes   300

Infection and sudden unexpected death in infancy: a systematic retrospective case review   302

Sudden Infant Death Syndrome: Changing Epidemiologic Patterns in California 1989-2004   304

Use of a Fan During Sleep and the Risk of Sudden Infant Death Syndrome   307

Quality of Care of Children in the Emergency Department: Association with Hospital Setting and Physician Training   309

Performance during Internal Medicine Residency Training and Subsequent Disciplinary Action by State Licensing Boards   311

Clinical Inactivity Among Pediatricians: Prevalence and Perspectives   313

Protecting the Public: State Medical Board Licensure Policies for Active and Inactive Physicians   316

Alcohol consumption and alcohol counselling behaviour among US medical students: cohort study   319

Five year outcomes in a cohort study of physicians treated for substance use disorders in the United States   321

Educational Debt and Reported Career Plans among Internal Medicine Residents 323

Handedness Effects on Procedural Training in Pediatrics   325

Effect of 80-Hour Workweek on Continuity of Care   326

Pediatric surgery workforce: population and economic issues   328

Electromagnetic Interference From Radio Frequency Identification Inducing Potentially Hazardous Incidents in Critical Care Medical Equipment   330

Chapter 12: Musculoskeletal

Age-related patterns of injury in children involved in all-terrain vehicle accidents   335

Mechanical supports for acute, severe ankle sprain: a pragmatic, multicentre, randomised controlled trial   337

Patterns of skeletal fractures in child abuse: systematic review   339

Pediatric Heelys injuries   340

Ultrasound hip evaluation in achondroplasia   342

Age-appropriate body mass index in children with achondroplasia: interpretation in relation to indexes of height   344

Asymmetric loads and pain associated with backpack carrying by children   345

Changing trends in acute osteomyelitis in children: impact of methicillin-resistant Staphylococcus aureus infections   347

Abatacept in children with juvenile idiopathic arthritis: a randomised, double-blind, placebo-controlled withdrawal trial   349

Autologous bone marrow transplantation in autoimmune arthritis restores immune homeostasis through CD4+CD25+Foxp3+ regulatory T cells   352

Differentation of Post-Streptococcal Reactive Arthritis from Acute Rheumatic Fever   353

Bone Metabolism in Adolescent Athletes With Amenorrhea, Athletes With Eumenorrhea, and Control Subjects   356

Chronic fatigue syndrome in children aged 11 years old and younger   358

Chapter 13: Neurology and Psychiatry

Low Iron Storage in Children and Adolescents with Neurally Mediated Syncope   361

The influence of different food and drink on tics in Tourette syndrome   363

A case-control evaluation of the ketogenic diet versus ACTH for new-onset infantile spasms   365

Hypothermia Therapy after Traumatic Brain Injury in Children   367

Nonsurgical treatment of deformational plagiocephaly: a systematic review   370

Effect of Simvastatin on Cognitive Functioning in Children With Neurofibromatosis Type 1: A Randomized Controlled Trial   372

Differential diagnosis of congenital muscular dystrophies   374

Prevalence of enuresis and its association with attention-deficit/hyperactivity disorder among U.S. children: results from a nationally representative study   375

Childhood Attention-Deficit/Hyperactivity Disorder and the Emergence of Personality Disorders in Adolescence: A Prospective Follow-Up Study   377

Stimulant Therapy and Risk for Subsequent Substance Use Disorders in Male Adults With ADHD: A Naturalistic Controlled 10-Year Follow-Up Study   379

Hypericum perforatum (St John's Wort) for Attention-Deficit/Hyperactivity Disorder in Children and Adolescents: A Randomized Controlled Trial   381

Absence of Preferential Looking to the Eyes of Approaching Adults Predicts Level of Social Disability in 2-Year-Old Toddlers With Autism Spectrum Disorder   384

Correlates of Accommodation of Pediatric Obsessive-Compulsive Disorder: Parent, Child, and Family Characteristics   387

Cognitive Behavioral Therapy, Sertraline, or a Combination in Childhood Anxiety   388

Cost-Effectiveness of Treatments for Adolescent Depression: Results From TADS   390

Burnout and Suicidal Ideation among U.S. Medical Students   392

Common genetic determinants of schizophrenia and bipolar disorder in Swedish families: a population-based study   394

Enuresis as a premorbid developmental marker of schizophrenia   396

Chapter 14: Newborn

Cumulative Live-Birth Rates after In Vitro Fertilization   399

Effects of technology or maternal factors on perinatal outcome after assisted fertilisation: a population-based cohort study   401

Clomifene citrate or unstimulated intrauterine insemination compared with expectant management for unexplained infertility: pragmatic randomised controlled trial   403

Intensive Care for Extreme Prematurity — Moving Beyond Gestational Age   405

Long-Term Medical and Social Consequences of Preterm Birth   407

Increased Risk of Adverse Neurological Development for Late Preterm Infants   411

Aggressive vs. Conservative Phototherapy for Infants with Extremely Low Birth Weight   412

Early Insulin Therapy in Very-Low-Birth-Weight Infants   414

A Randomized, Controlled Trial of Magnesium Sulfate for the Prevention of Cerebral Palsy   417

Neuroprotective Effects of the Nonpsychoactive Cannabinoid Cannabidiol in Hypoxic-Ischemic Newborn Piglets   418

Childhood outcomes after prescription of antibiotics to pregnant women with spontaneous preterm labour: 7-year follow up of the ORACLE II trial   420

Neurodevelopmental Outcomes of Preterm Infants Fed High-Dose Docosahexaenoic Acid: A Randomized Controlled Trial   422

Maternal caffeine intake during pregnancy and risk of fetal growth restriction: a large prospective observational study   424

Epidemiology and Treatment of Painful Procedures in Neonates in Intensive Care Units   425

Traumatic lumbar punctures in neonates: test performance of the cerebrospinal fluid white blood cell count   428

Maternal and paternal contribution to intergenerational recurrence of breech delivery: population based cohort study   429

Increasing Prevalence of Gastroschisis: Population-based Study in California   431

Newborn weight charts underestimate the incidence of low birthweight in preterm infants   433

Duration of meconium passage in preterm and term infants   434

Spousal violence and potentially preventable single and recurrent spontaneous fetal loss in an African setting: cross-sectional study   436

Granulocyte-macrophage colony stimulating factor administered as prophylaxis for reduction of sepsis in extremely preterm, small for gestational age neonates (the PROGRAMS trial): a single-blind, multicentre, randomised controlled trial   438

Timing of Elective Repeat Cesarean Delivery at Term and Neonatal Outcomes   440

Chapter 15: Nutrition and Metabolism

Misperceptions and misuse of Bear Brand coffee creamer as infant food: national cross sectional survey of consumers and paediatricians in Laos   443

High Body Mass Index for Age Among US Children and Adolescents, 2003-2006   444

Comparison of the Prevalence of Shortness, Underweight, and Overweight among US Children Aged 0 to 59 Months by Using the CDC 2000 and the WHO 2006 Growth Charts   446

An Obesity-Associated *FTO* Gene Variant and Increased Energy Intake in Children   449

Maternal Overweight and Obesity and the Risk of Congenital Anomalies: A Systematic Review and Meta-Analysis   451

Childhood Sleep Time and Long-Term Risk for Obesity: A 32-Year Prospective Birth Cohort Study   453

Obesity and Excessive Daytime Sleepiness in Prepubertal Children With
Obstructive Sleep Apnea   455

Prevalence and Predictors of Abnormal Liver Enzymes in Young Women with
Anorexia Nervosa   456

Intra-abdominal Adiposity and Individual Components of the Metabolic Syndrome
in Adolescence: Sex Differences and Underlying Mechanisms   458

Aliskiren Combined with Losartan in Type 2 Diabetes and Nephropathy   460

Effects of Intensive Glucose Lowering in Type 2 Diabetes   462

Risk of microalbuminuria and progression to macroalbuminuria in a cohort with
childhood onset type 1 diabetes: prospective observational study   464

Nasal insulin to prevent type 1 diabetes in children with HLA genotypes and
autoantibodies conferring increased risk of disease: a double-blind, randomized
controlled trial   466

Vitamin D supplementation in early childhood and risk of type 1 diabetes:
a systematic review and meta-analysis   468

Hypovitaminosis D among healthy children in the United States: a review of the
current evidence   469

Diagnosis, symptoms, frequency and mortality of 260 patients with urea cycle
disorders from a 21-year, multicentre study of acute hyperammonaemic episodes   471

Chapter 16: Oncology

Childhood cancer in the offspring born in 1921–1984 to US radiologic
technologists   475

Computed tomography before transfer to a level I pediatric trauma center risks
duplication with associated increased radiation exposure   476

Breast Cancer Surveillance Practices Among Women Previously Treated With
Chest Radiation for a Childhood Cancer   478

Male reproductive health after childhood cancer   480

Do doctors discuss fertility issues before they treat young patients with cancer? 482

Deletion of *IKZF1* and Prognosis in Acute Lymphoblastic leukemia   483

Clinical significance of minimal residual disease in childhood acute lymphoblastic
leukemia and its relationship to other prognostic factors: a Children's Oncology
Group study   485

Genome-wide Interrogation of Germline Genetic Variation Associated with
Treatment Response in Childhood Acute Lymphoblastic Leukemia   487

Twenty-five–year follow-up among survivors of childhood acute lymphoblastic
leukemia: a report from the Childhood Cancer Survivor Study   488

Mutations of *JAK2* in acute lymphoblastic leukaemias associated with Down's
syndrome   490

SFCE (Société Française de Lutte contre les Cancers et Leucémies de l'Enfant et de
l'Adolescent) Recommendations for the Management of Tumor Lysis Syndrome
(TLS) With Rasburicase: An Observational Survey   492

Retrospective Study of Childhood Ganglioneuroma   493

Effectiveness of screening for neuroblastoma at 6 months of age: a retrospective
population-based cohort study   495

Chromosome 6p22 Locus Associated with Clinically Aggressive Neuroblastoma   498

Stool DNA and Occult Blood Testing for Screen Detection of Colorectal Neoplasia 499

The Gist of literature on pediatric GIST: review of clinical presentation   501

Chapter 17: Ophthalmology

Outdoor Activity Reduces the Prevalence of Myopia in Children   505

Mental Illness in Young Adults Who Had Strabismus as Children   507

Pediatric Golf-Related Ophthalmic Injuries   509

A survey of ophthalmology residents' attitudes toward pediatric ophthalmology   511

Chapter 18: Respiratory Tract

Oral Prednisolone for Preschool Children with Acute Virus-Induced Wheezing   515

Effectiveness of PTC124 treatment of cystic fibrosis caused by nonsense mutations:
a prospective phase II trial   518

Sweat Chloride Testing in Infants Identified as Heterozygote Carriers by Newborn
Screening   521

Diagnosis of Cystic Fibrosis by Sweat Testing: Age-Specific Reference Intervals 522

Sweat test in patients with glucose-6-phosphate-1-dehydrogenase deficiency   523

Silver-Coated Endotracheal Tubes and Incidence of Ventilator-Associated
Pneumonia: The NASCENT Randomized Trial   525

Prevalence and Time Course of Acute Mountain Sickness in Older Children and
Adolescents After Rapid Ascent to 3450 Meters   527

When should oxygen be given to children at high altitude? A systematic review to
define altitude-specific hypoxaemia   530

Chapter 19: Therapeutics and Toxicology

Adverse Events From Cough and Cold Medications in Children   535

Pseudoephedrine Use Among US Children, 1999–2006: Results From the Slone
Survey   537

Medicines for Children: A Matter of Taste   539

News Media Coverage of Medication Research: Reporting Pharmaceutical
Company Funding and Use of Generic Medication Names   540

Paracetamol plus ibuprofen for the treatment of fever in children (PITCH):
randomised controlled trial   543

Paracetamol plus ibuprofen for the treatment of fever in children (PITCH):
economic evaluation of a randomised controlled trial   545

Alternating Antipyretics: Antipyretic Efficacy of Acetaminophen Versus
Acetaminophen Alternated With Ibuprofen in Children   547

Association between paracetamol use in infancy and childhood, and risk of asthma, rhinoconjunctivitis, and eczema in children aged 6–7 years: analysis from Phase Three of the ISAAC programme 549

Antiemetic Medications in Children with Presumed Infectious Gastroenteritis— Pharmacoepidemiology in Europe and Northern America 551

Safety and efficacy of acupuncture in children: a review of the evidence 553

Transdermal Patch Medication Delivery Systems and Pediatric Poisonings, 2002-2006 556

Fetal alcohol syndrome: a prospective national surveillance study 558

Association of Urinary Bisphenol A Concentration With Medical Disorders and Laboratory Abnormalities in Adults 560

Caustic ingestion in children: is endoscopy always indicated? The results of an Italian multicenter observational study 563

Arsenic Exposure and Prevalence of Type 2 Diabetes in US Adults 564

Fine-Particulate Air Pollution and Life Expectancy in the United States 567

Author Index

A

Aarons C, 340
Aarsen FK, 372
Abbassy AA, 232
Abdulkerim H, 22
Abraham L, 316
Abrahamowicz M, 458
Abrahams BS, 79
Ache KA, 230
Adilov N, 77
Afessa B, 525
Afsar FS, 39
Ahlquist DA, 499
Ahmad N, 347
Aiuti A, 281
Akobeng AK, 468
Albano AM, 388
Albrechtsen S, 429
Alexander BH, 475
Alfonseda Rojas JD, 24
Alio AP, 436
Alvarez FJ, 418
Amin R, 214, 464
Anderson RA, 482
Andriatahina T, 443
Anzueto A, 525
Appaswamy G, 64
Arifeen SE, 209
Armoni S, 518
Armstrong L, 251
Arnold GK, 311
Arnold JH, 139
Arola M, 480
Ashikov A, 64
Aylward RB, 234

B

Bachur RG, 272
Baker C, 300
Bales CB, 100
Barash J, 353
Barendse RM, 139
Barennes H, 443
Beardsall K, 414
Beasley R, 549
Beausoleil JL, 121
Beavers DP, 84
Bedogni G, 150
Bekkali N, 434
Bekmezian A, 296
Bell R, 451
Belmont JM, 170

Benninga M, 148
Bercovich D, 490
Berger G, 141
Bergman RL, 387
Berkovitch M, 205
Berterö C, 9
Bertrand Y, 492
Betalli P, 563
Bhattacharya S, 403
Biederman J, 379
Björk C, 394
Blank LL, 311
Bloch J, 527
Bloom KA, 21
Boguniewicz M, 30
Boon L, 352
Bor D, 540
Borowitz MJ, 485
Borys D, 556
Bost JE, 155
Boudewyns A, 102
Boztug K, 64
Bradfield JP, 498
Bradley EA, 75
Bradley RH, 14
Brethon B, 492
Brügmann-Pieper S, 173
Brieu N, 225
Brocklehurst P, 438
Brooke BS, 191
Brown-Whitehorn TF, 121
Brusilow S, 471
Bryson SE, 75
Buchanan GR, 66
Buddensiek N, 363
Burgess JA, 28
Burkhardt T, 433
Burns BJ, 390
Burton DC, 264
Bussel JB, 67
Buti M, 237
Butler C, 46
Byrnes GB, 28

C

Campbell M, 321
Capablo A, 197
Capo JA, 507
Capraro AJ, 270
Carbajal R, 425
Carbo C, 69
Carr K, 384
Carr R, 438

Carroll MD, 444
Cartwright L, 164
Casaulta C, 523
Casey JR, 96
Castanes MS, 511
Castro-Rodriguez JA, 24
Cattaneo F, 281
Ceccanti S, 127
Cecil JE, 449
Cemeroglu AP, 105
Chahine C, 92
Chalmers J, 124
Chambers H, 345
Chang LC, 37
Chang R-KR, 304
Chang RK, 178
Cheng C, 487
Cheung MS, 92
Christen-Zaech S, 39
Christo K, 356
Chung PJ, 293, 296
Chwals WJ, 476
Clark AL, 138
Clark AT, 19
Clark C, 12, 159
Clement E, 374
Clement MR, 164
Coats DK, 511
Codoñer-Franch P, 200
Cohen AL, 535
Coleman-Phox K, 307
Cord J, 17
Costelloe C, 543, 545
Cotten CM, 428
Cotton MF, 243
Coviello S, 223
Cozzi DA, 127
Craig ME, 110
Crawley E, 358
Creek A, 335
Croft NM, 136
Czarnetzki C, 93
Czyzewski DI, 133

D

Daikos GL, 151
Damore D, 325
Danan C, 425
Daniel M, 105
Darden PM, 326
Davies EH, 539
Davies S, 358
Davis AM, 170

Davis MM, 291
Dawkins R, 335
Deberail A, 87
De Bernardi B, 493
Declau F, 102
Deep-Soboslay A, 396
DeFoor W, 159
de Goede-Bolder A, 372
de Jager W, 352
De-la-Cruz J, 53
Delgado MF, 223
De Pellegrin M, 342
Devidas M, 485
De Wachter S, 82
de-Wahl Granelli A, 176
Dhara R, 207
Dharmage SC, 28
Dharmar M, 309
Dias T, 411
Di Martino L, 131
DiFabio D, 456
DiVasta AD, 456
Djeddi D, 195
Dobbelaere D, 471
Dockery DW, 567
Domino ME, 390
Donohue JE, 182
Doody MM, 475
Doré CJ, 438
Dover DC, 488
Drack AV, 509
Drolet BA, 37
Due R Jr, 173
Duke T, 530
Dunbar J, 2
Dunham KM, 313, 316
Dunstan F, 339
Duplain H, 527
Dy BA, 61
Dyrbye LN, 392
Dzakovic A, 129

E

Eakin MN, 133
Eaton S, 126
Eder AF, 61
Eduardo R, 253
Edwards JR, 264
Eggermont AMM, 43
Ehrlich HJ, 219
Eichenfield LF, 30
Eissenberg T, 11
El-Gamal Y, 232
El-Sayed N, 232

Elia N, 93
Elliman D, 228
Elliott EJ, 558
Elliott MN, 293
Elmerstig E, 9
Elon L, 319
Elward A, 266
Ewan PW, 19
Ezzati M, 567

F

Feins NR, 129
Felner EI, 109
Feng Z, 216
Ferlin A, 162
Finelli L, 207
Fiore A, 207
Firmansyah A, 119
Fisher SG, 193
Flegal KM, 444, 446
Fleischer AB Jr, 32
Flores SA, 249
Flory JD, 377
Foley R, 160
Fong H-F, 456
Ford AC, 135
Ford JS, 478
Ford-Jones E, 214
Forman RF, 6
Foster MM, 521
Frank E, 319
Freed GL, 313, 316
Fritz SA, 266
Fukase K, 122

G

Galimberti S, 281
Galinier P, 87
Gallego PH, 110
Galloway TS, 560
Gambini C, 493
Ganmore I, 490
Garbutt J, 266
Garcia-Marcos L, 24
Garnett EA, 138
Gasasira A, 234
Ge A, 553
Geomelas M, 363
Gerber MA, 258
Gibb DM, 243
Gibson RA, 422
Gillies C, 287

Goerge T, 69
Gold DR, 22
Gomara RE, 146
Gozal D, 455
Greaves R, 522
Green M, 136
Greenbaum LA, 157
Greenberg RG, 428
Gurney JG, 182
Gurofsky RC, 202
Gustafson KK, 326
Guyon G, 225

H

Habashi JP, 191
Hacker MR, 399
Haggstrom AN, 37
Hait EJ, 139
Hakim MD, 39
Halata MS, 146
Hall CB, 221
Hall GC, 81
Hall HI, 239
Hall NJ, 126
Halonen M, 26
Hamers SL, 434
Harman J, 148
Harper MB, 276
Harrild K, 403
Harris MA, 1
Harrison S, 339
Hartley JC, 302
Hasan SJ, 511
Haupt R, 493
Hay AD, 543
He JP, 375
Head TW, 92
Heathcote EJ, 237
Hedderick EF, 365
Hegar B, 119
Heisler M, 291
Hello M, 35
Hensbroek R, 330
Hernell O, 143
Hey E, 90
Heyman E, 205
Hillyer CD, 61
Hing S, 110
Hink EM, 509
Hirawat S, 518
Hirsch JC, 182
Hiyama E, 495
Hladik A, 49
Hoberman A, 96

Hochman M, 540
Hochman S, 540
Hollinghurst S, 545
Hoover DR, 245
Hoover-Fong JE, 344
Horan TC, 264
Hörnell A, 143
Ho-Tin-Noe B, 69
Houts RM, 14
Hsu HE, 255
Hummel D, 270
Hunger SP, 485
Hutchison JS, 367
Hutton JL, 337
Hyde TM, 396

I

Ibrahim HN, 160
Ichara I, 195
Iglesias B, 396
Imbach P, 66
Iobst C, 340
Ip J, 505
Irby CE, 32
Iwane MK, 221

J

Jackson E, 159
Jagger C, 287
Jarjour IT, 361
Jarjour LK, 361
Jenkins HE, 234
Jenkins P, 50
Jeyaratnam D, 262
Jindal V, 553
Johnson KJ, 475
Jones DR, 420
Jones R, 7
Jones W, 384
Judge DP, 191

K

Kabat W, 258
Kaemmer DA, 501
Kalaydjian A, 375
Kanter KR, 180
Katzman DK, 17
Kaufman DW, 537
Kaye SJ, 115
Keenan HT, 81

Keens TG, 304
Kellum E, 335
Kelly JP, 537
Kemp AM, 339
Kennedy KA, 370
Kenyon S, 420
Kerem E, 518
Kern SJ, 60
Keyhani S, 98
Kheirandish-Gozal L, 455
Kimia AA, 270
Kimura H, 213
Kirshbom PM, 180
Klein A, 374
Klein NJ, 302
Kleinman LC, 98
Kleis L, 105
Klin A, 384
Klitzner TS, 178
Klootwijk W, 107
Koehoorn M, 1
Kollef MH, 525
Kolon TF, 164
Kongolo G, 195
Kossoff EH, 365
Kostev K, 551
Krab LC, 372
Kramer LC, 547
Kuhn L, 247
Kump T, 157
Kumwenda NI, 245
Kupila A, 466
Kupper LL, 84
Kurlan R, 260

L

Lafuente H, 418
Lähteenmäki PM, 480
Lakhanpaul M, 515
Lam K, 298
Lamb SE, 337
Lambert PC, 515
Lamparello B, 356
Lande MB, 193
Landhuis CE, 453
Landon MB, 440
Lang IA, 560
Langley A, 387
Lanzkron S, 56
Larsson P, 202
Lassay L, 501
Latthaphasavang V, 443
Laurent C, 431
Law C, 228

Léauté-Labrèze C, 35
Lefaix C, 195
Leonard GT, 458
Lezotte D, 2
Li D-K, 307
Li S, 488
Lichtenstein P, 394
Lie RT, 407
Liem O, 148
Lighter J, 253
Limperopoulos C, 184
Lindberg LD, 7
Lopez M, 340
López-Jaén AB, 200
López-Laso E, 53
Loprinzi CL, 499
Lurie P, 60
Lynshue K, 49
Lysakowski C, 93

M

Macias BR, 345
Mackenbach JP, 289
Mahle WT, 180
Majnemer A, 184
Makrides M, 422
Malizia BA, 399
Manco M, 150
Maulhiot C, 202
Manolaki N, 151
Mansky PJ, 553
Marcellin P, 237
Marcellini M, 150
Marcin JP, 309
Maris JM, 498
Markestad T, 407
Marks G, 249
Marlowe DB, 6
Marsh JL, 337
Marshall SW, 81
Mashiach E, 353
Massie FS, 392
Mateos ME, 53
Mattioli LF, 170
McBurney PG, 326
McCarty RL, 381
McCormick MC, 411
McDonald FS, 323
McGrath M, 109
McGready J, 344
McKenzie JA, 507
McLellan AT, 321
McPhee AJ, 422
Meagher CC, 193

Meberg A, 173
Mechinaud F, 492
Meehan WP 3rd, 272
Mefford HC, 300
Mei Z, 446
Mejías A, 347
Mele E, 127
Melve KK, 429
Menesses A, 188
Mercuri E, 374
Mezoff AG, 235
Miller CJ, 377
Miller MA, 556
Miller SR, 377
Millett GA, 249
Millichap JG, 269
Millichap JJ, 269
Mishra A, 522
Misra M, 17
Mody R, 488
Mofenson LM, 245
Moharamzadeh D, 342
Mohney BG, 507
Mollison J, 403
Monsalvo AC, 223
Monuteaux MC, 379
Moore MR, 255
Moreno JC, 107
Moreno MA, 3, 5
Morgan IG, 505
Morgan WJ, 26
Morishima T, 213
Morita H, 188
Morone NE, 155
Morris A, 558
Morris BH, 412
Moscone F, 287
Moskowitz CS, 478
Mosse YP, 498
Moster D, 407
Muñiz P, 200
Müller M, 219
Müller-Vahl KR, 363
Mulligan CG, 483
Murthy G, 345
Muscat M, 226

N

Nader PR, 14
Nagao T, 213
Naimi T, 319
Nakayama DK, 328
Nana PN, 436
Näntö-Salonen K, 466
Natanson C, 60

Navas-Acien A, 564
Navon-Elkan P, 353
Neuman MI, 276
Neunert CE, 66
Newbury DF, 79
Newby EA, 136
Newman KD, 328
Newman LJ, 146
Newman NB, 521
Nicholson S, 77
Nieminen T, 95
Nilkolopoulou G, 151
Nobuhara KK, 431
Nordtveit TI, 429
Nowak-Wegrzyn A, 21
Nunez O, 54

O

O'Brien KO, 469
Odouli R, 307
Oeffinger KC, 478
Ogden CL, 444, 446
Ogilvy-Stuart AL, 414
Oh HML, 219
Oh W, 412
Okumura MJ, 291
Oliver SCN, 509
Olsson C, 143
Onslow M, 73
Otto J, 501
Owen CG, 115

P

Pacilli M, 126
Packman A, 73
Pahwa S, 242
Pais PJ, 157
Pan S, 325
Panickar J, 515
Papadakis K, 129
Papadakis MA, 311
Parekh D, 556
Parks MR, 3, 5
Parving H-H, 460
Pastor-Barriuso R, 564
Payne J, 558
Pearce A, 228
Pensabene L, 131
Penzias AS, 399
Peris TS, 387
Petrini JR, 411
Pfeil N, 551
Phillips K, 262

Piacentini J, 388
Pichichero ME, 96
Pickering LK, 277
Pike K, 420
Pistiner M, 22
Plagnol V, 113
Pope CA III, 567
Popkave C, 323
Poulton R, 453
Prabhakaran R, 356
Pratt R, 251
Prevost AT, 464
Prey S, 35
Prior JC, 1
Provan D, 67
Pucci N, 197

R

Rantos R, 119
Read JS, 242
Redmond NM, 543, 545
Rehm HL, 188
Reilly S, 73
Reller MD, 167
Rey-Santano MC, 418
Rhodes P, 239
Richards PA, 547
Richardson SE, 214
Riehle-Colarusso T, 167
Rigaud M, 253
Rihkanen H, 95
Rimoldi SF, 527
Robinson AV, 476
Rodière M, 225
Rodriguez S, 178, 304
Romano PS, 309
Romundstad LB, 401
Romundstad PR, 401
Rönkkö E, 95
Roord STA, 352
Rose KA, 505
Roskam A-JR, 289
Rothschild M, 98
Rouse DJ, 417
Rousset A, 425
Rovner AJ, 469
Roy E, 209
Ruperto N, 349
Rutledge J, 325

S

Saavedra-Lozano J, 347
Salazard B, 87

Salihu HM, 436
Sandberg K, 176
Santelli JS, 7
Saps M, 131
Sargent DJ, 499
Scarlett A, 560
Schäffer L, 433
Schaefer MK, 535
Scheinberg P, 54
Schepis TS, 6
Schipperus MR, 434
Schoeni MH, 523
Schulze KJ, 344
Schuster MA, 293
Scott LM, 490
Shah NS, 251
Shaikh N, 155
Shaker M, 50
Shamsi T, 67
Sharp AJ, 300
Sheeder J, 2
Shehab N, 535
Shevell M, 184
Shreeram S, 375
Shu Y, 216
Shulman RJ, 133
Shutt KA, 255
Sicherer SH, 21
Silbergeld EK, 564
Silva SG, 390
Simell S, 466
Sinnreich U, 141
Sivit CJ, 476
Skipper GS, 321
Smith K, 522, 530
Smith PB, 428
Smith-Simone S, 11
Smyth DJ, 113
Sobol S, 100
Sofi F, 197
Sommerfield T, 124
Song R, 239
Soultan ZN, 521
Spencer T, 379
Spergel JM, 121
Spiegel BMR, 135
Spong CY, 440
Spoudeas HA, 482
Staat MA, 235
Stadler LP, 235
Stephens D, 298
Stern DA, 26
Stirbu I, 289
Stirnimann A, 523
Stothard KJ, 451
Strickland MJ, 167

Strouse JJ, 56
Subhi R, 530
Sugimoto T, 495
Summar ML, 471
Sunde A, 401
Suominen J, 480
Sutherland LA, 84
Switalski KE, 313
Syme C, 458
Szilagyi PG, 211

T

Talley NJ, 135
Tan L, 160
Tanz RR, 258
Tavendale R, 449
Taylor SJC, 12
Teichgraeber JF, 370
Tennant PWG, 451
Therrien J, 185
Thomas MR, 392
Thompson A, 75
Thompson AM, 547
Tita ATN, 440
Tolford S, 276
Tucker A, 46
Tuleu C, 539
Turabelidze G, 46
Turner Z, 365
Tyson JE, 405, 412
Tzemos N, 185

U

Uhlig U, 551
Ullrich C, 50

V

Van den Ende J, 102
van der Togt R, 330
VanderStoep A, 3
Vander Stoep A, 381
Vanhaesebrouck S, 414
van Lieshout EJ, 330
van Toor H, 107
Vermandel A, 82
Vernacchio L, 537
Vernes SC, 79
Viner RM, 12
Violari A, 243
Vu LT, 431

W

Wagner G, 141
Waldman M, 77
Walker NM, 113
Walkup JT, 388
Wallace LS, 230
Wang H, 216
Ward KD, 11
Watt P, 449
Weber MA, 302
Weber W, 381
Weddell A, 482
Weinberg GA, 221
Welch D, 453
Wennergren M, 176
Wesson DE, 298
West CP, 323
Wetmore R, 100
Weyler J, 82
Whincup PH, 115
Whitty CJM, 262
Widmer B, 464
Wijma B, 9
Wilson R, 56
Wong AP, 138
Wu CO, 54

X

Xia JJ, 370

Y

Yang JJ, 487
Yang W, 487
Yazdani SA, 296
Yentzer BA, 32
Yin W, 242
Yip BH, 394
Yip J, 185
Youngson G, 124
Youngster I, 205

Z

Zaman K, 209
Zeichner JA, 30
Zimmerman FJ, 5
Zimmermann R, 433
Zipitis CS, 468
Zuccarello B, 162
Zuccarello D, 162